Movement Disorders Curricula

Cristian Falup-Pecurariu
Joaquim Ferreira • Pablo Martinez-Martin
Kallol Ray Chaudhuri
Editors

Movement Disorders Curricula

Springer

Editors
Cristian Falup-Pecurariu
Faculty of Medicine
Transilvania University
Brasov
Romania

Joaquim Ferreira
Laboratory of Clinical Pharmacology and Therapeutics
Faculty of Medicine
Lisbon
Portugal

Pablo Martinez-Martin
National Center of Epidemiology and CIBERNED
Carlos III Institute of Health
Madrid
Spain

Kallol Ray Chaudhuri
Centre of Excellence, King's College London
National Parkinson Foundation
Centre of Excellence
King's College
London
UK

ISBN 978-3-7091-1627-2 ISBN 978-3-7091-1628-9 (eBook)
DOI 10.1007/978-3-7091-1628-9

Library of Congress Control Number: 2017933455

Printed on acid-free paper

This Springer imprint is published by Springer Nature
The registered company is Springer-Verlag GmbH Austria
The registered company address is: Prinz-Eugen-Strasse 8-10, 1040 Wien, Austria

Preface

This book offers a comprehensive approach to the wide range of movement disorders, guiding readers from the phenomenology to diagnosis and management. Reflecting the latest developments in the field, it offers a unique summary of this dynamic area by pursuing a uniform approach to movement disorders curricula.

Divided into three parts, *Movement Disorders Curricula* provides an authoritative overview of this growing branch of neurology written by prominent experts from Europe, North and South America and Asia.

Part I presents the basic elements of movement disorders, including modern approach of computational physiology of the basal ganglia, epidemiological methods, animal models, genetics and neuropathology. It also features sections on clinical trials for movement disorders, phenomenology, rating scales and practical skills on how to record a video of a movement disorders patient.

Part II is dedicated to Parkinson's disease and cover important topics of etiology, pathogenesis, clinical features, non-motor problems, pharmacological and surgical treatment.

Part III deals with movement disorders and covers the whole range of this field.

The chapters were written by a panel of international experts whose authorities are well established in the movement disorders field. The Editors are extremely grateful to all the distinguished authors who contributed to this book.

Special thanks goes to Springer staff who has been working very professional: Barbara Zöhrer (Pfeifer) Editor Clinical Medicine, Wilma McHugh, Project Coordinator, Book Production; Priya Vairamani, Project Manager; Andrea Ridolfi, Editor, Clinical Medicine Books.

Equipping readers with the practical and research skills needed in the movement disorders field, the book offers a valuable tool to help them prepare for board examinations on general neurology, as well as for fellowships in movement disorders, being also a practical tool on bedside experience.

Brasov, Romania — Cristian Falup-Pecurariu
Lisbon, Portugal — Joaquim Ferreira
Madrid, Spain — Pablo Martinez-Martin
London, UK — Kallol Ray Chaudhuri

Contents

List of Videos

with mandibular deviation to the right and blepharospasm. You can hear the laryngeal stridor that interrupts her speech

Video 39.2 Facial tics. The young woman shows brief, rapid, repetitive left depressor anguli oris and platysma contractions, as well as increased blinking that increase when she talks. When asked to be quiet, the movements improve, almost disappearing. When she relaxes, the tics reappear. She explains that she can control the tics to a certain extent with a lot of concentration. She demonstrates the lower facial tics that also appear less often on the contralateral side

Video 39.3 Edentulous dyskinesias. Patient with loose dentures showing jaw deviation and jaw-closing stereotypic movement. He is explaining that he tends to remove the denture with his finger, as a habit. After removing the upper dentures, the movements almost completely disappear

Videos can be found in the electronic supplementary material in the online version of the book. On http://springerlink.com enter the DOI number given on the bottom of the chapter opening page. Scroll down to the Supplementary material tab and click on the respective videos link. In addition, all videos to this book can be downloaded from http://extras.springer.com. Enter the ISBN number and download all videos.

Part I

Overview

1 Computational Physiology of the Basal Ganglia, Movement Disorders, and Their Therapy

Liliya Iskhakova, Pnina Rappel, David Arkadir, Renana Eitan, Zvi Israel, and Hagai Bergman

1.1 The Classic D1/D2 Direct/Indirect Model of the Basal Ganglia Networks

Today, neurology textbooks (e.g., Adams and Victor's *Principles of Neurology* 10th Edition, 2014) depict the basal ganglia (BG) as the feed-forward part of a closed loop connecting all cortical areas sequentially through the BG direct and indirect pathways back to the motor cortex [1, 5]. The motor cortex projects to the spinal level through the corticospinal pathway and controls muscle activation and movements (Fig. 1.1).

This BG model emphasizes the structure of the two segregated internal BG pathways. Both pathways start in the projection neurons of the striatum and converge on the output structures of the basal ganglia (the internal segment of the globus pallidus – the GPi; the substantia nigra pars reticulata – the SNr). The striatal projection neurons in the direct pathway are medium spiny neurons (MSNs) that express D1 dopamine receptors, whereas those in the indirect pathway express D2 dopamine receptors [11]. Both D1 and D2 MSNs use GABA as their main neurotransmitter. The "direct pathway" is a monosynaptic GABAergic inhibitory projection from the striatum to the GPi/SNr, whereas the "indirect pathway" projection is polysynaptic and disinhibitory through the external segment of the globus pallidus (GPe) and the glutamatergic (excitatory) subthalamic nucleus (STN). Dopamine has differential effects on the two striato-pallidal pathways. It excites and facilitates transmission along the direct pathway via activation of D1 receptors and inhibits transmission along the indirect pathway via the D2 receptors.

The classical D1/D2 direct/indirect rate model of the basal ganglia has been one of the most influential models in the history of clinical neuroscience. It provides a general framework for the finding of physiological studies of Parkinsonian

L. Iskhakova, PhD • P. Rappel, BA
H. Bergman, MD, DSc (✉)
Department of Medical Neurobiology (Physiology), Institute of Medical Research – Israel-Canada (IMRIC), The Hebrew University Hadassah Medical School, Jerusalem, Israel

The Edmond and Lily Safra Center for Brain Research (ELSC), The Hebrew University, Jerusalem, Israel
e-mail: lilyai@ekmd.huji.ac.il; pnina.rappel@gmail.com; hagaibe@ekmd.huji.ac.il

D. Arkadir, MD, PhD
Department of Neurology, Hadassah-Hebrew University Medical Center, Jerusalem, Israel
e-mail: Arkadir@hadassah.orgda.il

R. Eitan, MD
Department of Psychiatry, Hadassah-Hebrew University Medical Center, Jerusalem, Israel
e-mail: renanaeitan@gmail.com

Z. Israel, BSc, MBBS
Department of Neurosurgery, Hadassah-Hebrew University Medical Center, Jerusalem, Israel
e-mail: israelz@hadassah.org.il

C. Falup-Pecurariu et al. (eds.), *Movement Disorders Curricula*,
DOI 10.1007/978-3-7091-1628-9_1

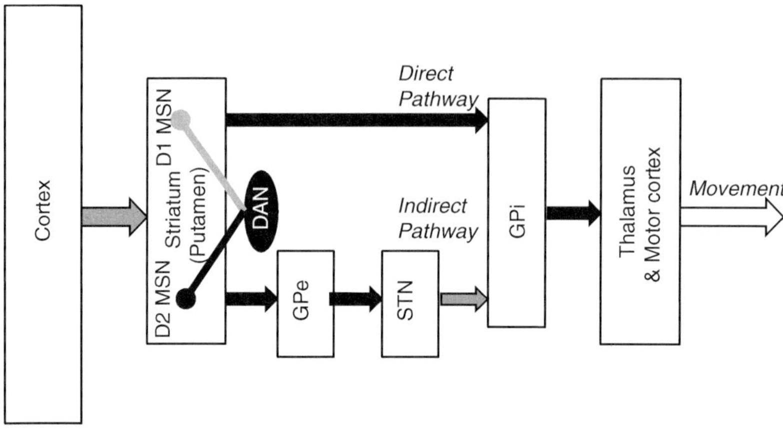

Fig. 1.1 The classical D1/D2 direct/indirect model of the basal ganglia. *Gray* and *black arrows* represent excitatory (glutamate) and inhibitory (GABA) connections, respectively. *Gray* and *black round shape arrows* represent excitatory and inhibitory effects of dopamine on MSNs expressing D1 and D2 receptors, respectively. *Abbreviations*: *DAN* midbrain dopaminergic neurons, *GPe, GPi* external and internal segments of the globus pallidus, *MSN* striatal medium spiny (projection) neurons, *SNr* substantia nigra pars reticulata, *STN* subthalamic nucleus

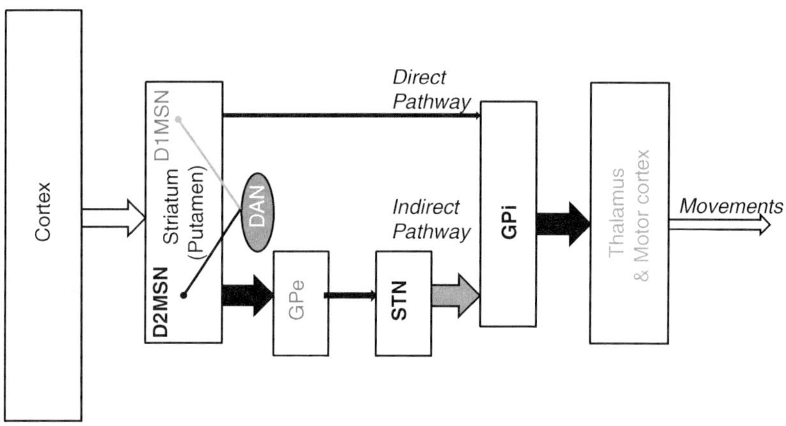

Fig. 1.2 The classical D1/D2 direct/indirect model of the basal ganglia in the dopamine depleted Parkinsonian animal. Conventions and abbreviations as in Fig. 1.1. Increase/decrease width of *arrows* (in comparison with Fig. 1.1) represent increase/decrease activity. *Black bold/gray* characters represent neuronal structures with increase/decrease of their discharge rate

MPTP-treated monkeys (Fig. 1.2). These studies found that following dopamine depletion, there was a decrease in the average discharge rate of GPe neurons and an increase in the GPi [9, 19] and the STN [6] discharge rate. Reverse trends of pallidal discharge rates in response to dopamine replacement therapy have been reported in both human patients [13, 15, 18] and primates [10, 12, 21].

The classical D1/D2 direct/indirect model can also explain the physiological mechanisms of dopamine replacement therapy for Parkinson's disease. Postsynaptic dopamine agonists enable the restoration of the normal dopamine tone to the striatum, and therefore raise the level of excitability of the motor cortex and ameliorate Parkinsonian akinesia. Similarly, STN and GPi inactivation, by GABA agonists, by lesions [5, 32], or by deep brain stimulation (under the assumption that deep brain stimulation mimics inactivation, see below), lead to a reduction in the over-activation of BG inhibitory output to the motor thalamocortical networks.

However, recent anatomical, physiological, and theoretical studies have revealed that the basal ganglia connectivity is more complex than the simple connectivity depicted by the D1/D2 direct/indirect model (e.g., back projections from STN to GPe and from GPe to striatum, hyperdirect cortex–STN pathway, etc.). Secondly, the model is falling short in explaining the dynamic patterns of basal ganglia activity and Parkinson's disease. A common finding of physiological recording in MPTP-treated monkeys [9, 19] [6, 7, 23, 31] and human patients with Parkinson's disease [16, 17, 29, 30, 33] is an increase in the fraction of basal ganglia neurons that discharge in periodic bursts at the tremor (3–7 Hz) frequency and at double tremor and beta range (12–30 Hz) frequency. Finally, this classical D1/D2 direct/indirect rate model ignores the emerging roles of the basal ganglia in reinforcement learning (see below) and behavioral adaptions to the changing environment.

1.2 The Reinforcement Learning Model of the Basal Ganglia

More modern computational models of the basal ganglia [27] treat the basal ganglia as an actor/critic reinforcement learning network (Fig. 1.3). The main axis or the actor part implements the behavioral policy or the mapping between states and actions (behavioral policy), and the critic calculates the mismatch between predictions and the actual state (prediction error). The prediction error is used to update the agent's predictions and for optimization of the behavioral policy (by reinforcing those actions that led to the state of affairs better than predictions and by weakening the associations between state and actions that led to a state worse than predictions). Rewards can be either positive or negative in these models, and the computational goal is to maximize the cumulative (future discounted) reward.

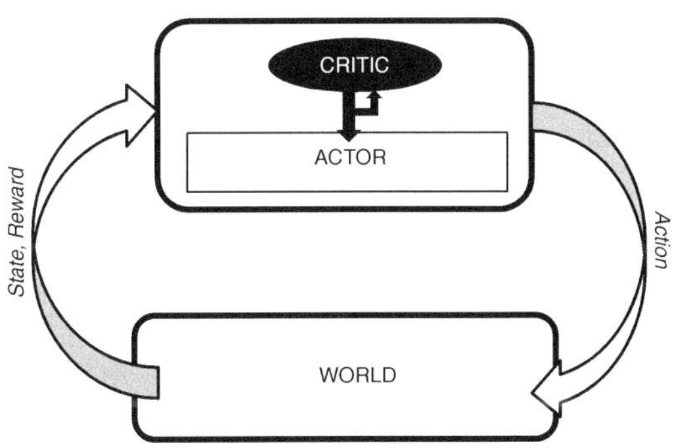

Fig. 1.3 Schematic actor/critic model of a reinforcement learning agent

In terms of BG anatomy (Fig. 1.4), the neural networks of the BG main axis (actor) connect the state encoding cortical domains with the cortical and brainstem motor centers. The midbrain dopaminergic neurons (located mainly at the substantia nigra pars compacta and in the ventral tegmental area, SNc and VTA, respectively) are the critics of the basal ganglia. Their normal background activity (~4–5 spikes/s) encodes the mismatch between predictions and reality. Positive prediction errors (reality better than predictions) are encoded by bursts of the dopamine neurons. On the other hand, omission of the expected reward, prediction of aversive events, and other cases of negative prediction error (reality worse than predictions) are encoded by depression (pause) of the spiking activity [26, 28]. These changes in dopamine activity and the coinciding cortical and striatal discharge lead to plastic changes in the efficacy of the corticostriatal synapses (long-term potentiation or depression accordingly), and therefore to modulation of the association between states (encoded by the cortical activity) and action (encoded by BG output activity).

The reinforcement actor/critic model of the basal ganglia has revolutionized current understanding of physiological mechanisms of model-free (procedural, implicit) learning and may provide insights into certain basal ganglia-related disorders such as akinesia and levodopa-induced dyskinesia. However, as for the classical D1/D2 direct/indirect model, this model has its own pitfalls. For example, the reinforcement learning BG model fails to provide a mechanism for the ultrafast action of dopamine agonists and antagonists (such as apomorphine or haloperidol). There is an ongoing debate in the electrophysiological literature on the ability of dopaminergic neurons

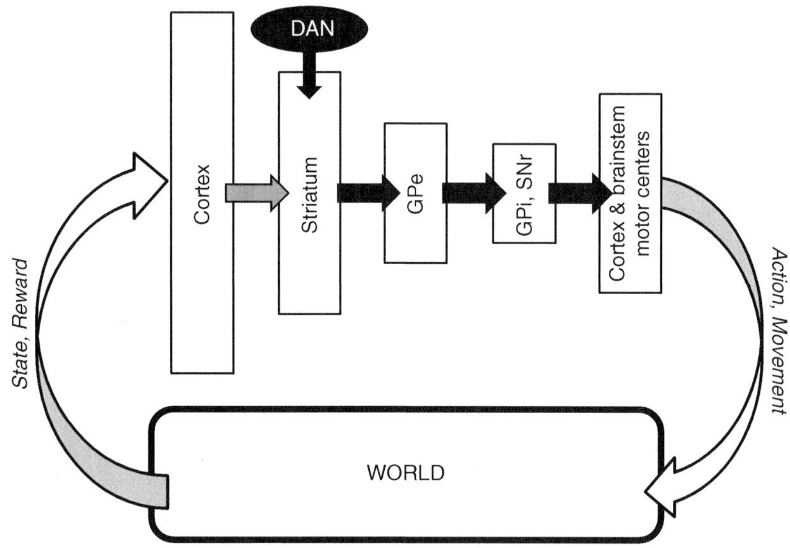

Fig. 1.4 Anatomical description of the actor/critic reinforcement model of the basal ganglia. Abbreviations and conventions as in Fig. 1.1

to encode the negative domain of pleasure prediction [14]. Finally, the model assumes a single final currency (pleasure or its absence) to control behavior, and thus probably does not describe the multidimensional emotional repertoire of humans and animals.

1.3 The Multi-objective Optimization Model of the Basal Ganglia

There are other neuromodulators of the basal ganglia in addition to the midbrain dopaminergic neurons. The striatum is highly enriched with cholinergic, serotonergic, and histaminergic markers, and many anatomical and physiological studies have suggested that the striatal cholinergic interneurons, dorsal raphe serotonin (5-HT) neurons, and tubero-mamillary histamine neurons are part of the basal ganglia critic system. We recently hypothesized [22] that the computational goal of the basal ganglia is to optimize the trade-off between the orthogonal goals of maximizing future cumulative gain and minimizing the behavioral (information) cost (i.e., multi- rather than single-objective optimization). This multi-objective optimization goal naturally leads to a soft-max like behavioral policy where each of the BG critic plays a dual role. First, and as in previous reinforcement models, the BG critics affect the efficacy of the cortico-striatal synapses [2, 24, 27]. Second, the BG critics also affect the excitability of the striatal projection neurons (as in the classical D1/D2 direct/indirect BG model), and therefore act as a pseudo-temperature soft-max parameter. This pseudo-temperature parameter controls the trade-off between gain and cost and the continuum between exploratory (gambling) and greedy (akinetic) behavioral policies (the motor vigor [8, 20]). The different critics have differential effects on state-to-action coupling and the pseudo-temperature (excitability) of the basal ganglia network (Fig. 1.5 and Table 1.1). At present, we assume that dopamine and serotonin increase the temperature, whereas the other two critics reduce the temperature. Similarly, dopamine and histamine increase the coupling between state and action, whereas serotonin and acetylcholine reduce it. The reason for this heterogeneity is the variability of the environment and the optimal responses of the agent. Both appetitive and aversive predictive cues and events should increase the pseudo-temperature to enable approach and escape. However, appetitive events should increase the state-to-action coupling leading to reinforcement of the behavior that has resulted in better than predicted state. Conversely, aversive events should lead to reduction in the state-to-action coupling. Dopamine

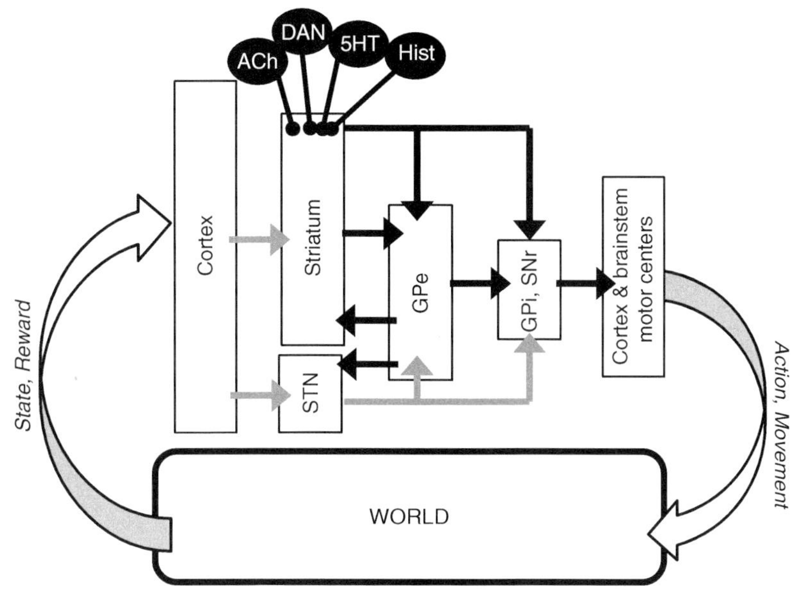

Fig. 1.5 Anatomical description of the multi-objective optimization model of the basal ganglia. Abbreviations and conventions as in Fig. 1.1

Table 1.1 Multiple and differential effects of BG critics on BG pseudo-temperature (through modulation of the excitability of striatal projection neurons) and state-to-action coupling (through modulation of the efficacy of cortico-striatal synapses)

	DA	ACh	5-HT	Histamine
Pseudo-temperature	↑	↓	↑	↓
State-to-action association	↑	↓	↓	↑

DA dopamine, *ACh* acetylcholine, *5-HT* serotonin, ↑ increase, ↓ decrease

released for appetitive events and serotonin for aversive events have similar effects on the pseudo-temperature, and opposite effects on the state-to-action coupling (Table 1.1) are therefore ideally suited for these demands. Similar reasoning can be applied for the role of acetylcholine and histamine in BG information processing.

Finally, the unique features of funneling along the main axis of the basal ganglia [4] are included in this new model. In the nonhuman primate, there are 10^9 neurons in the cortex that project to the striatum, 10^7 projection neurons in the striatum, and 10^5 neurons in the output structure of the basal ganglia (GPi and SNr). This funneling structure (schematically illustrated by the box size in Fig. 1.5) enables the basal ganglia to extract the features of the current state that are important for the ongoing and future movements. For example, when you unexpectedly meet your grandmother in the corridor of your department, the most relevant feature is that this is your grandmother and not the white–blue dress or the new hairstyle. Your next action is to approach and kiss your grandmother, and this does not depend on her specific dress and hairstyle.

The multi objective optimization model better captures the multifaceted organization of the actor/critic network of the basal ganglia. The combined effects of the critics on striatal excitability and on cortico-striatal synaptic efficacy enable the model to account for both ultrafast effects (e.g., apomorphine) and slow procedural learning kinetics. Furthermore, the model provides insights into the role of the non-dopaminergic critics in the basal ganglia physiology and pathophysiology (e.g., dopamine–acetylcholine motor balance and serotonin-related depression in Parkinson's disease).

The first step in the treatment of Parkinson's disease today is dopamine replacement therapy (DRT). This treatment is aimed at restoring the normal function of the BG critics. The first goal of DRT is to restore the full dynamic range of dopamine physiology, including phasic and environment-related changes at the dopamine level. However, the increased sprouting of dopaminergic axons, the over-sensitization of dopamine receptors, and other pathophysiological changes occurring over the many years of DRT lead to abnormal dynamics of dopamine in the striatum of these patients. This is clearly augmented by the use of dopamine agonists which directly affect postsynaptic receptors. Hence, striatal dopamine concentration and effects are no longer dependent on the environment and the behavior of the patient [3]. After five to ten years of years of treatment with DRT, Parkinsonian patients can no longer experience the benefits of DRT generated at the start of treatment, and side effects such as levodopa-induced dyskinesia affect their quality of life.

The D1/D2 direct/indirect model and the physiological recordings in the MPTP primate model of Parkinson's disease have led to a shift in focus of therapy from the critic to the actor part of the basal ganglia. Physiological and metabolic studies have revealed changes in the discharge rate, pattern, and synchronization of neurons in the STN and GPi of MPTP-treated monkeys. Inactivation of these overactive BG nuclei in monkey and humans leads to an amelioration of Parkinsonian symptoms and to new therapeutic methods that can be applied after DRT failure. We hypothesized that the basal ganglia network is the default, fast, and unconscious link between the neural structures encoding the current state and action (e.g., System 1 of Daniel Kahneman's Thinking, Fast and Slow, 2011). However, there are many additional networks, for example, amygdala – hypothalamic–pituitary–adrenal (HPA) axis and cortico-cortical networks. These networks provide parallel connectivity between state and action (Fig. 1.6); however, since the BG is the default connection between state and action, the other networks cannot compensate for abnormal BG activity. Silencing the BG abnormal activity enables the other networks to compensate and to reestablish close-to-normal state-to-action coupling.

However, permanent inactivation of a BG target is only achieved by lesioning, and hence is not recommended as a therapy of choice. Deep brain stimulation (DBS) is a reversible and adjustable procedure, and thus better suits current demands for efficient and ethical therapy. DBS effects mimic inactivation effects. Today, there is still an active debate concerning the mechanism governing DBS (e.g., by depolarization block or activation of afferent inhibitory projections); however, there is a general consensus that STN and GPi DBS provides effective treatment of late and even early-stage Parkinson's disease. Thus, the modern therapy of Parkinson's disease and other BG

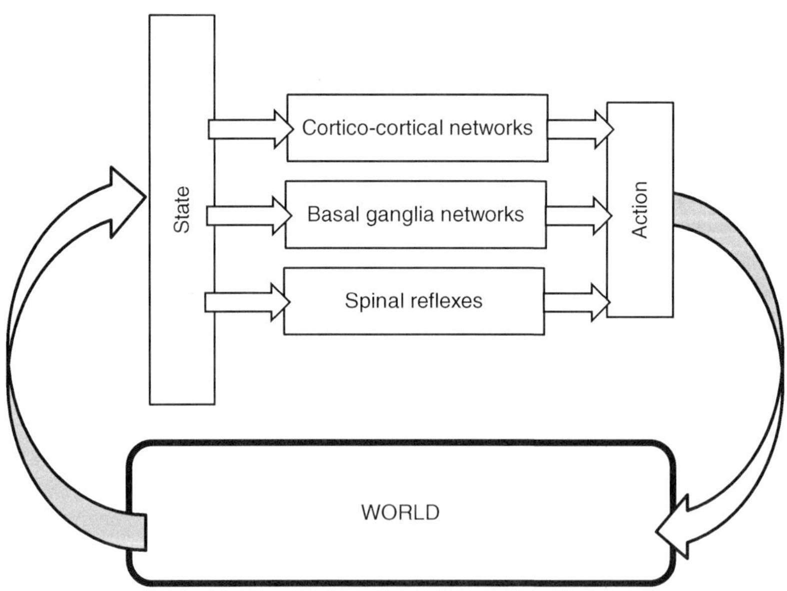

Fig. 1.6 The basal ganglia network is one of many neural networks connecting state-to-action association in the nervous system

disorders has shifted from chemical manipulation of the neurotransmitter level of the BG critic to manipulation of spiking activity in the BG actor. DBS treatments are also effective in other basal ganglia-related movement disorders such as dystonia and essential tremor and are currently being tested for mental disorders such as obsessive–compulsive and major depression disorders.

We predict that next generation of DBS devices will exploit BG actor/critic multi-objective optimization algorithms and will provide even better therapy for human patients. Today, DBS adjustments must be made by a physician every 2–10 weeks. However, the dynamic and complex nature of Parkinson's disease calls for more frequent and more sophisticated adjustment of the DBS parameters. This can be achieved by closed-loop DBS methods [25]. These future closed-loop DBS devices will be modulated by the BG neural activity, the objective telemetry of the patient's symptoms, and the subjective evaluation by the patient and caregivers of quality of life. This closed-loop modulation is aiming at achievement of multi-objective optimization of the patient's motor and nonmotor symptoms, along with minimization of the side effects of DBS therapy. Better understanding of the computational physiology of the basal ganglia in health and disease is therefore the first step in the long path for better treatment of human patients with basal ganglia disorders.

Acknowledgments This study was supported by the Simone and Bernard Guttman chair of Brain Research and by the Rosetrees and Vorst foundations (to HB).

References

1. Albin RL, Young AB, Penney JB. The functional anatomy of basal ganglia disorders. Trends Neurosci. 1989;12:366–75.
2. Arbuthnott GW, Wickens J. Space, time and dopamine. Trends Neurosci. 2007;30:62–9.
3. Arkadir D, Bergman H, Fahn S. Redundant dopaminergic activity may enable compensatory axonal sprouting in Parkinson disease. Neurology. 2014;82:1093–8.
4. Bar-Gad I, Morris G, Bergman H. Information processing, dimensionality reduction and reinforcement learning in the basal ganglia. Prog Neurobiol. 2003;71:439–73.
5. Bergman H, Wichmann T, DeLong MR. Reversal of experimental parkinsonism by lesions of the subthalamic nucleus. Science. 1990;249:1436–8.
6. Bergman H, Wichmann T, Karmon B, DeLong MR. The primate subthalamic nucleus. II. Neuronal activity in the MPTP model of parkinsonism. J Neurophysiol. 1994;72:507–20.
7. Bezard E, Boraud T, Chalon S, Brotchie JM, Guilloteau D, Gross CE. Pallidal border cells: an anatomical and electrophysiological study in the 1-methyl-4-phenyl-1,2,3,6-tetrahydropyridine-treated monkey. Neuroscience. 2001;103:117–23.
8. Cools R, Nakamura K, Daw ND. Serotonin and dopamine: unifying affective, activational, and decision functions. Neuropsychopharmacology. 2011;36:98–113.
9. Filion M, Tremblay L. Abnormal spontaneous activity of globus pallidus neurons in monkeys with MPTP-induced parkinsonism. Brain Res. 1991;547:142–51.
10. Filion M, Tremblay L, Bedard PJ. Effects of dopamine agonists on the spontaneous activity of globus pallidus neurons in monkeys with MPTP-induced parkinsonism. Brain Res. 1991;547:152–61.
11. Gerfen CR, Engber TM, Mahan LC, Susel Z, Chase TN, Monsma Jr FJ, Sibley DR. D1 and D2 dopamine receptor-regulated gene expression of striatonigral and striatopallidal neurons. Science. 1990;250:1429–32.
12. Heimer G, Rivlin-Etzion M, Bar-Gad I, Goldberg JA, Haber SN, Bergman H. Dopamine replacement therapy does not restore the full spectrum of normal pallidal activity in the 1-methyl-4-phenyl-1,2,3,6-tetra-hydropyridine primate model of Parkinsonism. J Neurosci. 2006;26:8101–14.
13. Hutchinson WD, Levy R, Dostrovsky JO, Lozano AM, Lang AE. Effects of apomorphine on globus pallidus neurons in parkinsonian patients. Ann Neurol. 1997;42:767–75.
14. Joshua M, Adler A, Mitelman R, Vaadia E, Bergman H. Midbrain dopaminergic neurons and striatal cholinergic interneurons encode the difference between reward and aversive events at different epochs of probabilistic classical conditioning trials. J Neurosci. 2008;28:11673–84.
15. Lee JI, Verhagen ML, Ohara S, Dougherty PM, Kim JH, Lenz FA. Internal pallidal neuronal activity during mild drug-related dyskinesias in Parkinson's disease: decreased firing rates and altered firing patterns. J Neurophysiol. 2007;97:2627–41.
16. Levy R, Hutchison WD, Lozano AM, Dostrovsky JO. Synchronized neuronal discharge in the basal ganglia of parkinsonian patients is limited to oscillatory activity. J Neurosci. 2002;22:2855–61.
17. Levy R, Ashby P, Hutchison WD, Lang AE, Lozano AM, Dostrovsky JO. Dependence of subthalamic nucleus oscillations on movement and dopamine in Parkinson's disease. Brain. 2002;125:1196–209.
18. Merello M, Balej J, Delfino M, Cammarota A, Betti O, Leiguarda R. Apomorphine induces changes in

GPi spontaneous outflow in patients with Parkinson's disease. Mov Disord. 1999;14:45–9.
19. Miller WC, DeLong MR. Altered tonic activity of neurons in the globus pallidus and subthalamic nucleus in the primate MPTP model of parkinsonism. In: Carpenter MB, Jayaraman A, editors. The basal ganglia II. New York: Plenum Press; 1987. p. 415–27.
20. Niv Y, Daw ND, Joel D, Dayan P. Tonic dopamine: opportunity costs and the control of response vigor. Psychopharmacol (Berl). 2007;191:507–20.
21. Papa SM, DeSimone R, Fiorani M, Oldfield EH. Internal globus pallidus discharge is nearly suppressed during levodopa-induced dyskinesias. Ann Neurol. 1999;46:732–8.
22. Parush N, Tishby N, Bergman H. Dopaminergic balance between reward maximization and policy complexity. Front Syst Neurosci. 2011;5:22.
23. Raz A, Vaadia E, Bergman H. Firing patterns and correlations of spontaneous discharge of pallidal neurons in the normal and the tremulous 1-methyl-4-phenyl-1,2,3,6-tetrahydropyridine vervet model of parkinsonism. J Neurosci. 2000;20:8559–71.
24. Reynolds JN, Wickens JR. Dopamine-dependent plasticity of corticostriatal synapses. Neural Netw. 2002;15:507–21.
25. Rosin B, Slovik M, Mitelman R, Rivlin-Etzion M, Haber SN, Israel Z, Vaadia E, Bergman H. Closed-loop deep brain stimulation is superior in ameliorating parkinsonism. Neuron. 2011;72:370–84.
26. Schultz W. Reward signaling by dopamine neurons. Neuroscientist. 2001;7:293–302.
27. Schultz W, Dayan P, Montague PR. A neural substrate of prediction and reward. Science. 1997;275:1593–9.
28. Tobler PN, Fiorillo CD, Schultz W. Adaptive coding of reward value by dopamine neurons. Science. 2005;307:1642–5.
29. Weinberger M, Hutchison WD, Lozano AM, Hodaie M, Dostrovsky JO. Increased gamma oscillatory activity in the subthalamic nucleus during tremor in Parkinson's disease patients. J Neurophysiol. 2009;101:789–802.
30. Weinberger M, Mahant N, Hutchison WD, Lozano AM, Moro E, Hodaie M, Lang AE, Dostrovsky JO. Beta oscillatory activity in the subthalamic nucleus and its relation to dopaminergic response in Parkinson's disease. J Neurophysiol. 2006;96: 3248–56.
31. Wichmann T, Soares J. Neuronal firing before and after burst discharges in the monkey basal ganglia is predictably patterned in the normal state and altered in parkinsonism. J Neurophysiol. 2006;95: 2120–33.
32. Wichmann T, Bergman H, DeLong MR. The primate subthalamic nucleus. III. Changes in motor behavior and neuronal activity in the internal pallidum induced by subthalamic inactivation in the MPTP model of parkinsonism. J Neurophysiol. 1994;72: 521–30.
33. Zaidel A, Spivak A, Grieb B, Bergman H, Israel Z. Subthalamic span of beta oscillations predicts deep brain stimulation efficacy for patients with Parkinson's disease. Brain. 2010;133:2007–21.

Animal Models of Movement Disorders

2

Susan Duty and Peter Jenner

2.1 Introduction

A wide and varied range of neurological diseases falls under the heading of movement disorders with a wide array of symptoms that can involve decreased, increased and involuntary abnormal motor function. Movement disorders can be sporadic, familial or drug/toxin induced and can affect either the peripheral or central nervous system or both. There can be clear evidence of pathology as occurs in Parkinson's disease (PD) or in Huntington's disease (HD) or no obvious neuronal loss as seen in restless leg syndrome (RLS) or in dystonia, where biochemical abnormalities and altered firing within neuronal circuitry appear to prevail. As a gross generalisation, a clear understanding of the aetiology of neuronal loss or biochemical abnormality is not available for most movement disorders and as a consequence prevention and treatment remains poor. Whilst pharmacological control of motor function has been a priority for some movement disorders, most notably PD, for others attempting to arrest aggressive neuronal loss, has been key, for example, in amyotrophic lateral sclerosis (ALS). The unmet need in the treatment of movement disorders is high, and it is the reason why the study of animal models of these illnesses has received much attention.

In this chapter, we look at a variety of animal models that has helped shape our understanding of the pathogenesis and treatment of movement disorders. It is not possible within the space available to deal with the full spectrum of movement disorders and the array of experimental approaches used. Individual movement disorders could be, and have been, the subject of complete reviews in their own right. Rather, we have chosen to be selective and to deal with examples that provide a flavour of the laboratory-based research that is contributing to the knowledge base. For this reason (and because of our own expertise), we have focussed on PD where toxins and gene manipulation have led to a plethora of animal models relevant to pathogenic mechanisms and to the symptomatology of PD. In addition, we have looked at the related Parkinson-plus syndromes (multiple system atrophy [MSA], progressive supranuclear palsy [PSP]) which are rarer, less well studied and poorly treated. As examples of aggressive diseases with evidence of genetic linkage, we have included animal models of HD and ALS where the emphasis is on prevention and neuroprotection as opposed to symptomatic treatment. Finally, we deal with dystonia as a

S. Duty
Wolfson Centre for Age-Related Diseases,
Institute of Psychiatry, Psychology and Neuroscience,
King's College London, London, UK
e-mail: susan.duty@kcl.ac.uk

P. Jenner (✉)
Neurodegenerative Diseases Research Group,
Institute of Pharmaceutical Sciences, School of
Biomedical Sciences, King's College, London, UK
e-mail: peter.jenner@kcl.ac.uk

C. Falup-Pecurariu et al. (eds.), *Movement Disorders Curricula*,
DOI 10.1007/978-3-7091-1628-9_2

group of disabling illnesses where pathological change is rare and where treatment is sparse but where animal models based on gene defects underlying some forms of dystonia are enabling progress to be made.

2.2 Parkinson's Disease

Parkinson's disease (PD) is the most common neurodegenerative movement disorder in which progressive pathology in the dopaminergic neurones of the substantia nigra pars compacta (SNpc) brings about symptoms of resting tremor, bradykinesia, rigidity and postural instability. Accompanying pathology in serotoninergic, noradrenergic and cholinergic brain regions may underlie some of the nonmotor symptoms that accompany this disease, including bladder hyperreflexia, sleep disturbances and cognitive decline. Animal models of PD range from multicellular organisms to primates and offer insight into disease mechanisms as well as serving as test beds for new treatment strategies. These models have been extensively reviewed elsewhere [25].

2.2.1 Modelling PD Motor Symptoms

For early preclinical testing of acute relief of motor symptoms, the rodent models of reserpine-induced akinesia and haloperidol-induced catalepsy, and rigidity may suffice. Most drugs in clinical use today for PD show efficacy in these models [25], supporting their predictive validity, and they remain popular for screening acute effects of potential symptomatic agents [14]. However, alternative models bearing a toxin-induced SNpc lesion are used for assessing longer-term symptomatic relief. Most commonly used are the 6-hydroxydopamine (6-OHDA)-lesioned rat or mouse and the 1-methyl-4-phenyl-1,2,3,6-tetrahydropyridine (MPTP)-treated mouse or non-human primate. MPTP and 6-OHDA induce apoptosis in dopaminergic neurones in the SNpc through a range of mechanisms known to occur in PD brain including oxidative stress, mitochondrial complex I dysfunction and inflammation. These models also mimic biochemical features of PD, including reduced striatal dopamine and show some impairment of motor function, thereby displaying both construct and face validity. The 6-OHDA rodent model has good predictive validity too, with most drugs in clinical use today against PD motor symptoms showing efficacy in behavioural tests in this model [25]. However, 3–5 days MPTP treatment in monkeys and marmosets induces a parkinsonian syndrome that more faithfully reproduces most of the cardinal signs of human PD (e.g. bradykinesia, rigidity and postural abnormalities but no resting tremor) [37, 44], making this the gold-standard model for studies preceding clinical trials. Again, all drugs used to treat motor symptoms in PD patients have shown efficacy in the MPTP-treated primate model [25], and this model has been key to validating new dopaminergic drugs for clinical use as well as concepts like sustained delivery systems such as the rotigotine transdermal patch [71]. However, there have been notable failures in translation, for example, the A2a antagonist, istradefylline [35, 40].

2.2.2 Modelling Nonmotor Symptoms

Alongside their motor impairment, PD patients also exhibit a range of nonmotor symptoms [7] that are somewhat less well understood and inadequately treated. However, some of these signs are exhibited by the established animal models of PD, offering an opportunity to explore the mechanisms behind their appearance and routes for potential pharmacological intervention. For example, both 6-OHDA-lesioned rats and MPTP-treated monkeys develop bladder hyperreflexia [3, 80], as occurs in PD [10], this being responsive to treatment with D1 receptor agonists [81]. Moreover, MPTP treatment induces sleep disturbance [6] and, in the case of low doses, cognitive impairment [21], providing platforms for identifying effective treatments for a number of nonmotor symptoms in the future.

2.2.3 Modelling Levodopa-Induced Dyskinesia

Excessive involuntary movements or dyskinesia emerge in around a third of PD patients following 3–5 years of levodopa treatment. Whilst past investigation of new drugs to treat this levodopa-induced dyskinesia (LID) relied upon preclinical testing in primates expressing LID, exploratory studies are now increasingly conducted in newer rodent models. Daily treatment of 6-OHDA-lesioned rats or mice with levodopa, for 14–21 days, induces stable abnormal involuntary movements (AIMs) that mirror, to some extent, LID in primates, forelimb dyskinesia or jerkiness, axial dystonia or twisting and orolingual dyskinesia [16]. Agents known to display antidyskinetic efficacy in MPTP-treated primates, such as 5-HT_{1A} receptor agonists [48], are effective against AIMs. Indeed, this model has good predictive validity of future efficacy in the primate model. For example, $mGlu_5$ receptor antagonists, identified as anti-dyskinetic in the rodent AIMs model [51], were subsequently shown to be effective in the MPTP-treated primate model of LID [38, 53, 64]. LID expressed in MPTP-treated primates is treated repeatedly with levodopa closely mirrors that seen in PD patients (chorea, dystonia and athetosis), albeit over a much reduced timescale and is reduced by amantadine, the only drug known to be effective in the control of LID in man [13]. Indeed, the primate LID model has been used to identify many candidates worthy of clinical trials, but whilst some treatments have shown good translation through to man like the aforementioned $mGlu_5$ receptor antagonists [9, 42, 70], this has not been the case for others including the 5-HT_{1A} receptor agonists [12, 32, 57]. MPTP-treated primates also display other treatment-related complications of a motor ('wearing off', 'on-off' and freezing) [43] or non-motor (neuropsychiatric-like behaviours) [29] phenotype, opening up avenues for exploring the mechanisms behind, and potential treatments for, these complications.

2.2.4 Modelling PD Pathology

These rodent and primate models have been successfully used to identify potential neurorestorative strategies such as neurotrophic factors, cell-based therapies and gene therapies [30, 41, 67]. However, a vast array of potential neuroprotective or disease-modifying agents has failed to demonstrate clinical efficacy, despite good outcomes in the models, even encompassing additional rotenone, lipopolysaccharide and proteasome models expanded on elsewhere [25]. These translational barriers serve to remind us that available models remain flawed. The degeneration produced in animals is largely rapid (days rather than years), nonprogressive and specific to dopaminergic neurones rather than extending to noradrenergic and serotonergic systems as per human PD. Moreover, the Lewy body pathology is absent. The hope that newer rodent genetic models recapitulating gene mutations associated with PD (e.g. alpha-synuclein, LRRK2, DJ-1 parkin or PINK1) might help bridge this gap has not yet been realised since many of these fail to display robust nigral pathology [20]. Nevertheless, these genetic mouse models, along with emerging genetic models in multicellular organisms including *Drosophila*, *C. elegans* and zebrafish [22, 55, 77], are powerful tools for disentangling the molecular pathways involved in PD pathogenesis and revealing novel targets for potential disease modification that may yet prove effective in man.

2.3 Multiple System Atrophy (MSA) and Progressive Supranuclear Palsy (PSP)

Parkinson-plus syndromes, represented by MSA and PSP, are complex movement disorders with more widespread pathological change, different pathological markers and more diverse symptomatology than occurs in PD. They can be confused with PD in their early stages, but with disease progression, a distinct pattern of clinical signs becomes apparent, and there is a lack of responsiveness to dopaminergic drug treatment.

MSA is characterised by pathological damage in the substantia nigra, cerebellum, brainstem and spinal cord. It is thought to be a synucleinopathy-like PD, but the protein accumulations are found in oligodendrocytes. Two forms of MSA are recognised – MSA with a dominance of PD features (MSA-P; formerly known as strio-nigral degeneration) and MSA with dominant cerebellar symptoms (MSA-C; formerly known as olivopontocerebellar degeneration) – both are accompanied by autonomic dysfunction [31]. Models of MSA have largely been based on the stereotaxic administration of toxins in rodents (6-OHDA into the medial forebrain bundle or striatum combined with quinolinic acid into the striatum, or either MPP+ or 3-nitropropionic acid [3-NP] alone into the striatum) or systemic administration of toxins to rodents and primates (MPTP and 3-NP) [28]. All result in varying degrees of loss of nigral and striatal neurones with decreased motor function, and sometimes transient dystonia, that is unresponsive to levodopa treatment. None of these models reflect the widespread pathology of MSA or its subtypes (MSA-P and MSA-C) or its diverse symptomatology in man, and none have been utilised to develop novel pharmacological treatments.

Transgenic mice models of human wild-type α-synuclein expression under the control of oligodendrocyte promoters have been used to produce genetic-based models bearing the pathological hallmark of MSA [39, 66, 79]. However, whilst oligodendrocyte accumulation of α synuclein was achieved, the overall pathology observed was limited with some neuronal loss in substantia nigra and the striatum but none in the cerebellum, and this was accompanied by limited disruption of motor function. As a consequence, toxin administration (3-NP) was combined with genetic manipulation resulting in pathology in both basal ganglia and olivopontocerebellar networks and more marked motor deficits [69, 75]. Whilst this may seem a more robust model of MSA, an improvement in nigrostriatal function seen in these mice when treated with the MAO-B inhibitor rasagiline [68] failed to translate into an effect in clinical trial in man.

PSP is characterised by marked parkinsonism and vertical supranuclear palsy with prominent postural instability and gait disturbance, falls and dementia [46] – although a number of variants have been described. Some initial response to dopaminergic therapy may occur, but this rapidly disappears with disease progression. Pathological change occurs in the brainstem, basal ganglia and cerebral cortex, and neuronal loss is marked in the substantia nigra, globus pallidus, subthalamic nucleus and pontine reticular formation [4]. PSP is representative of a group of tauopathies, and both neuronal and glial accumulations of hyperphosphorylated tau are found [47]. Linkage of PSP to mutations of the tau gene MAPT has led to the development of transgenic mouse models. Abundant hyperphosphorylated tau filaments were found in mice expressing four-repeat P301S mutant human tau in a similar way to human PSP, and non-apoptotic nerve cell loss and a pronounced inflammatory reaction were present along with impaired motor function [5, 8]. Some evaluation of agents that are able to prevent tau-related pathology has been undertaken in these mice although much is directed at other tau pathologies notably frontotemporal dementia. Anti-tau antibodies and passive vaccination reduce hyper-phosphorylation and aggregation of tau [17, 78]. Enhancing autophagy using trehalose or rapamycin reduces the tau burden and enhances neuronal survival in some brain regions in P301S mice although improvement in motor function may not occur [59, 65]. The PPAR agonist bezafibrate administration improves behavioural deficits and tau pathology in P301S mice [24]. Coenzyme Q10 improves survival and reduces behavioural deficits, but only a small reduction in hyperphosphorylated tau is seen [26], although preliminary studies suggest this may be reflected in man. A range of other agents have also been tested, but most now require clinical evaluation in PSP to evaluate the predictive validity of this model. Some are already entering the clinical trial phase of development. Preventing tau phosphorylation using the GSK-3 inhibitor tideglusib is under investigation in phase II studies in PSP. Davunetide, which is thought to stabilise microtubules and so reduce tau phosphorylation and aggregation, is also now undergoing clinical evaluation in PSP [33]. Although not extensively studied, systemic administration of the complex I inhibitor rotenone is reported to produce diffuse brain pathology with extensive tau deposition that more closely resembles PSP than PD and so might provide an alternative approach [36].

2.4 Huntington's Disease

Huntington's disease (HD) is an autosomal dominant neurodegenerative disorder of the polyglutamine (polyQ) class in which expansion of the CAG repeat in the N-terminal of the huntingtin (HTT) protein leads to its misfolding and aggregation as well as nuclear accumulation. A combination of events, including altered transcriptional regulation, excitotoxicity, inflammation and mitochondrial dysfunction leads to degeneration primarily of the medium spiny neurones in the striatum. This degeneration, notably of the striatopallidal pathway, disrupts basal ganglia function, leading to the characteristic motor symptoms of dystonia and chorea. Before the motor symptoms emerge, patients exhibit cognitive dysfunction, encompassing deficits in attention, working memory and executive function [7]. These symptoms are thought to reflect the early pathology in a number of cortical regions, witnessed by a reduction in cortical volume seen with MRI [62], as well as dysfunction in the hippocampus. A number of animal models of HD are available which reproduce the pathology and symptoms to varying degrees. These models have been the subject of some excellent reviews [52, 61].

The earliest models which appeared in the late 1970s were toxin-based models in which selective lesion of the striatopallidal pathway was induced either by intrastriatal injection of excitotoxins such as quinolinic acid or by intrastriatal or systemic injection of the succinate dehydrogenase inhibitor, 3-NP, which led to cell death via mitochondrial impairment. These models, constructed in rodents and non-human primates, exhibited clear pathology within the striatum and produced motor symptoms as well as cognitive deficits [61]. However, the cell loss was both extremely rapid and too regionally restricted (within the striatum), and the construct validity of toxin models was also questionable. It is therefore not surprising that, following isolation of the CAG repeat mutation of HD in 1993 [1], efforts were directed towards the generation of transgenic mouse models of HD replicating this CAG repeat. The earliest R6/1 and R6/2 models which expressed an additional fragment of the human HTT gene (116 and 144 CAG repeats, respectively) exhibited a progressive HD phenotype incorporating cell loss and inclusions in striatum, cortex and hippocampus, thereby better reproducing the widespread pathology seen in HD patients. Starting around 4 weeks of age, these mice exhibited motor (rotarod deficits, clasping behaviour, chorea-like movements) and cognitive (deficits in the Morris water maze and T-maze tasks) impairments alongside lowered body weight and a significantly reduced lifespan of around 14 weeks [49]. Similar phenotypes were induced in transgenic mice expressing full-length human HTT gene (YAC128 and BACHD), albeit with much milder behavioural deficits and a longer lifespan [52, 61]. In order to avoid the non-physiological expression of three copies of the HTT gene (two normal and one introduced human mutant copy) and potential problems of random integration in these transgenic models, newer knock-in models in which a single-mutated copy of human HTT is expressed alongside a single normal copy of mouse HTT (including HdhQ111 and CAG140) have been generated. Whilst these have better constructed validity and certainly expressed a more protracted pathology, in line with the human condition, their behavioural phenotype is far milder and more variably expressed [52, 72], making them less ideal for examining therapeutic interventions.

As far as the contribution of these animal models have made to HD research, each (toxin-based, transgenic and knock-in) has played a significant role in increasing our understanding of disease pathogenesis in HD. They have also been used to develop ideas for new therapeutic approaches to treating HD [72] such as those targeting excitotoxicity, abnormal protein degradation, neurodegeneration (with, e.g. neurotrophic factors like BDNF and GDNF) and transcriptional deregulation (with, e.g. histone deacetylase [HDAC] inhibitors). Nevertheless, it is the transgenic models that remain most often used. The rapidity in which these models are induced may diverge from the human condition, but this timescale is most efficient from the point of screening for potential therapeutic agents. In fact, almost 50 % of therapeutic studies still use the originally described R6/2 model, whilst a further 40 % use either R6/1, YAC128 or another transgenic model (N171-82Q). With restrictions on funding, it is anticipated that these models will continue to dominate for some years, especially in early preclinical therapeutic investigations. What remains uncertain is how strong their predictive validity is. With so few clinical trials conducted thus far [72], it is too early to establish the success rate for translation through to the clinic.

2.5 Dystonia

Dystonia is a general term covering a range of disorders involving focal, segmental or generalised torsion of the limbs, trunk or other body parts [2, 11, 27]. It can be primary or secondary and either sporadic in nature, familial or drug (levodopa or neuroleptics) or toxin (3-NP or manganese exposure) induced and can affect children or adults. There is seldom clear evidence of any pathological change (although discrete lesions in basal ganglia can induce dystonia), and both alterations in the basal ganglia and cerebellum are implicated in its pathogenesis based on imaging, surgical and biochemical markers. Dystonia is largely considered to be a dysfunction of neuronal networks (cortico-strio-pallido-thalamo-cortical or cerebello-thalamic-cortical) [15, 56] – this suggests its cause (or causes) is poorly understood. Altered presynaptic and postsynaptic dopaminergic function has been shown in basal ganglia – largely altered D-2 receptor density along with changes in markers of GABAergic transmission [76]. The ability of dopaminergic drugs to both induce and control dystonia also argues for the role of basal ganglia. In the cerebellum, the Purkinje fibre function appears central and glutamatergic and, GABAergic function can be changed [76]. Perhaps, not surprisingly, the treatment of dystonia is also poor and limited to surgery, deep brain stimulation, botulinum toxin, GABAergic agents, dopaminergic drugs and anticholinergic drugs – the latter being the only pharmacological approach of proven efficacy. Animal models have been developed largely on a genotypic and phenotypic basis with only some overlap between the two [45, 58, 60, 73, 76].

Phenotypic models in rodents and primates have involved lesioning, toxin treatment and/or drug administration. In basal ganglia, dystonia can be induced by toxin treatment alone, by the administration of levodopa to 6-OHDA lesioned rats or MPTP-treated primates, by the chronic administration of neuroleptic drugs or by acute administration of cholinergic agonists, such a pilocarpine [76]. 3-NP lesioning of striatal output fibres with or without 6-OHDA lesioning of the nigrostriatal pathway can induce dystonia. The focal injection of GABAergic drugs into the globus pallidus, substantia nigra pars reticulata or thalamus induces dystonia in both rodents and primates. Indeed, a variety of manipulations of basal ganglia circuitry lead to the expression of various forms of dystonia. In the cerebellum, the focal injection of kainic acid induces dystonia, and pharmacological manipulation suggests involvement of AMPA-type glutamate receptors. Spontaneous mutations in rodents have also proven a valuable source of models of dystonia, and these have been extensively reviewed, so only specific examples will be used in this article [45, 60, 73]. The hph-1 mouse is deficient in GTP cyclohydrolase that affects presynaptic dopaminergic function and provides a model of levodopa-responsive dystonia (the Segawa disease). In contrast, the dt^{sz} hamster shows generalised dystonia that seems linked to altered striatal GABAergic outflow, as dystonic movements are decreased by GABA agonists but increased by GABA antagonists, yet appears devoid of pathology. The tottering mouse has mutations in Cav2.1 calcium channels associated with a decline in the Purkinje fibre density. Perhaps, the most informative is the dt-rat that develops marked dystonia and has mutations affecting the protein caytaxin that is essential for cerebellar cortex development. Again, there is no obvious pathology, but there is an altered GABAergic function affecting cerebellar nuclei. In fact, a generalisation is that spontaneous mutations leading to dystonia are commonly associated with the Purkinje cell calcium signalling.

However, the greatest interest has been in animal models related to genes known to induce dystonia in man – there are at least 20 forms of inherited dystonia, but those related to DYT-1, 11 and 12 have attracted the most attention – of which DYT-1 has been the most studied [58]. DYT-1 dystonia is characterised by early-onset, generalised torsion dystonia linked to mutations in the protein torsin A that is involved in chaperone mediated protein folding and vesicular trafficking. DYT-1 knock-in, knock-down and knockout mice have been generated along with over-expressers of wild-type and mutant torsin A. Overexpression of human torsin A leads to alterations in motor function (such as beam walking, limb clasping) but whether these reflect dystonia as it occurs in man is not clear. As does occur in man, there is some evidence for morphological change in basal ganglia with the presence of ubiquitin and torsin A containing inclusions and alterations in pre- and postsynaptic dopaminergic function in the striatum together with change in cholinergic transmission and altered long-term potentiation and long-term depression (LTP and LTD). Altered cerebellar signalling has been found in DYT-1 dystonia, and this can also occur following genetic manipulation in mice. Whilst the model has been very formative in understanding pathogenic processes underlying DYT-1 dystonia, it does not seem to have been widely applied to the search for new pharmacological treatments, perhaps, because these animals do not exhibit overt dystonia.

2.6 Amyotrophic Lateral Sclerosis (ALS)

ALS is characterised by a loss of upper and lower motor neurones with gliosis, muscle wasting and spasticity leading to paralysis and rapid death. Characteristic cytoplasmic protein aggregations are found in affected motor neurones. Although symptomatic treatments exist, there is no disease-modifying therapy available with the possible exception of the glutamate antagonist, riluzole. Most cases of ALS are sporadic (SALS), but approximately 5–10 % are inherited familial (FALS), usually in an autosomal dominant manner [19]. It was the discovery of gene defects in this population that has led to the development of animal models of ALS. Missense mutations in SOD1 were the first identified cause of FALS [63]. Although it is still not understood how these lead to motor neurone degeneration, a toxic gain of function seems likely. A transgenic mouse, and later a transgenic rat, model (SOD1-G93A) was subsequently developed that exhibits key features of ALS – progressive motor dysfunction, motor neurone loss, gliosis, axonal abnormalities and mitochondrial impairment [34]. Many substances have been tested as potential disease-modifying agents for ALS, but to date, there has been no translation into man. Recently, S-(+)-apomorphine (the isomer inactive at dopamine receptors) was shown to attenuate motor dysfunction in SOD1-G93A mice and may offer an opportunity for clinical investigation. Indeed, previously, the R-(+)-enantiomer of the dopamine agonist pramipexole was suggested as modifying ALS perhaps through a mitochondrially mediated mechanism, but it was ineffective in clinical trial. However, SOD1 mutations only account for a small percentage of all FALS cases, and other gene mutations/proteins have been identified (including TDP-43, FUS, VCP, CD90RF72) that may have greater importance to the overall patient population. TAR DNA-binding protein 43 (TDP-43) has been identified as the major protein occurring in cytoplasmic inclusions in FALS and mutations in its encoding appear to be a major cause of FALS [54]. TDP-43 appears to regulate RNA processing but whether a loss of function or a gain of function of TDP-43 is responsible is not known. A variety of transgenic models based on manipulation of TDP-43 have been produced, and these show many of the characteristics of ALS although with mainly axonal phenotypes, whilst motor neurone degeneration appears variable [50, 74]. So far, these new models are being used to explore pathogenic mechanisms in ALS, but no doubt, they will be utilised to uncover new approaches to potential disease-modifying therapies. For example, at least in *Drosophila*, TDP-43 alters the expression of mRNA for the glutamate transporters EAAT1/2 [23].

Conclusions

This chapter has emphasised the important role played by animal models in attempting to reproduce the clinical symptoms and pathogenic mechanisms underlying a selected group of neurological diseases where altered control of motor function occurs. Through the use of toxins and genetic manipulation in animals, there has been a marked expansion of knowledge of human disease. In those diseases with a clear familial basis, such as HD and those where gene defects are increasingly held responsible for a large proportion of cases, such as ALS, the use of genetic manipulation in mice has come to dominate research. However, the same approach has not so far proved as fruitful in other movement disorders, for example, PD where gene defects clearly identified as dominant or recessive causes of the disease do not reproduce the symptomatology or pathology seen in man. Here, toxin-based models still play an important role either alone or in combination with genetic manipulation. In orphan diseases, such as MSA, PSP and dystonia, much more needs to be done to produce animal models that are truly reflective of the human condition as the unmet clinical need is high. What is striking, however, is that despite the effort put into modelling movement disorders in animals, we have not in recent times made the progress in the development of new therapeutic agents for symptomatic treatment that might be expected. Even more disappointingly, despite considerable progress in understanding pathogenic mechanisms underlying a variety of movement disorders, we have not so far uncovered any means of preventing or slowing neuronal loss that has translated into a clinically effective treatment. Nevertheless, the unravelling of the complex events that lead to the onset and progression of movement disorders would not have progressed, and will not progress further, without the use of existing and new animal models.

References

1. A novel gene containing a trinucleotide repeat that is expanded and unstable on Huntington's disease chromosomes. The Huntington's Disease Collaborative Research Group. Cell. 1993;72(6):971–83.
2. Albanese A, Bhatia K, Bressman SB, Delong MR, Fahn S, Fung VS, et al. Phenomenology and classification of dystonia: a consensus update. Mov Disord Off J Mov Disord Soc. 2013;28(7):863–73.
3. Albanese A, Jenner P, Marsden CD, Stephenson JD. Bladder hyperreflexia induced in marmosets by 1-methyl-4-phenyl-1,2,3,6-tetrahydropyridine. Neurosci Lett. 1988;87(1–2):46–50.
4. Albers DS, Augood SJ. New insights into progressive supranuclear palsy. Trends Neurosci. 2001;24(6):347–53.
5. Allen B, Ingram E, Takao M, Smith MJ, Jakes R, Virdee K, et al. Abundant tau filaments and nonapoptotic neurodegeneration in transgenic mice expressing human P301S tau protein. J Neurosci Off J Soc Neurosci. 2002;22(21):9340–51.
6. Barraud Q, Lambrecq V, Forni C, McGuire S, Hill M, Bioulac B, et al. Sleep disorders in Parkinson's disease: the contribution of the MPTP non-human primate model. Exp Neurol. 2009;219(2):574–82.
7. Bates GP, Dorsey R, Gusella JF, Hayden MR, Kay C, Leavitt BR, et al. Huntingon's disease. Nat Rev Dis Primers. 2015;1:1–21.
8. Bellucci A, Westwood AJ, Ingram E, Casamenti F, Goedert M, Spillantini MG. Induction of inflammatory mediators and microglial activation in mice transgenic for mutant human P301S tau protein. Am J Pathol. 2004;165(5):1643–52.
9. Berg D, Godau J, Trenkwalder C, Eggert K, Csoti I, Storch A, et al. AFQ056 treatment of levodopa-induced dyskinesias: results of 2 randomized controlled trials. Mov Disord. 2011;26(7):1243–50.
10. Berger Y, Blaivas JG, DeLaRocha ER, Salinas JM. Urodynamic findings in Parkinson's disease. J Urol. 1987;138(4):836–8.
11. Bertram KL, Williams DR. Diagnosis of dystonic syndromes – a new eight-question approach. Nat Rev Neurol. 2012;8(5):275–83.
12. Bibbiani F, Oh JD, Chase TN. Serotonin 5-HT1A agonist improves motor complications in rodent and primate parkinsonian models. Neurology. 2001;57(10):1829–34.
13. Blanchet PJ, Konitsiotis S, Chase TN. Amantadine reduces levodopa-induced dyskinesias in parkinsonian monkeys. Mov Disord Off J Mov Disord Soc. 1998;13(5):798–802.

14. Broadstock M, Austin PJ, Betts MJ, Duty S. Antiparkinsonian potential of targeting group III metabotropic glutamate receptor subtypes in the rodent substantia nigra pars reticulata. Br J Pharmacol. 2012;165(4b):1034–45.
15. Carbon M, Argyelan M, Habeck C, Ghilardi MF, Fitzpatrick T, Dhawan V, et al. Increased sensorimotor network activity in DYT1 dystonia: a functional imaging study. Brain J Neurol. 2010;133(Pt 3): 690–700.
16. Cenci MA, Lee CS, Bjorklund A. L-DOPA-induced dyskinesia in the rat is associated with striatal overexpression of prodynorphin- and glutamic acid decarboxylase mRNA. Eur J Neurosci. 1998;10(8): 2694–706.
17. Chai X, Wu S, Murray TK, Kinley R, Cella CV, Sims H, et al. Passive immunization with anti-Tau antibodies in two transgenic models: reduction of Tau pathology and delay of disease progression. J Biol Chem. 2011;286(39):34457–67.
18. Chaudhuri KR, Schapira AH. Non-motor symptoms of Parkinson's disease: dopaminergic pathophysiology and treatment. Lancet Neurol. 2009;8(5): 464–74.
19. Cleveland DW, Rothstein JD. From Charcot to Lou Gehrig: deciphering selective motor neuron death in ALS. Nat Rev Neurosci. 2001;2(11):806–19.
20. Dawson TM, Ko HS, Dawson VL. Genetic animal models of Parkinson's disease. Neuron. 2010;66(5): 646–61.
21. Decamp E, Schneider JS. Attention and executive function deficits in chronic low-dose MPTP-treated non-human primates. Eur J Neurosci. 2004;20(5): 1371–8.
22. Dexter PM, Caldwell KA, Caldwell GA. A predictable worm: application of Caenorhabditis elegans for mechanistic investigation of movement disorders. Neurotherapeutics. 2012;9(2):393–404.
23. Diaper DC, Adachi Y, Lazarou L, Greenstein M, Simoes FA, Di Domenico A, et al. Drosophila TDP 43 dysfunction in glia and muscle cells cause cytological and behavioural phenotypes that characterize ALS and FTLD. Hum Mol Genet. 2013;22(19): 3883–93.
24. Dumont M, Stack C, Elipenahli C, Jainuddin S, Gerges M, Starkova N, et al. Bezafibrate administration improves behavioral deficits and tau pathology in P301S mice. Hum Mol Genet. 2012;21(23):5091–105.
25. Duty S, Jenner P. Animal models of Parkinson's disease: a source of novel treatments and clues to the cause of the disease. Br J Pharmacol. 2011;164(4): 1357–91.
26. Elipenahli C, Stack C, Jainuddin S, Gerges M, Yang L, Starkov A, et al. Behavioral improvement after chronic administration of coenzyme Q10 in P301S transgenic mice. J Alzheimer's Dis JAD. 2012;28(1): 173–82.
27. Fahn S, Eldridge R. Definition of dystonia and classification of the dystonic states. Adv Neurol. 1976;14:1–5.
28. Fernagut PO, Tison F. Animal models of multiple system atrophy. Neuroscience. 2012;211:77–82.
29. Fox SH, Visanji N, Reyes G, Huot P, Gomez-Ramirez J, Johnston T, et al. Neuropsychiatric behaviors in the MPTP marmoset model of Parkinson's disease. Can J Neurol Sci Le journal canadien des sciences neurologiques. 2010;37(1):86–95.
30. Gasmi M, Brandon EP, Herzog CD, Wilson A, Bishop KM, Hofer EK, et al. AAV2-mediated delivery of human neurturin to the rat nigrostriatal system: long-term efficacy and tolerability of CERE-120 for Parkinson's disease. Neurobiol Dis. 2007;27(1): 67–76.
31. Gilman S, Wenning GK, Low PA, Brooks DJ, Mathias CJ, Trojanowski JQ, et al. Second consensus statement on the diagnosis of multiple system atrophy. Neurology. 2008;71(9):670–6.
32. Goetz CG, Damier P, Hicking C, Laska E, Muller T, Olanow CW, et al. Sarizotan as a treatment for dyskinesias in Parkinson's disease: a double-blind placebo-controlled trial. Mov Disord Off J Mov Disord Soc. 2007;22(2):179–86.
33. Gold M, Lorenzl S, Stewart AJ, Morimoto BH, Williams DR, Gozes I. Critical appraisal of the role of davunetide in the treatment of progressive supranuclear palsy. Neuropsychiatr Dis Treat. 2012;8:85–93.
34. Gurney ME, Pu H, Chiu AY, Dal Canto MC, Polchow CY, Alexander DD, et al. Motor neuron degeneration in mice that express a human Cu, Zn superoxide dismutase mutation. Science. 1994;264(5166):1772–5.
35. Hauser RA, Shulman LM, Trugman JM, Roberts JW, Mori A, Ballerini R, et al. Study of istradefylline in patients with Parkinson's disease on levodopa with motor fluctuations. Mov Disord Off J Mov Disord Soc. 2008;23(15):2177–85.
36. Hoglinger GU, Lannuzel A, Khondiker ME, Michel PP, Duyckaerts C, Feger J, et al. The mitochondrial complex I inhibitor rotenone triggers a cerebral tauopathy. J Neurochem. 2005;95(4):930–9.
37. Jenner P, Rupniak NM, Rose S, Kelly E, Kilpatrick G, Lees A, et al. 1-Methyl-4-phenyl-1,2,3,6-tetrahydropyridine-induced parkinsonism in the common marmoset. Neurosci Lett. 1984;50(1–3):85–90.
38. Johnston TH, Fox SH, McIldowie MJ, Piggott MJ, Brotchie JM. Reduction of L-DOPA-induced dyskinesia by the selective metabotropic glutamate receptor 5 antagonist 3-[(2-methyl-1,3-thiazol-4-yl)ethynyl]pyridine in the 1-methyl-4-phenyl-1,2,3,6-tetrahydropyridine-lesioned macaque model of Parkinson's disease. J Pharmacol Exp Ther. 2010;333(3):865–73.
39. Kahle PJ, Neumann M, Ozmen L, Muller V, Jacobsen H, Spooren W, et al. Hyperphosphorylation and insolubility of alpha-synuclein in transgenic mouse oligodendrocytes. EMBO Rep. 2002;3(6):583–8.
40. Kanda T, Jackson MJ, Smith LA, Pearce RK, Nakamura J, Kase H, et al. Combined use of the adenosine A(2A) antagonist KW-6002 with L-DOPA or with selective D1 or D2 dopamine agonists increases antiparkinsonian activity but not dyskinesia in MPTP-treated monkeys. Exp Neurol. 2000;162(2):321–7.

41. Kordower JH, Herzog CD, Dass B, Bakay RA, Stansell 3rd J, Gasmi M, et al. Delivery of neurturin by AAV2 (CERE-120)-mediated gene transfer provides structural and functional neuroprotection and neurorestoration in MPTP-treated monkeys. Ann Neurol. 2006;60(6):706–15.
42. Kumar R, Hauser RA, Mostillo J, Dronamraju N, Graf A, Merschhemke M, et al. Mavoglurant (AFQ056) in combination with increased levodopa dosages in Parkinson's disease patients. Int J Neurosci. 2016;126(1):20–4.
43. Kuoppamaki M, Al-Barghouthy G, Jackson M, Smith L, Zeng BY, Quinn N, et al. Beginning-of-dose and rebound worsening in MPTP-treated common marmosets treated with levodopa. Mov Disord Off J Mov Disord Soc. 2002;17(6):1312–7.
44. Langston JW, Forno LS, Rebert CS, Irwin I. Selective nigral toxicity after systemic administration of 1-methyl-4-phenyl-1,2,5,6-tetrahydropyrine (MPTP) in the squirrel monkey. Brain Res. 1984;292(2): 390–4.
45. LeDoux MS. Animal models of dystonia: lessons from a mutant rat. Neurobiol Dis. 2011;42(2): 152–61.
46. Litvan I, Agid Y, Calne D, Campbell G, Dubois B, Duvoisin RC, et al. Clinical research criteria for the diagnosis of progressive supranuclear palsy (Steele-Richardson-Olszewski syndrome): report of the NINDS-SPSP international workshop. Neurology. 1996;47(1):1–9.
47. Ludolph AC, Kassubek J, Landwehrmeyer BG, Mandelkow E, Mandelkow EM, Burn DJ, et al. Tauopathies with parkinsonism: clinical spectrum, neuropathologic basis, biological markers, and treatment options. Eur J Neurol Off J Eur Fed Neurol Soc. 2009;16(3):297–309.
48. Lundblad M, Andersson M, Winkler C, Kirik D, Wierup N, Cenci MA. Pharmacological validation of behavioural measures of akinesia and dyskinesia in a rat model of Parkinson's disease. Eur J Neurosci. 2002;15(1):120–32.
49. Mangiarini L, Sathasivam K, Seller M, Cozens B, Harper A, Hetherington C, et al. Exon 1 of the HD gene with an expanded CAG repeat is sufficient to cause a progressive neurological phenotype in transgenic mice. Cell. 1996;87(3):493–506.
50. McGoldrick P, Joyce PI, Fisher EM, Greensmith L. Rodent models of amyotrophic lateral sclerosis. Biochim Biophys Acta. 2013;1832(9):1421–36.
51. Mela F, Marti M, Dekundy A, Danysz W, Morari M, Cenci MA. Antagonism of metabotropic glutamate receptor type 5 attenuates l-DOPA-induced dyskinesia and its molecular and neurochemical correlates in a rat model of Parkinson's disease. J Neurochem. 2007;101(2):483–97.
52. Menalled L, El-Khodor BF, Patry M, Suarez-Farinas M, Orenstein SJ, Zahasky B, et al. Systematic behavioral evaluation of Huntington's disease transgenic and knock-in mouse models. Neurobiol Dis. 2009;35(3):319–36.
53. Morin N, Gregoire L, Gomez-Mancilla B, Gasparini F, Di Paolo T. Effect of the metabotropic glutamate receptor type 5 antagonists MPEP and MTEP in parkinsonian monkeys. Neuropharmacology. 2010;58(7): 981–6.
54. Neumann M, Sampathu DM, Kwong LK, Truax AC, Micsenyi MC, Chou TT, et al. Ubiquitinated TDP-43 in frontotemporal lobar degeneration and amyotrophic lateral sclerosis. Science. 2006;314(5796): 130–3.
55. Newman T, Sinadinos C, Johnston A, Sealey M, Mudher A. Using Drosophila models of neurodegenerative diseases for drug discovery. Expert Opin Drug Discovery. 2011;6(2):129–40.
56. Niethammer M, Carbon M, Argyelan M, Eidelberg D. Hereditary dystonia as a neurodevelopmental circuit disorder: evidence from neuroimaging. Neurobiol Dis. 2011;42(2):202–9.
57. Olanow CW, Damier P, Goetz CG, Mueller T, Nutt J, Rascol O, et al. Multicenter, open-label, trial of sarizotan in Parkinson disease patients with levodopa-induced dyskinesias (the SPLENDID Study). Clin Neuropharmacol. 2004;27(2):58–62.
58. Oleas J, Yokoi F, Deandrade MP, Pisani A, Li Y. Engineering animal models of dystonia. Mov Disord Off J Mov Disord Soc. 2013;28(7): 990–1000.
59. Ozcelik S, Fraser G, Castets P, Schaeffer V, Skachokova Z, Breu K, et al. Rapamycin attenuates the progression of tau pathology in P301S tau transgenic mice. PLoS ONE. 2013;8(5), e62459.
60. Raike RS, Jinnah HA, Hess EJ. Animal models of generalized dystonia. NeuroRx J Am Soc Exp Neurol Ther. 2005;2(3):504–12.
61. Ramaswamy S, McBride JL, Kordower JH. Animal models of Huntington's disease. ILAR J Natl Res Coun Inst Lab Anim Resour. 2007;48(4):356–73.
62. Rosas HD, Hevelone ND, Zaleta AK, Greve DN, Salat DH, Fischl B. Regional cortical thinning in preclinical Huntington disease and its relationship to cognition. Neurology. 2005;65(5):745–7.
63. Rosen DR, Siddique T, Patterson D, Figlewicz DA, Sapp P, Hentati A, et al. Mutations in Cu/Zn superoxide dismutase gene are associated with familial amyotrophic lateral sclerosis. Nature. 1993;362(6415):59–62.
64. Rylander D, Iderberg H, Li Q, Dekundy A, Zhang J, Li H, et al. A mGluR5 antagonist under clinical development improves L-DOPA-induced dyskinesia in parkinsonian rats and monkeys. Neurobiol Dis. 2010;39(3):352–61.
65. Schaeffer V, Goedert M. Stimulation of autophagy is neuroprotective in a mouse model of human tauopathy. Autophagy. 2012;8(11):1686–7.
66. Shults CW, Rockenstein E, Crews L, Adame A, Mante M, Larrea G, et al. Neurological and neurodegenerative alterations in a transgenic mouse model expressing human alpha-synuclein under oligodendrocyte promoter: implications for multiple system atrophy. J Neurosci Off J Soc Neurosci. 2005;25(46): 10689–99.

67. Sleeman IJ, Boshoff EL, Duty S. Fibroblast growth factor-20 protects against dopamine neuron loss in vitro and provides functional protection in the 6-hydroxydopamine-lesioned rat model of Parkinson's disease. Neuropharmacology. 2012;63(7):1268–77.
68. Stefanova N, Poewe W, Wenning GK. Rasagiline is neuroprotective in a transgenic model of multiple system atrophy. Exp Neurol. 2008;210(2):421–7.
69. Stefanova N, Reindl M, Neumann M, Haass C, Poewe W, Kahle PJ, et al. Oxidative stress in transgenic mice with oligodendroglial alpha-synuclein overexpression replicates the characteristic neuropathology of multiple system atrophy. Am J Pathol. 2005;166(3):869–76.
70. Stocchi F, Rascol O, Destee A, Hattori N, Hauser RA, Lang AE, et al. AFQ056 in Parkinson patients with levodopa-induced dyskinesia: 13-week, randomized, dose-finding study. Mov Disord. 2013;28: 1838–46.
71. Stockwell KA, Scheller D, Rose S, Jackson MJ, Tayarani-Binazir K, Iravani MM, et al. Continuous administration of rotigotine to MPTP-treated common marmosets enhances anti-parkinsonian activity and reduces dyskinesia induction. Exp Neurol. 2009;219(2):533–42.
72. Switonski PM, Szlachcic WJ, Gabka A, Krzyzosiak WJ, Figiel M. Mouse models of polyglutamine diseases in therapeutic approaches: review and data table. Part II. Mol Neurobiol. 2012;46(2):430–66.
73. Tassone A, Sciamanna G, Bonsi P, Martella G, Pisani A. Experimental models of dystonia. Int Rev Neurobiol. 2011;98:551–72.
74. Tsao W, Jeong YH, Lin S, Ling J, Price DL, Chiang PM, et al. Rodent models of TDP-43: recent advances. Brain Res. 2012;1462:26–39
75. Ubhi K, Lee PH, Adame A, Inglis C, Mante M, Rockenstein E, et al. Mitochondrial inhibitor 3-nitroproprionic acid enhances oxidative modification of alpha-synuclein in a transgenic mouse model of multiple system atrophy. J Neurosci Res. 2009;87(12):2728–39.
76. Wilson BK, Hess EJ. Animal models for dystonia. Mov Disord Off J Mov Disord Soc. 2013;28(7): 982–9.
77. Xi Y, Noble S, Ekker M. Modeling neurodegeneration in zebrafish. Curr Neurol Neurosci Rep. 2011;11(3): 274–82.
78. Yanamandra K, Kfoury N, Jiang H, Mahan TE, Ma S, Maloney SE, et al. Anti-tau antibodies that block tau aggregate seeding in vitro markedly decrease pathology and improve cognition in vivo. Neuron. 2013;80(2):402–14.
79. Yazawa I, Giasson BI, Sasaki R, Zhang B, Joyce S, Uryu K, et al. Mouse model of multiple system atrophy alpha-synuclein expression in oligodendrocytes causes glial and neuronal degeneration. Neuron. 2005;45(6):847–59.
80. Yoshimura N, Kuno S, Chancellor MB, De Groat WC, Seki S. Dopaminergic mechanisms underlying bladder hyperactivity in rats with a unilateral 6-hydroxydopamine (6-OHDA) lesion of the nigrostriatal pathway. Br J Pharmacol. 2003;139(8): 1425–32.
81. Yoshimura N, Mizuta E, Kuno S, Sasa M, Yoshida O. The dopamine D1 receptor agonist SKF 38393 suppresses detrusor hyperreflexia in the monkey with parkinsonism induced by 1-methyl-4-phenyl-1,2,3,6-tetrahydropyridine (MPTP). Neuropharmacology. 1993,32(4):315–21.

Epidemiological Methods for Studying Movement Disorders

3

Yoav Ben-Shlomo

3.1 What Is Epidemiology?

Epidemiology is the application of methods to the study of the distribution and determinants of diseases with the aim of providing evidence-based health care and identifying interventions that may prevent onset (primary or secondary prevention) or slow disease progression (tertiary prevention) (see the following textbooks for more and less detailed explanations of epidemiological methods [1, 2]). It encompasses descriptive epidemiology (measuring prevalence and incidence and describing patterns by time, place and person) as well as aetiological epidemiology to identify risk or protective factors, usually using ecological, case-control or cohort studies. Clinical epidemiology will also look at diagnosis, prognosis and treatments, through the use of clinical cohorts of patients and randomised controlled trials, though this chapter will not cover these elements (see Chap. 6 for randomised controlled trials).

This chapter will provide a brief overview of epidemiological methods used in observational studies and will mainly use Parkinson's disease (PD) as the exemplar movement disorder.

Y. Ben-Shlomo, MB, BS, PhD, FFPH
School of Social and Community Medicine,
University of Bristol, 39 Whatley Road,
Bristol, Avon BS8 2PS, UK
e-mail: y.ben-shlomo@bristol.ac.uk

3.2 Case Definition

All research studies start off with a research question or hypothesis which usually revolves around a specific condition or syndrome. This necessitates having some operational definition of what is a case ("case definition"). This may be as simple as a clinical diagnosis or complex research criteria. One must always consider the reliability (both inter-rate and intra-rater) and validity of any case definition and how this may influence the results (bias). A reliable measure may still be incorrect. For Parkinson's Disease (PD), the validity varies, depending on whether the diagnosis is made by a general practitioner [3], neurologist or geriatrician [4] or movement disorder specialist [5]. In each case the positive predictive of a clinical diagnosis improves with greater expertise but such a process adds to the cost and complexity of the study design. Even with expert diagnosis, errors can occur early in the natural history of the disease when newly diagnosed cases may be wrongly diagnosed as atypical feature may take to time to emerge resulting to a revised diagnosis [6]. The intensity of the method used to identify cases and the size of the population will have an influence. A meta-regression of prevalence rates for Tourette's syndrome [7] found that study size was the strongest predictor of prevalence rates with smaller population having higher rates.

C. Falup-Pecurariu et al. (eds.), *Movement Disorders Curricula*,
DOI 10.1007/978-3-7091-1628-9_3

3.3 Descriptive Epidemiology: Time, Place and Person

Descriptive epidemiology is essential for healthcare planning purposes (how many specialist clinics do we need?) as well as generating hypotheses that require more detailed investigations. One of the most obvious questions to ask is whether a disease is getting more common or less common or is not changing over time. This can be resolved by examining the incidence (number of new cases per time period/population at risk) over time. However, in the absence of good data on incidence, it is not uncommon to examine prevalence (number of existing cases at one moment or period/population at risk) instead. The interpretation of such data is more complex as in a closed population; the prevalence rate is a function of the number of new cases (input) and the average survival of cases (output) as death removes cases from the population. So, for example, a meta-analysis of prevalence rates of PD in the United Kingdom over time [8] found that the prevalence was remarkably similar over a 40-year period (1966–2009), but this may mask a decline in the risk of developing PD if survival has improved and greater diagnostic awareness of other parkinsonian disorders such as multiple system atrophy means that such cases were wrongly attributed as PD in the past as compared to today. The best long-term data on the incidence of PD in one population comes from Olmsted County, Minnesota [9], which found stable incidence rates, suggesting no major environmental risk factors for PD were introduced or removed from this population during these periods. This is in contrast to secular trends in smoking behaviour which show a steady decline in midlife smoking and might have been expected to increase PD incidence (see below for further explanation). Racial or ethnic differences in disease risk are important both as potential clues to aetiology and also as a measure of health care. A study of PD amongst Whites, African American and Hispanics in the USA found that whilst Black men had the highest incidence, they had the lowest prevalence and hence worst survival [10]. In this case, as Black men are more likely to be poorer, the differences in survival are probably related to socioeconomic status and worse access to health care. The consistent finding that men have a greater PD risk than women [11] has generated a hypothesis that female hormones may be protective for PD, and a historical cohort study [12] lends further support to this hypothesis as it found that both unilateral oophorectomy and bilateral oophorectomy prior to menopause were associated with increased PD risk.

3.4 Aetiological Epidemiology

In order to determine risk or protective factors for disease, it is self-obvious that any exposure must precede disease onset. This time period is known as the induction period, but for many diseases, pathology begins before clinical manifestation or diagnosis ("subclinical phase"). The latter is a harder milestone to measure and hence it is more common to measure the "latency period". This is complicated by the fact that there may be systematic variations in time between symptom onset and clinical diagnosis, for example, by educational level. In the case of PD, it is now recognised that the classical motor symptoms are often if not always preceded by a variety of non-motor features such as hyposmia, constipation and psychological morbidity [13], often decades before clinical diagnosis. The danger of not truly understanding the latency period is that any exposure may be measured after disease onset and then if one observes an association, it is either due to the disease process itself, e.g. reverse causation (see below), or the exposure which may be important in the progression of the disease rather than initiation itself.

When a researcher observes an association between an exposure and an outcome, it is sensible to consider the influence of chance, bias, confounding and reverse causation before concluding that such an association is causal. Most researchers are familiar with the concept of probability expressed as "*p*-values" and are gratified when their associations lie below the magical "$p<0.05$" or are dismayed when $p=0.06$ or more. This reflects a failure of understanding what p-values actually tell us as compared to 95% confidence intervals which provide more meaningful clinical or public health information (see this reference for an excellent explanation [14]). However, this situation is generally worse than most researchers appreciate if the prior probability of the hypothesis being tested is low. This issue is not limited to observational studies but also covers randomised controlled trials and meta-analyses. Under these circumstances, observations that appear unlikely to have occurred by chance are still likely to be false positives [15] resulting in misleading evidence. Other major problems in observational studies lie within the realm of confounding and biases. Whilst we now have sophisticated statistical methods, simple adjustment for covariates may make things worse if one conditions on variables without considering the appropriate causal model through the use of directed acyclic graphs [16].

There are a large variety of different biases that may distort the true "causal" association between an exposure and an outcome. These may be non-differential (random) or differential (selective) and may operate in either direction so that a true association is attenuated or masked (false negative) or accentuated or created when no causal association exists (false positive). For example, it has long been thought that PD may be related to early exposure to an infectious agent analogous to the encephalitis lethargica experience. However, early case-control studies where subjects were asked to recall past childhood infections many years earlier were essentially negative [17]. This is unsurprising given the difficulty of accurately recalling these past exposures over several decades, and any misclassification is likely to have been equally difficult for both cases and controls, hence attenuating any true association. The one case-control study that has examined this exposure (Harvard and Pennsylvania alumni study) with less bias found an apparent "protective effect" of measles based on self-report of childhood infections at time of entry to college which could not have been biased by future disease risk and required a much shorter recall period [18]. An infectious agent exposure has received recent renewed attention [19] since the discovery of Lewy body pathology in the olfactory bulb and enteric plexus of the stomach consistent with the role of a neurotropic viral infection. Imaginative epidemiological studies can then be used to provide further supportive evidence. For example, a record linkage study in Denmark was able to create a cohort of patients who had undergone vagotomy, hence preventing retrograde infection via the vagus nerve, and found a reduced risk of future PD though risk estimates were imprecise [20].

A classic example of differential misclassification can be demonstrated with recall of head injuries which is more likely to be reported by PD cases than controls ("recall bias") as cases have a stronger reason to report a prior injury producing an artefactual association or overestimating any true causal association. This problem can be reduced to some degree by limiting exposure to those head injuries that are serious enough that they cause concussion or hospital admission. A recent systematic review and meta-analysis demonstrates this problem as well as introduces us to the further issue of "publication bias" [21]. This review identified 22 studies, 19 of which were case-control studies, 2 nested case-control studies and 1 cohort study, and concluded that a history of head trauma that results in concussion is associated with a higher risk of developing PD. Based on data from 18,344 cases and 79,028 controls, the authors found a pooled odds ratio of 1.57 (95% CI 1.35, 1.83) which was highly unlikely to have occurred by chance and concluded a causal role for head injuries. However, they also found marked publication bias, so that there was an absence of smaller negative or null studies as would be expected by chance (see the funnel plot in Fig. 3 of this publication), suggesting that either authors or journals are less likely to submit and/or publish such papers favouring those with an apparent statistically significant finding (they failed to quantify this with a formal Egger test). However, the two largest contributing studies were nested case-control studies both done in Scandinavian countries whereby hospital records could be used to select cases and controls nested within a much larger cohort of subjects [22, 23]. In both these studies, where there is no recall bias as exposure is ascertained via hospital diagnosis codes created by medical and/or administrative staff, the increased risks are only seen with a latency period between the head injury and hospital-based contact for PD of between 1 and 4 years in the Swedish study and up to 9 years in the Danish study. The relatively short latency suggests that at best head injuries may accelerate disease progression possibly through altering the blood-brain barrier but are unlikely to be the initiator. Alternatively reverse causation must again be considered as impaired gait or bradykinesia may have contributed to the head injury. A similar argument has been made for the inverse association between smoking and PD whereby never smokers and ex-smokers have a greater risk of PD than current smokers and this is observed in both case-control and cohort studies [24]. This most likely represents a prodromal PD phenotype so that addictive prone behaviours are less likely to be expressed in people who will develop PD due to preclinical dopamine deficiency [25].

Selection bias is another issue with hospital-based case-control studies. So, for example, well water has been postulated to be a risk factor for PD (see reference [26] for an excellent review of PD epidemiology). However, cases in such studies are usually ascertained from specialist units, who receive referrals from both urban and rural populations, whilst hospital controls will oversample urban subjects. This will result in any rural exposure such as well water or farming being over-represented in the case population and an artefactual association. This example can also be used to illustrate the issue of "confounding", when a third variable is the antecedent or parent of both the exposure and the outcome. If we find that well water is associated with a greater risk of PD, then one must consider if another factor could be creating this association under the assumption that well water is not causally associated with PD. In this case it is likely that well water consumption is itself determined by rural residence which also increase the risk of exposure to pesticides and perhaps this is the causal factor. In this scenario mutual adjustment for both variables should determine if one or both are "independent risk factors". This appears to be unclear [26], but to further complicate matters, one must consider the degree of measurement error in each exposure. So if well water is better reported than pesticide exposure, it may appear to be a stronger risk factor even when it is not associated (known as "residual confounding").

Finally, where appropriate natural experiments exist, they can provide powerful tests of hypotheses if the change in exposure is unrelated to other potential confounders. For example, it has been argued that neuropsychiatric complications may occur after a streptococcal infection due to secondary autoimmune pathology resulting in Tourette's syndrome or tics though a population-based primary care study failed to find convincing evidence for such an association [27]. This same dataset failed to show any change in the incidence of Tourette's syndrome over time despite the natural experiment of a marked reduction in antibiotic prescribed over the same period in the United Kingdom because of concerns around antibiotic resistance (unpublished observation).

Epidemiological methods provide powerful approaches to generate hypotheses and test existing ideas about pathophysiology. Observational studies must be interpreted with caution but if undertaken with rigour and used imaginatively can provide powerful evidence concerning potentially causal or prodromal risk factors for movement disorders.

References

1. Rothman KJ, Greenland S, Lash TL. Modern epidemiology. Philadelphia: Wolters Kluwer Health/Lippincott Williams & Wilkins; 2008.
2. Ben-Shlomo Y, Brookes S, Hickman M, Farmer RDT. Lecture notes. Epidemiology, evidence-based medicine, and public health. Chichester: Wiley; 2013.
3. Schrag A, Ben Shlomo Y, Quinn N. How valid is the clinical diagnosis of Parkinson's disease in the community? J Neurol Neurosurg Psychiatry. 2002;73:529–34.
4. Hughes AJ, Daniel SE, Blankson S, Lees AJ. A clinicopathologic study of 100 cases of Parkinson's disease. Arch Neurol. 1993;50:140–8.
5. Hughes AJ, Daniel SE, Ben Shlomo Y, Lees AJ. The accuracy of diagnosis of parkinsonian syndromes in a specialist movement disorder service. Brain. 2002;125:861–70.

6. Caslake R, Taylor K, Scott N, Gordon J, Harris C, Wilde K, Murray A, Counsell C. Age-, gender-, and socioeconomic status-specific incidence of Parkinson's disease and parkinsonism in North East Scotland: the PINE study. Parkinsonism Relat Disord. 2013;19:515–21.
7. Scharf JM, Miller LL, Gauvin CA, Alabiso J, Mathews CA, Ben-Shlomo Y. Population prevalence of Tourette syndrome: a systematic review and meta-analysis. Mov Disord. 2015;30:221–8.
8. Wickremaratchi MM, Perera D, O'Loghlen C, Sastry D, Morgan E, Jones A, Edwards P, Robertson NP, Butler C, Morris HR, Ben-Shlomo Y. Prevalence and age of onset of Parkinson's disease in Cardiff: a community based cross sectional study and meta-analysis. J Neurol Neurosurg Psychiatry. 2009;80:805–7.
9. Rocca WA, Bower JH, McDonnell SK, Peterson BJ, Maraganore DM. Time trends in the incidence of parkinsonism in Olmsted County, Minnesota. Neurology. 2001;57:462–7.
10. Mayeux R, Marder K, Cote LJ, Hemenegildo N, Mejia H, Tang MX, Lantigua R, Wilder D, Gurland B, Hauser A. The frequency of idiopathic Parkinson's disease by age, ethnic group, and sex in Northern Manhattan, 1988–1993. Am J Epidemiol. 1995;142:820–7.
11. Wooten GF, Currie LJ, Bovbjerg VE, Lee JK, Patrie J. Are men at greater risk for Parkinson's disease than women? J Neurol Neurosurg Psychiatry. 2004;75:637–9.
12. Rocca WA, Bower JH, Maraganore DM, Ahlskog JE, Grossardt BR, de Andrade M, Melton LJ. Increased risk of parkinsonism in women who underwent oophorectomy before menopause. Neurology. 2008;70:200–9.
13. Savica R, Rocca WA, Ahlskog JE. When does Parkinson disease start? Arch Neurol. 2010;67:798–801.
14. Sterne JA, Davey SG. Sifting the evidence-what's wrong with significance tests? BMJ. 2001;322:226–31.
15. Ioannidis JPA. Why most published research findings are false. PLoS Med. 2005;2:696–701.
16. Hernan MA, Hernandez-Diaz S, Werler MM, Mitchell AA. Causal knowledge as a prerequisite for confounding evaluation: an application to birth defects epidemiology. Am J Epidemiol. 2002;155:176–84.
17. Kessler II. Epidemiologic studies of Parkinson's disease. III. A community based survey. Am J Epidemiol. 1972;96:242–54.
18. Sasco AJ, Paffenbarger RS. Measles infection and Parkinson's disease. Am J Epidemiol. 1985;122:1017–31.
19. Hawkes CH, Del Tredici K, Braak H. Parkinson's disease: a dual-hit hypothesis. Neuropathol Appl Neurobiol. 2007;33:599–614.
20. Svensson E, Horvath-Puho E, Thomsen RW, Djurhuus JC, Pedersen L, Borghammer P, Sorensen HT. Vagotomy and subsequent risk of Parkinson's disease. Ann Neurol. 2015;78:522–9.
21. Jafari S, Etminan M, Aminzadeh F, Samii A. Head injury and risk of Parkinson disease: a systematic review and meta-analysis. Mov Disord. 2013;28:1222–9.
22. Rugbjerg K, Ritz B, Korbo L, Martinussen N, Olsen JH. Risk of Parkinson's disease after hospital contact for head injury: population based case-control study. BMJ. 2008;337:a2494.
23. Fang F, Chen HL, Feldman AL, Kamel F, Ye WM, Wirdefeldt K. Head injury and Parkinson's disease: a population-based study. Mov Disord. 2012;27:1632–5.
24. Hernan MD, Takkouche B, Caamano-Isorna F, Gestal-Otero JJ. A meta-analysis of coffee-drinking, cigarette smoking, and the risk of Parkinson's disease. Ann Neurol. 2002;52:276–84.
25. Ritz B, Lee PC, Lassen CF, Arah OA. Parkinson disease and smoking revisited ease of quitting is an early sign of the disease. Neurology. 2014;83:1396–402.
26. Wirdefeldt K, Adami HO, Cole P, Trichopoulos D, Mandel J. Epidemiology and etiology of Parkinson's disease: a review of the evidence. Eur J Epidemiol. 2011;26:S1–58.
27. Schrag A, Gilbert R, Giovannoni G, Robertson MM, Metcalfe C, Ben-Shlomo Y. Streptococcal infection, Tourette syndrome, and OCD is there a connection? Neurology. 2009;73:1256–63.

The Phenomenology of Movement Disorders

4

Andrew P. Duker and Alberto J. Espay

4.1 Introduction

Although advances in neuropathology and molecular genetics provide increasingly more complex classification schemes for the conditions we define as movement disorders, it is the phenomenological clues that should guide a clinician's initial impression and tailored work-up of an individual patient. Indeed, the characteristics of the abnormal movement provide a framework upon which to construct a differential diagnosis, guide ancillary testing, and consider therapeutic interventions. Movement disorders emerge by impairments in planning, controlling, or executing movement [1] and are classically divided into those causing an excess of movement (hyperkinetic) or a paucity of voluntary and automatic movements (hypokinetic) [2]. The label of "movement disorder" can refer to the specific phenomenology of a movement (e.g., dystonia) or to a syndrome combining several different abnormal movements (e.g., Huntington's disease which can contain chorea, dystonia, etc). We will focus this chapter on the former, the characterization of the phenomenology of individual movements, in order to provide the basic building blocks upon which to define the more complex syndromes detailed in subsequent chapters.

A.P. Duker, MD • A.J. Espay, MD, MSc (✉)
James J. and Joan A. Gardner Family Center for Parkinson's Disease and Movement Disorders, Department of Neurology, Movement Disorders Center, University of Cincinnati Academic Health Center, 260 Stetson St., Suite 2300, Cincinnati, OH 45267-0525, USA

Department of Neurology and Rehabilitation Medicine, Cincinnati, OH, USA
e-mail: Andrew.Duker@uc.edu; Alberto.Espay@uc.edu

4.2 History

Most conditions which are now termed "movement disorders" were initially grouped under the heading of "extrapyramidal disorders," collectively assumed to correlate with dysfunction in the basal ganglia and connecting structures [3, 4]. This is the case with "classic" movement disorders, whereby there was pathological support for initially exclusive degeneration in structures of the basal ganglia (e.g., nigral degeneration in parkinsonism, caudate atrophy in Huntington's disease). It later became evident that pathology in locations outside the basal ganglia (e.g., cortical myoclonus or cerebellar ataxia) also caused disorders of movement. The field of movement disorders was born from the keen observations made by C. David Marsden in Queen Square and Stanley Fahn in Columbia beginning in the late 1960s [2]. There is no common localization and

C. Falup-Pecurariu et al. (eds.), *Movement Disorders Curricula*,
DOI 10.1007/978-3-7091-1628-9_4

no common pathology or etiology for the vast majority of the movement disorders. Rather, similar phenotypes may be due to a range of pathologies, as the chapters ahead will illustrate. Nevertheless, an organized approach to phenomenological clues is critical to elucidating the localization and possible pathology of abnormal movements.

4.3 Hypokinetic Movement Disorders

4.3.1 Parkinsonism

Parkinsonism is the prototypic hypokinetic movement disorder. The invariable (core) element of this phenomenological construct is the reduction in amplitude and/or speed of movements. The reduction in amplitude is referred to as *hypo*kinesia; the reduction of speed, *brady*kinesia; and the end result of both, *akinesia*. A variable element is *dysrhythmia* or changes in the movement periodicity. Most commonly, and sometimes confusingly, the term bradykinesia is used as a more general term to refer to all three of these characteristics. Variable additional components of parkinsonism include rigidity (the most common combination, often encompassed as "akinetic-rigid" syndrome to distinguish from the rare nonrigid variant, "pure akinesia"), tremor, reduction in gait stride (evolving, in increasing severity of impairment, into festination, trembling in place, and freezing of gait), and postural instability. Recognition of the subtleties between the various parkinsonian elements permits the clinical distinction between Parkinson's disease (PD) and other PD-like disorders, collectively referred to as atypical parkinsonisms.

4.3.1.1 Bradykinesia and the Sequence Effect

Bradykinesia, used in the broadest sense, can include deficits in the initiation and maintenance of movement, a disruption of the fluidity of previously semiconscious movement patterns such as gait or handwriting. The common feature, however, is the so-called sequence effect, defined as a decrement in amplitude and/or speed over the performance of a task [5]. This is observed as increasingly smaller excursions of movement in a finger tapping exercise, the trailing off with progressive shrinkage of letters in a handwritten sentence (ending in micrographia), or the decreasing stride length during gait (shuffling with festination). In PD, levodopa improves the speed of movement more than the amplitude of movement [6] but does not seem to improve the sequence effect, suggestive that it may be a non-dopaminergic disease feature [7]. A phenomenon shown by a subset of patients is the significant reduction of amplitude without concomitant impairment of speed (*pure* hypokinesia). When very small amplitude finger excursions in a tapping task are associated with rapid movements, the term *hastening* has been applied [8]. Pure hypokinesia tends to be more common in patients with atypical parkinsonisms, such as multiple system atrophy and progressive supranuclear palsy, but it is certainly within the broad phenotypic spectrum of PD. The hastening phenomenon of finger movements is equivalent to *festination* in the legs, the progressively decreasing stride length with increasing cadence during gait. Extreme impairments result in arrests of movement at initiation (*start hesitation* [9]) or during their performance (freezing). These latter phenomena are of paroxysmal appearance in advanced PD.

Bradykinesia is also manifested in slowness and paucity of facial movements (masked facies, decreased blink rate), associated or automatic movements (e.g., decreased arm swing), and overall reduction in the range of axial and appendicular movements. To fully appreciate the distribution and extent of the spectrum of bradykinesia, one must observe patients' automatic and externally cued movements and ask them to perform repetitive hand movements (finger tapping, pronation/supination, etc.) as "quickly and as fully as possible" [10] in order to evaluate for their speed, amplitude, and rhythm. Finally, patients may exhibit the phenomenon of "kinesia paradoxica," the sudden normalization of movement speed when faced with startling or threatening stimuli.

4.3.1.2 Rigidity

Rigidity refers to increased resistance when stretching a muscle passively, independent of the speed at which such passive excursion occurs (which distinguishes this abnormality from the velocity-dependent resistance of *spasticity*). It may be appreciated as "lead pipe" whereby the increase in tone is consistent and uniform in both flexion and extension, or as "cogwheel," in which the increased tone is interrupted in a rhythmic fashion, presumably due to superimposed beats of underlying tremor, even when such feature may not be overtly present. Lead pipe rigidity is more common in secondary or lesional forms of parkinsonism affecting the basal ganglia (e.g., carbon monoxide poisoning) as well as iatrogenic disorders (e.g., neuroleptic malignant syndrome). Cogwheel rigidity is far more common in PD, though by no means specific to this form of parkinsonism. Rigidity may be difficult to distinguish from "gegenhalten" or paratonia, where the resistance to passive movements is more variable than in rigidity due to difficulty in relaxation associated with dementing disorders affecting the frontal lobe. While rigidity may be associated with an increase in the magnitude and duration of the long-latency component of the stretch reflex [11], there likely is an involvement of higher corticospinal pathways as demonstrated by the enhancement of rigidity induced by contralateral activation maneuvers (the Froment's maneuver) [12], achieved by asking the patient to open and close the hand opposite to that being assessed for tone. Examination techniques require manipulating the wrist and elbow joints to ascertain arm rigidity, hip and knee joints to evaluate for leg rigidity, and neck to determine extent of axial rigidity. In PD, appendicular rigidity (arms > legs) tends to be greater than axial (neck) rigidity. In atypical parkinsonisms, most commonly progressive supranuclear palsy, there is a predominance of axial over appendicular rigidity. The more severe the rigidity, the less range of motion can be achieved. Stiff-person syndrome is a syndrome of rigidity due to an autoimmune encephalomyelopathy, consisting of predominantly axial rigidity due to continuous muscle contractions and superimposed stimulus-induced episodic muscle spasms often associated with an abrupt jerk and tonic contractions lasting seconds [13].

4.3.1.3 Parkinsonian Tremor

Tremor is classically categorized as a hyperkinetic intrusion in the otherwise hypokinetic disorder of parkinsonism. The typical parkinsonian tremor is at rest, although postural and action tremors are frequently present, albeit of lesser magnitude. Rest tremor occurs in a body part not voluntarily activated and completely supported against gravity [14]. Similar to bradykinesia and rigidity, rest tremor in PD affects the body asymmetrically. It can involve the upper extremities, jaw, and, less commonly but highly characteristic, the lower extremities. In the upper extremity, rest tremor is often described as "pill-rolling" due to the distinctive flexion then extension of the thumb and index finger, rubbing against each other at a 4–6 Hz frequency. The tremor is also associated with pronation-supination movements of the forearm, observed at the wrist and elbow. If not readily observable, classic arm or leg rest tremor may emerge during gait, mental tasks, or when performing a complex task with an unaffected body part. Rest tremor tends to be suppressed during initiation of a voluntary movement, such as raising the arms, but reappears when a steady position is achieved, such as when holding the arms outstretched, a phenomenon termed "reemergent" rest tremor. This transient suppressibility with movement onset can reliably differentiate the rest tremor of PD from an apparent rest tremor in essential tremor [15].

4.3.1.4 Postural Instability

Rather than an individual phenomenology, the postural instability of parkinsonism is a complex manifestation whereby an impairment of postural reflexes leads to excessive postural displacements following a force, tested at the bedside by the pull test or push and release test [16]. Early postural instability is more common in atypical parkinsonisms, particularly progressive supranuclear palsy and multiple system atrophy. In the former, this phenomenon is associated with backward falls and a patient perception that the center of gravity is shifted backward.

4.3.1.5 Freezing of Gait

Freezing of gait is a characteristic but poorly understood phenomenon in parkinsonism. It is defined [17] as an episodic inability, measured in seconds, to generate effective stepping, disproportionate to the extent of rigidity or other motor deficits. It is considered one of the "high-level" gait disorders because it is tightly interconnected with cognitive processes, particularly executive dysfunction. It is most commonly experienced during turning and step initiation (often described as *gait ignition failure*) but also when faced with spatial constraint, stress, and distraction. Freezing can be considered part of the spectrum of disorders whereby there is an abnormal stride length-cadence relationship, including festination (progressively decreasing stride length at the expense of increasing cadence), hesitation, and "trembling in place" (Fig. 4.1). Focused attention and sensory, visual, or auditory cues are capable of resolving freezing episodes. Freezing of gait may be related to gait asymmetry [18, 19] or possibly a manifestation of the sequence effect [20]. Freezing can be documented by observing gait initiation from the sitting position and having patients walk in tight spaces such as a doorway or corner. It may occur more commonly when turning in one direction, typically toward the less affected side in PD patients (such turns require greater stride from the more affected and therefore shorter-stride side); for this reason it is helpful to ask the patient to turn in both directions to test for freezing.

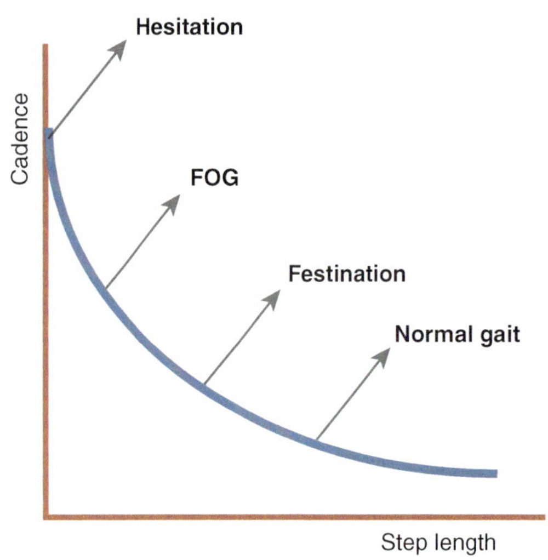

Fig. 4.1 Freezing of gait (*FOG*). The spectrum of FOG can be understood as an altered relationship between cadence and step length with a continuum from hesitations (impairment to start or change gait pattern) to FOG and festination. Interestingly, trembling in place is characterized by a rhythmic muscular contraction of about 4 Hz in the absence of effective stepping ("cadence without step"). This is probably the highest cadence that humans can perform (240 steps/min). These phenomena may coexist in the same patient and follow a gradient of severity: turning hesitation (especially toward the least affected side in PD patients), followed by narrow hesitation, festination, and FOG while walking (Adapted with permission from Fasano and Bloem, *Continuum (Minneap Minn)*. 2013 Oct; 19(5):1344–82)

4.3.2 Catatonia

While it can be considered a movement disorder, from a phenomenological standpoint catatonia is a neuropsychiatric syndrome describing patients that make few voluntary or responsive movements, in the setting of normal blinking, swallowing, and apparent lack of distress. The range of manifestations include catalepsy ("passive obedience," tendency to hold passive positions, particularly against gravity), waxy flexibility (limbs are kept in the same posture they were last placed by an examiner), mutism, posturing, mannerisms, echolalia, and echopraxia [21]. Psychiatric conditions associated with catatonia include schizophrenia and other psychotic disorders, major depression, and bipolar disorder. Catatonia has been reported after focal lesions to the pallidum or thalamus, particularly in encephalitis (limbic, anti-NMDA, viral [encephalitis lethargica]).

4.4 Hyperkinetic Movement Disorders

4.4.1 Tremor

Although tremor can be a feature of a hypokinetic (parkinsonian) disorder, in which it is predominantly present at rest, it is technically a hyperkinetic movement disorder, with the "excess" movement manifesting in the form of rhythmical, involuntary oscillatory activity of any body part [14]. This action-induced phenomenon can be subdivided into *postural* and *action* tremor, depending on whether the largest amplitude of the oscillatory activity is appreciated, respectively, when the affected limb is held outstretched or when it moves between targets, perpendicular to the direction of limb movement. A special component of action tremor is *intention* tremor, whereby the tremor is most prominent when the affected limb approaches a target. Tremor syndromes can be further characterized by their frequency, amplitude, location, and exacerbating factors. Physiologic tremor is a high-frequency, low-amplitude postural tremor that can be elicited in most of us in the context of stress, sleep deprivation, or the excessive caffeine that may be required to, say, get through reading this chapter. With surface electromyography, the frequency of physiologic tremor can be documented at 8–12 Hz [22]. *Enhanced* physiologic tremor is the term applied to the overtly visible physiologic tremor, which to the naked eye appears as a fine but rapid tremor, sometimes interfering with the performance of fine motor tasks. Essential tremor (ET), probably a syndrome rather than a disease (much as PD is viewed in the hypokinetic realm), is suspected when a postural and kinetic tremor appears of larger amplitude and lower frequency than physiologic tremor, involving predominantly the arms, but potentially also the head. Gait ataxia and postural instability, as well as nonmotor features of decreased cognition, anxiety, and social phobia, can also occur [23], although the overt presence of other features should raise suspicion for a non-ET disorder (e.g., fragile X tremor-ataxia syndrome when ataxia is a clear accompaniment of tremor).

Two special brands of tremor need to be distinguished from the tremor disorders noted above: dystonic and cerebellar tremor. Dystonic tremor applies to the rather jerky oscillatory activity of a body part, particularly if associated with abnormal posturing of that part (dystonic tremor *proper*) or of another body region (*tremor associated with dystonia*). Dystonic tremor, in addition, may be uniquely magnified by particular positions and tasks, to the extent that a *position-dependent* and *task-specific* tremor can only be dystonic in nature. Although head or vocal tremor can be part of the ET syndrome, *isolated* head tremor is most often a phenotype of adult-onset cervical dystonia expressed as dystonic head tremor. The same can be said of isolated vocal tremor. Cerebellar outflow tremor (previously referred to as Holmes' tremor) is a slow-frequency tremor present at rest, growing in amplitude with posture and becoming even worse with action, especially when nearing a target. Such end-target increase, *intention* tremor, is the most sensitive manifestation of pathology in the ipsilateral cerebellar hemisphere or in cerebellar outflow regions of the midbrain or superior cerebellar peduncle.

An orphan tremor disorder is the so-called primary writing tremor, whereby the tremor occurs exclusively during handwriting. Although this tremor is exquisitely task specific and action induced, it is considered neither a form of dystonic nor essential tremor [24].

Finally, functional (psychogenic) tremor is diagnosed when an oscillatory activity is variable in frequency, amplitude, and distribution over a short period of observation, and it can be suppressible with complex motor tasks or entrainable to a rate distinct to the "native" one. Such a clinically definite functional tremor requires no further testing although it can be confirmed with surface electromyography (laboratory supported functional tremor), which can also serve to document the *coactivation* sign, an increase in EMG signal amplitude from antagonistic muscle sets prior to tremor activity [25]. Psychogenic tremor is the most common psychogenic movement disorder phenotype.

4.4.2 Dystonia

Dystonia applies to abnormally sustained or intermittent muscle contractions causing posturing of any body part, jerky tremor, or both. The movement is typically absent at rest (at least in the early phases) but brought on by voluntary actions of the affected or unaffected limb. The latter scenario is also conceptualized as the *overflow* phenomenon [26]. The movements can be partial or exclusively task specific, such as is the case in writer's cramp (i.e., focal, task-specific hand dystonia) or musician's dystonia (e.g., embouchure dystonia). A characteristic feature of dystonia is the attenuation of the motor phenotype by a sensory trick (*geste antagoniste*). In this case, patients lightly touch themselves in a specific body part, affected or unaffected, creating a closed-loop sensory feedback that brings transient relief. Dystonia results from the abnormal co-contraction of antagonistic set of muscle groups, which can be better appreciated with surface electromyography, a veritable extension of the clinical examination. It often affects somatotopically contiguous muscle groups but can also generalize. When the agonist-antagonist co-contraction is intermittent, the resulting dystonic tremor appears as "jerky" and irregular, owing to asymmetric contractions of a dominant muscle group and "corrective" contractions of the antagonistic muscle group. Limb dystonia with superimposed arrhythmic and jerky movements, often referred to as *myoclonic dystonia* [27], may develop months after recovering from combined vascular lesions in the striatum and posterior thalamus (Fig. 4.2). Myoclonic dystonia is not to be confused with a distinct autosomal dominant disorder, *myoclonus dystonia*, whereby dystonia and myoclonus coexist but in different body parts, with the "jerks" (myoclonus) predominantly affecting the neck and proximal upper limbs. Dystonic tremor can affect the head exclusively or predominantly, leading to a "no-no" tremor. This focal tremor tends to exhibit a null point in head rotation at which the agonist-antagonist forces are balanced, typically in the direction of the overwhelmingly dystonic muscle group. Cervical dystonia was previously descriptively referred to as spasmodic torticollis, in reference to the cervical turning (torticollis) associated with brief, irregular jerks. However, cervical dystonia can express with a variable combination of lateral tilting (laterocollis), neck flexion (anterocollis), and/or extension (retrocollis), among others. Although cervical dystonia of adult onset is often idiopathic, prominent anterocollis may be a feature of the parkinsonian type of multiple system atrophy, and prominent retrocollis can be a telltale sign of tardive dystonia. Focal dystonia can selectively affect isolated regions, most prominently, orbicularis oculi muscles (blepharospasm: excessive blinking, tonic eyelid closure, or a combination thereof), orofacial muscles (jaw-opening or jaw-closing oromandibular dystonia), and vocal cords (spasmodic dysphonia of adductor [strained voice] or abductor [whispering voice] type).

Functional (psychogenic) dystonia is suspected in anyone with a sudden or rapid onset dystonia in any focal distribution, most often the foot [28] and oromandibular [29] regions. The

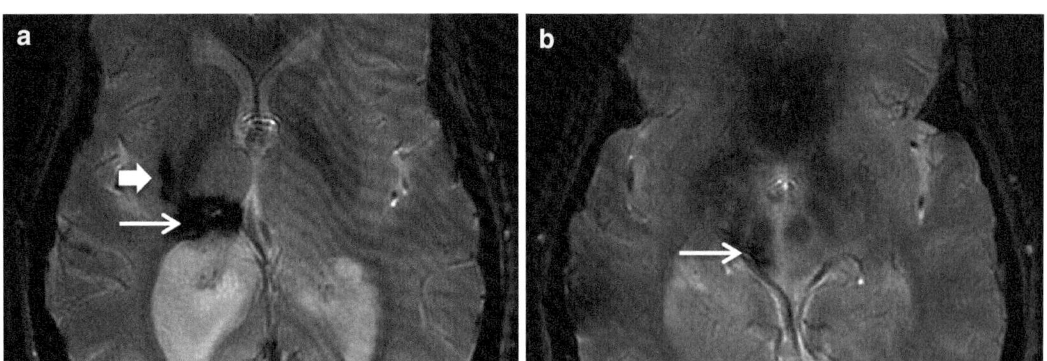

Fig. 4.2 Myoclonic dystonia. A hemorrhagic infarction in the dorsolateral putamen (*thick arrow*, **a**), posterior thalamus (*thick arrow*, **a**), and subthalamic connecting fibers (*thick arrow*, **b**) developed 6 months before the onset of rapid large-amplitude jerks in a 59-year-old woman

dystonia is fixed at onset, tends to be painful, and does not respond to sensory tricks [30]. Secondary autonomic changes in the foot region developing after prolonged tonic posturing can lead to the misdiagnosis of functional dystonia as complex regional pain syndrome type 1, formerly referred to as reflex sympathetic dystrophy.

4.4.3 Chorea

Chorea refers to involuntary semi-purposeful movements that are not patterned but rather seem to flow from one body part to another in a random or unpredictable fashion. It can resemble restlessness (see akathisia below) except for its clear lack of volitional control. Mild chorea can be masked by purposeful movement (parakinesia) or superseded by voluntary movements, but severe chorea can be enough to throw a patient out of a chair. Motor impersistence, sometimes called negative chorea, is an inability to sustain voluntary muscle contraction such as handgrip or tongue protrusion. It is typically associated with the chorea of Huntington's disease. The archaic term "dyskinesia" (literally, abnormal movements, the least intrinsically meaningful label for those interested in learning the phenomenological intricacies of movement disorders) is often used to denote chorea but in the sense of an identified trigger, most often a drug. The regional distribution of such understanding of dyskinesia, nevertheless, is used with an etiological-driven mind. For instance, orobucco-lingual *dyskinesia* (chorea, athetosis, or a combination of the two) is most likely to be tardive in nature; upper-body-predominant dyskinesia (true chorea) is most often a peak-dose, levodopa-induced hyperkinetic motor complication of PD, and lower-body dyskinesia (chorea or dystonia) can be a diphasic (beginning of dose and/or end of dose) levodopa-induced motor complication of PD.

4.4.4 Ballism

Ballism is a high-amplitude, "flinging" movement of the proximal extremities, which represents a severe end of the chorea spectrum. Hemiballismus is the most common presentation, although bilateral ballism and monoballism have been reported. The face can be involved. Although classically associated with a lesion in the contralateral subthalamic nucleus [31] (Fig. 4.3a), it is now recognized that lesions in other parts of the basal ganglia may be more common causes of hemiballismus [32]. A common trigger is nonketotic hyperglycemia, which is mysteriously unilateral in most (Fig. 4.3b) but bilateral in some. The hemi- and biballism that respectively ensue represent complications from these lesions that are often delayed by several weeks and associated with T1-weighted hyperintensity in the putamen. The natural history of poststroke or metabolic ballism is that of slow improvement. Such evolution typically replaces ballism with chorea, and eventually chorea with athetosis, before the movements disappear or a mild residual dystonia persists. Such progression suggests that the hyperkinetic spectrum of movement disorders is a continuum that ranges from ballism (most severe) to athetosis and dystonia (mildest).

4.4.5 Athetosis

To the extent that athetosis can be considered a "slow chorea," the speed and amplitude of movements that separate chorea and athetosis (and, when one is decisionally impaired, *choreoathetosis*) obey no strict boundaries. Athetotic movements, typically but by no means exclusively of distal limbs, are still as random as chorea but with a slower speed and lower amplitude, conveying a *writhing* demeanor. These can be thought of as a chorea played back in slow motion. They are often seen in the setting of cerebral palsy (*athetoid* type). A peripherally induced form of writhing hand or leg movements is well documented to occur among those with proprioceptive loss due to lesions anywhere in the sensory nerves or ganglia, posterior cord, or even contralateral parietal cortex. The movements thus generated are termed pseudoathetosis [33] and are qualitatively similar to the centrally generated form. The decrease in proprioception may prompt the increase in "search" movements in an attempt to enhance

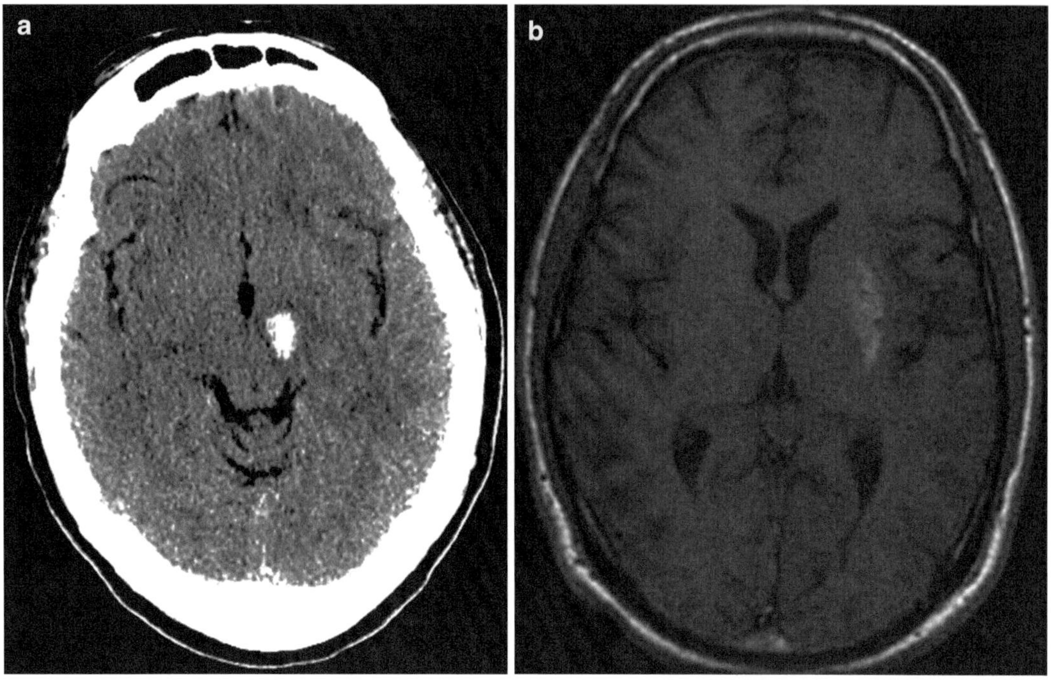

Fig. 4.3 Ballism. (**a**) Head CT demonstrating a hemorrhagic infarction in the left subthalamic nucleus in a 60-year-old woman who developed right hemiballism within 1 h of such event. (**b**) Axial T1-weighted brain MRI demonstrated an area of hyperintensity in the left posterior putamen documented during an episode of severe diabetic ketoacidosis, 3 weeks before the onset of right hemiballism in 37-year-old insulin-dependent diabetic man

feedback from the joints' location in space. A patient with pseudoathetosis of the hands may have "piano-playing" movements of the fingers when the arms are outstretched. A special form of rhythmic pseudoathetosis leading to flexor-extensor movements of the toes or fingers may develop in those with painful peripheral neuropathies of the legs (painful legs-moving toes or PLMT) [34] or arms (painful arms-moving fingers) [35].

4.4.6 Akathisia

Akathisia refers to a perception of inner restlessness rendering patients unable to remain still. There is an urge to move that can only be transiently relieved when the actual movement takes place. The most common form of akathisia is neuroleptic induced, which induces rocking, crossing and uncrossing of the legs, repetitive hand movements, and seemingly compulsive picking at items. A form of akathisia associated with paresthesia, particularly of the lower extremities, worse in the evening, and interfering with sleep initiation, is referred to as restless legs syndrome (RLS) or Willis-Ekbom disease [36].

4.4.7 Tics

Like akathisia, tics are abnormal movements born out of underlying sensory perceptions or *premonitory urges*. These urges precede the tic, and performing the stereotypic movement can result in their transient relief. They can be suppressible by the patient and easily distractible, which previously (and unfortunately) led to their miscategorization as functional or psychogenic. Prolonged volitional suppression of the movements can result in a "flurry" of tics once released, as if they return with a vengeance. Motor tics can be simple or complex in nature, sometimes encompassing long strings of patterned movement in just about any body part, including the head and neck. Vocal tics can consist of speech or other vocalizations, sniffs, coughs, grunts, etc. Individual tics can wax and wane over time, and new tics can replace old ones. In fact, in Tourette syndrome, the most common etiology of tics, a history of tics changing in appearance and distribution (e.g., sniffing in childhood, shoulder shrugging in adolescence), is reassuring. Tic movements involving sustained twisting or turning postures are sometimes termed dystonic tics, but this term can be as confusing as myoclonic dystonia, thus making it an unlikely descriptor in our medical records.

4.4.8 Stereotypy

Closely related to tics, stereotypies are non-goal-directed movement patterns that are repeated continuously for a period of time in the same form and on multiple occasions and which are typically distractible [37]. In contrast to tics, stereotypies have an earlier age of onset (often <2 years old); are usually performed at the expense of other movement; are more rhythmic, often less complex, and longer in duration; and remain constant over time with little change in the movement. They are not associated with a premonitory urge and are usually not suppressible (although as above they can be distractible) [38]. Using a report of urge or suppressibility as a distinction between stereotypy and tic is challenging as the term stereotypy is typically used to refer to these movements in developmentally disabled individuals, autistics, and patients with Rett syndrome. A distinct phenotype with localizing value is the "figure-of-eight" head-shaking stereotypies, which appear in young children with vestibulocerebellar impairment due to congenital hindbrain abnormalities, such as Dandy-Walker malformation, Joubert syndrome, and rhombencephalosynapsis [39]. Other stereotypies include body rocking, head banging, arm flapping, hand-wringing, and clapping.

4.4.9 Myoclonus

Myoclonus is the semiologic nomenclature corresponding to sudden, brief, quick, "shock-like" movements, distributed in the extremities, face, or trunk. Positive myoclonus is caused by muscle contraction, whereas negative myoclonus by brief lapses in muscle tone. Negative myoclonus is termed asterixis and is often associated with metabolic encephalopathies. Myoclonus can be classified by distribution (focal, multifocal, segmental, generalized), by etiology (primary or secondary), or by localization (cortical, subcortical, brainstem, spinal). Cortical myoclonus is usually focal, located in the face and hands, present on action, and induced or worsened by tactile stimulation or by stretching distal limbs, whereas subcortical myoclonus is more likely to be segmental or generalized, present with rest and action, and sensitive to auditory stimuli [40]. Brainstem myoclonus causes bilateral, synchronous flexor movements, induced by auditory or tactile stimuli (e.g., tapping on the face) [41]. Electrophysiological studies can confirm the short duration of myoclonic bursts, usually less than 200 ms (Fig. 4.4), and surface EMG with EEG back-averaging can help to identify the cortical origin, whenever present [42].

4.4.10 Ataxia

Ataxia refers to a breakdown in the coordination of voluntary movement. Ataxia is most commonly the result of dysfunction in the cerebellum or cerebellar efferent (cerebellar-thalamic) pathways, causing either a vermal cerebellar syndrome, with predominant abnormalities of gait (staggering, "drunk-like" gait), speech, and poor postural control of the head (titubation), or a hemispheric cerebellar syndrome, with appendicular incoordination of goal-directed movements (*dysdiadochokinesia*). Accompaniments to the vermal cerebellar syndrome include hypometric saccades, which localize to the dorsal vermis, and hypermetric saccades, which result from fastigial nucleus lesions. The nonrhythmic oscillations of ataxia, not to be confused with cerebellar outflow tremor (a true oscillation), result from the straying of a movement from its intended course and the subsequent voluntary corrections. These corrections worsen closer to the target (dysmetria) where they may generate a rhythmic oscillation (*intention* tremor).

Sensory ataxia, a non-cerebellar form of ataxia, refers to incoordination caused by a

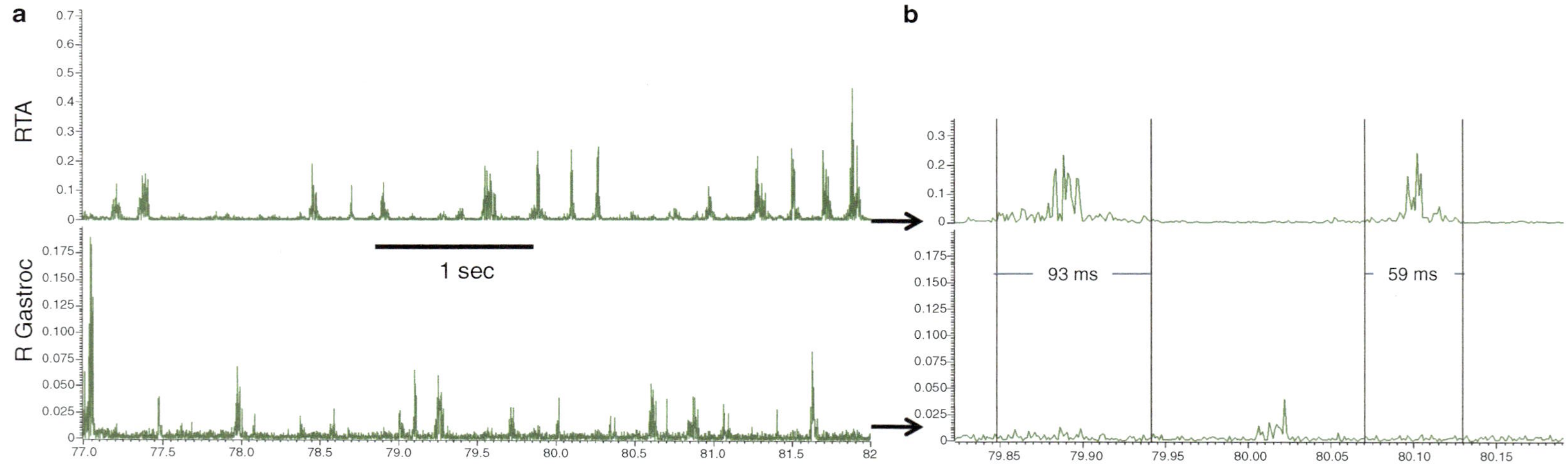

Fig. 4.4 Surface electromyography in myoclonus – electrophysiologic study of an 82-year-old woman with orthostatic myoclonus. Closer inspection of raw data (**a**) of the right tibialis anterior (R TA) and right gastrocnemius revealed nonrhythmic activity, with individual bursts (**b**) lasting <150 ms, within the range for myoclonus (Adapted with permission from Espay and Chen [40])

decrease in afferent proprioceptive input, often seen as a wide-based steppage gait associated with large-fiber peripheral neuropathy or dorsal column impairment. Friedreich's ataxia, the most common autosomal recessive ataxia, is truly a form of sensory ataxia. The demonstration of prominent early cerebellar atrophy in a patient with wide-based gait ataxia is a strong argument against Friedreich's ataxia and any other sensory ataxias.

The vermal cerebellar ataxia is best suggested by the observation of sidestepping during tandem or inability to perform such task altogether. Appendicular ataxia is uncovered during such clinical tests as the finger-nose-finger, heel-knee-shin, and sudden and forceful displacement of an outstretched limb. The latter elicits a rebound due to over correction when attempting to return the limb to the original position.

Conclusions

A systematic approach to the evaluation of a patient with a movement disorder includes careful history and observation of the characteristics of the abnormal movements. Factors such as speed (Fig. 4.5), complexity (Fig. 4.6), response to maneuvers, variability with position, and others help to describe and classify the movement. Once the phenomenological category (or categories) is decided upon, then

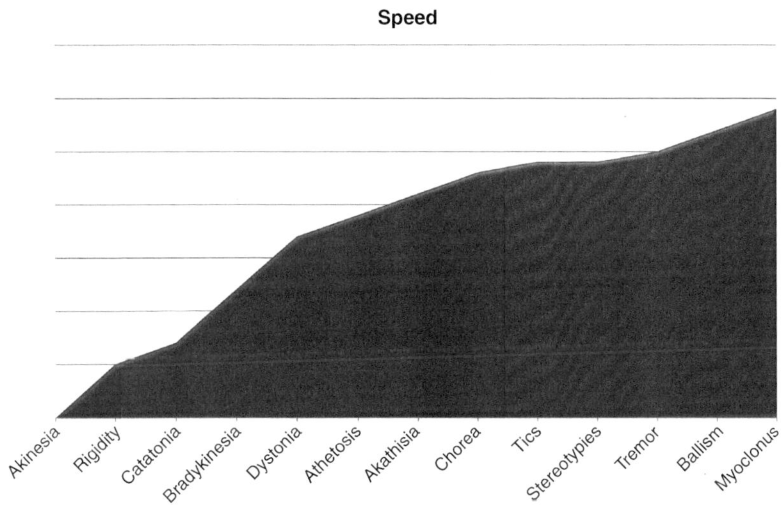

Fig. 4.5 A graphical representation of the movement disorders organized by the speed of movement

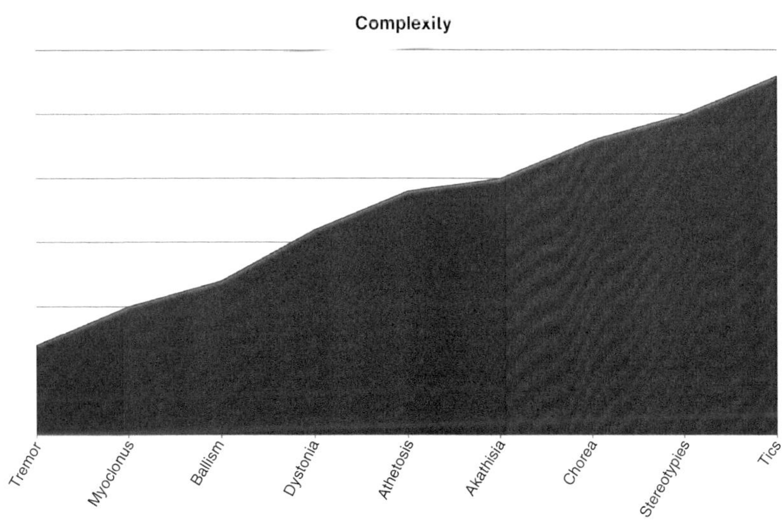

Fig. 4.6 A graphical representation of the movement disorders organized by the complexity of movement

a logical start can be made toward the differential etiologic diagnosis, about which the following chapters will indulge.

References

1. Klein C. Movement disorders: classifications. J Inherit Metab Dis. 2005;28(3):425–39.
2. Fahn S. Classification of movement disorders. Mov Disord. 2011;26(6):947–57.
3. Goetz CG, Chmura TA, Lanska DJ. History of movement disorders as a neurological specialty: part 14 of the MDS-sponsored History of Movement Disorders exhibit, Barcelona, June 2000. Mov Disord. 2001;16(5): 954–9.
4. Goetz CG, McGhiey A. The movement disorder society and movement disorders: a modern history. Mov Disord. 2011;26(6):939–46.
5. Benecke R, Rothwell JC, Dick JP, Day BL, Marsden CD. Disturbance of sequential movements in patients with Parkinson's disease. Brain. 1987;110:361–79.
6. Espay AJ, Giuffrida JP, Chen R, Payne M, Mazzella F, Dunn E, et al. Differential response of speed, amplitude, and rhythm to dopaminergic medications in Parkinson's disease. Mov Disord. 2011;26(14): 2504–8.
7. Kang SY, Wasaka T, Shamim EA, Auh S, Ueki Y, Lopez GJ, et al. Characteristics of the sequence effect in Parkinson's disease. Mov Disord. 2010;25(13): 2148–55.
8. Nakamura R, Nagasaki H, Narabayashi H. Disturbances of rhythm formation in patients with Parkinson's disease: part I. Characteristics of tapping response to the periodic signals. Percept Mot Skills. 1978;46(1): 63–75.
9. Giladi N, McMahon D, Przedborski S, Flaster E, Guillory S, Kostic V, et al. Motor blocks in Parkinson's disease. Neurology. 1992;42(2):333–9.
10. Goetz CG, Tilley BC, Shaftman SR, Stebbins GT, Fahn S, Martinez-Martin P, et al. Movement Disorder Society-sponsored revision of the Unified Parkinson's Disease Rating Scale (MDS-UPDRS): scale presentation and clinimetric testing results. Mov Disord. 2008;23(15):2129–70.
11. Berardelli A, Sabra AF, Hallett M. Physiological mechanisms of rigidity in Parkinson's disease. J Neurol Neurosurg Psychiatry. 1983;46(1):45–53.
12. Powell D, Hanson N, Threlkeld AJ, Fang X, Xia R. Enhancement of parkinsonian rigidity with contralateral hand activation. Clin Neurophysiol. 2011;122(8): 1595–601.
13. Espay AJ, Chen R. Rigidity and spasms from autoimmune encephalomyelopathies: stiff-person syndrome. Muscle Nerve. 2006;34(6):677–90.
14. Deuschl G, Bain P, Brin M. Consensus statement of the movement disorder society on tremor. Ad Hoc Sci Comm. 1998;13 Suppl 3:2–23.
15. Papengut F, Raethjen J, Binder A, Deuschl G. Rest tremor suppression may separate essential from parkinsonian rest tremor. Parkinsonism Relat Disord. 2013;19(7):693–7.
16. Jacobs JV, Horak FB, Van Tran K, Nutt JG. An alternative clinical postural stability test for patients with Parkinson's disease. J Neurol. 2006;253(11): 1404–13.
17. Giladi N, Nieuwboer A. Understanding and treating freezing of gait in parkinsonism, proposed working definition, and setting the stage. Mov Disord. 2008;23 Suppl 2:S423–5.
18. Fasano A, Herzog J, Seifert E, Stolze H, Falk D, Reese R, et al. Modulation of gait coordination by subthalamic stimulation improves freezing of gait. Mov Disord. 2011;26(5):844–51.
19. Frazzitta G, Pezzoli G, Bertotti G, Maestri R. Asymmetry and freezing of gait in parkinsonian patients. J Neurol. 2013;260(1):71–6.
20. Chee R, Murphy A, Danoudis M, Georgiou-Karistianis N, Iansek R. Gait freezing in Parkinson's disease and the stride length sequence effect interaction. Brain. 2009;132(Pt 8):2151–60.
21. Tandon R, Heckers S, Bustillo J, Barch DM, Gaebel W, Gur RE, et al. Catatonia in DSM-5. Schizophr Res. 2013;150(1):26–30.
22. Hallett M. Overview of human tremor physiology. Mov Disord. 1998;13 Suppl 3:43–8.
23. Teive HAG. Essential tremor: phenotypes. Parkinsonism Relat Disord. 2012;18 Suppl 1:S140–2.
24. Espay AJ, Chen R. Primary writing tremor and writer's cramp: distinct phenomenology, diverging pathophysiology. Clin Neurophysiol. 2011;122(1):5–6.
25. Deuschl G, Köster B, Lücking CH, Scheidt C. Diagnostic and pathophysiological aspects of psychogenic tremors. Mov Disord. 1998;13(2):294–302.
26. Albanese A, Bhatia K, Bressman SB, Delong MR, Fahn S, Fung VSC, et al. Phenomenology and classification of dystonia: a consensus update. Mov Disord. 2013;28(7):863–73.
27. Gonzalez-Usigli H, Espay AJ. Semiology and localization of ballistic movements. Neurology. 83(4):e56-7.
28. Fahn S, Williams DT. Psychogenic dystonia. Adv Neurol. 1988;50:431–55.
29. Fasano A, Valadas A, Bhatia KP, Prashanth LK, Lang AE, Munhoz RP, et al. Psychogenic facial movement disorders: clinical features and associated conditions. Mov Disord. 2012;27(12):3–5.
30. Schrag A, Trimble M, Quinn N, Bhatia K. The syndrome of fixed dystonia: an evaluation of 103 patients. Brain. 2004;127(Pt 10):2360–72.
31. Martin J. Hemichorea resulting from a local lesion of the brain. (The syndrome of the body of Luys.). Brain. 1927;50:637–51.
32. Postuma R, Lang A. Hemiballism: revisiting a classic disorder. Lancet Neurol. 2003;2(November):661–8.
33. Sharp FR, Rando TA, Greenberg SA, Brown L, Sagar SM. Pseudochoreoathetosis. Movements associated with loss of proprioception. Arch Neurol. 1994;51(11): 1103–9.

34. Spillane JD, Nathan PW, Kelly RE, Marsden CD. Painful legs and moving toes. Brain. 1971;94(3):541–56.
35. Verhagen WI, Horstink MW, Notermans SL. Painful arm and moving fingers. J Neurol Neurosurg Psychiatry. 1985;48(4):384–5.
36. Trenkwalder C, Paulus W. Restless legs syndrome: pathophysiology, clinical presentation and management. Nat Rev Neurol. 2010;6(6):337–46.
37. Edwards MJ, Lang AE, Bhatia KP. Stereotypies: a critical appraisal and suggestion of a clinically useful definition. Mov Disord. 2012;27(2):179–85.
38. Mahone EM, Bridges D, Prahme C, Singer HS. Repetitive arm and hand movements (complex motor stereotypies) in children. J Pediatr. 2004;145(3):391–5.
39. Tully HM, Dempsey JC, Ishak GE, Adam MP, Mink JW, Dobyns WB, et al. Persistent figure-eight and side-to-side head shaking is a marker for rhombencephalosynapsis. Mov Disord. 2013;28(14):2019–23.
40. Espay AJ, Chen R. Myoclonus. Continuum (Minneap Minn). 2013;19(5 Movement Disorders):1264–86.
41. Shibasaki H, Kakigi R, Oda K, Masukawa S. Somatosensory and acoustic brain stem reflex myoclonus. J Neurol Neurosurg Psychiatry. 1988;51(4):572–5.
42. Shibasaki H, Hallett M. Electrophysiological studies of myoclonus. Muscle Nerve. 2005;31(2):157–74.

Neuropathology of Movement Disorders

5

Kurt A. Jellinger

5.1 Introduction

Most movement disorders related to basal ganglia dysfunction are characterized by neuronal degeneration/loss in the nervous system associated with protein deposits as diagnostic hallmarks. Classification: (1) α-synucleinopathies, caused by misfolded α-synuclein (αSyn) forming inclusions in the nervous system and extraneuronal organs, include Lewy body (LB) disorders, e.g., Parkinson's disease (PD), dementia with Lewy bodies (DLBs), and multiple system atrophy (MSA). LBs are found in many disorders, e.g., in 2–75 % of aged and Alzheimer's disease (AD). (2) Frontotemporal lobe degenerations including tauopathies with neuronal/glial inclusions composed of three and/or four repeat (3R/4R) triplets of tau protein, e.g., progressive supranuclear palsy (PSP). (3) Polyglutamine repeat (CAG) disorders, e.g., Huntington's disease (HD). (4) Other degenerative disorders without specific markers, e.g., pallidal atrophy and dyskinesias [1]. Only major neurodegenerative forms of movement disorders are reviewed.

K.A. Jellinger, MD
Institute of Clinical Neurobiology,
Medical University Vienna, Alberichgasse 5/13,
Vienna 1150, Austria
e-mail: kurt.jellinger@univie.ac.at

5.2 Hypokinetic-Rigid Movement Disorders

They include various forms of parkinsonism, most frequent LB-related sporadic PD, DLB, etc.

5.2.1 Sporadic Parkinson's Disease

PD or brain stem type of LB disease is a progressive multi-organ proteinopathy caused by a misfolded αSyn with variegated motor and non-motor symptoms owing to a spreading process of αSyn deposition [2, 3]. It occurs first in synaptic terminals causing neuronal loss and disturbance of many neurotransmitter systems, cellular dysfunction preceding Lewy pathology [4]. Brains show pallor of the substantia nigra (SN) and locus ceruleus (LC), neuronal loss in many subcortical nuclei, predominantly the SN compacta (SNc) and LC, with αSyn+ deposits in neurons (LB) and dystrophic neurites (LN) throughout the nervous system. Nigrostriatal degeneration causes denervation of the striatum with dopamine loss, which, together with other biochemical deficits, governs the clinical picture. Degrees of SNc cell loss and striatal hypofunction are correlated with disease duration and severity of motor dysfunction. This first appears at loss of 30 % of SN neurons but 50–60 % of their axon terminals, with a substantial loss of dopamine markers in nigros-

C. Falup-Pecurariu et al. (eds.), *Movement Disorders Curricula*,
DOI 10.1007/978-3-7091-1628-9_5

triatal terminals in early PD [5]. The end-stage PD shows a massive loss of SN neurons.

Hallmark lesions are cytoplasmic inclusions (LBs) and LNs. Classical brain stem and cortical LBs, although morphologically different, share biochemical features. The major components are αSyn, ubiquitin, and phosphorylated neurofilaments, associated with proteins and enzymes implicated in cellular (dys) functions [6]. Although LBs are not specific to PD, the diagnosis of PD can be made by inspecting two or more sections from the mid-part of SN showing LBs. If none are found in either SN or LC, this diagnosis can be excluded [7].

Biochemical increase of phosphorylated αSyn precedes aggregation and formation of LBs [8]. Their significance for neurodegeneration or neuroprotection is poorly understood. While αSyn deposits are related to neuronal damage, they may represent end products of elimination of toxic molecules as a cell-protective mechanism [9].

The severity and extent of αSyn pathology are scored semiquantitatively in specific brain regions [10]. Staging of their spread was proposed to predict the sequence of lesions [3]. LB pathology begins in the lower brain stem – the dorsal nucleus of the vagus – and anterior olfactory nucleus (stage 1), extending to the caudal raphe nuclei and coeruleus-subcoeruleus complex (stage 2). The initial stages are presymptomatic and may explain early non-motor symptoms [11]. Later, SNc and LC are involved (stage 3), followed by the anteromedial limbic cortex and amygdala (stage 4). In stages 5 and 6, the pathological process involves the neocortex. Stages 3 and 4 have been correlated with motor symptoms; stages 5 and 6 showing transition between PD and DLB are frequently associated with cognitive impairment. The validity of this scheme, which corresponds to the classification of LB disorders into three phenotypes – brain stem predominant, limbic/transitional, diffuse neocortical – is under debate, since 6.3–47% of autopsy-proven PD cases did not follow this spread, while 50% of individuals with widespread αSyn pathology lacked clinical symptoms or were unclassifiable [2]. The Braak staging often shows acceptable correlations between morphological and clinical data [12], while a recently proposed unifying system for LB disorders distinguishing four stages correlates αSyn pathology well with nigrostriatal degeneration and motor dysfunction [13].

The clinical subtypes of PD – rigid akinetic and tremor dominant – show specific morphologic patterns of pathophysiological importance, with different involvement of striato-cortical and cerebello-thalamocortical pathways [2].

Cognitive deficits are common in PD, particularly in later disease stages. Their correlates are variable: involvement of subcortical and brain stem structures, LB pathology in limbic and neocortical areas, concurrent AD pathology, or a combination of Lewy and AD changes recently confirmed as a robust correlate of dementia in PD [14]. Parkinson's disease dementia (PDD) and DLB, arbitrarily separated by early or late onset of dementia, both show a variable mixture of Lewy and AD pathologies [2, 15]. Despite morphological similarities, more severe αSyn load in hippocampal CA 2/3 areas and more severe Aβ plaques in the striatum differentiate DLB from PDD [2, 16].

5.2.2 Multiple System Atrophy

This sporadic multisystem synucleinopathy involves the nigrostriatal and olivopontocerebellar systems underlying its clinical variants [17]. Brains reveal discoloration of the atrophic striatum, depigmented SN and LC (MSA-P), and atrophy of the pontine basis and cerebellum (MSA-C). Neuronal loss and gliosis in these areas are associated with widespread αSyn+ glial cytoplasmic inclusions (GCIs) in oligodendroglia (Papp-Lantos bodies, diagnostic hallmarks), less frequent neuronal and glial nuclear inclusions, and myelin depletion [18, 19]. GCIs, nonmembrane-bound aggregations of αSyn+ tubules/filaments, contain many proteins and enzymes that differ from LBs, although these occur in around 20% of MSA cases. Staging schemes of the severity and distribution of lesions show overlapping forms. Progression of MSA pathology differs from PD [2, 19].

5.2.3 Neurodegeneration with Brain Iron Accumulation

NBIA, 1, previously Hallervorden-Spatz disease, a rare autosomal recessive disorder (dystonia, rigidity, choreoathetosis) caused by mutations of the pantothenate kinase gene (PANK 1), shows discolorated globus pallidus due to iron accumulation, axonal swellings (spheroids) in the entire nervous system, and LBs [20]. PKAN 2, caused by PANK2 mutations with similar phenotypes, is not a synucleinopathy [21].

5.2.4 Frontotemporal Lobar Degenerations (Including Tauopathies)

FTDLs are characterized by cellular inclusions composed of tau, TDP-43, or FUS proteins. FTDL-tau is frequently listed in the group of tauopathies – PSP, etc. (see [22]). Pick's disease (PiD) is a specific form of tauopathy consisting of spherical intraneuronal tau inclusion (Pick bodies) composed predominantly of 3R-tau isoforms. PiD is a member of FTLD tau forms possibly originating in limbic/paralimbic cortices and showing neuropathological subtypes [23].

5.2.5 Progressive Supranuclear Palsy

PSP or Steele-Richardson-Olszewski syndrome, a sporadic parkinsonian disorder with various subtypes, shows affection of the basal ganglia, subthalamic nucleus (STN), SN, and dentate nucleus with atrophy of superior cerebellar peduncles. Characteristic neuronal lesions are globose tangles composed of 4R-tau (straight filaments) in the brain stem, flame-shaped tangles, and "tufted" astrocytes in gray and white matter. The severity and distribution of tau pathology vary in the different subtypes – PSP or Richardson's syndrome, and atypical forms [7].

5.2.6 Corticobasal Degeneration

Previous corticodentatonigral degeneration with neuronal achromatism, a rare parkinsonian disorder, shows highly variable neuropathology: asymmetrical frontoparietal cortical atrophy, discolorated globus pallidus, depigmented SN, widespread accumulation of 4R-tau in swollen "ballooned" neurons, astrocytes, and astrocytic plaques (unique to CBD) differing from neuritic AD plaques by the absence of Aβ accumulation [7]. Pretangles show ultrastructural differences between AD and CBD [24].

5.2.7 Frontotemporal Dementia with Parkinsonism Linked to Chromosome 17-Tau

FTDP-17 due to mutations of the MAPT gene for tau protein, presenting behavioral disturbances and parkinsonism, shows temporal atrophy, discolorated globus pallidus, neuronal loss in cortical and subcortical gray matter, with tau+ NFTs, or globose tangles resembling those of other 4R tauopathies (twisted or straight tubules). FTDP-17 shows similarities to FTLD-tau but no relationship to FTLD-TDP-43 or FUS [25].

5.3 Hyperkinetic Movement Disorders

Neuropathology of hyperkinetic movement disorders is challenging. The most important are Huntington's disease, neuroacanthocytosis, dystonia, and tremor syndromes [1].

5.3.1 Huntington's Disease

This autosomal dominant hereditary disease is due to repeat expansion to >35 CAG (cytosine-adenine-guanine) trinucleotide in a gene located at chromosome 4p.16.3 that codes for huntingtin (HTT). Cortical and neostriatal atrophy is classified into four degrees. In progressed stages the thalamus, hippocampus, and white matter are affected. HTT aggregates involve cellular processes (neurites), neuronal cytoplasm and nuclei in the neostriatum and cortex, the latter correlating with CAG length [26]. The causes of neostriatal vulnerability are not clear.

5.3.2 Neuroacanthocytosis and HD-Like Syndromes

Rare genetically determined neuroacanthocytosis, a combination of erythrocytic acanthocytosis with chorea, dystonia, and parkinsonism, due to several genetic loci (VPS13A gene), shows atrophy of the striopallidum and other subcortical nuclei. The absence of cortical and subthalamic lesions differs from HD. HD-like syndromes are rare (about 1%) [27]. Autosomal dominant Huntington disease-like 2 shows degeneration of neostriatum and neocortices associated with anti-TAT-box-binding neuronal inclusions.

5.3.3 Dentatorubral-Pallidoluysian Atrophy

Rare autosomal dominant disorder largely confined to Japanese population caused by an abnormally expanded CAG triplet in the DRLPA gene (atrophin-1) at chromosome 12p.13.31. Atrophy, discoloration, and neuronal loss/gliosis affect the dentate nucleus, globus pallidus, SN, and nucleus ruber, with disruption of dendatorubral, pallidofugal, spinocerebellar, and motor systems. CAG repeat-dependent accumulation of mutant atrophin-1 in neuronal nuclei and intranuclear and cytoplasmic inclusions are widespread in the nervous system [28].

5.3.4 Progressive Pallidal Degeneration

This rare autosomal recessive or sporadic disorder, manifested as dystonia, choreoathetosis, rigid akinesia, etc., shows symmetric atrophy of globus pallidus alone or associated with degeneration of SN, STN, or other systems [1, 29].

5.3.5 Wilson's Disease (Hepatolenticular Degeneration) and Menkes' Disease

Autosomal recessive Wilson's disease with dystonia, parkinsonism and psychotic symptoms, liver cirrhosis, cerebral degeneration, and abnormal hepatic copper metabolism due to a defect in P-type ATPase, is caused by ATPB gene on chromosome 13q.14.3. It results in abnormal copper accumulation in the liver and brain and involves the basal ganglia with cavitation and neuronal loss in the deep frontal cortex [30].

Menkes' disease, an X-linked recessive disorder due to mutations in the copper transporter ATP7A, associated with abnormal hair, mental retardation, hypotonia, and cerebellar symptoms, shows cerebral atrophy, multilocal neuronal degeneration, and cerebellar lesions [1].

5.4 Other Movement Disorders

5.4.1 Dystonias

The syndrome of sustained muscle contractions and repetitive movements comprises a heterogenous group of hereditary or metabolic disorders. Only limited morphological data are available. Primary dystonias (autosomal dominant and recessive) show interaction between the torsinA (TOR1A) gene responsible for DYT1 and thanatos-associated domain-containing apoptosis-associated protein 1 (THAP1) gene for DYT 6 [31–33]. A patchy pattern of neuronal loss and gliosis in caudate and putamen, occasional NFTs and LBs in the brain stem, and loss of Purkinje cells suggest corticostriate and cerebellar dysfunctions.

5.4.2 Tremor Syndromes

Tremor entities and their classification have been reviewed [34]. Essential tremor (ET), the most common form, a heterogenous disorder, shows various morphologies: LBs in the brain stem and loss of cerebellar Purkinje cells with increased numbers of axon torpedoes without LBs, suggesting synergetic effects. The molecular basis of these structural changes is unknown [35, 36].

Conclusion

Despite clinical and morphological overlapping, most neurodegenerative movement disorders show characteristic pathomorphology with specific protein markers, which, together with modern molecular genetic and biochemical methods, allow a correct diagnosis and classification of disease entities and give insight into their pathogenesis. However, their etiology awaits further elucidation as a basis for future preventive and therapeutic strategies.

References

1. Jellinger KA. Neuropathology of movement disorders. In: Winn HR, editor. Youmans neurological surgery, vol. 1. 7th ed. Philadelphia: Elsevier-Saunders; 2016. p. e83.1–41.
2. Jellinger KA. Neuropathology of sporadic Parkinson's disease: evaluation and changes of concepts. Mov Disord. 2012;27:8–30.
3. Del Tredici K, Braak H. Review: sporadic Parkinson's disease: development and distribution of alpha-synuclein pathology. Neuropathol Appl Neurobiol. 2016;42:33–50.
4. Bellucci A, Mercuri NB, Venneri A, Faustini G, Longhena F, Pizzi M, et al. Review: Parkinson's disease: from synaptic loss to connectome dysfunction. Neuropathol Appl Neurobiol. 2016;42:77–94.
5. Kordower JH, Olanow CW, Dodiya HB, Chu Y, Beach TG, Adler CH, et al. Disease duration and the integrity of the nigrostriatal system in Parkinson's disease. Brain. 2013;136:2419–31.
6. Wakabayashi K, Tanji K, Odagiri S, Miki Y, Mori F, Takahashi H. The Lewy body in Parkinson's disease and related neurodegenerative disorders. Mol Neurobiol. 2013;47:495–508.
7. Dickson DW. Parkinson's disease and parkinsonism: neuropathology. Cold Spring Harb Perspect Med. 2012;2, a009258.
8. Lue L-F, Walker DG, Adler CH, Shill H, Tran H, Akiyama H, et al. Biochemical increase in phosphorylated a-synuclein precedes histopathology of Lewy-type synucleinopathies. Brain Pathol. 2012;22: 745–56.
9. Jellinger KA. Synuclein and Parkinson's disease: an update. In: Martinez A, Gil C, editors. Emerging drugs and targets for Parkinson's disease. London: The Royal Society of Chemistry; 2013. p. 175–216.
10. Alafuzoff I, Ince PG, Arzberger T, Al-Sarraj S, Bell J, Bodi I, et al. Staging/typing of Lewy body related alpha-synuclein pathology: a study of the BrainNet Europe Consortium. Acta Neuropathol. 2009;117: 635–52.
11. Jellinger KA. Neuropathobiology of non-motor symptoms in Parkinson disease. J Neural Transm (Vienna). 2015;122:1429–40.
12. Halliday G, McCann H, Shepherd C. Evaluation of the Braak hypothesis: how far can it explain the pathogenesis of Parkinson's disease? Expert Rev Neurother. 2012;12:673–86.
13. Beach TG, Adler CH, Lue L, Sue LI, Bachalakuri J, Henry-Watson J, et al. Unified staging system for Lewy body disorders: correlation with nigrostriatal degeneration, cognitive impairment and motor dysfunction. Acta Neuropathol. 2009;117:613–34.
14. Walker Z, Possin KL, Boeve BF, Aarsland D. Lewy body dementias. Lancet. 2015;386:1683–97.
15. Walker L, McAleese KE, Thomas AJ, Johnson M, Martin-Ruiz C, Parker C, et al. Neuropathologically mixed Alzheimer's and Lewy body disease: burden of pathological protein aggregates differs between clinical phenotypes. Acta Neuropathol. 2015;129:729–48.
16. Halliday GM, Song YJ, Harding AJ. Striatal beta-amyloid in dementia with Lewy bodies but not Parkinson's disease. J Neural Transm. 2011;118: 713–9.
17. Fanciulli A, Wenning GK. Multiple-system atrophy. N Engl J Med. 2015;372:249–63.
18. Ahmed Z, Asi YT, Sailer A, Lees AJ, Houlden H, Revesz T, et al. The neuropathology, pathophysiology and genetics of multiple system atrophy. Neuropathol Appl Neurobiol. 2012;38:4–24.
19. Jellinger KA. Neuropathology of multiple system atrophy: new thoughts about pathogenesis. Mov Disord. 2014;29:1720–41.
20. Kruer MC. The neuropathology of neurodegeneration with brain iron accumulation. Int Rev Neurobiol. 2013;110:165–94.
21. Li A, Paudel R, Johnson R, Courtney R, Lees AJ, Holton JL, et al. Pantothenate kinase-associated neurodegeneration is not a synucleinopathy. Neuropathol Appl Neurobiol. 2013;39:121–31.
22. Lashley T, Rohrer JD, Mead S, Revesz T. Review: an update on clinical, genetic and pathological aspects of frontotemporal lobar degenerations. Neuropathol Appl Neurobiol. 2015;41:858–81.
23. Irwin DJ, Brettschneider J, McMillan CT, Cooper F, Olm C, Arnold SE, et al. Deep clinical and neuropathological phenotyping of Pick disease. Ann Neurol. 2016;79:272–87.
24. Tatsumi S, Uchihara T, Aiba I, Iwasaki Y, Mimuro M, Takahashi R, et al. Ultrastructural differences in pretangles between Alzheimer disease and corticobasal degeneration revealed by comparative light and electron microscopy. Acta Neuropathol Commun. 2014;2:161.
25. Halliday G, Bigio EH, Cairns NJ, Neumann M, Mackenzie IR, Mann DM. Mechanisms of disease in

frontotemporal lobar degeneration: gain of function versus loss of function effects. Acta Neuropathol. 2012;124:373–82.
26. Rub U, Vonsattel JP, Heinsen H, Korf HW. The Neuropathology of Huntington s disease: classical findings, recent developments and correlation to functional neuroanatomy. Adv Anat Embryol Cell Biol. 2015;217:1–146.
27. Govert F, Schneider SA. Huntington's disease and Huntington's disease-like syndromes: an overview. Curr Opin Neurol. 2013;26:420–7.
28. Tsuji S. Dentatorubral-pallidoluysian atrophy. Handb Clin Neurol. 2012;103:587–94.
29. Kara E, Hardy J, Houlden H. The pallidopyramidal syndromes: nosology, aetiology and pathogenesis. Curr Opin Neurol. 2013;26:381–94.
30. Bandmann O, Weiss KH, Kaler SG. Wilson's disease and other neurological copper disorders. Lancet Neurol. 2015;14:103–13.
31. Jinnah HA, Teller JK, Galpern WR. Recent developments in dystonia. Curr Opin Neurol. 2015;28:400–5.
32. Paudel R, Hardy J, Revesz T, Holton JL, Houlden H. Review: genetics and neuropathology of primary pure dystonia. Neuropathol Appl Neurobiol. 2012;38:520–34.
33. Albanese A, Bhatia K, Bressman SB, Delong MR, Fahn S, Fung VS, et al. Phenomenology and classification of dystonia: a consensus update. Mov Disord. 2013;28:863–73.
34. Govert F, Deuschl G. Tremor entities and their classification: an update. Curr Opin Neurol. 2015;28:393–9.
35. Louis ED. Essential tremor: from bedside to bench and back to bedside. Curr Opin Neurol. 2014;27:461–7.
36. Jellinger KA. Neuropathology of essential tremor. J Mult Scler. 2016;3:165.

Rational and Methodology for the Appraisal of Clinical Trials in Movement Disorders

6

R. Bouça-Machado and Joaquim J. Ferreira

6.1 Why Should We Appraise the Quality of Clinical Trials?

In the past few decades, the number of clinical trials published in various biomedical domains has increased substantially. However, despite an increase in the quantity of trials, systematic reviews have shown that the quality of these clinical trials has not increased in the same way [1, 2].

The methodological quality of studies, a concept that has undergone several changes since its inception, comprises the evaluation of internal and external study validity. Internal validity refers to the degree to which observations accurately reflect what they are intended to measure. External validity is the extent to which internally valid research findings can be inferred back to the population of interest and other populations. The key to correctly translating the results from a single piece of research to the population of interest rests on the ability to verify that the study was devised with proper planning, design, and analysis and that it was conducted in a sample that accurately reflected the target population [3, 4].

Nowadays, there are a wide range of therapeutic interventions available and the results of randomised controlled trials (RCT), the gold standard for evaluating efficacy and effectiveness of health-care interventions, are crucial for informing patients, clinicians and decision/policymakers about the best treatments for improving patient outcomes and the efficiency of health-care systems. The presence of bias, a systematic error or deviation from the truth, which predisposes towards the experimental or control group and may overestimate or underestimate the true benefits and harms of an intervention, poses a threat to the capacity of RCTs in establishing the efficacy of an intervention [5, 6]. Therefore, an accurate quality assessment is imperative to ensure that the best available evidence is used to inform clinical and policy decisions [2, 7, 8].

6.2 Which Tools Can Be Used to Evaluate the Quality of Clinical Trials?

Many tools, in different health areas, have been used to assess the quality of trials. However, they can be grouped into three principal methods of

R. Bouça-Machado
Clinical Pharmacology Unit, Neurological Clinical Research Unit, Instituto de Medicina Molecular, Lisbon, Portugal

J.J. Ferreira (✉)
Clinical Pharmacology Unit, Neurological Clinical Research Unit, Instituto de Medicina Molecular, Lisbon, Portugal

Laboratory of Clinical Pharmacology and Therapeutics, Faculty of Medicine, University of Lisbon, Lisbon, Portugal

Department of Neurology, Hospital de Santa Maria, Lisbon, Portugal
e-mail: joaquimjferreira@gmail.com

C. Falup-Pecurariu et al. (eds.), *Movement Disorders Curricula*,
DOI 10.1007/978-3-7091-1628-9_6

quality assessment: individual factors, checklists and scales. Scales differ from the other methods as they provide quantitative estimates of quality that can be easily replicated and formally incorporated into the peer review process and into systematic reviews. Currently, there is no agreement regarding which tools are best for the accurate determination of trial quality, and it has been shown that the use of more than one tool to assess a single piece of primary research may lead to different results. Most of the tools have not been developed using scientifically rigorous methods, lack reliability and/or have not been fully validated. Despite these limitations, however, clinical trials included in systematic reviews or meta-analyses should be evaluated.

In 1995, Moher and colleagues identified 25 scales and 9 checklists which could be used to assess the quality of RCTs [4, 6, 9], and in 1996, in order to enhance the quality of RCT reporting, the Consolidated Standards of Reporting Trials (CONSORT) statement was introduced which consisted of a checklist that identified 21 essential elements that should be present in the methods, results and discussion sections to enable internal and external validity to be evaluated and thereby to determine the study's quality [1, 10].

Since then further tools have been developed to aid both trial design and assessment. The 33-item SPIRIT checklist applies to protocols for all clinical trials and aims to facilitate high-quality drafts, but in addition, the SPIRIT documents can also serve as a practical resource for trial investigators and personnel to draft and understand the key elements of a protocol [11].

In a review from 2013, the Jadad scale was, by far, the most cited and used tool. This is a five-item short and simple scale, with three domains: randomisation, blinding and account of all patients. This instrument has been validated to assess the quality of studies in pain relief, but given that none of the three items included in the final version of the instrument is specific to pain reports, it has been used extensively in other clinical areas. Its main advantages include its ease of use, the fact that it contains many of the important elements that have been shown empirically to correlate with bias and that it has known reliability and external validity [4, 9, 12].

The Cochrane Collaboration has led a shift in the approach to quality assessment in which the concept of trial quality is linked to the internal validity of the study, referred to as the risk of bias (RoB). This concept was developed following a growing body of empirical evidence quantifying the association between certain design features and estimates of treatment effects (TEs). The RoB tool is a two-part process and includes the following areas: sequence generation, allocation concealment, blinding (of participants, personnel and outcome assessment), incomplete outcome data, selective outcome reporting and 'other issues'. The first part concerns the description of what was reported in the trial, ensuring it is detailed enough for the trial judgement to be made. The second part appraises the risk of bias for each of the analysed areas and classifies them into one of the three categories: low, high or unclear risk of bias [13].

The International Parkinson and Movement Disorder Society's (MDS) therapeutic reviews apply the 'Checklists for Critical Appraisal. The Evidence Based Medicine Workbook checklist' from 1997, which is a list of the key methodologically relevant topics required to determine the methodological soundness of a trial. A percentage score, based on descriptive variables, can be calculated and used as an indicator of overall quality for each study and also allows the stratification of multiple trials based on their quality. There are five domains in the scale: results, selection validity, measurement, statistical analysis and utility. In the first domain, results, the estimated treatment effect and clinical importance are assessed. The validity domain analyses eligible criteria and sample issues, and the measurement domain assesses randomisation, blinding, dropouts and side effects. The type of analysis and statistical method used is evaluated in the statistical analysis domain, and the utility domain examines the usefulness of the results to aid clinical decisions [8].

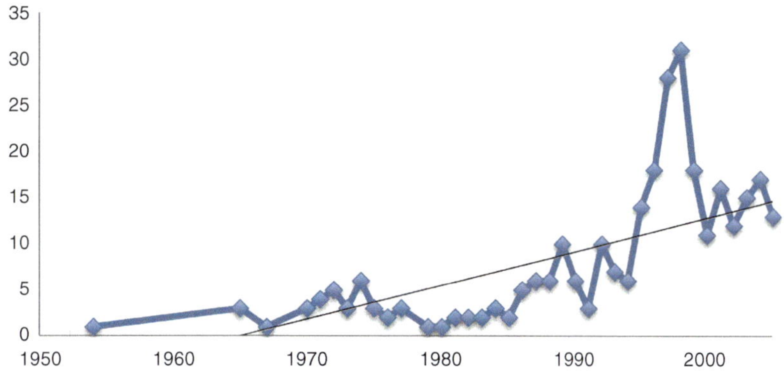

Fig. 6.1 Number of clinical trials published over time

6.3 Quality of Clinical Trials in MDS Systematic Reviews

Since 2002, the International Parkinson and Movement Disorder Society (MDS) has published one EBM review and six updates of treatments for Parkinson's disease (PD). All used the same inclusion criteria for selecting clinical trials: interventions in PD patients (not other types of parkinsonian disorders), use of established scales, a minimum of 20 subjects treated for a minimum of 4 weeks and reported in full-paper format in English. In some cases these criteria (especially sample size and duration) were not used, but these exceptions were noted with a justification for inclusion [8, 14].

The analysis of all studies in EBM reviews and updates shows that over the past decades, there has been a significant increase in the number of published clinical trials (Fig. 6.1). Of the 436 included studies, 4.5 % ($n=20$) were published between 1954 and 1973, 18.6 % ($n=80$) between 1974 and 1993 and 77 % ($n=336$) between 1994 and 2014.

The majority of studies have a parallel design (83.7 % ($n=365$), 16.3 % ($n=71$) crossover) and use a double-blind procedure (40.1 % ($n=175$), 8.3 % ($n=36$), single-blind or 8.3 % ($n=36$) open-label procedure). Sample size and follow-up duration differ significantly between studies. The median sample size is 49 subjects [Min-Max: 2–1,176] and median follow-up duration is 16 weeks [Min-Max: 0–480].

Table 6.1 Levels of evidence

Level of evidence	Definition
Level I studies	Randomised controlled trials
Level II studies	Controlled clinical trials or observational controlled studies
Level III studies	Non-controlled studies

The major limitations reported by authors are absence of a washout period in crossover trials, small samples and high attrition rates, lack of comparability between groups at baseline and a lack of a clearly stated primary outcome.

MDS EBM reviews are based on a hierarchical organisation of evidence, with clinical evidence classified into three levels (Table 6.1). If sufficient RCTs (level I studies) are available, studies with lower levels of evidence are only considered in order to support them [8]. Of the 436 included studies, 81.9 % ($n=357$) were level I studies, 5.5 % ($n=24$) level II and 12.6 % ($n=55$) level III studies. All level II and III studies belong to the original MDS EBM review, which dates from 2002. In respect to level I studies, the median quality score was 71.9 ([Min-Max: 21–100], SD: 15.7). Comparing the number of publications/year and quality score, we can see that in the past years that not only has the number of published clinical trials increased but that this was accompanied by an increase in the mean quality score (Fig. 6.2).

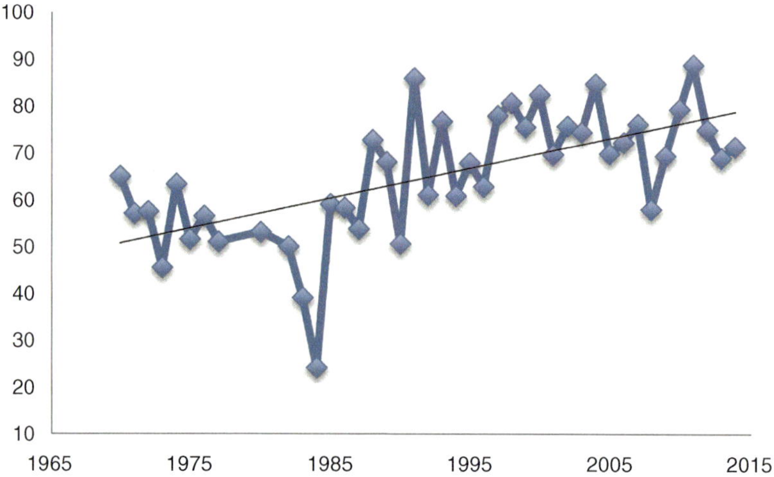

Fig. 6.2 Quality score of clinical trials published over time (mean)

6.4 Placebo Effect in Parkinson's Disease

Placebo treatment is a method utilised as a control condition in clinical trials. A positive placebo response is seen in up to 50 % of patients with PD [15]. Examples of this are clinical trials for oral anti-Parkinson medications where patients receiving placebo showed a significant clinical improvement, which was sustained for 6 months, as well as a meta-review in which 33.3 % (n = 12) of articles reported a 9–59 % improvement in patient motor symptoms following placebo. Surgical trials also demonstrate substantial placebo effects: patients with subthalamic nucleus deep brain stimulators (STN-DBS) as treatment for PD demonstrate improved motor performance when they believe their stimulators are turned on and perform worse than baseline when they believe their stimulators are turned off, compared to responses under conditions in which they were blind to stimulator function. In an elegant series of studies using an overt-covert experimental design, Benedetti and colleagues demonstrated that sham STN-DBS improves bradykinesia, as measured by hand velocity, and that this is also directly measurable as a neurochemical/neurophysiological response using [11C] raclopride positron emission tomography.

Several theories have been proposed to explain how the placebo effect is modulated in PD: first, placebo may be more effective in anxious PD subjects as its effects are often associated with patients' desire to reduce anxiety and suffering; second, placebo treatment induces positive expectations, a reward of clinical improvement; and third, this expectation induces direct or indirect neurochemical alterations in dopaminergic systems that consequently result in improved parkinsonism [15–17].

Since placebo has such a powerful effect, some authors encourage the use of placebo-control trials in interventions that have never been proven to be effective, and their use is based on anecdotal reports and/or physician preferences. In EBM reviews and updates, almost half of the included studies (46.8 %, n = 204) used placebo as a control group. The remaining studies used active controls (34,4 %, n = 150), no intervention (6.2 %, n = 27), and 12.6 % (n = 55) are uncontrolled studies.

6.5 Clinically Meaningful Outcomes

PD is associated with a variable clinical disease course, severity and combination of motor and non-motor features, and it is still largely unknown which factors influence PD progression or long-term outcomes [18].

Over the past few decades, there has been a noticeable discrepancy between the outcomes that patients, caregivers and clinicians crave and those that have been the focus of PD research. Patients frequently ask about the impact of the disease on their quality of life (e.g. the ability to continue living at home, work and drive a car), cognition and premature death or nursing home placement. From the caregiver's perspective, in addition to these aspects, the degree of dependence on a caregiver and the overall financial implications of the disease are also important issues [18]. To consider a study of quality, besides evaluating its methodological characteristics, it is also important to consider its utility in clinical practice.

Table 6.2 Outcome tools to evaluate meaningful progression

Outcome	Assessment tool
Motor function/progression	MDS-UPDRS
	Hoehn and Yahr (H&Y) scale
Cognitive function	Montreal Cognitive Assessment (MoCA) and DSM-V dementia definition
Depression and anxiety	Hamilton depression rating scale (Ham-D) and Beck depression inventory (BDI)
	Geriatric Depression Scale (GDS)
	Zung Self-Rating Depression scale (SDS) UPDRS part I
Autonomic dysfunction	SCOPA-AUT, OHQ and COMPASS
	UPDRS part IV
	Blood pressure and pulse measurements supine or sitting and after 3 min standing
Quality of life	39-item PD Questionnaire (PDQ-39)
	Schwab and England Independence Scale (S&E)
	NeuroQOL
Suggestion of a panel of rating scales to a routine office visit	UPDRS (parts I–IV) at the time of the office visit, documenting the patient's on, partial on or off state, despite its weaknesses described above, the H&Y scale, the MoCA-score, the 15-item version of the GDS and the S&E scale. Blood pressure and pulse measurements with the patient supine or sitting and after standing for 3 min should be performed when possible

To this end, the Geo-PD consortium has suggested a group of tools to capture clinically meaningful progression and outcomes (Table 6.2).

As mentioned above, the primary goals of studies do not always coincide with patients' expectations. In the same way, trials with statistical differences in the outcome measures may not represent an improvement from the patient's perspective. The Movement Disorder Society Task Force for Rating Scales for Parkinson's disease has encouraged the identification of cutoffs on the UPDRS with statistical significant differences that actually represent an improvement in the patient's experience (minimal clinically relevant differences), as this scale is one of the most used primary outcomes in trials.

Schrag and Hauser, in 2006 and 2014, used two pivotal, double-blind, parallel-group trials of the dopamine agonists pramipexole ER and ropinirole, to study the minimal clinically important changes (MCIC) in the UPDRS (parts II and III) and the off time. To quantify the threshold effect size that should be met to conclude that an intervention has a meaningful clinical impact, the authors used the Clinician-Rated Global Impression of Improvement (CGI-I) scale and Patient-Rated Global Impression of Improvement (PGI-I) as anchors [19, 20]. The authors proposed that the lower limit of MCIC for total UPDRS score (I + II + III) be 3.8, and the change in off time be 1.0 h (Tables 6.3 and 6.4). They also emphasised the usefulness of MCIC to

Table 6.3 Minimal clinically important changes in early and advanced PD

	Early PD		Advanced PD	
	ER	IR	ER	IR
UPDRS II	−1.8	−2.0	−1.8	−2.3
UPDRS III	−6.2	−6.1	−5.2	−6.5
UPDRS II + III	−8.0	−8.1	−7.1	−8.8
Off duration		−1.0 H	−1.3 H	

Table 6.4 EMA recommendations for design of PD clinical trials

Goal	Stage of disease	Treatment[b]	Study design	Duration of trial[e]	Main efficacy variable
Symptomatic relief	Early stage	Before L-dopa	Double-blind placebo-controlled studies	6 months	Improvement of the core symptoms, i.e. motor symptoms
Symptomatic relief	Early stage – de novo patients[a]	Before L-dopa	Three-arm randomised double-blind placebo- and active-controlled studies	6 months	Improvement of the core symptoms, i.e. motor symptoms
Symptomatic relief	Some form of advance stage, with insufficient control of motor symptoms	L-Dopa+	Three-arm placebo- and active-controlled trials	3 months	Improvement of motor symptoms and activities of daily living
Symptomatic relief	'End stage', with motor fluctuations	L-Dopa+	Three arm randomised double-blind placebo-controlled studies wherein a test drug arm, a standard drug arm and a placebo arm, all in addition to L-dopa+[d]	3 months	Decrease in number, duration and/or intensity of 'off' periods and 'on' time with and without dyskinesia
Symptomatic relief	Highly advanced PD, with severe and highly unpredictable motor fluctuations that succeed each other rapidly during the day	Continuous delivery devices of L-dopa+ or dopamine-agonist subcutaneously, intravenously or by a duodenal catheter	Randomised blinded comparative studies or alternative study designs, like number of trials. Superiority should be shown against placebo in the add-on setting or against a treatment regime with the conventional route of administration	No detailed recommendations can be made as this also depends on the substance and device used	Reduction of the motor fluctuations
Modify disease progression	Postponing late motor complications	L-Dopa+[c]	Long-term double-blind, placebo-controlled add-on studies wherein the test drug or placebo is added to L-dopa+	Sufficient to show an effect. May last for years	Time to late motor complications as pre-specified in the protocol

Modify disease progression – to slow the progression of motor symptoms	Early stage – de novo patients[a]	Untreated PD	Randomised, placebo-controlled and long-term studies	Up to 24 months	Change in UPDRS or time to L-dopa+/ DA-agonists
Modify disease progression to slow further decline of motor impairment, progression of disability, prevent motor and non-motor complications	Stable-treated PD	L-Dopa+	Randomised, placebo-controlled and long-term studies	2–5 years	Emergence of axial symptoms: freezing of gait, loss of balance or Hoehn and Yahr stage III
Modify disease progression – prevention of disability	Advanced PD	L-Dopa+	Randomised, placebo-controlled and long-term studies	5 years	Autonomic failure, falls, cognitive symptoms and possibly 'time to' dementia and 'time to' nursing home placement

[a]Defined as patients with recently diagnosed PD (3–6 months) and no previous dopaminergic treatment except for a short period (<30 days)

[b]In all conditions concomitant L-dopa+ and other relevant medication should be kept constant during the trial and recorded for validation of the study design to provide reassurance that treatment effects are not due to dose reductions in L-dopa+. In the same way, before the test drug/placebo is added, L-dopa+ therapy should be optimised in order to distinguish between an effect of the test drug and an increased efficacy due to the optimised L-dopa+ dose regime

[c]The reduction in L-dopa+ doses as primary efficacy variable is not recommended. However, it is necessary to take into account L-dopa+ reductions when evaluating other efficacy variables in the light of these reductions

[d]The term treatment regime is used here to capture different formulations as well as different devices with the same agents. As an example a slow release L-dopa+ should be compared to an immediate release L-dopa+ formulation. A benefit of the new treatment regime as compared to the standard treatment regime should be established

[e]Excluding the titration period, where dose adaptations of the test drug are allowed

enable the performance of power calculations and to understand meaning, from a patient's perspective, of the magnitude of change observed in a clinical trial [19].

6.6 Genetic Testing in Clinical Trials

Over the past 15 years, important discoveries have been made in the genetics of PD. A recent meta-analysis revealed that 24 loci, including GBA and other monogenic forms like LRRK2 and SNCA, have clinically significant associations with disease risk. Other studies have revealed, in atypical parkinsonian syndromes and more rarely in typical PD, unexpected mutations in genes that are more often associated with other inherited diseases, such as spinocerebellar ataxias of frontotemporal dementias. Unfortunately, this knowledge is only useful in a very limited proportion of PD cases where one of the rare forms of the disease with Mendelian inheritance is suspected based on family history or age to start [21, 22].

Performing a genetic test is not a risk-free procedure. Clinicians and researchers should be aware that the diagnosis or confirmation of a genetic disorder affects not only the patient or at-risk individual but also the entire family, and therefore counselling should be given concerning the risk of transmission, penetrance and expressivity issues and possible therapeutic or preventive aspects [21].

According to the European Federation of Neurological Societies (EFNS) and the Movement Disorder Society – European Section (MDS-ES), in Gasser, 2015, clinical genetic testing in PD should be limited to testing for mutations in SNCA and LRRK2 in patients with typical PD and a clear dominant family history. In recessive genes – parkin, PINK1 and DJ-1 – this test should only be undertaken in two situations: in patients with typical PD and those with a family history consistent with recessive inheritance (affected siblings, parents unaffected) and/or in patients with age of onset under 50 or sporadic PD patients with typical age of onset under 40. Other scenarios must be considered on a case-by-case basis, according to patient and family benefit or in research setting [21].

In clinical trials which test strategies for disease course modification, targeting specific molecular pathways and genetic stratification, with or without awareness of participants, may be an important tool to reduce heterogeneity of samples and would allow researchers to test interventions in mutation carrier-only groups, enrich target populations and might also help uncover future interventions for the presymptomatic disease stage [21].

6.7 Recommendations for the Design of Parkinson's Disease Clinical Trials

In 2012, the European Medicines Agency (EMA) published a general guidance on the development of medicinal products for the treatment of PD [23].

These studies are hampered not only by the long duration and slow progressive course of the disease, the variability and heterogeneity of symptoms and signs, cyclic episodes in severity of the symptoms/signs over the day related to the time of medication and polytherapy, but also by misdiagnosis, co-morbidity and co-medication adding to the heterogeneity of the patient population [23].

The EMA guidelines presented a set of six study objectives: two associated to symptomatic relief, three related to disease progression and one with substitution of neuronal loss. For each objective they proposed a study design and some recommendations, like duration of protocol and the main efficacy variables (Table 6.4) [23].

In some study designs, the incorporation of a placebo arm beyond the active control arm is recommended. When comparisons between placebo and other interventions are performed, placebo treatment outcomes may mask, diminish or increase the calculated treatment effect [15, 23].

Another recommendation of the EMA guidelines concerns imaging. Biomarkers measuring the cerebral dopamine uptake (SPECT-β-CIT) or dopamine-receptor density (PET-F-dopa), although associated to nigrostriatal function, cannot yet be considered sufficient surrogate biomarkers as it is not established that they correlate to a meaningful, measurable and persistent changes in clinical function.

Simultaneous assessment of clinical outcomes and biomarkers is recommended in order to evaluate whether both are causally associated with treatment and to assess the potential predictive value of a biomarker for clinical outcome. The ELLDOPA study can be used to illustrate this point. The Earlier versus Later L-dopa Therapy in Parkinson's disease (ELLDOPA) study was a multicentre, placebo-controlled, randomised, dose-ranging, double-blind clinical trial conducted by the Parkinson Study Group. Results from clinical data suggest that levodopa is not 'neurotoxic' and may even be neuroprotective. Conversely, findings of β-CIT SPECT imaging were discordant with these clinical results, showing that levodopa may hasten the progression of PD. In reality, it is thought that the observed change in the levels of uptake of this marker reflected a pharmacological effect of levodopa on DAT activity, rather than evidence of injury to dopaminergic neurons [23, 24].

Substitution of neuronal loss as a therapy in PD is currently confined to the experimental stage, as it is still full of uncertainties, e.g. the source of tissue, the selection of patients, number of cells required, need for immunosuppressant and/or growth factors, most effective surgical procedure, need and feasibility of sham surgery and so on. Therefore, no detailed recommendations have been made [23].

References

1. Falagas ME, Grigori T, Ioannidou E. A systematic review of trends in the methodological quality of randomized controlled trials in various research fields. J Clin Epidemiol. 2009;62(3):227–31.e9. doi:10.1016/j.jclinepi.2008.07.012.
2. Dechartres A, Charles P, Hopewell S, Ravaud P, Altman DG. Reviews assessing the quality or the reporting of randomized controlled trials are increasing over time but raised questions about how quality is assessed. J Clin Epidemiol. 2011;64(2):136–44. doi:10.1016/j.jclinepi.2010.04.015.
3. Hartung D, Touchette D. Overview of clinical research design. Am J Health Syst Pharm. 2009;66:398–408. doi:10.2146/ajhp080300.
4. Armijo-olivo S, Stiles CR, Bn RN, Frcpc NAH, Biondo PD, Rn GGC. Assessment of study quality for systematic reviews : a comparison of the cochrane collaboration risk of bias tool and the effective public health practice project quality assessment tool : methodological research. J Eval Clin Pract. 2012;18:12–8. doi:10.1111/j.1365-2753.2010.01516.x.
5. Gurusamy KS, Gluud C, Nikolova D, Davidson BR. Assessment of risk of bias in randomized clinical trials in surgery. Br J Surg. 2009;96(4):342–9. doi:10.1002/bjs.6558.
6. Higgins J, Green S. Cochrane handbook for systematic reviews of interventions 4.2.6 [Updated Sept 2006]; 2006. doi:10.3233/PRM-2010-0129.
7. Armijo-Olivo S, Fuentes J, Ospina M, Saltaji H, Hartling L. Inconsistency in the items included in tools used in general health research and physical therapy to evaluate the methodological quality of randomized controlled trials: a descriptive analysis. BMC Med Res Methodol. 2013;13(1):116. doi:10.1186/1471-2288-13-116.
8. Lang AE, Lees AJ. Management of Parkinson's disease: an evidence-based review. Mov Disord. 2002;17(Suppl 4). doi:10.1002/mds.5554.
9. Jadad AR, Moore RA, Carroll D, et al. Assessing the quality of reports of randomized clinical trials : is blinding necessary ? Control Clin Trials. 1996;17:1–12.
10. Kane RL, Wang J, Garrard J. Reporting in randomized clinical trials improved after adoption of the CONSORT statement. J Clin Epidemiol. 2007;60(3):241–9. doi:10.1016/j.jclinepi.2006.06.016.
11. Chan A-W, Tetzlaff JM, Gøtzsche PC, et al. SPIRIT 2013 explanation and elaboration: guidance for protocols of clinical trials. BMJ. 2013;346:e7586 doi:10.1136/bmj.e7586.
12. Halpern SH, Douglas MJ. Jadad scale for reporting randomized controlled trials. Evid Based Obstet Anesth. BMJ Books;2005:237–8.
13. Armijo Olivo S, Fuentes CJ, Rogers T, Hartling L, Saltaji H, Cummings G. How should we evaluate the risk of bias of physical therapy trials? A psychometric and meta-epidemiological approach towards developing guidelines for the design, conduct, and reporting of RCTs in Physical Therapy (PT) area: a study protocol. Syst Rev. 2013;2(1):88. doi:2046-4053-2-88 [pii] 10.1186/2046-4053-2-88.
14. Goetz CG, Poewe W, Rascol O, Sampaio C. Evidence-based medical review update : pharmacological and surgical treatments of Parkinson' s disease : 2001–2004. Mov Disord. 2005;20(5):523–39. doi:10.1002/mds.20464.
15. Diederich NJ, Goetz CG. The placebo treatments in neurosciences: new insights from clinical and neuroimaging studies. Neurology. 2008;71(9):677–84. doi:10.1212/01.wnl.0000324635.49971.3d.

16. Lidstone SC. Great expectations: the placebo effect in Parkinson's disease. In: Benedetti F, Enck P, Frisaldi E, Schedlowski M, (ed). Placebo, handbook of experimental pharmacology. Heidelberg: Springer Berlin; 2014:139–47.
17. Shetty N, Friedman JH, Kieburtz K, Marshall F, Oakes D, Parkinson Study Group. The palcebo response in Parkinson's disease. Clin Neuropharmacol. 1999;22(4):207–12.
18. Puschmann A, Brighina L, Markopoulou K, et al. Clinically meaningful parameters of progression and long-term outcome of Parkinson disease: An international consensus statement. Parkinsonism Relat Disord. 2015;21. doi:10.1016/j.parkreldis.2015.04.029.
19. Hauser RA, Gordon MF, Mizuno Y, et al. Minimal clinically important difference in parkinson's disease as assessed in pivotal trials of pramipexole extended release. Parkinsons Dis. 2014;2014. doi:10.1155/2014/467131.
20. Schrag A, Sampaio C, Counsell N, Poewe W. Minimal clinically important change on the unified Parkinson's disease rating scale. Mov Disord. 2006;21(8):1200–7. doi:10.1002/mds.20914.
21. Gasser T. Usefulness of genetic testing in PD and PD trials: a balanced review. J Park Dis. 2015;5(2):209–15. doi:10.3233/JPD-140507.
22. Kalia LV, Lang AE. Parkinson's disease. Lancet. 2015;6736(14):1–17. doi:10.1016/S0140-6736(14)61393-3.
23. Ema. Guideline on clinical investigation of medicinal products in the treatment of Parkinson' s disease. 2012;44(June):1–16.
24. Fahn S. A new look at levodopa based on the ELLDOPA study. J Neural Transm Suppl. 2006;70:419–26.

7 How to Record a Video of a Movement Disorder Patient

Brandon Barton and Esther Cubo

7.1 Introduction

Video recordings of patients have been used for many purposes including education of patients or health-care providers, documentation of physical examinations, assessing quality and accuracy of patient care, monitoring operative procedures, telemedicine, and as a diagnostic procedure such as with epilepsy monitoring [1, 2]. In the field of movement disorders, video recordings help to document the phenomenology of the movements and provide the opportunity to view, review, and discuss the clinical case's diagnosis with one's peers or specialty colleagues. Documentation of a movement disorder by visual methods is critical in a field where the correct semiologic definition of the different conditions is one of the most important but problematic steps in the diagnostic workup [3]. Words are inadequate to fully match the descriptive and diagnostic power of watching a movement disorder patient in a visual media. In addition, a video record may help the physician to provide better care by documenting the response to treatment or disease progression, to rate the severity of the movements by using standardized video rating scales, to train participants in clinical trials to uniformly and accurately administer rating scales, and to better define long-term evolution of a chronic disorder [4]. When video recordings are used prospectively for research, they have proven invaluable for the blinded rating of the study subjects. Unique or informative videos may be published in academic journals or textbooks. Historical videos have a value in understanding disorders that may later become uncommon such as Kuru [5] or that document case histories of early patients in the history of neurology [6]. Video case presentations of patients serve as a core of educational presentations at movement disorder teaching conferences, invaluable for learning the common and rare manifestations of each disorder.

7.2 Prior to Filming the Patient

It is necessary to explain the rationale for the video recording to the patient and to obtain a written consent form from the patient or legal representative. This consent form is obligatory, addressing confidentiality and the proposed uses for the video.

B. Barton, MD, MS
Department of Neurological Sciences, Rush University Medical Center, Chicago, IL, USA

Neurology Service, Jesse Brown VA Medical Center, Chicago, IL, USA

E. Cubo, MD, PhD (✉)
Neurology Department, Hospital Universitario Burgos, Avda Islas Baleares 3, Burgos 09006, Spain

Department of Neurology, Complejo Asistencial Universitario, Burgos, Spain
e-mail: esthercubo@gmail.com

Received: September 18th, 2013.

C. Falup-Pecurariu et al. (eds.), *Movement Disorders Curricula*,
DOI 10.1007/978-3-7091-1628-9_7

A consent is required for any clinical presentation of the video outside the patient encounter, and the patient has the right to refuse the video. If the video is to be published in any form, further special consent and documentation are usually required. It is important to collect the following information: patient's identification (name, last name, medical record number, date of birth, and protocol number and time duration) and date of the video recording. This information could be written and displayed as a title screen at the beginning of the video and then should be kept for storage.

7.3 General Guidelines

Patients should be filmed in a quiet room with adequate lighting from angles that will not obscure any part of the body in shadow [7]. A clean, non-reflective, light blue background is recommended because it allows for the best neutral contrast for skin tones. For those that see movement disorder patients frequently, a special video room dedicated to filming patients is ideal. If videotaping is anticipated at the visit, instruct patients beforehand to wear solid colors without patterns and avoid bulky clothing that obscures the neck or limbs. If possible, a trained staff member can serve as a videographer, allowing for consistency in camera operation and completing full video protocols. Suggested equipment for the video room should contain the following:

1. An armless chair in which to observe the patient in a seated position and observe how they can rise without using their arms to push up.
2. A lab coat, which the patient may be asked to put on and button up, in order to test motor coordination and dexterity.
3. A table where the patient can write or draw or perform any other motor act which is affected by abnormal movements. This table should be without drawers and allow good visibility of the patient's upper and lower body while being observed. A good example of such a table is a portable bedside hospital tray with adjustable height.
4. Paper and pens or pencils for writing and drawing.
5. Plastic glasses, towels, and water to demonstrate severity of tremor while pouring water from glass to glass.
6. Backup assistance to help unstable patients with severe gait and balance issues ambulate. Even if a patient feels that they cannot walk, every attempt to evaluate their ability to try to stand and walk should be used since this is a key part of the examination.

Whenever recording a particular aspect of the natural history of the disease or response to treatment is needed, the same video recording protocol must be used (see Table 7.1). A universally defined standard for video protocols is not yet published, but internal consistency is important when filming a patient at multiple times with the same health-care providers. It is important to avoid common mistakes (see Table 7.2) to enhance the quality of the video recording. If a patient's explanation of the history is succinct, she/he can be asked it at the start of the recording, which is particularly useful when speech or language impairments are part of the neurologic

Table 7.1 Key elements for any video protocol

Position	Phenomenology to observe
Seated at rest	Parkinsonian rest tremor, hyperkinetic disorders (chorea, ataxia, dystonia)
Standing	Parkinsonism, ataxia, dystonia
Rapid movements of the limbs (finger tapping, hand opening, foot stomping)	Action dystonia, tremors, bradykinesia, ataxia, myoclonus
Speech	Dysarthria, hypophonia, tremor, dysphonia
Eye movements	Supranuclear ophthalmoplegia, square wave jerks, saccadic pursuit, apraxia
Limbs sustained against gravity	Tremor, myoclonus, ataxia
Gait: forward, backward, tandem	Parkinsonism, dystonia, ataxia, gait disorders
Coordination: finger to nose, heel to shin	Ataxia, tremor

Table 7.2 Common mistakes

Video too brief to ascertain overall pattern of movements
Inadequate lighting
Only one angle used to view the patient
Not observing the limbs in multiple positions including rest
Focusing on one small element of the exam without the context of the general examination of voluntary and involuntary movements
Omitting gait or attempts at gait
Shaky camera technique (lacking tripod or image stabilization)
Neglecting to collect important identifier data (e.g., date/medical record number)

deficit. Otherwise a speech sample could be obtained by asking the patient to read a specific text passage or, if the patient cannot read, to describe a story that might stem from a narrative-style drawing or cartoon. After video recording, insert a note in the medical chart documenting when the patient was video recorded. It is a good practice to videotape a complete protocol of an individual at the first examination in order to have a baseline audiovisual record with which to compare future clinical evaluations.

Regardless of this ideal, some patients will of necessity be video recorded under suboptimal conditions such as in the emergency room, intensive care unit, or while having an acute event in the examination room. In such cases the videographer should attempt to expose the parts of the body being examined as best possible while positioning the patient safely.

7.4 Protocols

Specific movement disorder video recording protocols have been developed by some clinical groups for parkinsonism, dystonia, chorea, myoclonus, tremor, gait, and tic disorders, although universal videotaping protocols have not been adopted. Standardized rating scales for some types of movement such as dyskinesias, parkinsonism, and tics have been validated and are now widely accepted as useful clinical assessment tools, and these protocols can be performed while being videotaped and serve as a useful framework to capture the key elements of the disorder [8–12]. The following general protocols should be observed for specific disorders: (1) In general, it is common to elicit movement characteristics of each disorder while recording. Listen to the history and have the patients perform the actions which bring out or display the movements most reliably. (2) For dystonia, it is important to demonstrate any sensory tricks which temporarily control their dystonia. Perform a bend-over test for scoliosis, eating for eating dystonia, or speech for spasmodic dysphonia. (3) For tremor, it is also important to add a writing section, activity such as pouring water from a full cup to another cup without touching with the dominant and nondominant hand, and spiral drawing. (4) For parkinsonism, to demonstrate parkinsonian signs, it is important to film full body, upper body, lower body, standing up, posture and walking, and pull test, following the Unified Parkinson's Disease Rating Scale (UPDRS) [12] motor items and to demonstrate resting tremor, bradykinesia, and gait problems. (5) To demonstrate levodopa-induced dyskinesias, validated scales such as the Unified Dyskinesia Rating Scale (UDysRS) [8] or the video-based dyskinesia severity score (SVS) can be utilized [13]. The UDysRS video training protocol [8] is based on videotapes of the patient while performing activities of daily living such as the communication task, putting on a lab coat, and walking. The SVS [13] is specific for the communication task where the patient is asked to read while seated on a chair. (6) For myoclonus, it is important to include a loud noise to startle subject such as clapping hands together or dropping a heavy book on the floor. (7) For chorea, it is important to elicit orolingual movement and to ask to fully protrude tongue as long as possible and to observe the choreiform movements at rest and while doing motor acts such as walking. (8) For tics, the most common protocol is the Rush Video-Based Tic Rating Scale [11]. Here, the videotape protocol involves a 10-min film of patients placed in front of a video camera in a quiet room. Two body views are recorded, full frontal view (far) and head and shoulder (near), under two conditions: relaxed while the examiner is in the room and relaxed while the patient is alone. The severity of the tic disorder has been shown to worsen with the patient alone.

7.5 Hardware Considerations

Video technology has rapidly advanced in the last decade, and ease of use has been vastly improved for most casual users [4]. Most video cameras can record and transfer the video directly to a computer file via USB connection for editing and storage. A dedicated clinic camcorder for clinical videos can provide much better quality as compared to pocket camcorders such as smartphones, largely due to image stabilization and wider angle of view. One does not need to invest in highly expensive video cameras given the very good quality of low-to-mid range price digital cameras on the market. The use of a tripod is recommended to reduce jitter inevitable in handheld recording devices. A small detachable microphone can greatly enhance the speech comprehension and reduce background noise without interfering with the patient's movements.

7.6 Software Considerations

High-definition (HD) video generally provides relatively small file sizes with acceptable quality [4]. The ideal format in which the digital output is stored is a complex question that depends on the user and the capabilities of available software and storage. Current common video file output formats include MEPG2 (.mpg), MPEG4 (.mp4), Windows Media Video (.wmv), QuickTime (.mov), and Flash Video (.flv). In general, playback in multiple formats are supported by video player programs (e.g., Windows Media Player, QuickTime) although one should carefully test that the files play back correctly on the desired computers and presentation software. Videos can be saved or converted in many formats or edited by one of many editing programs that may be purchased separately, provided with the computer's operating system (e.g., Windows Movie Maker) or provided by the video camera manufacturer.

7.7 Long-Term Storage

Given the confidential and private nature of patient videos and their long-term value in patient care, education, and research, quality and security of file storage are important [4]. File backup and accessibility of the correct files through proper labeling (using patient identifiers, corresponding diagnoses, and file numbers) is critical. A backup of all files on a separate hard drive is highly recommended since digital or taped media is highly susceptible to damage, corruption, or physical loss. This may be accomplished by having redundant backup drives on the same storage device, having another alternative storage on a remotely accessed password-protected server, or sharing part of a network with a larger secure server (such as a common university server) that has remote backup capabilities. Many databases are already "web enabled," allowing for the data to be accessed from any computer that has the ability to access a web browser.

References

1. Taylor K, Mayell A, Vandenberg S, Blanchard N, Parshuram CS. Prevalence and indications for video recording in the health care setting in north American and British pediatric hospitals. Paediatr Child Health. 2011;16:e57–60.
2. Barboi AC, Goetz CG, Musetoiu R. The origins of scientific cinematography and early medical applications. Neurology. 2004;62:2082–6.
3. Jog MS, Grantier L. Methods for digital video recording, storage, and communication of movement disorders. Mov Disord. 2001;16:1196–200.
4. Duker AP. Video recording in movement disorders: practical issues. Continuum (Minneap Minn). 2013;19:1401–5.
5. Kompoliti K, Goetz CG, Gajdusek DC, Cubo E. Movement disorders in kuru. Mov Disord. 1999;14:800–4.

6. Hornyak M, Rovit RL, Simon AS, Couldwell WT. Irving s. Cooper and the early surgical management of movement disorders. Video history. Neurosurg Focus. 2001;11:E6.
7. de Leon D, Moskowitz CB, Stewart C. Proposed guidelines for videotaping individuals with movement disorders. J Neurosci Nurs. 1991;23:191–3.
8. Goetz CG, Nutt JG, Stebbins GT, Chmura TA. Teaching program for the unified dyskinesia rating scale. Mov Disord. 2009;24:1296–8.
9. Goetz CG, Stebbins GT, Chmura TA, Fahn S, Poewe W, Tanner CM. Teaching program for the movement disorder society-sponsored revision of the unified Parkinson's disease rating scale: (MDS-UPDRS). Mov Disord. 2010;25:1190–4.
10. Comella CL, Stebbins GT, Goetz CG, Chmura TA, Bressman SB, Lang AE. Teaching tape for the motor section of the Toronto western spasmodic torticollis scale. Mov Disord. 1997;12:570–5.
11. Goetz CG, Pappert EJ, Louis ED, Raman R, Leurgans S. Advantages of a modified scoring method for the rush video-based tic rating scale. Mov Disord. 1999;14:502–6.
12. Goetz CG, Tilley BC, Shaftman SR, Stebbins GT, Fahn S, Martinez-Martin P, Poewe W, Sampaio C, Stern MB, Dodel R, Dubois B, Holloway R, Jankovic J, Kulisevsky J, Lang AE, Lees A, Leurgans S, LeWitt PA, Nyenhuis D, Olanow CW, Rascol O, Schrag A, Teresi JA, van Hilten JJ, LaPelle N. Movement disorder society-sponsored revision of the unified Parkinson's disease rating scale (MDS-UPDRS): scale presentation and clinimetric testing results. Mov Disord. 2008;23:2129–70.
13. Rao AS, Dawant BM, Bodenheimer RE, Li R, Fang J, Phibbs F, Hedera P, Davis T. Validating an objective video-based dyskinesia severity score in Parkinson's disease patients. Parkinsonism Relat Disord. 2013;19:232–7.

Rating Scales in Movement Disorders

8

Carmen Rodriguez-Blazquez, Maria João Forjaz, and Pablo Martinez-Martin

8.1 Introduction

Rating scales are basic tools for measurement in neurology. Their goals include the quantification of clinical and directly observable behaviors, such as tremor, and of not directly observable and subjective aspects ("constructs") of the condition, such as fatigue. Their simplicity and the quality and quantity of information they provide at a low cost make rating scales a useful and widely used tool in clinical and research settings. Rating scales allow clinician and researchers to identify and evaluate signs and symptoms, document the disease course and severity, determine the treatment efficacy, evaluate the impact of the disease, compare between different health states and populations, and assess public health policies and resource allocation.

In recent years, a plethora of rating scales for movement disorders has been developed and published, making the selection of an appropriate tool a complex task for clinicians and health researchers. In the field of the movement disorders, rating scales can be rater based, usually for the assessment of motor and non-motor manifestations, functional status, complications, and treatment effects, or self-administered, instruments globally known as "patient-reported outcomes" or PRO [1]. The information furnished by PRO includes a wide range of subjective aspects of the disease: symptoms, functional status, psychological well-being, quality of life, perceived change, satisfaction with treatment, etc.

In addition to the objectives and characteristics of the study, available information on the development and validation processes of a rating scale should guide the selection of scales. During the validation process, the scales attributes are tested following agreed principles and norms and applying a strict methodology that guarantee the quality and accuracy of the data the scale provides. In this field, two main approaches exist: the classical test theory (CTT) [2, 3] and the latent trait theories (LTT), which includes the item response theory (IRT) and the Rasch measurement theory. The advantages and disadvantages of each approach can be found in the literature [2, 3].

C. Rodriguez-Blazquez • P. Martinez-Martin (✉)
National Centre of Epidemiology and CIBERNED, Carlos III Institute of Health, Madrid, Spain
e-mail: crodb@isciii.es; pmartinez@isciii.es

M.J. Forjaz
National School of Public Health and REDISSEC, Carlos III Institute of Health, Madrid, Spain
e-mail: jforjaz@isciii.es

C. Falup-Pecurariu et al. (eds.), *Movement Disorders Curricula*,
DOI 10.1007/978-3-7091-1628-9_8

According to the CTT, the main properties to be tested during the validation study are the following [4, 5]: feasibility and acceptability, scaling assumptions, reliability, validity, precision,

Table 8.1 Examples of psychometric attributes and standard values

Attribute and definition	Standard criteria	References
Feasibility The extent to which the measure can be used in the intended context	*Missing data* <5–10 %	Smith et al. *Health Technol Assess*. 2005;9(10):1–93
Acceptability How acceptable is the scale for the target population	*Observed vs. theoretical range* coincident	
	Mean vs. median coincident	
	Floor and ceiling effects <15 %	McHorney and Tarlov. *Qual Life Res*. 1995;4(4):293–307
	Skewness −1 to +1	Van der Linden et al. *J Neurol Neurosurg Psychiatry*. 2005;76(12):1677–81
Reliability: degree to which a scale is free of random error		
Internal consistency The extent to which the items measure the same construct	*Cronbach's alpha* >0.70 (group); 0.90–0.95 (individual)	McHorney and Tarlov. *Qual Life Res*. 1995;4(4):293–307
	Inter-item correlation: *r* >0.20 and <0.75	Eisen and Ware. *Med Care*. 1979;17(9):902–21
	Item-total correlation: *r*=0.20–0.40	Smith et al. *Health Technol Assess*. 2005;9(10):1–93
	Homogeneity coefficient: >0.30	Ware and Gandek. *J Clin Epidemiol*. 1998;51(11):945–52
		Eisen et al. *Med Care*. 1979;17(9):902–21
Reproducibility Stability of scores over time or across different raters	*Inter-observer and test-retest reliability*:	
	Kappa (nominal/ordinal data) >0.60 or >0.70	Landis and Koch. *Biometrics*. 1977;33(1):159–74
	Intraclass correlation coefficient (continuous data) >0.70	Terwee et al. *J Clin Epidemiol*. 2007;60(1):34–42
Validity: the extent to which an instrument measures the construct is intended to measure		
Content validity The degree to which the content of an instrument covers the main aspects of the construct to be measured	*Expert opinion*	Terwee et al. *J Clin Epidemiol*. 2007;60(1):34–42
	Lynn's content validity index	Lynn. *Nurs Res*. 1986;35(6):382–5
Construct validity (hypothesis testing) The extent to which the scale's scores are consistent with hypotheses regarding the construct	*Convergent validity*: *r* >0.60	Chassany et al. *Drug Inf J*. 2002;36(1):209–38
	Divergent validity: *r* <0.30	Fitzpatrick et al. *Health Technol Assess*. 1998;2(14):i–iv, 1–74
	Internal validity: *r*=0.30–0.70	Hobart et al. *Brain*. 2001;124(Pt 5):962–73
	Known-group validity: Significant difference between groups	Fayers and Machin 2000
Criterion validity The degree of relationship of a scale with a "gold standard"	*r* >0.60	Terwee et al. *J Clin Epidemiol*. 2007;60(1):34–42

responsiveness, and interpretability (although the latter is not considered a measurement property). The definition and standard criteria for assessment of each one are described in Table 8.1.

8.2 Rating Scales for Movement Disorders

This section describes the most widely used, relevant, and valid instruments, mainly those recommended by the Movement Disorders Society Task Force (MDS-TF) [6]. Information on less used rating scales or those with incomplete validation data is displayed in Table 8.2. This chapter does not review health-related quality-of-life measures, as it is the scope of another chapter in this book, or rating scales aimed at assessing non-motor manifestations.

8.2.1 Ataxias

The most frequently used scales to assess ataxia manifestations are the *International Cooperative Ataxia Rating Scale* (ICARS) [7], the *Friedreich Ataxia Rating Scale* (FARS) [8], and the *scale for the assessment and rating of ataxia* (SARA) [9]. The three scales have demonstrated good psychometric properties and responsiveness [10]. The FARS also includes information about activities of daily living.

8.2.2 Choreas

Several scales have been developed to assess choreas: the *UFMG Sydenham's Chorea Rating Scale* (*USCRS*) [11], the *Shoulson and Fahn Functional Disability Scale for Huntington's Disease* [12], the *Huntington's Disease Activities of Daily Living Scale* (*HD-ADL*) [13], the *Behavior Observation Scale Huntington* (*BOSH*) [14], and the *Unified Huntington's Disease Rating Scale* (*UHDRS*) [15]. There is complete reliability and validity data on the UHDRS, and it has been used as a major outcome measure in clinical trials. It is a complex scale that assesses clinical and functional manifestations of Huntington's disease in four domains: motor function, cognitive function, behavioral abnormalities, and functional capacity. There is a shortened version of the motor section of the UHDRS, which is a teaching videotape [16], and a version for advanced patients (UHDRS-FAP) [17].

8.2.3 Drug-Induced Movement Disorders

The *Simpson-Angus Scale* (*SAS*) [18] and the *Extrapyramidal Symptom Rating Scale* (*ESRS*) [19] are the most frequently used scales for the assessment of drug-induced movement disorders. The SAS is the shortest and among its advantages, it is easy to administer, several studies have assessed its psychometric properties, and there is a cutoff value established for parkinsonism [20]. The ESRS has shown satisfactory inter-rater reliability, convergent validity, and sensitivity to change in antipsychotic-induced movement disorders and idiopathic Parkinson's disease (PD) [20]. The *Abnormal Involuntary Movement Scale (AIMS)* [21] is also used to assess drug-induced dyskinesia in a quick and easy way.

8.2.4 Dyskinesia

The MDS-TF for dyskinesia [22] has recommended the use of the *Abnormal Involuntary Movement Scale (AIMS)* [21] and the *Rush Dyskinesia Rating Scale* [23].

The *AIMS* shows satisfactory psychometric properties and is widely used in clinical trials and research. It contains ten items for assessing the severity of dyskinesia in different parts of the body (face and mouth, limbs, and trunk) and the global severity and the disability due to the abnormal movements. The *Rush Dyskinesia Rating Scale* is aimed at assessing dyskinesia during three standardized motor tasks: walking, drinking from a cup, and dressing. Severity of dyskinesia is rated from 0 (absent) to 4 (violent dyskinesia, incompatible with any normal motor task). Its clinimetric properties, despite some limitations, can be deemed as adequate. The *Unified Dyskinesia Rating Scale* (*UDysRS*) [24], specifically addressed to be used in Parkinson's disease, incorporates the *Rush Dyskinesia Rating Scale*. It will be describe in the paragraph on Parkinson's disease.

Table 8.2 Other scales for movement disorders

Movement disorder	Scale name	Reference
Akathisia	Akathisia Ratings of Movement Scale (ARMS)	Bodfish et al. *Am J Ment Retard.* 1997;101:413–23
	Barnes Akathisia Rating Scale (BARS)	Barnes TR. *Br J Psychiatry.* 1989;154:672–6
Ataxia	Brief Ataxia Rating Scale (BARS)	Schmahmann et al. *Mov Disord.* 2009;24:1820–1828
	Modified ICARS (MICARS)	Schmahmann et al. *Mov Disord.* 2009;24:1820–8
	Cerebellar Ataxia Scale	Klockgether et al. *J Neurol Neurosurg Psychiatry.* 1990;53:297–305
	Nobile-Orazio Ataxia Scale	Nobile-Orazio et al. *Ann Neurol.* 1988;24:93–7
Choreas	Problem Behaviors Assessment for Huntington Disease (PBA-HD)	Craufurd et al. *Neuropsychiatry Neuropsychol Behav Neurol.* 2001;14(4):219–26
Drug-induced movement disorders	St. Hans Rating Scale for extrapyramidal syndromes	Gerlach et al. *Acta Psychiatr Scand.* 1993;87:244–52
	Schedule for the Assessment of Drug-Induced Movement Disorders (SADIMoD)	Loonen et al. *Int J Neuropsychopharmacol.* 2000;3(4):285–96
	Liverpool University Neuroleptic Side-Effect Rating Scale (LUNSERS)	Jung et al. *Hum Psychopharmacol.* 2005 Jan;20(1):41–5
Dystonia	Barry-Albright Dystonia (BAD) Scale	Barry et al. *Dev Med Child Neuro.* 1999;41:404–11
	Blepharospasm Rating Scale (BRS)	Fahn S. In: *Quantification of neurological deficit.* Boston: Butterworths; 1989
	Blepharospasm Disability Scale	Lindeboom et al. *Mov Disord.* 1995;10:444–9
	Cervical Dystonia Severity Scale (CDSS)	O'Brien et al. *Mov Disord.* 2001;16:1086–90
	Spasmodic Torticollis Rating Scale	Tsui et al. *Lancet.* 1986;2:245–7
	Torticollis Rating Scale	Fahn S. In: *Quantification of neurological deficit.* Boston: Butterworths; 1989
	Arm Dystonia Disability Scale (ADDS)	Fahn S. In: *Quantification of neurological deficit.* Boston: Butterworths; 1989
	Writer's Cramp Rating Scale (WCRS)	Wissel et al. *J Neurol Neurosurg Psychiatry.* 1996;61:172–5
	Frequency of Abnormal Movements Scale (FAM Scale)	Spector and Brandfonbrener. *Med Probl Perform Art.* 2005;20:157–62
	Leg Dystonia Disability Scale	Fahn S. In: *Quantification of neurological deficit.* Boston: Butterworths; 1989
	Oromandibular Dystonia Rating Scale	Fahn S. In: Munsat T, ed. *Quantification of neurological deficit.* Boston: Butterworths; 1989
	Unified Dystonia Rating Scale (UDRS)	Comella et al. *Mov Disord.* 2003;18(3):303–12
	Dystonia Discomfort Scale (DDS)	Dressler et al. *Eur J Neurol.* 2014;21(3):459–62
	Comprehensive Cervical Dystonia Rating Scale	Comella et al. *Mov Disord.* 2016;31(4):563–9
Hemifacial spasm	Martí and Tolosa Scale	Martí et al. In: *New trends in clinical neuropharmacology: calcium antagonists, acute neurology, headache and movement disorders.* London: John Libbey & Co.; 1988

Table 8.2 (continued)

Movement disorder	Scale name	Reference
Myoclonus	Opsoclonus-Myoclonus Syndrome Evaluation Scale	Pranzatelli et al. *Clin Neuropharmacol.* 2001;24:352–7
	Myoclonus Evaluation Scale	Chadwick et al. *Brain.* 1977;100:455–87
	Unified Myoclonus Rating Scale (UMRS)	Frucht et al. *Adv Neurol.* 2002;89:361–76
Parkinson's disease	Rapid Assessment of Disability Scale (RADS)	Martinez-Martin et al. *Gac Sanit.* 2005;19 (Suppl 1):68; *J Neurol* 2013;260:228–236
	Short Parkinson's Evaluation Scale (SPES)	Rabey et al. *Clin Neuropharmacol.* 1997;20:322–37
	Columbia University Rating Scale (CURS)	Yahr et al. *Arch Neurol.* 1969;21:343–54
	Intermediate Scale for Assessment of Parkinson's Disease (ISAPD)	Martínez-Martin et al. *Parkinsonism Relat Disord.* 1995;1:97–102
	Rating Scale for Gait Evaluation (RSGE)	Martínez-Martín et al. *Clin Neuropharmacol.* 1997;20:183–94
	Clinical Gait and Balance Scale (GABS)	Thomas et al. *J Neurol Sci.* 2004;217:89–99
	Clinical Dyskinesia Rating Scale (CDRS)	Hagell and Widner. *Mov Disord.* 1999;14:448–55
Restless legs syndrome	RLS-6 Severity Scales	Kohnen et al. *Sleep.* 2003;26:A342
	Augmentation Severity Rating Scale (ASRS)	García-Borregero et al. *Sleep Med.* 2007;8:455–63
Tics and Tourette syndrome	Hopkins Motor and Vocal Tic Scale (HMVTS)	Walkup et al. *J Am Acad Child Adolesc Psychiatry.* 1992;31:472–7
	The Tourette's Disorder Scale (TODS)	Shytle et al. *Assessment.* 2003;10:273–87
	Tourette Syndrome Questionnaire (TSQ)	Jagger et al. *Schizophr Bull.* 1982;8:267–78
	Motor tic, Obsessions and compulsions, Vocal tic Evaluation Survey (MOVES)	Gaffney et al. *J Child Adolesc Psychopharmacol.* 1994;4:269–80
Tremor	Essential Tremor Screening Questionnaire	Lorenz et al. *Mov Disord.* 2008;23:1006–12
	MDS-UPDRS Tremor Scale	Forjaz et al. *Mov Disord.* 2015;30(8):1139–43

8.2.5 Dystonia

The recently published MDS-TF in dystonia [25] has recommended seven scales for the assessment of dystonia: the *Fahn-Marsden Dystonia Rating Scale* (*F-M Scale*) [26], for generalized dystonia; the *Cervical Dystonia Impact Scale* (*CDIP-58*) [27] and the *Toronto Western Spasmodic Torticollis Rating Scale* (*TWSTRS*) [28] for cervical dystonia; the *Blepharospasm Disability Index* (*BSDI*) [29] for blepharospasm; the *Craniocervical Dystonia Questionnaire* (*CDQ-24*) [30] for blepharospasm and cervical dystonia; and the *Voice Handicap Index* (*VHI*) [31] and the *Vocal Performance Questionnaire* (*VPQ*) [32] for laryngeal dystonia.

The *F-M Scale* assesses severity of dystonia and includes a patient-reported questionnaire assessing difficulties in activities of daily living. It is the standard instrument for assessing dystonia in clinical studies [25]. The *CDIP-58* measures the health impact of cervical dystonia, and it has validated using Rasch analysis. The *TWSTRS* is a complex but very widely used scale for assessing cervical dystonia in clinical practice and research. It consists of three subscales evaluating motor severity, disability, and pain, and it shows satisfactory reliability, validity, and responsiveness [25]. The *BSDI* is an easy scale to measure disability in blepharospasm due to dystonic movements that affect vision. It has six items rating the severity of impairment in specific activities, scored for from 0 to 4. The *CDQ-24* measures the impact of craniocervical dystonia on five domains, and it has good psychometric properties. Finally, the *VHI* and the *VPQ* are two similar, short, useful scales addressed to assess the level of disability experienced by patients with different voice disorders.

8.2.6 Parkinsonisms

8.2.6.1 Multiple System Atrophy (MSA) and Progressive Supranuclear Palsy (PSP)

The main tool to assess MSA is the *Unified Multiple System Atrophy Rating Scale* (*UMSARS*) [33]. It is a scale designed by the European MSA-Study Group task force to assess motor and autonomic manifestations and disability in multiple system atrophy. Psychometric properties are adequate and the scale captures disease progression and changes over time. It is owned and licensed by the MDS [34].

The *Neuroprotection and Natural History in Parkinson Plus Syndromes Scale* (*NNIPPS*) [35] is a comprehensive tool for assessing MSA and PSP that can be applied in the early stages. It has 83 items grouped in 15 dimensions assessing activity of daily living/mobility, axial bradykinesia, limb bradykinesia, rigidity, oculomotor, cerebellar, bulbar/pseudo-bulbar, mental, orthostatic, urinary, limb dystonia, axial dystonia, pyramidal, myoclonus, and tremor. It has good internal consistency and inter-rater reliability in total scores and most dimensions. Responsiveness was higher for PSP than for MSA.

8.2.6.2 Parkinson's Disease (PD)

There is a wide range of rating scales specifically addressed to assess PD motor manifestations: multi-domain scales, such as the *Unified Parkinson's Disease Rating Scale* (*UPDRS*) [36] and the *MDS-sponsored version of the UPDRS* (*MDS-UPDRS*) [37]; global severity assessment tools such as the *Hoehn and Yahr staging* (*HY*) [38] and the *Clinical Impression of Severity Index* (*CISI-PD*) [39]; motor manifestations and functional status measures such as the *Scales for Outcomes in Parkinson's Disease* (*SCOPA*)-*Motor* [40] and the *Schwab and England Scale* (*SES*) [41]; and scales to assess motor complications and fluctuations, like the series of *Wearing-off Questionnaires* (*WOQ*) [42–44] and the *Unified Dyskinesia Rating Scale* (*UDysRS*) [24].

The *UPDRS* has been the most widely used scale for assessing Parkinson's disease severity. It is composed by four subscales: mentation, behavior, and mood; activities of daily living (ADL); motor examination; and complications. It also includes the Hoehn and Yahr staging system. The clinimetric properties of the UPDRS have been extensively tested [45], and it is a reference measure for regulatory agencies due to its responsiveness.

The *MDS-UPDRS* is designed to overcome the limitations of the UPDRS and is recommended by the Movement Disorder Society. It maintains the UPDRS structure in four sections: Part I, non-motor experiences of daily living; Part II, motor experiences of daily living; Part III, motor examination; and Part IV, motor complications. Items are scored for severity and presence of symptoms. The MDS-UPDRS has been carefully designed to be applicable to PD patients across all levels of severity and disability, with an adapted vocabulary that avoids medical jargon. Its psychometric properties are satisfactory and it seems to be responsive, and its use in clinical trials is progressively increasing. Translations and certificated rater training are available through the MDS [34].

Among the scales for global severity ratings, the *HY* is the reference system to classify the course of PD. It consists of a 5-point scale that rates the clinical global impression on the functional and clinical status of the patient. A modification with seven stages, included in the UPDRS, is also frequently used. A revision of its clinimetric properties, advantages, and disadvantages has been published [46].

The *CISI-PD* is a global severity index formed by four items: motor signs, disability, cognitive status, and motor complications. The CISI-PD displays satisfactory reliability and validity. However, it lacks information about responsiveness.

The *SCOPA-Motor* is a scale with 21 items developed for assessing motor signs, difficulties in activities of daily living, and motor complications. It shows adequate internal consistency, inter-rater reliability, and construct validity but there is scarce information on test-retest reliability and responsiveness.

The *SES* is a single-item measure that has become a standard measure for assessment of disability in PD. It was included in the UPDRS due to its simplicity, but was not specifically designed for PD patients, and the information on its reliability and validity in this population is still limited. Despite these limitations, it has been commonly used in clinical trials and it shows sensitivity to change due to treatment.

The set of *Wearing-off Questionnaires* were designed as self-completed screening tools for wearing-off. There are four versions, with 9 (WOQ-9), 10 (Q10), 19 (WOQ-19 or *Patient Card Questionnaire* or the *QUICK Questionnaire*), or 32 items (WOQ-32 or *Patient Questionnaire*). WOQ-19 and WOQ-9 are recommended scales by the MDS-TF, whereas the WOQ-32 is suggested for screening of wearing-off in PD [47].

The *UDysRS* is a scale with two sections: historical (on dyskinesia and off dystonia) and objective (impairment and disability). It contains both self-assessed and clinician-based rated questions, possesses good clinimetric properties, and is able to detect treatment effects. Clinically important change has been calculated as 11.1 points in the *UDysRS* Part III for remission of dyskinesia [48]. A standardized training program is also available [49].

8.2.7 Psychogenic Movement Disorders

The *Rating Scale for Psychogenic Movement Disorders* (*PMD Scale*) [50] is the most widely used scale to assess psychogenic movement disorders. It contains 10 types of manifestations (rest tremor, action tremor, dystonia, chorea, bradykinesia, myoclonus, tics, athetosis, ballism, and cerebellar ataxia), 2 functions (gait, speech), and 14 body regions. Some clinimetric properties (inter-rater reliability, construct validity, and responsiveness) have been studied, with satisfactory results.

8.2.8 Restless Legs Syndrome (RLS)

Among the scales available to assess RLS severity, the *Johns Hopkins Restless Legs Syndrome Severity Scale* (*JHRLSS*) [51] was the first to be published. It is a single-item scale that rates the presence, duration, and severity of RLS symptoms and has been validated against objective measures of RLS. A telephone-based interview version has been derived from the *JHRLSS* (*Johns Hopkins telephone diagnostic interview, TDI*) [52], with good clinimetric properties.

The *International Restless Legs Syndrome Study Group* (*IRLS*) *Rating Scale* [53], a ten-item self-administered scale, has become the gold standard to measure severity and impact of RLS in clinical trials [54]. Clinimetric properties have been extensively analyzed, using both CTT and IRT approaches, and they have been found adequate, with a minimal clinically significant change of three points [55–57]. A MDS-TF review on RLS instruments is ongoing.

8.2.9 Tics and Tourette Syndrome

Some of the most used rating scales to assess tics and Tourette syndrome are the *Yale Global Tic Severity Scale* (*YGTSS*) [58], the *Rush Video-Based Tic Rating Scale* [59], and the *Tourette Syndrome Global Scale* (*TSGS*) [60].

The *YGTSS* is a complex scale that rates the clinical global impression on the symptoms. It assesses motor and phonic symptoms severity, complexity, and interference. Satisfactory results in terms of reliability, validity, and responsiveness have been reported [61].

The *Rush Video-Based Tic Rating Scale* is an objective method to assign ratings on five disability categories: number of body areas, frequency of motor tics, frequency of phonic tics, severity of motor tics, and severity of phonic tics. It seems to be responsive to changes and is one of the MDS-owned rating scales for movement disorders [34, 62].

The *TSGS* is a complex multidimensional scale which assesses symptoms and social functioning. It shows several weaknesses (e.g., complexity, failing to assess tic types, lack of full validation studies), but it has been used as a primary outcome variable in clinical trials with good inter-rater reliability.

8.2.10 Tremor

The MDS Task Force on scales for tremor [63] has identified five tremor severity scales that deserve to be listed as "recommended": the *Fahn-Tolosa-Marin Tremor Rating Scale* [64], the *Bain and Findley Clinical Tremor Rating Scale* and the *Bain and Findley Spirography Scale* [65], the *Washington Heights-Inwood Genetic Study of Essential Tremor Rating Scale* (*WHIGET*) [66], and the *Tremor Research Group Essential Tremor Rating Assessment Scale* (*TETRAS*) [67].

The *Fahn-Tolosa-Marin scale* is widely used in research and clinical trials. It includes rater- and patient-based ratings and disability aspects of tremor and shows good overall psychometric properties. The *Bain and Findley scale*, which assesses rest, postural and kinetic tremor severity in the head, voice, and limbs, is also broadly used due to its easiness and good attributes. The *Bain and Findley Spirography Scale* rates the drawing of spirals from 0 to 10. It shows good reliability and face and construct validity, but training of raters is required. The *WHIGET*, made up of 26 items, evaluates severity and persistence of essential tremor in a variety of tasks, distinguishing among rest, kinetic, and postural tremors. However, this scale is limited to the upper extremity essential tremor and requires training and standardization to ensure reliability. Finally, the *TETRAS* includes an activity of daily living subscale with 12 items, rated from 0 to 4, and a performance subscale with nine items, rated from 0 to 4 in half-point intervals. It is a short, easy to apply scale with good reliability and validity.

Conclusions

There is available a wide variety of rating scales for assessment of movement disorders. These instruments are indispensable in clinical practice and research and, therefore, have to be properly designed, validated, and applied. Furthermore, the interpretation of the rating scales-based outcomes should allow extracting consistent conclusions on the real status of the evaluated patients and the importance of changes subsequent to evolutionary changes in the condition or effect of interventions. However, central aspects of the procedures for validation of these measures are, in some way, arbitrary or controversial, and there is no agreement with respect to some apparently elementary concepts (e.g., responsiveness) [5, 68–70].

When there are several rating scales available for the same goal, selection should be guided by the accumulated experience on those scales, the administration and respondent burden, and the quality of the psychometric properties. The recommendations made in systematic reviews, such as those published by the MDS Task Force [6], and experts consensus guidelines [70] should be also taken into account.

Clearly, the field of the rating scales is a dynamic one and demands attention for developing and using appropriately the instruments on which is based a part of the current knowledge related with the course of the diseases, comparison of groups, and outcomes of interventions.

References

1. Acquadro C, Berzon R, Dubois D, Leidy NK, Marquis P, Revicki D, et al. Incorporating the patient's perspective into drug development and communication: an ad hoc task force report of the Patient-Reported Outcomes (PRO) harmonization group meeting at the food and drug administration, February 16, 2001. Value Health. 2003;6(5):522–31.
2. Streiner DL, Norman GR. Health measurement scales. A practical guide to their development and use. 4th ed. Oxford: Oxford University Press; 2008.

3. Nunnally JC, Bernstein IH. Psychometric theory. New York: McGraw Hill; 1994.
4. Scientific Advisory Committee of the Medical Outcomes Trust. Assessing health status and quality-of-life instruments: attributes and review criteria. Qual Life Res. 2002;11(3):193–205.
5. Mokkink LB, Terwee CB, Patrick DL, Alonso J, Stratford PW, Knol DL, et al. The COSMIN checklist for assessing the methodological quality of studies on measurement properties of health status measurement instruments: an international Delphi study. Qual Life Res. 2010;19(4):539–49.
6. Movement Disorders Society. Committee on rating scales development. URL: http://www.movementdisorders.org/MDS/About/Committees--Other-Groups/MDS-Committees/Committee-on-Rating-Scales-Development.htm. Retrieved: 7 Apr 2016.
7. Trouillas P, Takayanagi T, Hallett M, Currier RD, Subramony SH, Wessel K, et al. International cooperative ataxia rating scale for pharmacological assessment of the cerebellar syndrome. The ataxia neuropharmacology committee of the world federation of neurology. J Neurol Sci. 1997;145(2):205–11.
8. Subramony SH, May W, Lynch D, Gomez C, Fischbeck K, Hallett M, et al. Measuring friedreich ataxia: interrater reliability of a neurologic rating scale. Neurology. 2005;64(7):1261–2.
9. Schmitz-Hübsch T, du Montcel ST, Baliko L, Berciano J, Boesch S, Depondt C, et al. Scale for the assessment and rating of ataxia: development of a new clinical scale. Neurology. 2006;66(11):1717–20.
10. Bürk K, Schulz SR, Schulz JB. Monitoring progression in Friedreich ataxia (FRDA): the use of clinical scales. J Neurochem. 2013;126 Suppl 1:118–24.
11. Teixeira Jr AL, Maia DP, Cardoso F. UFMG Sydenham's chorea rating scale (USCRS): reliability and consistency. Mov Disord. 2005;20(5):585–91.
12. Shoulson I, Fahn S. Huntington disease: clinical care and evaluation. Neurology. 1979;29(1):1–3.
13. Bylsma FW, Rothlind J, Hall MR, Folstein SE, Brandt J. Assessment of adaptive functioning in Huntington's disease. Mov Disord. 1993;8(2):183–90.
14. Timman R, Claus H, Slingerland H, van der Schalk M, Demeulenaere S, Roos RAC, et al. Nature and development of Huntington disease in a nursing home population: the Behavior Observation Scale Huntington (BOSH). Cogn Behav Neurol. 2005;18(4):215–22.
15. Unified Huntington's disease rating scale: reliability and consistency. Huntington Study Group. Mov Disord. 1996;11(2):136–42.
16. Siesling S, Zwinderman AH, van Vugt JP, Kieburtz K, Roos RA. A shortened version of the motor section of the unified Huntington's disease rating scale. Mov Disord. 1997;12(2):229–34.
17. Youssov K, Dolbeau G, Maison P, Boissé M-F, de Langavant LC, Roos RAC, et al. The unified huntington's disease rating scale for advanced patients: validation and follow-up study. Mov Disord. 2013;28:1717–23.
18. Simpson GM, Angus JW. A rating scale for extrapyramidal side effects. Acta Psychiatr Scand Suppl. 1970;212:11–9.
19. Chouinard G, Margolese HC. Manual for the extrapyramidal symptom rating scale (ESRS). Schizophr Res. 2005;76(2–3):247–65.
20. Knol W, Keijsers CJPW, Jansen PAF, van Marum RJ. Systematic evaluation of rating scales for drug-induced parkinsonism and recommendations for future research. J Clin Psychopharmacol. 2010;30(1):57–63.
21. Guy W. Abnormal involuntary movement scale. ECDEU assessment manual for psychopharmacology. Washington, DC: US Government Printing Office; 1976. p. 534–7.
22. Colosimo C, Martínez-Martín P, Fabbrini G, Hauser RA, Merello M, Miyasaki J, et al. Task force report on scales to assess dyskinesia in Parkinson's disease: critique and recommendations. Mov Disord. 2010;25(9):1131–42.
23. Goetz CG, Stebbins GT, Shale HM, Lang AE, Chernik DA, Chmura TA, et al. Utility of an objective dyskinesia rating scale for Parkinson's disease: inter- and intrarater reliability assessment. Mov Disord. 1994;9(4):390–4.
24. Goetz CG, Nutt JG, Stebbins GT. The unified dyskinesia rating scale: presentation and clinimetric profile. Mov Disord. 2008;23(16):2398–403.
25. Albanese A, Sorbo FD, Comella C, Jinnah HA, Mink JW, Post B, et al. Dystonia rating scales: critique and recommendations. Mov Disord. 2013;28(7):874–83.
26. Burke RE, Fahn S, Marsden CD, Bressman SB, Moskowitz C, Friedman J. Validity and reliability of a rating scale for the primary torsion dystonias. Neurology. 1985;35(1):73–7.
27. Cano SJ, Warner TT, Linacre JM, Bhatia KP, Thompson AJ, Fitzpatrick R, et al. Capturing the true burden of dystonia on patients: the Cervical Dystonia Impact Profile (CDIP-58). Neurology. 2004;63(9):1629–33.
28. Consky ES, Lang AE. Clinical assessments of patients with cervical dystonia. In: Jankovic J, Hallett M, editors. Therapy with botulinum toxin. New York: Marcel Dekker; 1994. p. 211–37.
29. Jankovic J, Kenney C, Grafe S, Goertelmeyer R, Comes G. Relationship between various clinical outcome assessments in patients with blepharospasm. Mov Disord. 2009;24(3):407–13.
30. Müller J, Wissel J, Kemmler G, Voller B, Bodner T, Schneider A, et al. Craniocervical dystonia questionnaire (CDQ-24): development and validation of a disease-specific quality of life instrument. J Neurol Neurosurg Psychiatry. 2004;75(5):749–53.
31. Jacobson BH, Johnson A, Grywalski C, Silbergleit A, Jacobson G, Benninger MS, et al. The Voice Handicap Index (VHI): development and validation. Am J Speech Lang Pathol. 1997;6(3):66–70.
32. Carding PN, Horsley IA, Docherty GJ. A study of the effectiveness of voice therapy in the treatment of 45 patients with nonorganic dysphonia. J Voice. 1999;13(1):72–104.

33. Wenning GK, Tison F, Seppi K, Sampaio C, Diem A, Yekhlef F, et al. Development and validation of the Unified Multiple System Atrophy Rating Scale (UMSARS). Mov Disord. 2004;19(12):1391–402.
34. Movement Disorders Society. MDS rating scales. URL: http://www.movementdisorders.org/MDS/Education/Rating-Scales.htm. Retrieved: 7 Apr 2016.
35. Payan CAM, Viallet F, Landwehrmeyer BG, Bonnet A-M, Borg M, Durif F, et al. Disease severity and progression in progressive supranuclear palsy and multiplesystematrophy: validation of the NNIPPS–Parkinson plus scale. PLoS One. 2011;6(8):e22293.
36. Fahn S, Elton R. UPDRS program members. Unified Parkinson's disease rating scale. In: Fahn S, Marsden C, Goldstein M, Calne D, editors. Recent developments in Parkinson's disease. Florham Park: Macmillan Healthcare Information; 1987. p. 153–63.
37. Goetz CG, Fahn S, Martinez-Martin P, Poewe W, Sampaio C, Stebbins GT, et al. Movement disorder society-sponsored revision of the unified Parkinson's disease rating scale (MDS-UPDRS): process, format, and clinimetric testing plan. Mov Disord. 2007; 22(1):41–7.
38. Hoehn MM, Yahr MD. Parkinsonism: onset, progression and mortality. Neurology. 1967;17(5):427–42.
39. Martínez-Martín P, Rodríguez-Blázquez C, Forjaz MJ, de Pedro J. The clinical impression of severity index for Parkinson's disease: international validation study. Mov Disord. 2009;24(2):211–7.
40. Marinus J, Visser M, Stiggelbout AM, Rabey JM, Martínez-Martín P, Bonuccelli U, et al. A short scale for the assessment of motor impairments and disabilities in Parkinson's disease: the SPES/SCOPA. J Neurol Neurosurg Psychiatry. 2004;75(3):388–95.
41. Schwab R, England A. Third symposium for Parkinson's disease. Edingburg: Livingstone; 1969. p. 152–7.
42. Stacy M, Hauser R. Development of a patient questionnaire to facilitate recognition of motor and non-motor wearing-off in Parkinson's disease. J Neural Transm. 2007;114(2):211–7.
43. Stacy MA, Murphy JM, Greeley DR, Stewart RM, Murck H, Meng X. The sensitivity and specificity of the 9-item wearing-off questionnaire. Parkinsonism Relat Disord. 2008;14(3):205–12.
44. Martinez-Martin P, Hernandez B. The Q10 questionnaire for detection of wearing-off phenomena in Parkinson's disease. Parkinsonism Relat Disord. 2012;18(4):382–5.
45. The Unified Parkinson's Disease Rating Scale (UPDRS): status and recommendations. Mov Disord. 2003;18(7):738–50.
46. Goetz CG, Poewe W, Rascol O, Sampaio C, Stebbins GT, Counsell C, et al. Movement disorder society task force report on the hoehn and yahr staging scale: status and recommendations. Mov Disord. 2004;19(9):1020–8.
47. Antonini A, Martinez-Martin P, Chaudhuri RK, Merello M, Hauser R, Katzenschlager R, et al. Wearing-off scales in Parkinson's disease: critique and recommendations. Mov Disord J Mov Disord Soc. 2011;26(12):2169–75.
48. Mestre TA, Beaulieu-Boire I, Aquino CC, Phielipp N, Poon YY, Lui JP, et al. What is a clinically important change in the unified dyskinesia rating scale in Parkinson's disease? Parkinsonism Relat Disord. 2015;21(11):1349–54.
49. Goetz CG, Nutt JG, Stebbins GT, Chmura TA. Teaching program for the unified dyskinesia rating scale. Mov Disord. 2009;24(9):1296–8.
50. Hinson VK, Cubo E, Comella CL, Goetz CG, Leurgans S. Rating scale for psychogenic movement disorders: scale development and clinimetric testing. Mov Disord. 2005;20(12):1592–7.
51. Allen RP, Earley CJ. Validation of the Johns Hopkins restless legs severity scale. Sleep Med. 2001;2(3): 239–42.
52. Hening WA, Allen RP, Thanner S, Washburn T, Heckler D, Walters AS, et al. The Johns Hopkins telephone diagnostic interview for the restless legs syndrome: preliminary investigation for validation in a multi-center patient and control population. Sleep Med. 2003;4(2):137–41.
53. Walters AS, LeBrocq C, Dhar A, Hening W, Rosen R, Allen RP, et al. Validation of the international restless legs syndrome study group rating scale for restless legs syndrome. Sleep Med. 2003;4(2):121–32.
54. Kohnen R, Allen RP, Benes H, Garcia-Borreguero D, Hening WA, Stiasny-Kolster K, et al. Assessment of restless legs syndrome – methodological approaches for use in practice and clinical trials. Mov Disord. 2007;22 Suppl 18:S485–94.
55. Wunderlich GR, Evans KR, Sills T, Pollentier S, Reess J, Allen RP, et al. An item response analysis of the international restless legs syndrome study group rating scale for restless legs syndrome. Sleep Med. 2005;6(2):131–9.
56. Abetz L, Arbuckle R, Allen RP, Garcia-Borreguero D, Hening W, Walters AS, et al. The reliability, validity and responsiveness of the international restless legs syndrome study group rating scale and subscales in a clinical-trial setting. Sleep Med. 2006;7(4):340–9.
57. Allen RP. Minimal clinically significant change for the international restless legs syndrome study group rating scale in clinical trials is a score of 3. Sleep Med. 2013;14(11):1229.
58. Leckman JF, Riddle MA, Hardin MT, Ort SI, Swartz KL, Stevenson J, et al. The yale global tic severity scale: initial testing of a clinician-rated scale of tic severity. J Am Acad Child Adolesc Psychiatry. 1989;28(4):566–73.
59. Goetz CG, Pappert EJ, Louis ED, Raman R, Leurgans S. Advantages of a modified scoring method for the rush video-based tic rating scale. Mov Disord. 1999; 14(3):502–6.
60. Harcherik DF, Leckman JF, Detlor J, Cohen DJ. A new instrument for clinical studies of Tourette's syndrome. J Am Acad Child Adolesc Psychiatry. 1984; 23(2):153–60.

61. Jeon S, Walkup JT, Woods DW, Peterson A, Piacentini J, Wilhelm S, et al. Detecting a clinically meaningful change in tic severity in tourette syndrome: a comparison of three methods. Contemp Clin Trials. 2013;36(2):414–20.
62. Smeets AYJM, Duits AA, Plantinga BR, Leentjens AFG, Oosterloo M, Visser-Vandewalle V, et al. Deep brain stimulation of the internal globus pallidus in refractory tourette syndrome. Clin Neurol Neurosurg. 2016;142:54–9.
63. Elble R, Bain P, Forjaz MJ, Haubenberger D, Testa C, Goetz CG, et al. Task force report: scales for screening and evaluating tremor: critique and recommendations. Mov Disord. 2013;28(13):1793–800.
64. Fahn S, Tolosa E, Marín C. Clinical rating scale for tremor. In: Jankovic J, Tolosa E, editors. Parkinson's disease and movement disorders. Baltimore: Williams and Wilkins; 1993. p. 271–80.
65. Bain PG, Findley LJ, Atchison P, Behari M, Vidailhet M, Gresty M, et al. Assessing tremor severity. J Neurol Neurosurg Psychiatry. 1993;56(8):868–73.
66. Louis ED, Ottman R, Ford B, Pullman S, Martinez M, Fahn S, et al. The Washington heights-inwood genetic study of essential tremor: methodologic issues in essential-tremor research. Neuroepidemiology. 1997; 16(3):124–33.
67. Elble R, Comella C, Fahn S, Hallett M, Jankovic J, Juncos JL, et al. Reliability of a new scale for essential tremor. Mov Disord. 2012;27(12):1567–9.
68. Fayers P, Machin D. Quality of life. Chichester: Wiley; 2000. 51 p.
69. Terwee CB, Dekker FW, Wiersinga WM, Prummel MF, Bossuyt PMM. On assessing responsiveness of health-related quality of life instruments: guidelines for instrument evaluation. Qual Life Res. 2003; 12(4):349–62.
70. Mokkink LB, Terwee CB, Knol DL, Stratford PW, Alonso J, Patrick DL, et al. Protocol of the COSMIN study: consensus-based standards for the selection of health measurement instruments. BMC Med Res Methodol. 2006;6:2.

Genetics of Movement Disorders

9

Aloysius Domingo and Christine Klein

9.1 Introduction

It is no exaggeration to state that genetics has revolutionized the field of movement disorders in the past 25 years. Particularly groundbreaking milestones include, but are not limited to: the identification of the Huntingtin gene and of repeat expansion as a mechanism underlying many neurodegenerative diseases, revision of the previously held view that Parkinson's disease is a textbook example of a nonhereditary condition, and – more generally speaking – the finding of literally hundreds of genes that are causative for a broad range of different movement disorders. Although we are still far from a complete understanding of many, if not most, of the disease mechanisms underlying hereditary movement disorders, we have garnered a wealth of novel insights into pathophysiology by studying the respective genes, proteins, and pathways involved. For a few, albeit still rare, examples, molecular genetic studies have resulted in the development of new therapeutic strategies.

The degree of genetic contribution to the etiology of movement disorders is highly variable, ranging from fully penetrant causative mutations to low-penetrant mutations and risk factor alleles. Some disorders, such as Huntington's disease (HD), are by definition genetic and always caused by mutations in genes. Other movement disorders, such as Parkinson's disease or the dystonias, can be caused by mutations but appear largely sporadic in the overwhelming majority of cases (Fig. 9.1). Some other groups of movement disorders are commonly monogenic, such as the spinocerebellar ataxias and the hereditary spastic paraplegias, and have been linked to particularly long and still growing lists of different genes involved, mutations in which cause largely overlapping phenotypes. A detailed description of these latter two groups of movement disorders is beyond the scope of this chapter. For common movement disorders with reported frequencies of up to 10% in the general population, such as restless legs syndrome (RLS) and essential tremor (ET), no clearly causative gene has yet been identified and independently confirmed, despite the presence of numerous large pedigrees following a seemingly dominant mode of inheritance with multiple affected members in successive generations. Overall, there is an inverse relationship between the prevalence of a given movement disorder and the occurrence and identification of monogenic cases.

Other important and at least partially unexpected observations in the context of genetic movement disorders include the phenomenon of

A. Domingo, MD • C. Klein, MD (✉)
Institute of Neurogenetics, University of Luebeck, Maria Goeppert Str. 1, Luebeck 23562, Germany
e-mail: aloysius.domingo@neuro.uni-luebeck.de; christine.klein@neuro.uni-luebeck.de

C. Falup-Pecurariu et al. (eds.), *Movement Disorders Curricula*, DOI 10.1007/978-3-7091-1628-9_9

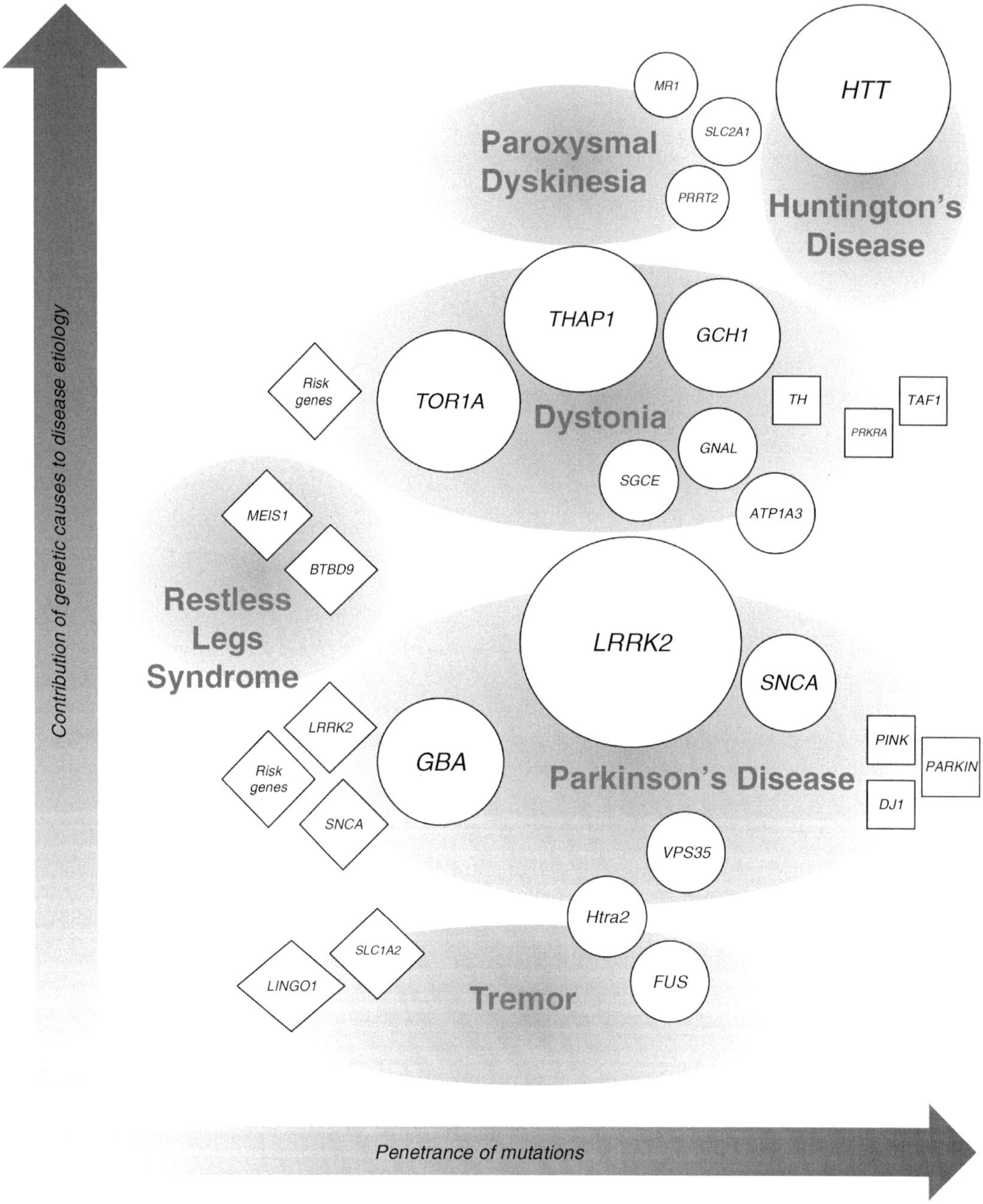

Fig. 9.1 The contribution and effect of genetic causes to the etiology of movement disorders are variable. At one extreme end is Huntington's disease, which is by definition genetic, and in which the causative allele is highly penetrant. At the other extreme are disorders such as essential tremor and restless legs syndrome, where genes discovered so far are mostly risk conferring. In Parkinson's disease and dystonia, both monogenic causes with high and with reduced penetrance, as well as risk-conferring genes, contribute to the etiology. These may overlap in Parkinson's disease (*SNCA*, *LRRK2*). In this figure, *circles* represent dominantly inherited genes, *squares* for recessively inherited genes, and *diamonds* represent risk-conferring genes

reduced penetrance (absence of disease in a mutation carrier which is found in many dominant disorders) and highly variable disease expression. The latter can sometimes be extreme, with the same gene being involved in distinct phenotypes and then referred to as pleiotropy. An illustrative example is mutations in the *ATP1A3* gene, first described to cause rapid-onset dystonia-parkinsonism and now also found as the underlying cause of alternating hemiplegia in childhood and cerebellar ataxia, pes cavus, optic atrophy, sensorineural hearing loss (CAPOS) syndrome.

In the following, we will review the genetics of Parkinson's disease and parkinsonism of dystonia, paroxysmal dyskinesia, HD, ET, and RLS.

9.2 Genetics of Parkinson's Disease and Parkinsonism

9.2.1 Definition and Classification

"Parkinsonism" encompasses the etiologically heterogeneous clinical syndromes that present with bradykinesia, rest tremor, rigidity, and postural instability [1]. The prototype is idiopathic Parkinson's disease (iPD), which is typically late-onset and progressive and has a good response to dopamine replacement therapy. Although largely not inherited in a Mendelian fashion, mutations in single genes may cause iPD, and about 2–3 % are in fact attributable to single genetic events, in syndromes hereafter referred to as "monogenic PD." In early-onset, familial, and ethnic cases, the probability of an underlying genetic cause is higher [2].

Genes that are confirmed to be linked with monogenic PD clinically resembling iPD include *SNCA*, *LRRK2*, *VPS35*, *PARKIN*, *PINK1*, and *DJ1*. The first three cause dominantly inherited or sporadic disease that closely resembles iPD; the recessive genes *PARKIN*, *PINK1*, and *DJ1* meanwhile cause early-onset PD (EOPD) (Table 9.1). "PARK" locus symbols, previously assigned to corresponding chromosomal loci in familial PD cases [3], have now been replaced by the more accurate, less-confusing, and more descriptive gene symbols.

9.2.2 Dominantly Inherited Monogenic PD

9.2.2.1 PARK-*SNCA*: Monogenic PD with Nonmotor Features and Lewy Body Pathology (PARK1/4)

Single nucleotide missense mutations and multiplications in the alpha-synuclein (*SNCA*) gene cause monogenic PD that is generally younger at onset compared to iPD. The decline of levodopa-responsive motor symptoms is also faster, and the development of motor fluctuations is typically earlier. *SNCA* encodes the alpha-synuclein protein, which regulates neurotransmitter release in dopaminergic neurons [4]. The aggregation of the protein in Lewy bodies is considered the pathological hallmark of PD [5], and the misprocessing of alpha-synuclein, either at the level of its amino acid sequence, its expression, post-translational modifications, or degradation, plays a central role in the development of most forms of PD and other degenerative diseases [6].

Table 9.1 Monogenic causes of Parkinson's disease

Designation and clinical subgroup	Additional phenotypic notes	Mode of transmission	Previous locus symbol
Typical PD			
PARK-*SNCA*	More aggressive, prominent nonmotor features	AD	PARK1 and 4
PARK-*LRRK2*	Sporadic, tremor-dominant PD	AD	PARK8
PARK-*VPS35*	May be sporadic, late-onset PD	AD	PARK17
PARK-*GBA*	Highly reduced penetrance	AD	None
Early-onset PD			
PARK-*PARKIN*	EOPD with dystonia as initial sign	AR	PARK2
PARK-*PINK1*	EOPD with nonmotor features	AR	PARK6
PARK-*DJ1*	Rare cause of EOPD	AR	PARK7

The first missense mutation described in *SNCA* codes for an A53T change [7]; it has since been found in many other families of European and Asian origin. Other substitutions have also been described, mostly in single families [8]. In general, however, missense mutations are rare in all populations and comprise only a small fraction of PARK-*SNCA* [9]. Locus multiplications (duplications, triplications) are more frequent and have been described in more ethnicities, as well as in other neurodegenerative diseases aside from PD. The first description of a triplication in fact was in a large family with autosomal dominant parkinsonism with prominent dementia [10]. Interestingly, patients carrying duplications manifest disease that is more similar to iPD, while triplication carriers typically suffer from a more aggressive phenotype. For example, debilitating nonmotor features tend to be invariably present in triplication carriers, and dementia manifests earlier compared to cases with duplication [8].

9.2.2.2 PARK-*LRRK2*: Sporadic, Tremor-Dominant PD (PARK8)

LRRK2 (leucine-rich repeat kinase 2) is the most frequently mutated gene in iPD. The most common mutation, G2019S, represents 4 % of familial and 1 % of sporadic PD across all populations; in North African Arabs, the discovery rate can be as high as 39 % of all cases [11]. Thus, PARK-*LRRK2* is the most important differential diagnosis when considering genetic PD, given also that the phenotype is often indistinguishable from nongenetic disease. The motor symptoms in PARK-*LRRK2* tend to be tremor-dominant at onset, and cognitive impairment and anosmia also appear to occur less frequently [11, 12].

LRRK2 is a large gene and as many as 80 different genetic variants appear in one database [9]. Unequivocally pathogenic substitutions are all rare and found only in a few families, with the exception of the G2019S mutation, which has been described in Europeans [13, 14], in North African Arabs, and in Ashkenazi Jews [15]. It is rarely observed in East Asia [16]. Furthermore, the expression of disease in G2019S mutation carriers is characterized by reduced penetrance [17] and varies according to country of origin [18], indicating that ancestral background contributes to *LRRK2* disease. Another G2385R missense change, for example, is associated with iPD but only in the Asian population [19].

9.2.2.3 PARK-*VPS35* (PARK17): Late-Onset Dominantly Inherited PD

The D620N substitution in *VPS35* (vacuolar protein sorting 35) was the first PD-causing variant identified via next-generation sequencing [20, 21]. A large multicenter study involving 15,000 individuals worldwide later estimated that PARK-*VPS35* represents 0.4 % of PD cases [22]. PARK-*VPS35* is dominantly inherited with reduced penetrance and has a phenotype that is very similar to iPD [23]. The protein is a component of the retromer complex and participates in retrograde trafficking pathways; a mutation that disrupts the interaction of VPS35 protein with others in the complex perturbs the recruitment of the retromer [24].

9.2.2.4 Recently Identified Genes That May Underlie Dominantly Inherited PD

Interestingly, mutations in the DnaJ homolog subfamily C member 13 gene (*DNAJC13*) – which also participates in the retromer complex – were recently identified in one Mennonite family with dominantly inherited PD and in two sporadic cases [25]. The gene *CHCHD2* (coiled-coil-helix—coiled-coil-helix domain-containing 2) has also been recently identified as a cause of dominantly inherited, late-onset PD [26]. Mutations in the gene either segregate with PD in pedigrees or have been found to be more frequent in PD than controls in association studies or databases.

9.2.3 Early-Onset, Recessively Inherited Monogenic PD

9.2.3.1 PARK-*PARKIN*: EOPD with Dystonia (PARK2)

PARKIN mutation carriers have an earlier age at onset but less aggressive disease compared to iPD [6]. It is the most common form of EOPD across all ethnic groups, representing about 10–20 % of cases of PD with age at onset within the fourth decade. Dystonia is a common-presenting sign in PARK-*PARKIN* and may even sometimes be seen as an isolated finding [27, 28]. On the other hand, dementia is almost always absent despite long disease duration [28, 29].

There are 183 different mutations in *PARKIN* in the literature according to one review, occurring in homozygous or compound heterozygous forms – with two-thirds carrying a copy number variation [28]. Most mutations are found in exons 1–3, which code for a critical ubiquitin-like domain [17]. The Parkin protein is an E3 ubiquitin ligase that participates in the process of ubiquitination, with target proteins that are involved in mitochondrial fission and fusion and mitophagy [30, 31].

9.2.3.2 PARK-*PINK1*: EOPD with Nonmotor Features (PARK6)

Mutations in phosphatase and tensin homolog-induced kinase 1 (*PINK1*) were first identified in three EOPD families with homozygous mutations [32]. Subsequently, PARK-*PINK1* was identified in more families and even late-onset sporadic cases [33] – in homozygous and compound heterozygous states – and it now represents 1–9 % of all genetic PD across all ethnicities [34]. The usual phenotype is indistinguishable from PARK-*PARKIN*, only with a higher rate of psychiatric symptoms and cognitive impairment [35]. Point mutations represent most mutations, the most common being a truncation at Q456 in exon 7 [17].

PINK1 protein and Parkin protein together participate in the regulation of mitophagy [36]. Under physiologic conditions, PINK1 localizes to the damaged mitochondria and recruits Parkin, initiating mitophagy. *PARKIN* mutants, however, show impaired ubiquitination, allowing the accumulation of the dysfunctional mitochondria [37] and resulting in decreased ATP production and abnormal mitochondrial morphology [38].

9.2.3.3 PARK-*DJ-1*: Recessively Inherited EOPD (PARK7)

DJ-1 was first identified using homozygosity mapping as the cause of PD in two consanguineous families from genetically isolated communities in the Netherlands and Italy [39]. PARK-*DJ-1* is significantly less common than either PARK-*PARKIN* or PARK-*PINK1* and accounts for only 1–2 % of cases [34]. Clinical and neuroimaging features are similar to the other two recessive PD syndromes. The DJ-1 protein acts as a sensor for oxidative stress and is thought to have protective properties in the cell; loss of function disables mutants from translocating to the mitochondria in response to oxidation, reducing its protective function [40].

9.2.4 Genes Implicated in Association Studies and PARK-*GBA*

Association studies and subsequent meta-analyses have recently been used to identify variations that confer a risk for iPD beyond monogenic cases. Although the risk is significantly lower compared to mutations causative for monogenic PD, there is an overlap in genes identified by genome-wide association studies (GWAS) and the monogenic syndromes. For example, some of the strongest and most consistent associations have been for variants in *SNCA* and *LRRK2* [41].

Of particular note are the consistently strong associations in GWAS for variants in the glucocerebrosidase (*GBA*) gene. Homozygous mutations in *GBA* cause Gaucher disease; heterozygous mutations meanwhile have been found to be significantly more frequent in iPD in Europeans [42], as well as in Ashkenazi Jews [43]. *GBA* mutations are also consistently more common in individuals with a family history of PD compared to sporadic cases, and there is an age-specific risk that increases from age 60 to 80 years for those carrying heterozygous mutations [44]. Thus, heterozygous *GBA* mutations may actually represent dominantly inherited PD with significantly reduced penetrance than merely a risk-conferring allele.

Table 9.2 Selected monogenic causes of atypical parkinsonism

Designation and clinical subgroup	Additional phenotypic notes	Mode of transmission	Previous locus symbol
Kufor-Rakeb syndrome, PARK-*ATP13A2*	Juvenile parkinsonism with supranuclear gaze palsy, brain iron accumulation	AR	PARK9
Parkinsonian-pyramidal syndrome, PARK-*FBXO7*	Juvenile parkinsonism with pyramidal signs	AR	PARK15
EOPD with atypical features, PARK-*DNAJC6*	Also with mental retardation and seizures	AR	PARK19
EOPD with atypical features, PARK-*SYNJ1*	With seizures, cognitive decline, dystonia	AR	PARK20

9.2.5 Atypical Parkinsonism

Despite overlapping with iPD in clinical presentation, neuropathology, and disease mechanism, the atypical parkinsonisms are considered clinically and genetically distinct from iPD (Table 9.2) [34]. Clinically, these forms present with nonclassical motor and nonmotor features and are rarely dopamine sensitive [45]; hence, they should not be confused with genetic forms of iPD despite the PARK symbols assigned to them. Genes associated with the atypical and juvenile parkinsonism syndromes are recessively inherited.

9.3 Genetics of Dystonia

9.3.1 Definition and Classification

While Hermann Oppenheim probably described the first cases of genetic dystonia in 1911 (i.e., DYT1) and coined the term "dystonia musculorum deformans" [46, 47], the modern history of dystonia genetics dates back to 1994 when mutations in the *GCH1* (GTP cyclohydrolase I) gene were discovered as the cause of dopa-responsive dystonia (DRD).

Dystonia is clinically defined as a movement disorder characterized by sustained or intermittent muscle contractions causing abnormal, often repetitive movements, postures, or both. Dystonic movements are typically patterned and twisting and may be tremulous. Dystonia is often initiated or worsened by voluntary action and associated with overflow muscle activation [48]. Dystonias can be classified phenomenologically by age of onset (infancy, childhood, adolescence, early and late adulthood), body distribution (focal, segmental, multifocal, and generalized), temporal pattern (static or progressive disease course; persistent, action-specific, diurnal, or paroxysmal presentation), and association with additional features (isolated or combined with other movement disorders [48, 49]. Formerly, isolated dystonia was referred to as "primary dystonia," combined dystonia (e.g., with parkinsonism or myoclonus) as "dystonia-plus," and complex dystonia – where dystonia is usually an inconsistent feature and only one of several disease manifestations – as "secondary dystonia." Although collectively the complex dystonias account for a large number of cases, it is beyond the scope of this chapter to discuss this highly heterogeneous group of disorders, which are reviewed elsewhere [50].

Genetic features used for classification comprise mode of transmission and molecular genetic data, such as linkage to a known gene locus or identification of a specific genetic defect. As in PD, this list of currently 25 "DYTs" represents an assortment of clinically and genetically heterogeneous disorders and includes erroneous assignments. Confirmed genes for isolated dystonias are *TOR1A*, *THAP1*, and *GNAL*. In the combined forms, dystonia is accompanied by parkinsonism (*GCH1*, *TH*, *ATP1A3*, *PRKRA*, *TAF1*) or myoclonus (*SGCE*) (Table 9.3).

Table 9.3 Confirmed monogenic causes of dystonia

Designation and clinical subgroup	Additional phenotypic notes	Mode of transmission	Previous locus symbol
Isolated dystonias			
DYT-*TOR1A*	Early-onset generalized dystonia	AD	DYT1
DYT-*THAP1*	Adolescent-onset dystonia of mixed type	AD	DYT6
DYT-*GNAL*	Adult-onset cranial-cervical dystonia	AD	DYT25
Combined dystonias			
Dystonia plus parkinsonism			
DYT-*GCH1*	Dopa-responsive dystonia	AD	DYT5a
DYT-*TH*	Dopa-responsive dystonia	AR	DYT5b
DYT-*ATP1A3*	Rapid-onset dystonia-parkinsonism	AD	DYT12
DYT-*PRKRA*	Dystonia-parkinsonism	AR	DYT16
DYT-*TAF1*[a]	Dystonia-parkinsonism	X-linked	DYT3
Dystonia plus myoclonus			
DYT-*SGCE*	Myoclonus-dystonia	AD	DYT11

[a]Due to a founder effect, genetic testing is possible. The pathogenicity of the *TAF1* gene is, however, not absolutely confirmed

9.3.2 Monogenic Isolated Dystonia

9.3.2.1 DYT-*TOR1A*: Early-Onset Generalized Dystonia; Oppenheim Dystonia (DYT1)

The mean age of onset is at 13 years with twisting of an arm or leg, and progression to involve other limbs and the torso, but usually sparing the face and neck [51]. Almost all cases are caused by the same three-base pair deletion (GAG) in the coding region of the torsin (*TOR1A*) gene that accounts for about 60% of cases with generalized dystonia in the non-Jewish population and about 90% of patients of Ashkenazi Jewish origin due to a founder effect [52]. DYT-*TOR1A* is inherited in an autosomal dominant fashion with reduced penetrance (30%) and variable expressivity with respect to age and site of onset and progression. If symptoms do not occur prior to 28 years of age in mutation carriers, they usually remain unaffected for the rest of their life.

9.3.2.2 DYT-*THAP1*: Adolescent-Onset Dystonia with Mixed Phenotype (DYT6)

THAP1-associated dystonia combines features of focal and generalized primary dystonia and is also inherited in an autosomal dominant manner with penetrance estimated at 40%. The onset is later (mean 19 years) than in *TOR1A*-associated dystonia, and there is more prominent cranial involvement with dysphonia being a predominant feature. Mutations in the THAP domain-containing, apoptosis-associated protein 1 (*THAP1*) gene underlie this form of dystonia [53]. *THAP1* shows significant mutational heterogeneity with currently over 60 different missense, and truncating *THAP1* mutations reported mainly in European but also in patients of other ethnicities [54].

9.3.2.3 DYT-*GNAL*: Adult-Onset Segmental Dystonia (DYT25)

Mutations in the Guanine nucleotide-binding protein (G protein), alpha-activating activity polypeptide, and olfactory type (*GNAL*) gene cause cervical or cranial dystonia with onset most commonly in the third decade of life [55]. Although additional studies in larger samples are needed, *GNAL* mutations probably account for about 1% of all cases of focal or segmental dystonia involving the craniocervical region [56], making *GNAL* the first-known gene that explains a (small) subset of cases with the most common form of isolated dystonia.

9.3.2.4 Recently Identified Genes That May Underlie Isolated Dystonia

Four genes have recently been implicated in adult-onset segmental (mostly craniocervical) dystonia, namely, *CIZ1* [57], *ANO3* [58], *HPCA* [59], and *COL6A3* [60]. Importantly, mutations in all four were detected only very recently and via next-generation sequencing approaches and all still await independent confirmation in other studies. The *TUBB4* gene [61, 62] likewise awaits confirmation in conjunction with dystonia; mutations in the gene have otherwise been found to underlie hypomyelination and atrophy of the basal ganglia and cerebellum (H-ABC) [63].

9.3.3 Monogenic Combined Dystonias

9.3.3.1 DYT-*GCH1* and DYT-*TH*: Dopa-Responsive Dystonia; Segawa Syndrome (DYT5a and DYT5b)

Dopa-responsive dystonia (DRD) is characterized by a childhood onset of dystonia, a diurnal fluctuation of symptoms, and a dramatic response to L-dopa therapy [64]. Later in the course of the disease, parkinsonian features may occur and may, in rare cases, be the only sign of the condition [65]. While rare autosomal recessive forms of DRD are mostly associated with mutations in the tyrosine hydroxylase (*TH*) gene, the more frequent form of DRD (DYT5a) is caused by dominant mutations in the GTP cyclohydrolase 1 (*GCH1*) gene. Penetrance is lower among men than women. Although the disorder is exquisitely treatable and long known, there is still considerable diagnostic delay of about 13 years. Many mutation carriers display some residual (dystonic and/or Parkinsonian) features. In addition, non-motor features (sleep disturbances, mood disorders, migraine) are reported in a considerable subset of patients [66].

9.3.3.2 DYT-*ATP1A3*: Rapid-Onset Dystonia-Parkinsonism (DYT12)

ATP1A3-associated dystonia has a sudden onset within hours to weeks, typically in adolescence or young adulthood, in response to physical or mental stress. It is inherited in an autosomal dominant fashion with reduced penetrance. Typical features include dystonic spasms predominantly in the upper limbs, orofacial dystonia, dysarthria, and dysphagia, along with symptoms of parkinsonism. Several different missense mutations, including de novo mutations, were identified in the *ATP1A3* gene encoding Na^+/K^+ ATPase alpha 3 [67]. As mentioned above, the spectrum of phenotypes associated with mutations in *ATP1A3* has been expanded to include alternating hemiplegia of childhood [68] and CAPOS syndrome [69].

9.3.3.3 DYT-*PRKRA*: Dystonia-Parkinsonism (DYT16)

PRKRA-linked dystonia-parkinsonism is a rare, recessively inherited form of early-onset generalized dystonia, which is accompanied by parkinsonism and caused by mutations in the *PRKRA* gene [70]. Initially only described in patients of Brazilian descent, a homozygous mutation was recently also found in a Polish family with a similar clinical presentation of combined dystonia and mild parkinsonism [71]. The possible role of heterozygous mutations in this gene as a risk factor for dystonia currently remains a matter of debate [72].

9.3.3.4 DYT-*TAF1*: Dystonia-Parkinsonism, Lubag Disease (DYT3)

X-linked dystonia-parkinsonism (XDP) is endemic to the Philippines and inherited in an X-linked recessive fashion [73]. Patients present in adulthood with dystonia, most pronounced in the craniofacial region. The dystonia subsequently generalizes and patients develop parkinsonian features, which predominate in late disease stages. XDP is the only condition among the isolated and combined dystonias with overt neurodegeneration of the striatum. The underlying genetic cause has not yet been unequivocally identified [74]; however, patients of Filipino origin can be tested for this condition based on a founder haplotype. Furthermore, there is at least evidence that the

TAF1 gene is dysregulated in pathologic and cellular models of the disease [75, 76].

9.3.3.5 DYT-*SGCE*: Myoclonus-Dystonia (DYT11)

Myoclonus-dystonia (M-D) is characterized by a combination of myoclonus and dystonia with onset usually in childhood or early adolescence. In most affected individuals, myoclonic jerks are dramatically but transiently ameliorated by intake of alcohol. Approximately half of the affected individuals have cervical dystonia and/or writer's cramp. The disease is inherited as an autosomal dominant trait with reduced penetrance and caused by loss-of-function mutations in the Epsilon-sarcoglycan (*SGCE*) gene [77]. Reduced penetrance upon maternal transmission of the disease allele is caused by maternal genomic imprinting of the *SGCE* gene [78]. Interestingly, large deletions of the entire *SGCE* gene are frequently accompanied by a deletion of the neighboring gene(s) and may thus have associated, albeit seemingly unrelated phenotypes such as delayed skeletal development and severe osteoporosis. *CACNA1B* mutations have been linked to an M-D syndrome with cardiac arrhythmias [79] but have not yet been independently confirmed, as with a mutation in the *KCTD17* gene, which has been reported to underlie M-D with prominent dystonia [80].

9.3.4 Genetic Risk Factors for Dystonia

Dystonia has a high heritability and it is tempting to speculate that yet undescribed genetic factors contribute to the disease in at least a subset of cases. Numerous and overall small candidate association studies have investigated a possible association with variants in known dystonia-linked genes (e.g., *TOR1A*) or plausible candidates (e.g., dopamine receptor genes) and have led to inconclusive results. The only unequivocally confirmed association is of protective nature and was found in carriers of the *TOR1A* GAG deletion. If mutation carriers harbor the D2016H polymorphism of *TOR1A* in trans with the GAG deletion (i.e., on the other allele), penetrance of dystonia is reduced to about 3 % [81, 82]. More recently, two small GWAS have been performed in patients with cervical dystonia [83] and musician's dystonia [84], identifying possible associations with a sodium leak channel (*NALCN*) and *Arylsulfatase G*, respectively. A recent replication study in cervical dystonia patients was, however, unable to confirm the *NALCN* association in a Spanish dystonia and control population [85], indicating the need for more highly powered, multiethnic association studies in dystonia.

9.4 Genetics of Paroxysmal Dyskinesia

The paroxysmal dyskinesias present with a mixed pattern of hyperkinetic movement disorders and have previously been grouped under the inherited dystonias (*PRRT2*/DYT10, *MR-1*/DYT8, *SLC2A1*/DYT18) (Table 9.4). While dystonia is indeed a common feature of paroxysmal dyskinesia, other hyperkinetic involuntary movements, such as chorea, athetosis or ballism, are often equally present and may even predominate. All of the paroxysmal dyskinesias are elicited by specific triggers.

9.4.1 DYT-*PRRT2*: Paroxysmal Kinesigenic Dyskinesia (DYT10)

Paroxysmal kinesigenic dyskinesia (PKD) usually starts in childhood or adolescence and is triggered by sudden movements. Attacks typically last only seconds or minutes and may appear up to 100 times per day. They mostly consist of dystonic and choreoathetotic movements, which are highly responsive to small doses of antiepileptics, such as carbamazepine. PKD has been clinically and genetically linked to a variety of related conditions, most importantly benign familial infantile seizures (BFIS), which may co-occur in the same patient or present as isolated features [86]. Missense and truncating mutations

Table 9.4 Monogenic causes of paroxysmal dyskinesias

Designation and clinical subgroup	Additional phenotypic notes	Mode of transmission	Previous locus symbol
DYT-*PRRT2*	Paroxysmal kinesigenic dyskinesia	AD	DYT10
DYT-*MR1*	Paroxysmal nonkinesigenic dyskinesia	AD	DYT8
DYT-*SLC2A1*	Paroxysmal exertion-induced dyskinesia	AD	DYT18

in the proline-rich transmembrane protein 2 (*PRRT2*) gene were identified as the cause of PKD [87].

9.4.2 DYT-*MR1*: Paroxysmal Nonkinesigenic Dyskinesia (DYT8)

Attacks of paroxysmal nonkinesigenic dyskinesia (PNKD) can be precipitated by alcohol, caffeine, stress, hunger, fatigue, and tobacco. They usually consist of a combination of dystonia, chorea, athetosis or ballism, last from minutes to hours, and in severe cases may occur several times per day. Two missense mutations (A7V and A9V) in the Myofibrillogenesis regulator 1 (*MR-1*) gene are the cause of the disease [88].

9.4.3 DYT-*SLC2A1*: Paroxysmal Exertion-Induced Dyskinesia (DYT18)

The *SLC2A1* gene, previously linked to GLUT1 (i.e., the glucose transporter of the blood-brain barrier) deficiency syndrome, was identified to also cause paroxysmal exertion-induced dyskinesia [89, 90]. Attacks consist of chorea, athetosis, and dystonia in excessively exercised body regions with the legs being most frequently affected. A single attack lasts from a few minutes to an hour and occurs after prolonged physical exercise. Several patients have other disease manifestations, such as epilepsy, hemolytic anemia, and migraine. A ketogenic diet is an effective therapeutic option.

9.5 Genetics of Huntington's Disease

The diagnosis of HD is established clinically by involuntary chorea, behavioral and psychiatric disturbances, and dementia. The disease is confirmed genetically by family history consistent with autosomal dominant inheritance and the finding of unstable CAG repeats in the Huntingtin (*HTT*) gene [91]. So far, *HTT* is the only gene known to cause the disease. The c.52CAG (<26) allele (i.e., less than 26 trinucleotide repeats) is classified as benign, 27–35 CAG repeats are termed intermediate, while the c.52CAG (36_39) allele is considered HD causing but with reduced penetrance. An individual carrying more than 40 repeats will almost certainly manifest with HD symptoms [92].

Intermediate alleles are not considered disease causing but have the potential to expand within one generation, and thus children of carriers of 27–35 CAG repeats risk having trinucleotide repeats at the >36 range and developing HD [93]. Recent studies however detect behavioral manifestations in carriers of intermediate alleles, although motor performance and cognition in these individuals were similar to controls. It is unknown whether the symptoms thus represent a prodromal stage of HD or a distinct phenotype caused by carrying 27–35 CAG repeats [94].

The molecular effects of mutant huntingtin protein seem to be manifold, and multiple cellular processes have been shown in studies to be deranged in HD, including the expression of brain-derived neurotrophic factor, transcription of protein kinases in striatal neurons, mitochondrial respiration, N-methyl-D-aspartate (NMDA) receptor activation, the ubiquitin-proteasome and autophagy-lysosome clearance systems, and post-translational modification (reviewed in [95, 96]).

9.6 Genetics of Essential Tremor

ET is a hyperkinetic movement disorder characterized by action tremor in the upper limbs, especially the hands, and less frequently, of the head, tongue, trunk, or lower extremities. The etiology of ET is multifactorial, and advanced age appears to confer the most significant risk. However, as with other movement disorders, the existence of early-onset and familial cases exemplifies the contribution of genetic factors to the disease mechanism [97].

9.6.1 Familial ET Loci Identified by Linkage Studies

The ETM1 locus in 13q13 was first identified via linkage analyses at 16 families from Iceland [98], with a later study identifying an S9G variant in the Dopamine D3 receptor (*DRD3*) gene locus to be associated with the phenotype in French individuals with familial ET [99]. A recent meta-analysis of replication studies, however, failed to reach significance when the association between the allele and ET was tested and concluded that *DRD3* is likely not causative for monogenic ET nor does the S9G variant represent a major genetic risk factor [100].

The ETM2 locus in 2p24 meanwhile was initially mapped in a Czech/American family, with the putative causative variant (A265G) in the hematopoietic lineage cell-specific protein-binding protein 3 (*HS1BP3*) gene segregating in two other families with ET [101]. This and the ET3 locus in chromosome 6 have yet to be confirmed in more cases and replication studies.

9.6.2 Genes Identified via Next-Generation Sequencing

The fused in sarcoma (*FUS*) gene, which is also linked to amyotrophic lateral sclerosis (ALS) and atypical parkinsonism, was the first gene to be found to cause ET using exome sequencing. A stop mutation (Q290X) in *FUS* segregated in the original family; further screening in familial and sporadic ET cases identified two additional rare mutations [102]. Importantly, other studies and data from aggregation servers indicate that rare variants in the gene may be as common in control individuals [103], calling the pathogenicity of the gene into question.

In a consanguineous Turkish family with both ET and PD, exome sequencing identified heterozygous and homozygous G399S mutations in the Htra serine peptidase 2 (*Htra2*) gene to be causative for both phenotypes [104], possibly further substantiating previous studies asserting relationships between monogenic ET and PD. Interestingly, the same allele in the heterozygous state and other polymorphisms in *Htra2* have already been previously associated with PD and the PARK13 locus [105], although a later meta-analysis failed to detect a strong association between PD and the common variants in the gene [106].

9.6.3 Genes Implicated by Association Studies and Their Meta-analyses

Two genes have been associated to genetically complex ET via GWAS: *LINGO1* (leucine-rich repeat and immunoglobulin domain-containing 1) and *SLC1A2* (solute-carrier family 1 member 2) [107, 108]. Although discovered polymorphisms in both achieve genome-wide significance in some analyses, further replication studies reveal heterogeneous results. A recent meta-analysis considers both to be possible susceptibility genes for ET, while also noting that accurate phenotyping and case description may confound statistical results, especially as tremor may be a component of other movement disorders [100].

9.7 Genetics of Restless Legs Syndrome

RLS is clinically diagnosed using four main criteria: urge to move the legs, induction or exacerbation of the movement disorder at rest, relief of symptoms with activity, and worsening at night or during sleep [109]. The disease is characterized by high familial aggregation, thus suggesting a genetic component to its etiology [110]. Association studies implicate susceptibility loci in *BTBD9* and *MEIS1*, which are both involved in iron metabolism and availability [111], with variants in both 5′ and 3′ untranslated regions of *MEIS1* (Meis homeobox 1) carrying the strongest association and functional signals [112]. So far, no monogenic causes have been identified.

9.8 Genetic Testing in Movement Disorders

We have attempted to simplify the genetic causes of PD, dystonia, and other movement disorders in this chapter; however, it is nonetheless obvious that the nuances of heritable neurologic disorders are complex. Thus, consultation with a geneticist is recommended prior to embarking on "gene hunting" for a suspected case. The decision to undergo genetic testing involves many different factors, including the indication for the test, the implication of the results based on the stage of disease, the feasibility, the sensitivity-specificity, the accuracy of the test, and the general lack of neuroprotection in PD and other movement disorders, among others [34]. Furthermore, several cases of false-positive findings exist in the literature – a phenomenon that has been increasing in this age of next-generation sequencing [113] – so that a careful assessment of the diagnostic value of any variant discovered by genetic testing cannot be overemphasized. Detecting HD-causing CAG repeats in clinically compatible HD is probably an exemption to this cautious rule, given that *HTT* is the only gene so far linked with HD, and the CAG repeats are the only pathologic variant associated with the disease.

At least for PD, dystonia, and Huntington's disease, guidelines on molecular diagnosis and clinical genetic testing have been established by the European Federation of Neurological Societies (EFNS) [114]. In PD, the guidelines recommend testing for *LRRK2* in familial cases with dominantly inherited PD and for *PARKIN*, *PINK1*, and *DJ-1* in EOPD and in those suggestive of recessive inheritance, emphasizing the role of history-taking and careful assessment of the family history and inheritance pattern prior to the genetic test. In dystonia, genetic testing for the GAG deletion in *TOR1A* and for *GCH1* and *SGCE* in clinically compatible cases is recommended. On the other hand, the guidelines clearly indicate that *no* genetic test can currently be recommended for the more common (adult-onset) focal dystonias and for individual diagnosis of essential tremor and restless legs syndrome, given that most genetic variants discovered for these disorders are either risk-conferring but not necessarily disease causing or are pending independent confirmation. Findings of recent studies identifying causative genes using next-generation sequencing would still have to be replicated in many studies and using different populations, and the frequency of mutations occurring in patients (and controls) would first have to established, before any sort of recommendation on these genes can be advocated.

Lastly, while genetic etiologies are likely only rare causes of movement disorders such as PD and dystonia, gene panel testing via next-generation sequencing technology has recently become available as an option that allows for accurate and final diagnosis in patients facing a long and expensive "diagnostic odyssey" [115]. As the technology transitions from research laboratories into the clinical and diagnostic setting – "from bench to bedside" – we expect more usage of neurogenetic requests and reports, clinical and diagnostic practice guidelines, variant databases and knowledge bases in genetically determined movement disorders.

Acknowledgments CK is supported by a career development award from the Hermann and Lilly Schilling Foundation, and AD is the recipient of a scholarship from the German Academic Exchange Service (DAAD).

References

1. Williams DR, Litvan I. Parkinsonian syndromes. Continuum. 2013;19(5, Movement Disorders): 1189–212.
2. Alcalay RN, Caccappolo E, Mejia-Santanaet H, et al. Frequency of known mutations in early-onset Parkinson disease: implication for genetic counseling. Arch Neurol. 2010;67(9):1116–22.

3. Marras C, Lang A, Lohmann K, et al. Fixing the broken system of genetic locus symbols: Parkinson disease and dystonia as examples. Neurology. 2012;78(13):1016–24.
4. Norris EH, Giasson BI, Lee VMY. α-Synuclein: normal function and role in neurodegenerative diseases. In: Schatten GP, editor. Current topics in developmental biology, vol 60, Stem cells in development and disease. Academic; 2004. p. 17–54. doi:10.1016/S0070-2153(04)60002-0.
5. Spillantini MG, Schmidt ML, Lee VM. [alpha]-Synuclein in Lewy bodies. Nature. 1997;388(6645):839–40.
6. Klein C, Schlossmacher MG. Parkinson disease, 10 years after its genetic revolution: multiple clues to a complex disorder. Neurology. 2007;69(22):2093–104.
7. Polymeropoulos MH, Lavedan C, Leroy E, et al. Mutation in the α-synuclein gene identified in families with Parkinson's disease. Science. 1997;276(5321):2045–7.
8. Kasten M, Klein C. The many faces of alpha-synuclein mutations. Mov Disord. 2013;28(6):697–701.
9. Nuytemans K, Theuns S, Cruts M, et al. Genetic etiology of Parkinson disease associated with mutations in the SNCA, PARK2, PINK1, PARK7, and LRRK2 genes: a mutation update. Hum Mutat. 2010;31(7):763–80.
10. Singleton AB, Farrer M, Johnson J, et al. α-Synuclein locus triplication causes Parkinson's disease. Science. 2003;302(5646):841.
11. Healy DG, Falchi M, O'Sullivan SS, et al. Phenotype, genotype, and worldwide genetic penetrance of LRRK2-associated Parkinson's disease: a case-control study. Lancet Neurol. 2008;7(7):583–90.
12. Saunders-Pullman R, Stanley K, Wang C, et al. Olfactory dysfunction in LRRK2 G2019S mutation carriers. Neurology. 2011;77(4):319–24.
13. Zimprich A, Biskup S, Leitner P, et al. Mutations in LRRK2 cause autosomal-dominant parkinsonism with pleomorphic pathology. Neuron. 2004;44(4):601–7.
14. Kachergus J, Mata IF, Hulihan M, et al. Identification of a novel LRRK2 mutation linked to autosomal dominant parkinsonism: evidence of a common founder across European populations. Am J Hum Genet. 2005;76(4):672–80.
15. Ozelius L, Senthil J, Saunders-Pullman R, et al. LRRK2 G2019S as a cause of Parkinson's disease in Ashkenazi jews. N Engl J Med. 2006;354(4):424–5.
16. Tan EK, Shena H, Tan LCS, et al. The G2019S LRRK2 mutation is uncommon in an Asian cohort of Parkinson's disease patients. Neurosci Lett. 2005;384(3):327–9.
17. Klein C, Westenberger A. Genetics of Parkinson's disease. Cold Spring Harb Perspect Med. 2012;2(1):a008888.
18. Hentati F, Trinh J, Thomson C, et al. Lrrk2 parkinsonism in Tunisia and Norway: a comparative analysis of disease penetrance. Neurology. 2014;83:568–9.
19. Funayama M, Li Y, Tomiyama H, et al. Leucine-rich repeat kinase 2 G2385R variant is a risk factor for Parkinson disease in Asian population. Neuroreport. 2007;18(3):273–5.
20. Vilariño-Güell C, Wider C, Ross OA, et al. VPS35 mutations in Parkinson disease. Am J Hum Genet. 2011;89(1):162–7.
21. Zimprich A, Benet-Pagès A, Struhal W. A mutation in VPS35, encoding a subunit of the retromer complex, causes late-onset Parkinson disease. Am J Hum Genet. 2011;89(1):168–75.
22. Sharma M, Ioannidis JPA, Aasly JO, et al. A multicentre clinico-genetic analysis of the VPS35 gene in Parkinson disease indicates reduced penetrance for disease-associated variants. J Med Genet. 2012;49(11):721–6.
23. Bonifati V. Genetics of Parkinson's disease – state of the art, 2013. Parkinsonism Relat Disord. 2014;20 Suppl 1:S23–8.
24. Priya A, Kalaidzidis IV, Kalaidzidis Y, Lambright D, Datta S. Molecular insights into rab7-mediated endosomal recruitment of core retromer: deciphering the role of vps26 and vps35. Traffic. 2015;16(1):68–84.
25. Vilariño-Güell C, Rajput A, Milnerwood AJ. DNAJC13 mutations in Parkinson disease. Hum Mol Genet. 2014;23(7):1794–801.
26. Funayama M, Ohe K, Amo T, et al. CHCHD2 mutations in autosomal dominant late-onset Parkinson's disease: a genome-wide linkage and sequencing study. Lancet Neurol. 2015;14:274–82.
27. Lohmann E, Periquet M, Bonifati V, et al. How much phenotypic variation can be attributed to parkin genotype? Ann Neurol. 2003;54(2):176–85.
28. Grünewald A, Kasten M, Ziegler A, et al. Next-generation phenotyping using the Parkin example: time to catch up with genetics. JAMA Neurol. 2013;70(9):1186–91.
29. Doherty KM, Silveira-Moriyama L, Parkkinen L, et al. Parkin disease: a clinicopathologic entity? JAMA Neurol. 2013;70(5):571–9.
30. Zanon A, Rakovic A, Blankenburg H, et al. Profiling of Parkin-binding partners using tandem affinity purification. PLoS One. 2013;8(11):e78648.
31. Hasson SA, Kane LA, Yamano K, et al. High-content genome-wide RNAi screens identify regulators of parkin upstream of mitophagy. Nature. 2013;504(7479):291–5.
32. Valente EM, Abou-Sleiman PM, Caputo V, et al. Hereditary early-onset Parkinson's disease caused by mutations in PINK1. Science. 2004;304(5674):1158–60.
33. Gelmetti V, Ferraris A, Brusa L, et al. Late onset sporadic Parkinson's disease caused by PINK1 mutations: clinical and functional study. Mov Disord. 2008;23(6):881–5.
34. Klein C, Schlossmacher MG. The genetics of Parkinson disease: implications for neurological care. Nat Clin Prac Neurol. 2006;2(3):136–46.
35. Kasten M, Weichert C, Lohmann K, Klein C. Clinical and demographic characteristics of PINK1 mutation

carriers – a meta-analysis. Mov Disord. 2010;25(7): 952–4.
36. Youle RJ, Narendra DP. Mechanisms of mitophagy. Nat Rev Mol Cell Biol. 2011;12(1):9–14.
37. Rakovic A, Grünewald A, Kottwitz J, et al. Mutations in PINK1 and Parkin impair ubiquitination of mitofusins in human fibroblasts. PLoS One. 2011;6(3):e16746.
38. Grünewald A, Voges L, Rakovic A, et al. Mutant Parkin impairs mitochondrial function and morphology in human fibroblasts. PLoS One. 2010;5(9):e12962.
39. Bonifati V, Rizzu P, van Baren MJ, et al. Mutations in the DJ-1 gene associated with autosomal recessive early-onset parkinsonism. Science. 2003;299(5604):256–9.
40. Canet-Avilés RM, Wilson M, Miller D, et al. The Parkinson's disease protein DJ-1 is neuroprotective due to cysteine-sulfinic acid-driven mitochondrial localization. Proc Natl Acad Sci U S A. 2004;101(24):9103–8.
41. Lill CM, Roehr JT, McQueen MB, et al. Comprehensive research synopsis and systematic meta-analyses in Parkinson's disease genetics: the PDGene database. PLoS Genet. 2012;8(3):e1002548.
42. Lesage S, Anheim M, Condroyer C, et al. Large-scale screening of the Gaucher's disease-related glucocerebrosidase gene in Europeans with Parkinson's disease. Human Mol Genet. 2011;20(1):202–10.
43. Sidransky E, Nalls MA, Aasly JO, et al. Multicenter analysis of glucocerebrosidase mutations in Parkinson's disease. N Engl J Med. 2009;361(17): 1651–61.
44. Alcalay RN, Dinur T, Quinn T, et al. Comparison of parkinson risk in Ashkenazi jewish patients with Gaucher disease and GBA heterozygotes. JAMA Neurol. 2014;71(6):752–7.
45. Stamelou M, Quinn NP, Bhatia K. "Atypical" atypical parkinsonism: new genetic conditions presenting with features of progressive supranuclear palsy, corticobasal degeneration, or multiple system atrophy – diagnostic guide. Mov Disord. 2013;28(9):1184–99.
46. Oppenheim H. Über eine eigenartige Krampfkrankheit des kindlichen und jugendlichen Alters (Dysbasia lordotica progressiva, Dystonia musculorum deformans). Neurol Cent. 1911;30:1090–107.
47. Klein C, Fahn S. Translation of Oppenheim's 1911 paper on dystonia. Mov Disord. 2013;28:851–62.
48. Albanese A, Bhatia K, Bressman SB, et al. Phenomenology and classification of dystonia: a consensus update. Mov Disord. 2013;28:863–73.
49. Klein C. Genetics in dystonia. Park Relat Disord. 2014;20(Suppl1):S137–42.
50. Klein C, Marras C, Münchau A. Dystonia overview. In: Pagon RA, Adam MP, Ardinger HH, et al., editors. GeneReviews. Seattle: University of Washington; 2014.
51. Bressman SB, Sabatti C, Raymond D, et al. The DYT1 phenotype and guidelines for diagnostic testing. Neurology. 2000;54:1746–52.
52. Ozelius LJ, Hewett JW, Page CE, et al. The early-onset torsion dystonia gene (DYT1) encodes an ATP-binding protein. Nat Genet. 1997;17:40–8.
53. Fuchs T, Gavarini S, Saunders-Pullman R, et al. Mutations in the THAP1 gene are responsible for DYT6 primary torsion dystonia. Nat Genet. 2009;41:286–8.
54. Blanchard A, Ea V, Roubertie A, et al. DYT6 dystonia: review of the literature and creation of the UMD Locus-Specific Database (LSDB) for mutations in the THAP1 gene. Hum Mutat. 2011;32:1213–24.
55. Vemula SR, Puschmann A, Xiao J. Role of Galpha(olf) in familial and sporadic adult-onset primary dystonia. Hum Mol Genet. 2013;22:2510–9.
56. Kumar KR, Lohmann K, Masuho I, et al. Phenotypic spectrum of mutations in GNAL: a novel cause of cranio-cervical dystonia. JAMA Neurol. 2013;71(4):490–4.
57. Xiao J, Uitti RJ, Zhao Y, et al. Mutations in CIZ1 cause adult onset primary cervical dystonia. Ann Neurol. 2012;71:458–69.
58. Charlesworth G, Plagnol V, Holmstrom KM, et al. Mutations in Ano3 cause dominant craniocervical dystonia: ion channel implicated in pathogenesis. Am J Hum Genet. 2012;91:1041–50.
59. Charlesworth G, Angelova PR, Bartolomé-Robledo F, et al. Mutations in HPCA cause autosomal-recessive primary isolated dystonia. Am J Hum Genet. 2015;96(4):657–65.
60. Zech M, Lam DD, Francescatto L. Recessive mutations in the α3 (VI) collagen gene COL6A3 cause early-onset isolated dystonia. Am J Hum Genet. 2015;96(6):883–93.
61. Lohmann K, Wilcox R, Winkler S, et al. Whispering dysphonia (DYT4 dystonia) is caused by a mutation in the TUBB4 gene. Ann Neurol. 2013;73(4): 537–45.
62. Hersheson J, Mencacci NE, Davis M, et al. Mutations in the autoregulatory domain of ß-tubulin 4a cause hereditary dystonia. Ann Neurol. 2013;73(4): 546–53.
63. Simons C, Wolf NI, McNeil N. A de novo mutation in the β-tubulin gene TUBB4A results in the leukoencephalopathy hypomyelination with atrophy of the basal ganglia and cerebellum. Am J Hum Genet. 2013;92(5):767–73.
64. Segawa M, Hosaka A, Miyagawa F, et al. Hereditary progressive dystonia with marked diurnal fluctuation. Adv Neurol. 1976;14:215–33.
65. Mencacci NE, Isaias IU, Reich MM, et al. Parkinson's disease in GTP cyclohydrolase 1 mutation carriers. Brain. 2014;137(Pt 9):2480–92.
66. Tadic V, Kasten M, Bruggemann N, et al. Dopa-responsive dystonia revisited: diagnostic delay, residual signs, and nonmotor signs. Arch Neurol. 2012;69(12):1558–62.
67. de Carvalho Aguiar P, Sweadner KJ, Penniston JT, et al. Mutations in the Na+/K+ -ATPase alpha3 gene ATP1A3 are associated with rapid-onset dystonia parkinsonism. Neuron. 2004;43:169–75.

68. Heinzen EL, Swoboda KJ, Hitomi Y, et al. De novo mutations in ATP1A3 cause alternating hemiplegia of childhood. Nat Genet. 2012;44:1030–4.
69. Demos MK, van Karnebeek CD, Ross CJ. A novel recurrent mutation in ATP1A3 causes CAPOS syndrome. Orphanet J Rare Dis. 2014;9:15.
70. Camargos S, Scholz S, Simón-Sánchez J, et al. DYT16, a novel young-onset dystonia-parkinsonism disorder: identification of a segregating mutation in the stress-response protein PRKRA. Lancet Neurol. 2008;7(3):207–15.
71. Zech M, Castrop F, Schormair B. DYT16 revisited: exome sequencing identifies PRKRA mutations in a European dystonia family. Mov Disord. 2014;29(12):1504–10.
72. Seibler P, Djarmati A, Langpap B, et al. A heterozygous frameshift mutation in PRKRA (DYT16) associated with generalised dystonia in a German patient. Lancet Neurol. 2008;7(5):380–1.
73. Lee LV, Rivera C, Teleg RA, et al. The unique phenomenology of sex-linked dystonia parkinsonism (XDP, DYT3, "Lubag"). Int J Neurosci. 2011;121 Suppl 1:3–11.
74. Domingo A, Westenberger A, Lee LV, et al. New insights on the genetics of X-linked dystonia-parkinsonism (XDP/DYT3). Eur J Hum Genet. 2015;23(10):1334–40.
75. Makino S, Kaji R, Ando S, et al. Reduced neuron-specific expression of the TAF1 gene is associated with X-linked dystonia-parkinsonism. Am J Hum Genet. 2007;80:393–406.
76. Domingo A, Amar D, Grütz K, et al. Evidence of TAF1 dysfunction in peripheral models of X-linked dystonia-parkinsonism. Cell Mol Life Sci. 2016. [Epub ahead of print].
77. Zimprich A, Grabowski M, Asmus F, et al. Mutations in the gene encoding epsilon-sarcoglycan cause myoclonus-dystonia syndrome. Nat Genet. 2001;29:66–9.
78. Müller B, Hedrich K, Kock N, et al. Evidence that paternal expression of the epsilon-sarcoglycan gene accounts for reduced penetrance in myoclonus-dystonia. Am J Hum Genet. 2002;71:1303–11.
79. Groen JL, Andrade A, Ritz K, et al. CACNA1B mutation is linked to unique myoclonus-dystonia syndrome. Hum Mol Genet. 2015;24(4):987–93.
80. Mencacci NE, Rubio-Agusti I, Zdebik A, et al. A missense mutation in KCTD17 causes autosomal dominant myoclonus-dystonia. Am J Hum Genet. 2015;96(6):938–47.
81. Risch NJ, Bressman SB, Senthil G, Ozelius LJ. Intragenic cis and trans modification of genetic susceptibility in DYT1 torsion dystonia. Am J Hum Genet. 2007;80(6):1188–93.
82. Kamm C, Fischer H, Garavaglia B, et al. Susceptibility to DYT1 dystonia in European patients is modified by the D216H polymorphism. Neurology. 2008;70(23):2261–2.
83. Mok KY, Schneider SA, Trabzuni D, et al. Genomewide association study in cervical dystonia demonstrates possible association with sodium leak channel. Mov Disord. 2014;29(2):245–51.
84. Lohmann K, Schmidt A, Schillert A, et al. Genome-wide association study in musician's dystonia: a risk variant at the arylsulfatase G locus? Mov Disord. 2014;29(7):921–7.
85. Gómez-Garre P, Huertas-Fernández I, Cáceres-Redondo MT, et al. Lack of validation of variants associated with cervical dystonia risk: a GWAS replication study. Mov Disord. 2014;29(14):1825–8.
86. Schmidt A, Kumar KR, Redyk K, et al. Two faces of the same coin: benign familial infantile seizures and paroxysmal kinesigenic dyskinesia caused by PRRT2 mutations. Arch Neurol. 2013;69(5):668–70.
87. Chen WJ, Lin Y, Xiong ZQ, et al. Exome sequencing identifies truncating mutations in PRRT2 that cause paroxysmal kinesigenic dyskinesia. Nat Genet. 2011;43:1252–5.
88. Lee HY, Xu Y, Huang Y, et al. The gene for paroxysmal non-kinesigenic dyskinesia encodes an enzyme in a stress response pathway. Hum Mol Genet. 2004;13:3161–70.
89. Weber YG, Storch A, Wuttke TV, et al. GLUT1 mutations are a cause of paroxysmal exertion-induced dyskinesias and induce hemolytic anemia by a cation leak. J Clin Invest. 2008;118:2157–68.
90. Weber YG, Kamm C, Suls A, et al. Paroxysmal choreoathetosis/spasticity (DYT9) is caused by a GLUT1 defect. Neurology. 2011;77:959–64.
91. MacDonald, Bates, Buckler, et al. A novel gene containing a trinucleotide repeat that is expanded and unstable on Huntington's disease chromosomes. Cell. 1993;72(6):971–83.
92. Warby S, Graham RK, Hayden MR. Huntington's disease. In: Pagon RA, Adam MP, Ardinger HH, et al., editors. GeneReviews. Seattle: University of Washington; 2014.
93. Semaka A, Creighton S, Warby S, Hayden MR. Predictive testing for Huntington disease: interpretation and significance of intermediate alleles. Clin Genet. 2006;70(4):283–94.
94. Killoran A, Biglan KM, Jankovic J, et al. Characterization of the Huntington intermediate CAG repeat expansion phenotype in PHAROS. Neurology. 2013;80:2022.
95. Ha AD, Fung V. Huntington's disease. Curr Opin Neurol. 2012;25(4):491–8.
96. Ross CA, Tabrizi SJ. Huntington's disease: from molecular pathogenesis to clinical treatment. Lancet Neurol. 2011;10:83–98.
97. Zeuner K, Deuschl G. An update on tremors. Curr Opin Neurol. 2012;25(4):475–82.
98. Gulcher JR, Jónsson P, Kong A, et al. Mapping of a familial essential tremor gene, FET1, to chromosome 3q13. Nat Genet. 1997;17(1):84–7. PubMed PMID: 9288103.
99. Jeanneteau F, Funalot B, Jankovic J, et al. A functional variant of the dopamine D3 receptor is associated with risk and age-at-onset of essential tremor. Proc Natl Acad Sci U S A. 2006;103(28):10753–8.

100. Kuhlenbäumer G, Hopfner F, Deuschl G. Genetics of essential tremor: meta-analysis and review. Neurology. 2014;82(11):1000–7.
101. Higgins JJ, Lombardi RQ, Pucilowska J, Jankovic J, Tan EK, Rooney JP. A variant in the HS1-BP3 gene is associated with familial essential tremor. Neurology. 2005;64(3):417–21.
102. Merner ND, Girard SL, Catoire H, et al. Exome sequencing identifies FUS mutations as a cause of essential tremor. Am J Hum Genet. 2012;91(2):313–9.
103. Hopfner F, Stevanin G, Müller SH, et al. The impact of rare variants in FUS in essential tremor. Mov Disord. 2015;30(5):721–4.
104. Gulsuner H, Gulsuner S, Mercan FN, et al. Mitochondrial serine protease HTRA2 p.G399S in a kindred with essential tremor and Parkinson disease. Proc Natl Acad Sci U S A. 2014. pii: 201419581. [Epub ahead of print].
105. Strauss KM, Martins LM, Plun-Favreau H, et al. Loss of function mutations in the gene encoding Omi/HtrA2 in Parkinson's disease. Hum Mol Genet. 2005;14(15):2099–111.
106. Krüger R, Sharma M, Reiss O, et al. A large-scale genetic association study to evaluate the contribution of Omi/HtrA2 (PARK13) to Parkinson's disease. Neurobiol Aging. 2011;32(3):548.e9–548.e18.
107. Stefansson H, Steinberg S, Petursson H, et al. Variant in the sequence of the LINGO1 gene confers risk of essential tremor. Nat Genet. 2009;41:277–9.
108. Thier S, Lorenz D, Nothnagel M, et al. Polymorphisms in the glial glutamate transporter SLC1A2 are associated with essential tremor. Neurology. 2012;79(3):243–8.
109. Trenkwalder C, Paulus W. Restless legs syndrome: pathophysiology, clinical presentation and management. Nat Rev Neurol. 2010;6(6):337–46.
110. Kumar KR, Lohmann K, Klein C. Genetics of Parkinson disease and other movement disorders. Curr Opin Neurol. 2012;25(4):466–74.
111. Winkelmann J, Schormair B, Lichtner P, et al. Genome-wide association study of restless legs syndrome identifies common variants in three genomic regions. Nat Genet. 2007;39(8):1000–6.
112. Schulte E, Kousi M, Tan PL, et al. Targeted resequencing and systematic in vivo functional testing identifies rare variants in MEIS1 as significant contributors to restless legs syndrome. Am J Hum Genet. 2014;95:85–95.
113. Domingo A, Erro R, Lohmann K. Novel Dystonia Genes: Clues on disease mechanisms and the complexities of high-throughput sequencing. Mov Disord. 2016;31(4):471–7.
114. Harbo HF, Finsterer J, Baets J, et al. EFNS guidelines on the molecular diagnosis of neurogenetic disorders: general issues, Huntington's disease, Parkinson's disease and dystonias. Eur J Neurol. 2009;16(7):777–85.
115. Lohmann K, Klein C. Next generation sequencing and the future of genetic diagnosis. Neurotherapeutics. 2014;11(4):699–707.

Part II

Parkinson's Disease

Etiology and Pathogenesis of Parkinson's Disease

10

Jonathan Timpka, Maria Angela Cenci, and Per Odin

10.1 Sporadic, Inherited, Idiopathic, or Familial?

The term Parkinson's disease (PD) has traditionally been earmarked for idiopathic forms of parkinsonism. Lately, the term has been widened to also cover familial or inherited forms of parkinsonism with a similar clinical course to idiopathic PD. Hence, there is an often made distinction between sporadic, i.e., idiopathic, and inherited or familial forms of PD. PD is differentiated from symptomatic parkinsonism, which may be drug induced or the result of vascular disease and parkinsonism caused by another neurodegenerative disorder, such as multiple system atrophy or dementia with Lewy bodies. Familial forms of PD make up approximately 5 % of PD patients [1]. However, 15 % of sporadic PD patients have a first-degree relative with the disease [2], which could suggest shared genetic or environmental risk factors.

10.2 Familial Forms of Parkinson's Disease

As the genetics of PD is discussed in a previous chapter, the subject is discussed only briefly in the setting of this chapter. In 1997, it was found that a mutation in SNCA, the gene coding for the protein α-synuclein, caused autosomal-dominant inherited PD in an Italian family [3]. Since then, it has been shown that also duplication and triplication mutations of SNCA cause autosomal-dominant PD through overexpression of the normal, wild-type α-synuclein [4]. α-synuclein is a protein normally localized presynaptically, functioning as a SNARE-complex chaperone [5], and is nowadays regarded as one of the main actors in the pathogenesis of PD. Although point mutations in SNCA are rarely seen in sporadic PD, α-synuclein is central also in these cases as it is the main component of Lewy bodies. The most common cause of familial PD as a result of autosomal-dominant mutation is a mutation in the *LRRK2* gene. *LRRK2* has been found to also be a risk factor for Crohn's disease, an association that is

J. Timpka, MSc
Department of Clinical Sciences Lund, Neurology, Lund University, Lund SE-221 85, Sweden
e-mail: jonathan.timpka@med.lu.se

M.A. Cenci, MD, PhD
Department of Experimental Medical Science, Lund University, Lund, Sweden
e-mail: Angela.Cenci_Nilsson@med.lu.se

P. Odin, MD, PhD (✉)
Department of Clinical Sciences Lund, Neurology, Lund University, Lund SE-221 85, Sweden

Department of Neurology, Klinikum-Bremerhaven, Postbrookstrasse 103, DE-27574 Bremerhaven, Germany
e-mail: per.odin@med.lu.se; per.odin@klinikum-bremerhaven.de

C. Falup-Pecurariu et al. (eds.), *Movement Disorders Curricula*,
DOI 10.1007/978-3-7091-1628-9_10

discussed later in this chapter. Several genes have also been linked to an autosomal-recessive inheritance of PD, particularly *PRKN*, *PINK1*, and *DJ-1*. With the emergence of genome-wide association studies at the beginning of the millennium came the possibility to effectively identify disease risk loci en masse. This has been the case also in PD, where a relatively recent, large meta-analysis found strong evidence that the loci *GBA*, *LRRK2*, *MAPT*, *PARK16*, and *SNCA*, among others, are PD risk loci [6].

10.3 Lewy Bodies

Lewy bodies were first described in 1912 by Friedrich H. Lewy. In advanced stages of PD, Lewy bodies can often be found throughout large parts of the central nervous system (CNS), including the cortex, olfactory bulb, hypothalamus, posterior pituitary, cerebellum, dorsal vagal nucleus, and spinal cord. Lewy bodies are an intracytoplasmic accumulation of proteins and are the consequence of an increased protein production, a decreased clearance, or, as is most likely, both. Interestingly, the olfactory bulb is the only structure with a primarily sensory function that is typically and significantly engaged by Lewy pathology at an early stage of the disease. Several structures outside of the CNS also exhibit Lewy bodies in PD, most notably the enteric nervous system of the gastrointestinal tract [7], sympathetic ganglia [8], and heart [9]. The ubiquitin-proteasome and lysosome systems that normally dispose of unwanted proteins in the affected neurons are either saturated or dysfunctional. Instead, the α-synuclein forms oligomers and fibrillary aggregations, making up the Lewy body inclusions together with ubiquitin, neurofilaments, and over 90 other identified proteins [10]. Neurons are thought to be particularly vulnerable to the increased proteolytic stress as they have a limited capacity to regenerate. The function of Lewy bodies is not entirely uncontroversial as it has been proposed that they may in fact be neuroprotective [11], although most publications view them as neurotoxic.

10.4 Braak Staging and the Propagation of α-Synuclein

On the basis of extensive neuropathological research, Braak et al. have developed a hypothesis for the spreading of Lewy bodies and a six-stage model for staging of the disease [12, 13]. The Braak staging model states that Lewy bodies first appear in the dorsal vagal nucleus of the medulla oblongata and the olfactory bulb, which is stage 1, and then spread in a predictable, caudo-rostral fashion. In stage 2, medullar structures such as the locus coeruleus and lower raphe nuclei are affected by the Lewy pathology. The involvement of the substantia nigra occurs first in stage 3, at which point the basal forebrain is also beginning to be affected. The degeneration of the substantia nigra pars compacta is manifest in stage 4, and at this point Lewy pathology begins to appear also in the cerebral cortex. In stage 4, the damage to the substantia nigra is significant, and the overt symptoms of parkinsonism arise. In stages 5 and 6, the degeneration of the substantia nigra is almost complete and the neocortical involvement is extensive. Over a time span of years, the histopathologic hallmark has spread throughout the significant parts of the mid- and forebrain. The gradual spreading proposed by Braak corresponds to a host of recent findings, showing that α-synuclein fibrillation may be propagated from one cell to another [14]. This is exemplified by the discovery that when the embryonal brain tissue is transplanted into a brain with PD, the transplanted tissue may exhibit LB pathology at a biological age of only 10–15 years [15, 16]. The Braak hypothesis is, however, not uncontested. It, for example, fails to comprehensively explain why some structures are spared by the progressing disease, why not all patients with characteristic Lewy pathology exhibit parkinsonism [17], or why the spreading of Lewy pathology is not always quite so predictable [18].

The preclinical period of the disease has traditionally been regarded as the 5–6 years prior to the development of the manifest symptoms that fulfill the criteria for a clinical diagnosis. This view has subsequently been somewhat altered, as it has been shown that sleep disorders, neuropsychiatric problems, and autonomic dysfunction, which are all common non-motor symptoms, may start to arise as early as 20 years prior to diagnosis [19].

10.5 Environmental Toxins and Pathogens

Environmental toxins are topical in current PD research, but it must be kept in mind that it is an oversimplification to view any of the currently discussed substances, here or elsewhere, as an independent cause of PD. Their influence is nonetheless interesting mainly of two reasons: there is a vast interest in producing effective animal models of PD, and one starting point has been to expose animals to various neurodegenerative substances and, most importantly, the role of environmental toxins in the pathogenesis of PD is still not fully clarified [20]. Several viruses have also been discussed in the setting of parkinsonism, especially since the influenza outbreak in 1918 was followed by cases of encephalitis lethargica which exhibited parkinsonism. These patients did react well to antiparkinsonistic medication for a period of time [21], but did not exhibit characteristic Lewy pathology during autopsy. It has been hypothesized that influenza virus infection is not a direct cause of PD, but may be a precipitating, first factor that paves way for a second stressor in a "dual hit" theory [22, 23].

Some studies have indicated that people living in rural areas have a higher risk of developing PD when compared to their counterparts living in urban areas [24]. This is hypothesized to be because of the more widespread use of insecticides and pesticides in rural areas. On the other hand, several other studies have found no significant difference in the prevalence between urban and rural areas [25] or, as in Taiwan, an even higher prevalence in urban areas [26]. A careful approach may be exemplified by a Thai study, which suggests that exposure to pesticides may indeed be a risk factor for PD, but so is some component of urban living [27].

Rotenone is a pesticide, insecticide, and piscicide naturally occurring in the roots or stems of several members of Fabaceae. Infusion of rotenone into the substantia nigra of mice or rats has been found to create PD-like characteristics. Both the dosage and administration of rotenone are of great importance, as systemic administration causes a multisystemic degeneration unlike the degeneration seen in PD [28], and high doses are selectively damaging to the striatum and globus pallidus, but spare the substantia nigra [29]. In two studies, rotenone was administered to the animals per os over a longer period of time to simulate a more natural exposure to environmental toxins and to possibly initiate even more PD-like features [30, 31]. A chronic, per oral exposure to rotenone was shown to give rise to a PD-like pathology that was not only originating in the enteric nervous system but also spreading to the substantia nigra, causing a loss of dopaminergic neurons and PD-like characteristics [31]. When the vagal nerve was resected in a later study, the disease progression to the central nervous system was interrupted [32]. The effect of rotenone has also been shown to be reduced through concurrent treatment with an oligomer modulator, thus preventing aggregation of α-synuclein [33].

10.6 The Olfactory Bulb and the Enteric Nervous System

In the hypothesis presented by Braak et al., it is proposed that the process of PD illness originates in the enteric nervous system of the gastrointestinal tract or the olfactory bulb and is propagated to the CNS [7, 34, 35], possibly via a prion-like mechanism [14, 36]. The previously mentioned work on rotenone has constituted one interesting approach, possibly strengthening a gut-to-brain hypothesis. Another angle may be demonstrated by an elegantly made, recent study showing retrograde transportation of aggregated α-synuclein along the vagal nerve. After injection of α-synuclein from human brain lysates into the intestinal wall of rats, the α-synuclein was transported toward the vagal nucleus at a rate of 20–30 mm per day [37].

In a study of three PD patients that had undergone a colon biopsy for unrelated reasons 2–5 years before the onset of motor symptoms, the stored biopsies were examined again, but this time with the goal of finding α-synuclein. The tissue did in fact show an intense staining for α-synuclein [38], a histopathological appearance that could not be seen in neither healthy individuals nor in patients with inflammatory bowel disease. Therefore it was not simply a consequence of inflammation or oxidative stress [39]. As a result, it was proposed that the finding of α-synuclein in colonic submucosa may be a useful premotor biomarker for PD. Besides the previously mentioned *LRRK2*, overlapping risk loci between enteric inflammation and PD can be further exemplified by *CARD15*, a locus that has been found to be associated to PD in genome-wide association studies. Mutations of *CARD15* were established in 2001 as the first genetic risk factor for Crohn's disease and still remains as one of the most significant. The causality and underlying mechanisms of the associations to PD are currently being studied. One hypothesis is that the enteric inflammation and subsequent impairment of barrier function increase the susceptibility for external stressors.

With the Braak staging concept in mind, it is logical that non-motor symptoms are predominant before the substantia nigra is significantly degenerated. These patients with very early stage PD are difficult to identify in the primary health care, as most of the early symptoms are both common and unspecific. Moreover, there are few effective clinical predictors of PD. As the olfactory bulb and the enteric nervous system are the structures that are known to first exhibit Lewy body pathology, it is not surprising that olfactory dysfunction and constipation may be two of the earliest symptoms of PD. As a matter of fact, smelling tests [40] and the frequency of bowel movements [41] have both been evaluated as possible predictors of PD with mildly positive results.

10.7 Oxidative Stress, Inflammation, and Iron

Toxicological studies have found that toxins resulting in mitochondrial damage may cause parkinsonism [42] and the previously mentioned forms of autosomal-recessive inherited PD all have in common that they alter mitochondrial function. It has been proposed that the dopaminergic neurons of the substantia nigra consume more energy than comparable neurons and thus would be more sensitive to an impaired mitochondrial function [43]. Cytosolic dopamine has been shown to be a potential source of oxidative stress [44, 45], which may be a significant factor in the setting of a more generalized neuronal stress. Cell survival rates within the substantia nigra pars compacta vary greatly in advanced PD, which could be the result of different protein profiles among neurons [46], making them unevenly vulnerable to oxidative stress. Melatonin is produced in the pineal gland and is mostly known for its central role in the establishing of a diurnal rhythm. Melatonin has been shown to be protective against mitochondrial damage induced by metabolites of the substance 1-methyl-4-phenyl-1,2,3,6-tetrahydropyridine (MPTP), a known oxidotoxin that causes PD-like symptoms [47, 48]. Furthermore, melatonin promotes cytoskeletal rearrangements and has an anti-oxidative and anti-inflammatory function [49], which makes it a potential therapeutic agent in PD. It has been hypothesized that a decrease in melatonin production is one of the reasons behind the increased oxidative stress and degenerative changes seen during aging [50]. All unknown pathogens and environmental agents aside, old age remains the principal risk factor for PD [51].

Low-grade neuroinflammation may be another key to the complex and widespread neurodegeneration in PD. Some epidemiological studies show that the use of nonsteroidal anti-inflammatory drugs (NSAIDs) seems to be protective against PD [52], but the effect is, at best, moderate. The human leukocyte antigen (HLA) is a group of genes that code for several cell-surface proteins that regulate the immune system. The HLA system is normally of great interest in autoimmune disorders and transplantation medicine, but it has been found that certain HLA types are overrepresented also in PD patients. Genetic variations in several other inflammatory pathways as well as in parts of both the adaptive and innate immune responses have also been found to affect the risk for developing PD [53]. The degree of activation of astrocytes and microglia is a central mechanism in neuronal death in PD. Dying neurons in the substantia nigra release neuromelanin [54]. Extraneuronal neuromelanin has been shown to cause a substantial microglial activation [55], which leads to further damage to the dopamine neurons. Consequently, the glial activation has been proposed as a potential drug target [56].

Patients with PD have been found to have an increased concentration of iron in the substantia nigra. The cause for this is unknown, but several factors have been suggested: an increased permeability of the blood-brain barrier, a pro-inflammatory state, an increase of lactoferrin receptors in neurons and microvessels, and alterations in iron transport and binding [57]. High serum concentrations of iron have on the contrary been reported to be protective against PD [58], likely because of iron's function as a cofactor in the production of dopamine and other neurotransmitters. The long-term treatment of PD patients with an iron chelator to reduce midbrain iron accumulation is still being evaluated, but a positive effect on motor symptoms has been noticed [59].

References

1. Samii A, Nutt JG, Ransom BR. Parkinson's disease. Lancet. 2004;363(9423):1783–93.
2. Lesage S, Brice A. Parkinson's disease: from monogenic forms to genetic susceptibility factors. Hum Mol Genet. 2009;18(R1):R48–59.
3. Polymeropoulos MH, Lavedan C, Leroy E, Ide SE, Dehejia A, Dutra A, et al. Mutation in the alpha-synuclein gene identified in families with Parkinson's disease. Science. 1997;276(5321):2045–7.
4. Ibanez P, Lesage S, Janin S, Lohmann E, Durif F, Destee A, et al. Alpha-synuclein gene rearrangements in dominantly inherited parkinsonism: frequency, phenotype, and mechanisms. Arch Neurol. 2009;66(1):102–8.
5. Burre J, Sharma M, Tsetsenis T, Buchman V, Etherton MR, Sudhof TC. Alpha-synuclein promotes SNARE-complex assembly in vivo and in vitro. Science. 2010;329(5999):1663–7.
6. Lill CM, Roehr JT, McQueen MB, Kavvoura FK, Bagade S, Schjeide BM, et al. Comprehensive research synopsis and systematic meta-analyses in Parkinson's disease genetics: the PDGene database. PLoS Genet. 2012;8(3):e1002548.
7. Braak H, de Vos RA, Bohl J, Del Tredici K. Gastric alpha-synuclein immunoreactive inclusions in Meissner's and Auerbach's plexuses in cases staged for Parkinson's disease-related brain pathology. Neurosci Lett. 2006;396(1):67–72.
8. Wakabayashi K, Takahashi H. Neuropathology of autonomic nervous system in Parkinson's disease. Eur Neurol. 1997;38 Suppl 2:2–7.
9. Orimo S, Amino T, Itoh Y, Takahashi A, Kojo T, Uchihara T, et al. Cardiac sympathetic denervation precedes neuronal loss in the sympathetic ganglia in Lewy body disease. Acta Neuropathol. 2005;109(6):583–8.
10. Wakabayashi K, Tanji K, Odagiri S, Miki Y, Mori F, Takahashi H. The Lewy body in Parkinson's disease and related neurodegenerative disorders. Mol Neurobiol. 2013;47(2):495–508.
11. Olanow CW, Perl DP, DeMartino GN, McNaught KS. Lewy-body formation is an aggresome-related process: a hypothesis. Lancet Neurol. 2004;3(8):496–503.
12. Braak H, Del Tredici K, Rub U, de Vos RA, Jansen Steur EN, Braak E. Staging of brain pathology related to sporadic Parkinson's disease. Neurobiol Aging. 2003;24(2):197–211.
13. Braak H, Ghebremedhin E, Rub U, Bratzke H, Del Tredici K. Stages in the development of Parkinson's disease-related pathology. Cell Tissue Res. 2004;318(1):121–34.
14. Dunning CJ, Reyes JF, Steiner JA, Brundin P. Can Parkinson's disease pathology be propagated from one neuron to another? Prog Neurobiol. 2012;97(2):205–19.
15. Li JY, Englund E, Holton JL, Soulet D, Hagell P, Lees AJ, et al. Lewy bodies in grafted neurons in subjects with Parkinson's disease suggest host-to-graft disease propagation. Nat Med. 2008;14(5):501–3.
16. Li JY, Englund E, Widner H, Rehncrona S, Bjorklund A, Lindvall O, et al. Characterization of Lewy body pathology in 12- and 16-year-old intrastriatal mesencephalic grafts surviving in a patient with Parkinson's disease. Mov Dis Off J Mov Dis Soc. 2010;25(8):1091–6.
17. Jellinger KA. Formation and development of Lewy pathology: a critical update. J Neurol. 2009;256 Suppl 3:270–9.
18. Attems J, Jellinger KA. The dorsal motor nucleus of the vagus is not an obligatory trigger site of Parkinson's disease. Neuropathol Appl Neurobiol. 2008;34(4):466–7.
19. Savica R, Rocca WA, Ahlskog JE. When does Parkinson disease start? Arch Neurol. 2010;67(7):798–801.
20. Pan-Montojo F, Reichmann H. Considerations on the role of environmental toxins in idiopathic

Parkinson's disease pathophysiology. Transl Neurodegener. 2014;3:10.
21. Sacks O. The origin of "Awakenings". Br Med J. 1983;287(6409):1968–9.
22. Jang H, Boltz DA, Webster RG, Smeyne RJ. Viral parkinsonism. Biochim Biophys Acta. 2009;1792(7):714–21.
23. Jang H, Boltz D, Sturm-Ramirez K, Shepherd KR, Jiao Y, Webster R, et al. Highly pathogenic H5N1 influenza virus can enter the central nervous system and induce neuroinflammation and neurodegeneration. Proc Natl Acad Sci U S A. 2009;106(33):14063–8.
24. Brown TP, Rumsby PC, Capleton AC, Rushton L, Levy LS. Pesticides and Parkinson's disease – is there a link? Environ Health Perspect. 2006;114(2):156–64.
25. Walker RW, Hand A, Jones C, Wood BH, Gray WK. The prevalence of Parkinson's disease in a rural area of North-East England. Parkinsonism Relat Disord. 2010;16(9):572–5.
26. Chen CC, Chen TF, Hwang YC, Wen YR, Chiu YH, Wu CY, et al. Different prevalence rates of Parkinson's disease in urban and rural areas: a population-based study in Taiwan. Neuroepidemiology. 2009;33(4):350–7.
27. Bhidayasiri R, Wannachai N, Limpabandhu S, Choeytim S, Suchonwanich Y, Tananyakul S, et al. A national registry to determine the distribution and prevalence of Parkinson's disease in Thailand: implications of urbanization and pesticides as risk factors for Parkinson's disease. Neuroepidemiology. 2011;37(3–4):222–30.
28. Hoglinger GU, Feger J, Prigent A, Michel PP, Parain K, Champy P, et al. Chronic systemic complex I inhibition induces a hypokinetic multisystem degeneration in rats. J Neurochem. 2003;84(3):491–502.
29. Ferrante RJ, Schulz JB, Kowall NW, Beal MF. Systemic administration of rotenone produces selective damage in the striatum and globus pallidus, but not in the substantia nigra. Brain Res. 1997;753(1):157–62.
30. Inden M, Kitamura Y, Takeuchi H, Yanagida T, Takata K, Kobayashi Y, et al. Neurodegeneration of mouse nigrostriatal dopaminergic system induced by repeated oral administration of rotenone is prevented by 4-phenylbutyrate, a chemical chaperone. J Neurochem. 2007;101(6):1491–504.
31. Pan-Montojo F, Anichtchik O, Dening Y, Knels L, Pursche S, Jung R, et al. Progression of Parkinson's disease pathology is reproduced by intragastric administration of rotenone in mice. PLoS One. 2010;5(1):e8762.
32. Pan-Montojo F, Schwarz M, Winkler C, Arnhold M, O'Sullivan GA, Pal A, et al. Environmental toxins trigger PD-like progression via increased alpha-synuclein release from enteric neurons in mice. Sci Rep. 2012;2:898.
33. Wagner J, Ryazanov S, Leonov A, Levin J, Shi S, Schmidt F, et al. Anle138b: a novel oligomer modulator for disease-modifying therapy of neurodegenerative diseases such as prion and Parkinson's disease. Acta Neuropathol. 2013;125(6):795–813.
34. Braak H, Del Tredici K. Neuroanatomy and pathology of sporadic Parkinson's disease. Adv Anat Embryol Cell Biol. 2009;201:1–119.
35. Hawkes CH, Del Tredici K, Braak H. Parkinson's disease: the dual hit theory revisited. Ann N Y Acad Sci. 2009;1170:615–22.
36. Olanow CW, Brundin P. Parkinson's disease and alpha synuclein: is Parkinson's disease a prion-like disorder? Mov Dis: Off J Mov Dis Soc. 2013;28(1):31–40.
37. Holmqvist S, Chutna O, Bousset L, Aldrin-Kirk P, Li W, Bjorklund T, et al. Direct evidence of Parkinson pathology spread from the gastrointestinal tract to the brain in rats. Acta Neuropathol. 2014;128(6):805–20.
38. Shannon KM, Keshavarzian A, Dodiya HB, Jakate S, Kordower JH. Is alpha-synuclein in the colon a biomarker for premotor Parkinson's disease? Evidence from 3 cases. Mov Dis: Off J Mov Dis Soc. 2012;27(6):716–9.
39. Shannon KM, Keshavarzian A, Mutlu E, Dodiya HB, Daian D, Jaglin JA, et al. Alpha-synuclein in colonic submucosa in early untreated Parkinson's disease. Mov Dis: Off J Mov Dis Soc. 2012;27(6):709–15.
40. Ross GW, Petrovitch H, Abbott RD, Tanner CM, Popper J, Masaki K, et al. Association of olfactory dysfunction with risk for future Parkinson's disease. Ann Neurol. 2008;63(2):167–73.
41. Abbott RD, Petrovitch H, White LR, Masaki KH, Tanner CM, Curb JD, et al. Frequency of bowel movements and the future risk of Parkinson's disease. Neurology. 2001;57(3):456–62.
42. Langston JW, Ballard P, Tetrud JW, Irwin I. Chronic Parkinsonism in humans due to a product of meperidine-analog synthesis. Science. 1983;219(4587):979–80.
43. Bolam JP, Pissadaki EK. Living on the edge with too many mouths to feed: why dopamine neurons die. Mov Dis: Off J Mov Dis Soc. 2012;27(12):1478–83.
44. Cantuti-Castelvetri I, Shukitt-Hale B, Joseph JA. Dopamine neurotoxicity: age-dependent behavioral and histological effects. Neurobiol Aging. 2003;24(5):697–706.
45. Asanuma M, Miyazaki I, Diaz-Corrales FJ, Ogawa N. Quinone formation as dopaminergic neuron-specific oxidative stress in the pathogenesis of sporadic Parkinson's disease and neurotoxin-induced parkinsonism. Acta Med Okayama. 2004;58(5):221–33.
46. Double KL, Reyes S, Werry EL, Halliday GM. Selective cell death in neurodegeneration: why are some neurons spared in vulnerable regions? Prog Neurobiol. 2010;92(3):316–29.
47. Hantraye P, Varastet M, Peschanski M, Riche D, Cesaro P, Willer JC, et al. Stable parkinsonian syndrome and uneven loss of striatal dopamine fibres following chronic MPTP administration in baboons. Neuroscience. 1993;53(1):169–78.

48. Chen LJ, Gao YQ, Li XJ, Shen DH, Sun FY. Melatonin protects against MPTP/MPP+ -induced mitochondrial DNA oxidative damage in vivo and in vitro. J Pineal Res. 2005;39(1):34–42.
49. Polimeni G, Esposito E, Bevelacqua V, Guarneri C, Cuzzocrea S. Role of melatonin supplementation in neurodegenerative disorders. Front Biosci. 2014;19:429–46.
50. Dowling GA, Mastick J, Colling E, Carter JH, Singer CM, Aminoff MJ. Melatonin for sleep disturbances in Parkinson's disease. Sleep Med. 2005;6(5):459–66.
51. Collier TJ, Kanaan NM, Kordower JH. Ageing as a primary risk factor for Parkinson's disease: evidence from studies of non-human primates. Nat Rev Neurosci. 2011;12(6):359–66.
52. Gao X, Chen H, Schwarzschild MA, Ascherio A. Use of ibuprofen and risk of Parkinson disease. Neurology. 2011;76(10):863–9.
53. Holmans P, Moskvina V, Jones L, Sharma M, Vedernikov A, International Parkinson's Disease Genomics C, et al. A pathway-based analysis provides additional support for an immune-related genetic susceptibility to Parkinson's disease. Hum Mol Genet. 2013;22(5):1039–49.
54. Langston JW, Forno LS, Tetrud J, Reeves AG, Kaplan JA, Karluk D. Evidence of active nerve cell degeneration in the substantia nigra of humans years after 1-methyl-4-phenyl-1,2,3,6-tetrahydropyridine exposure. Ann Neurol. 1999;46(4):598–605.
55. Zhang W, Phillips K, Wielgus AR, Liu J, Albertini A, Zucca FA, et al. Neuromelanin activates microglia and induces degeneration of dopaminergic neurons: implications for progression of Parkinson's disease. Neurotox Res. 2011;19(1):63–72.
56. Rappold PM, Tieu K. Astrocytes and therapeutics for Parkinson's disease. Neurother: J Am Soc Exp NeuroTherap. 2010;7(4):413–23.
57. Ward RJ, Zucca FA, Duyn JH, Crichton RR, Zecca L. The role of iron in brain ageing and neurodegenerative disorders. Lancet Neurol. 2014;13(10):1045–60.
58. Pichler I, Del Greco MF, Gogele M, Lill CM, Bertram L, Do CB, et al. Serum iron levels and the risk of Parkinson disease: a Mendelian randomization study. PLoS Med. 2013;10(6):e1001462.
59. Kwiatkowski A, Ryckewaert G, Jissendi Tchofo P, Moreau C, Vuillaume I, Chinnery PF, et al. Long-term improvement under deferiprone in a case of neurodegeneration with brain iron accumulation. Parkinsonism Relat Disord. 2012;18(1):110–2.

11 Clinical Features and Differential Diagnosis of Parkinson's Disease

Nadia Magdalinou and Huw R. Morris

11.1 Introduction

Parkinson's disease (PD) is a progressive neurodegenerative movement disorder defined pathologically by degeneration of the substantia nigra and by the formation of eosinophilic intracellular inclusions, containing α-synuclein. The typical clinical features of PD have been defined in the Queen Square Brain Bank clinical diagnostic criteria, which emphasise the importance of bradykinesia, treatment response to levodopa and asymmetry [1]. Parkinsonism or Parkinson's syndrome refers to diseases in which there are some features of bradykinesia, gait disturbance, tremor or rigidity without the supporting exclusion or inclusion features of PD. PD is an age-dependent condition with an average age at onset in the late 60s and PD becomes more common with advancing age. There is a broad differential diagnosis for PD, and the possible differential diagnoses relate to the age at onset, with a variety of Parkinson's mimics occurring in different age groups. In this chapter we will describe the typical features of PD and then discuss its differential diagnosis in relation to age at onset, encompassing juvenile/early-onset PD, PD in midlife and PD in the elderly. Age ranges are given as a guide and important clinical pointer, but these syndromes overlap and occur in different age groups.

11.2 Definition of PD

PD is a progressive neurological disorder initially described as a clinical entity by James Parkinson. It is a clinically defined disorder, based upon the presence of bradykinesia accompanied by at least one other characteristic feature, such as resting tremor, rigidity and impaired postural reflexes [2]. The signs and symptoms are usually asymmetric at onset, and typically there is a good response to levodopa treatment.

We now know that PD affects many different regions of the nervous system [3]. Non-motor features include anosmia, autonomic disturbance, speech/swallowing problems and cognitive decline, which eventually progresses to dementia in approximately 80 % of patients, over 20 years [4–7]. A useful clinical classifi-

N. Magdalinou
Reta Lila Weston Institute of Neurological disease, UCL Institute of Neurology, Queen Square Brain Bank, 1 Wakefield Street, London WC1N 3BG, UK

H.R. Morris (✉)
Department of Clinical Neuroscience, UCL Institute of Neurology, Upper 3rd Floor, Royal Free Hospital, Rowland Hill Street, London NW3 2PF, UK
e-mail: h.morris@ucl.ac.uk

C. Falup-Pecurariu et al. (eds.), *Movement Disorders Curricula*,
DOI 10.1007/978-3-7091-1628-9_11

cation is between the tremor dominant and non-tremor dominant motor phenotypes. Patients with the non-tremor dominant disease have more rapid cognitive impairment, earlier autonomic involvement and worse functional disability. Tremor dominant patients have a slower disease progression, but eventually also develop the typical motor and non-motor features of PD [8–10].

11.3 Pathology and Aetiology of PD

PD is caused by progressive loss of dopamine-secreting neurons that project from the substantia nigra pars compacta in the midbrain to the striatum (putamen and caudate nucleus) [11]. The pathological hallmarks of the disease are Lewy bodies and Lewy neurites, whose main component is an aggregated form of α-synuclein protein. In PD, Lewy bodies are found in the basal ganglia, brainstem and sometimes in the cortex.

A complex interaction between environmental and genetic risk factors is usually considered to be important in the aetiology of PD. Infectious (influenza, whooping cough), toxic (pesticides, solvents) and other exposures (rural residence, well water drinking) have been considered as possible environmental risk factors. However, the most consistent environmental finding is that non-smokers have a greater risk of disease [12].

Rare hereditary forms of typical PD can be caused by mutations affecting the genes coding for α-synuclein, LRRK2 and VPS35 [13]. Population studies have demonstrated a strong association between disease risk and distinct single nucleotide polymorphisms (SNPs) in the α-Syn-encoding gene in PD [14]. Other genetic variants that are important in typical/late-onset PD include an association with single heterozygous mutations in the glucocerebrosidase (*GBA*) gene, and the presence of the G2019S mutation, which occurs in about 1 % of patients with sporadic PD [15].

11.4 Typical Features of PD

11.4.1 History

The age of onset of PD varies, with most patients presenting between 60 and 75 years of age. Community-based incidence studies indicate that the average age of onset of PD is 68 years [16]. The overall prevalence in European populations is 1.6 in 100 [17]. The onset is gradual and there is often a 'premotor' phase of the disease, which may include hyposmia, constipation, depression or rapid eye movement (REM) sleep behaviour disorder [18]. These premotor features can sometimes occur several years prior to the onset of motor signs [19].

It is important to be aware that in early stage disease many clinical features may be intermittent, so a careful history is important. A common initial symptom is resting tremor (4–6 Hz) of one hand or leg. We routinely ask patients whether the tremor occurs with action or whether the tremor is present when at rest or relaxing, although examination is more important than history in defining rest tremor. Patients may complain of difficulty with manual tasks, particularly repetitive tasks, related to bradykinesia and stiffness. Common complaints include difficulty with brushing teeth, writing, doing up buttons or using a screwdriver. Gait disturbance is unusual as a primary presenting feature although many patients (and their families) will have noticed a change in posture, with an increase in stooping, slowing up of gait and occasional shuffling or stumbling. An asymmetric presentation is usual and some patients may be misdiagnosed as having had a stroke. However, as the disease progresses clinical features appear on the contralateral side, although the disease remains asymmetric. Non-motor symptoms, such as those related to neuropsychiatric, sensory, autonomic or sleep disturbance, are very common and perhaps under-diagnosed. They can occur in the early premotor stage, but also later in the disease course. At presentation patients may have disturbance of sense of smell, constipation, REM sleep behaviour disorder and mild urinary urgency and frequency.

PD is a progressive disorder and we carefully ask about a history of progressive worsening in symptoms over time. We also enquire about possible precipitants or aetiological factors such as head injury, infection or exposure to drugs known to cause parkinsonism.

Patients usually have an excellent response to dopamine replacement treatment and will report a >70 % improvement, provided that they are on adequate treatment and not limited by side effects. Some patients develop choreiform, involuntary movements (dyskinesias) as a side effect of long-term treatment, with about 40 % developing dyskinesia and 'wearing-off' 5 years after the diagnosis. The risk of dyskinesia is higher in patients with younger onset disease.

11.4.2 Examination

The process of examination starts from the moment the patient is called in from the waiting area and continues during the history. PD patients usually have reduced facial expression (hypomimia), a soft voice (hypophonia) and a generalised or lateralised loss of spontaneous and associative movement. As the patient gestures while speaking, it may become obvious that there is a marked paucity of movement of one side. Resting tremor should be sought with the patient sitting relaxing in a chair and while lying relaxed on the couch. Axial (neck) and limb rigidity should be examined both with the patient sitting and lying relaxed and also while carrying out reinforcement tasks (e.g. undertaking simultaneous movement with the contralateral arm – synkinesis).

The most important diagnostic feature in PD is bradykinesia. Bradykinesia involves slowness in the initiation and then speed and amplitude of movement. With many types of repetitive movement (finger taps, hand grips, alternating movements, handwriting spirals), there may be a progressive decrease in the speed and amplitude of movement, with arrests and 're-setting' movements. This form of decrement is relatively specific to PD and should be specifically sought and recorded. Patients with PD usually have a slightly stooped posture, with asymmetric reduced arm swing when walking. As the disease progresses, they develop a short-stepped, shuffling gait, with postural instability. Asking the patient to walk quickly may highlight or accentuate the gait disorder.

11.4.3 Investigations

PD remains essentially a clinical diagnosis and the majority of patients do not require specific investigations. However, if there are atypical features, particularly early prominent gait, autonomic or cognitive features, structural imaging should be carried out, with computerised tomography (CT) or ideally magnetic resonance imaging (MRI). Some conditions can cause parkinsonism or a parkinsonian-like condition without degeneration of dopaminergic nerve terminals, for example, dopa-responsive dystonia, essential tremor, dystonic tremor (DT) or drug-induced parkinsonism. SPECT tracers, which bind to dopamine transporter protein (DaTSCAN) in the nigrostriatal nerve endings, can directly determine loss of binding and degeneration of dopaminergic terminals in PD. However, these scans are abnormal in other types of neurodegenerative parkinsonism, such as progressive supranuclear palsy (PSP) and multiple system atrophy (MSA).

11.5 Differential Diagnosis: Early-Onset Parkinsonism (Age at Onset <45 Years)

Conventionally, juvenile parkinsonism refers to patients who develop parkinsonism before the age of 20, and early-onset parkinsonism refers to patients who develop symptoms before the age of 45. There is a paucity of pathological studies of early-onset parkinsonism/PD. Pathologically verified (Lewy body) PD is rare before the age of 20 [20], but becomes more common in patients in their 30s and 40s. There are a number of autosomal recessive parkinsonian conditions that may have clinical features, which are indistinguishable from late-onset PD, but are due to mutations in autosomal recessive genes. The differential diagnosis of PD in teenage and early adult life includes (i) autosomal recessive parkinsonism, (ii) neuro-metabolic conditions in which there is primary failure of dopamine biosynthesis or neurotransmission, (iii) pallido-pyramidal conditions in which there may be multisystem neurodegeneration with prominent L-DOPA responsiveness, (iv) dystonia-parkinsonism syndromes, such as Wilson's disease and (v) multisystem neurodegenerative syndromes in which parkinsonism may be one part of a broader clinical picture (Table 11.1).

Table 11.1 Selected causes of juvenile/early-onset parkinsonism

	Typical features	Investigations
PD-like		
Parkin, PINK1, DJ-1, FBXO7	Akinetic rigid	Bi-allelic mutations on genetic testing
	Prominent lower limb symptoms	
	Exercise-induced dystonia	
	Prominent L-DOPA-induced dyskinesia	
	Usually no cognitive involvement	
Pallido-pyramidal syndromes/neurodegeneration with brain iron syndromes		
SPG-11	Spasticity, parkinsonism and dystonia	MRI – atrophy of the corpus callosum
		Bi-allelic gene mutations
PANK2	Spasticity, parkinsonism and dystonia	MRI – low signal of T2 imaging in the putamen with 'eye of the tiger' sign
		Bi-allelic gene mutations
ATP13A2	Spasticity, parkinsonism and dystonia	Bi-allelic gene mutation
	Good initial response to L-DOPA	
	Upgaze palsy	
	Peri-faucial myoclonus	
PLA2G6	Spasticity, parkinsonism and dystonia	Bi-allelic gene mutation
Parkinsonism-dystonia		
Wilson's disease	Prominent bulbar and behavioural features	Low serum caeruloplasmin
		MRI
		Kayser-Fleischer ring
		Autosomal dominant gene mutation
Neuro-metabolic		
GTP-CH1	Diurnal variation with sleep benefit (although this can also occur in early onset PD)	Low CSF biopterins and neopterins
	Excellent response to ~300 mg/day of L-DOPA in childhood	Normal DaTSCAN
	Autosomal dominant family history	Autosomal dominant gene mutation
Multisystem degenerative diseases		
Juvenile Huntington disease	Family history of chorea and dementia	Genetic testing: HD gene expansion
Niemann-Pick type C	Vertical gaze palsy	Abnormal cholesterol staining on fibroblast studies
	Parkinsonism-dystonia	Genetic testing
	Hepatosplenomegaly	

11.5.1 History and Examination

The approach to a patient with juvenile/early-onset parkinsonism should include a careful history related to potential drug exposure, a detailed family history including an enquiry about parental consanguinity and a clinical assessment looking for concurrent parkinsonism, pyramidal signs, dystonia, eye movement abnormalities and cognitive impairment.

Autosomal recessive juvenile parkinsonism due to recessive mutations in parkin, PINK1 and DJ-1 is particularly common in patients with parkinsonism before the age of 20 and is usually considered to be a form of typical PD, although the pathological phenotype may not involve typical Lewy body formation [21–23]. Recently, mutations in FBX07 have been described as causing a similar syndrome to parkin disease [24]. Patients with both parkin disease and DRD can have sleep benefit, prominent lower limb dystonia and diurnal variation with relatively minimal symptoms in the early morning. Both patient groups usually have a very good response to L-DOPA and anticholinergic medication, although unlike DRD, *parkin* disease is often associated with early, severe L-DOPA-induced dyskinesia (LID). It has been suggested that *parkin* patients are distinguished from typical late-onset PD patients by the presence of slow disease progression, dystonia and LID although this may be a feature of all patients with early-onset parkinsonism, rather than a specific feature of *parkin* disease [21, 25, 26]. The different propensity to the development of LID in DRD and AR-JP means that it is important to distinguish between these conditions as carefully as possible. Dopamine transporter imaging, CSF neurotransmitter analysis and genetic analysis may all be helpful.

A number of pallido-pyramidal syndromes have been described which may involve brain iron accumulation, in which there is parkinsonism with an initial response to L-DOPA followed by loss of L-DOPA response accompanied by atypical features such as supranuclear gaze palsy, cognitive impairment, spasticity and severe dystonia. These include parkinsonism due to PANK2, PLA2G6, ATP13A2 (Kufor-Rakeb disease) and SPG11 [24].

The primary neuro-metabolic condition which can cause parkinsonism and dystonia is dopa-responsive dystonia (DRD), due to autosomal dominant mutations in the GTP cyclohydrolase 1 gene. Some patients may have prominent concurrent parkinsonism. In DRD striatal dopamine transporter imaging is normal and CSF neurotransmitter analysis shows reduced levels of total biopterins and neopterins in the CSF. About 60 % of patients with DRD have a mutation in the GTP cyclohydrolase 1 gene.

11.5.2 Investigations

All patients with early-onset parkinsonism should have brain imaging, ideally with MR and screening for Wilson's disease with serum caeruloplasmin. If there are features suggestive of Wilson's disease, 24 h urinary copper excretion and slit lamp examination looking for the presence of Kayser-Fleischer rings should be carried out. In patients in whom a complex parkinsonian disorder is suspected, MRI with T2*/gradient echo sequences is recommended, to optimally detect iron deposition in the basal ganglia. Patients with DRD have a normal DaTSCAN, and cerebrospinal fluid (CSF) neurotransmitter analysis shows a decrease in CSF biopterins and neopterins. These investigations will help in distinguishing a biosynthetic from a presynaptic deficit in dopaminergic transmission. Genetic analysis of parkin, PINK1 and DJ-1 is available, and positive results, with bi-allelic pathogenic mutations, will be identified in about 10 % of parkinsonism/PD patients identified with disease onset before the age of 45 [27]. However, many patients from consanguineous families and with a strong family history do not have mutations in known genes implying that there are further pathogenic genes to be identified in this group of patients.

11.6 Differential Diagnosis: Midlife Onset Parkinsonism (Age at Onset 45–74 Years of Age)

The commonest differential diagnoses of PD include essential/dystonic tremor, atypical parkinsonian conditions, particularly MSA, and secondary parkinsonism, most importantly due to dopamine-blocking medications.

11.7 Tremor

11.7.1 Essential Tremor

Essential tremor (ET) can sometimes be misdiagnosed as PD. ET is usually bilateral, symmetric and occurs when maintaining a posture and during action. There is a significant family history in 50 % of patients. Tremor of the head and neck is common. There is very slow progression, good response to alcohol and no association with parkinsonian features [28, 29].

11.7.2 Dystonic Tremor

Dystonic tremor (DT) is commonly misdiagnosed as PD. This may be associated with focal dystonia. Typically, there is postural tremor, but there is often a rest component with a prominent thumb tremor. Dystonic tremor is often asymmetric and unlike PD may be prominent with action and specific tasks. Unlike PD, patients often have prominent writing and cup-pouring tremor.

11.7.3 Atypical Parkinsonian Syndromes

Stanley Fahn first used the term 'Parkinson-plus or atypical parkinsonism' to characterise a heterogeneous group of neurodegenerative disorders that are different from PD, but share its central feature of akinetic rigidity [30]. The 'plus' or 'atypical' descriptor indicates the presence of additional characteristics not usual in patients with PD. Many patients in this group will have early postural instability and falls. There are also important specific diagnostic features, such as early autonomic failure and pyramidal signs in multiple system atrophy (MSA), supranuclear gaze palsy and frontal/dysexecutive syndrome with progressive supranuclear palsy (PSP) and dystonia, apraxia and myoclonus in corticobasal degeneration (CBD). Another important disease we classify as an atypical parkinsonian syndrome (APS) is dementia with Lewy bodies (DLB) where the dementia onset is before or within a year of onset of extrapyramidal features [31]. The earlier onset of dementia differentiates DLB from Parkinson's disease dementia (PDD). 'Red flags' in the clinical history can alert the physician to alternative diagnosis to PD [32] (see Table 11.2). APS account for less than 10 % of all parkinsonian disorders and rarely respond with sustained improvement to levodopa. They usually follow a much more aggressive disease course than PD and are characterised by atrophy in several cortical and subcortical networks. They sometimes present in a strikingly similar way to PD, especially in the early stages, and misdiagnosis can occur [2].

APS have further sub-classifications. PSP usually presents in its 'classical' form also known as Richardson's syndrome (PSP-RS) [33], but can also occur with asymmetric onset, tremor and moderate initial response to L-dopa (PSP-parkinsonism (PSP-P)) [34] or with a syndrome with freezing at the initial stages, called pure

Table 11.2 Red flags suggesting a diagnosis other than PD [32]

1. Early instability and falls	In the first 3 years of symptoms
2. Predominantly axial symptoms	Axial>limb rigidity
3. Symmetrical signs	Especially at onset
4. Early autonomic features and dementia	In the first 3 years of symptoms
5. Sudden onset of symptoms	Tempo not fitting with a slowly progressive neurodegenerative syndrome
6. Poor/non-sustained L-dopa response	At least 600 mg of L-dopa per day for 2 months
7. Rapid progression	Despite dopaminergic treatment

akinesia with gait freezing (PAGF) [35]. The yearly incidence of PSP is estimated to be 5.3 per 100,000, the average age of onset is 67 years and the median survival time is 6 years [36].

MSA is classified according to the predominance of parkinsonism versus ataxia to MSA-parkinsonism (MSA-P) or MSA-cerebellar type (MSA-C) [37]. Annual incidence rate of MSA is estimated to be 3.0 per 100,000, average age of symptom onset is 56 years of age and disease duration is approximately 9.8 years [38].

CBD is a very rare disease, with an estimated annual incidence of less than 1 in 100,000, an average age of symptom onset at 63 and an approximate disease duration of less than 10 years [39].

11.7.4 Other Neurodegenerative Diseases

Patients with frontotemporal dementia (FTD) and Alzheimer's disease (AD) can develop parkinsonian signs, although usually the cognitive syndrome will make the underlying diagnosis obvious. FTD can cause a PD like asymmetric PD-like akinetic-rigid syndrome or a gait disorder predominant PSP-like syndrome. AD most commonly causes a frontal gait disorder/gait apraxia. Very rarely, sporadic and familial parkinsonism is associated with motor neuron disease, with dementia as an additional feature in some patients [40].

11.7.5 Secondary Parkinsonism

11.7.5.1 Drugs

Dopamine receptor blocking drugs are the most common cause of drug-induced parkinsonism, which is more common with older, 'typical' neuroleptics (such as chlorpromazine and thioridazine). Almost all neuroleptics (including aripiprazole, risperidone and olanzapine) can cause parkinsonism, except quetiapine and clozapine. Antiemetics, like metoclopramide, and antiepileptic drugs, such as sodium valproate, can also cause parkinsonism in individuals with intact dopaminergic systems or patients with underlying asymptomatic PD [41, 42].

11.7.5.2 Toxins

Parkinsonism can be caused by several toxins, including manganese, cyanide, organophosphates, carbon monoxide and a variety of solvents [43–45]. Manganese (Mn) toxicity usually results from the consumption of Mn-containing water. It can present with symmetrical parkinsonism, dystonia and a characteristic 'cock walk' gait involving a high-stepping gait with an erect posture. Hallucinations and behavioural disturbance may be early features [46].

11.7.5.3 Infectious and Postinfectious

Post-encephalitic parkinsonism was observed several years after an influenza epidemic, although no clear link to influenza virus has been established. There is underlying tau pathology and a limited response to levodopa [47, 48]. In addition, parkinsonism has been associated with several infections, such as HIV, measles and Epstein-Barr virus [49].

11.8 Differential Diagnosis: Late-Life Parkinsonism (AAO>74 years of Age)

PD becomes more common in the elderly rising to a prevalence of 3.5 in 100 for those aged over 85 years [17]. However, PD is often confused with vascular parkinsonism and predominant gait disorders such as PSP, PAGF and NPH. Furthermore, parkinsonism can occur in other neurodegenerative conditions including DLB, CBS, AD and FTDP17. Comorbidity including arthritis and cerebrovascular disease can make PD more difficult to diagnose in elderly patients.

11.9 Gait Disorders

11.9.1 Vascular Parkinsonism

Vascular parkinsonism (VP) is a progressive motor disorder with balance difficulties, tremor, rigidity and bradykinesia typically affecting the legs more than the arms, often described as 'lower body parkinsonism' [50]. Vascular parkinsonism is a very important cause of gait disorders in the elderly and frequently misdiagnosed. The diagnostic criteria include a sudden or delayed progressive onset of parkinsonism/gait disorder with infarcts in or near the basal ganglia or subcortical white matter [50]. The development of a shuffling gait, minimal upper limb symptoms, bilateral symptoms at onset, poor response to levodopa and early cognitive decline points towards a vascular aetiology. Patients with vascular parkinsonism usually have an erect posture with retained and sometimes exaggerated arm swing. They usually have a short-stepped gait with or without gait freezing/gait ignition failure.

11.9.2 PAGF

PAGF presents with prominent difficulties in initiating gait and freezing during walking, writing and speaking. Typically, there is minimal limb rigidity and tremor and a lack of response to levodopa. The underlying pathology is usually PSP pathology, but PD has also been found [35].

11.9.3 Normal Pressure Hydrocephalus

Normal pressure hydrocephalus (NPH) is a controversial entity typically presenting with the triad of cognitive decline, urinary incontinence and gait disturbance. Brain imaging shows marked enlargement of cerebral ventricles and patients have a good initial response to cerebrospinal fluid large volume withdrawal [51]. Parkinsonism with a good levodopa response has been noted in some patients. Pathological studies have shown that the majority of patients have co-existing neurodegenerative or vascular pathologies [52].

11.9.4 Investigations in Mid- and Late-Life Parkinsonism

Multiple imaging modalities, such as different magnetic resonance imaging (MRI) techniques, single-photon emission computer tomography (SPECT), position emission tomography (PET) [53] and transcranial sonography [54], have been used to help in the diagnosis of PD and the discrimination between PD and similar disorders.

Conventional MRI has an important role in discriminating atypical parkinsonian syndromes [55, 56] (see Tables 11.3 and 11.4), detecting vascular load and radiological signs of NPH. Imaging presynaptic dopaminergic terminal function with a dopamine transporter (DAT) SPECT scan shows high sensitivity for detecting atypical parkinsonian syndromes, but poor specificity for discriminating them from PD [57]. DAT scan is usually normal in vascular and drug-induced parkinsonism, psychogenic and essential tremor, so it may be useful in differentiating these conditions from PD. The European Medicines Agency (EMA) and Food and Drug Administration (FDA) licences for DaTSCAN indicate that DaTSCAN can be useful in excluding essential tremor but not in differentiating PD from other parkinsonian disorders. Both NICE in the UK (www.nice.org.uk/guidance/cg35) and the American Academy of Neurology (AAN) [58] recommend the use of DaTSCAN scan in differentiating essential tremor from parkinsonian disorders.

Table 11.3 Selected causes of midlife parkinsonism

Causes	Typical features	Investigations
Neurodegenerative		
PD	Initially, asymmetric pill-rolling tremor, rigidity and bradykinesia	MRI: unremarkable
	Good and sustained levodopa response	
	Late-onset dementia	
MSA	Early falls	MRI: pontine 'hot-cross bun', cerebellar atrophy or putaminal abnormalities
	Early autonomic disturbance	
	Severe dysphonia	
	Inspiratory sighs	
	Orofacial dystonia	
	Polyminimyoclonus	
	No sustained levodopa response	
PSP	Early falls and postural instability	MRI: volume loss in the midbrain with relative preservation of pons
	Vertical slow saccades/supranuclear gaze palsy	
	Usually symmetric akinetic rigid syndrome	
	Frontal/executive impairment	
	Poor levodopa response	
CBS	Asymmetric presentation	MRI: may have asymmetric frontoparietal atrophy
	Dystonia	
	Myoclonus	
	Cognitive decline	
	Delayed initiation of saccades	
	Poor levodopa response	
DLB	Hallucinations/delusions	MRI: cortical atrophy with preservation of medial temporal structures
	Cognitive slowing	
	Visuospatial impairment	
	Behavioural and sleep disturbance	
	Fluctuating cognitive impairment	
	Good levodopa response in 50 % of patients	
FTD	Behavioural or personality changes	MRI: usually asymmetric frontal/temporal atrophy
	Dysexecutive syndrome	
	Language decline	
AD	Most common cause of dementia	MRI: disproportional hippocampal atrophy
	Cognitive decline with predominant episodic memory impairment	
	Possible myoclonus	
Tremor		
Essential tremor	Bilateral	MRI: normal
	Postural and action	DaTSCAN: normal
	Positive family history	
	Good response to alcohol	
Dystonic tremor	Tremor in a body part also displaying dystonia	MRI: normal
	Unilateral/asymmetrical	DaTSCAN: normal
	Jerky	
Psychogenic tremor	Variable amplitude/frequency	MRI: normal
	Worse when examined	
	Distractible/entrainable	

(continued)

Table 11.3 (continued)

Causes	Typical features	Investigations
Secondary parkinsonism		
Manganese toxicity	Symmetrical parkinsonism	MRI T1 hypointensity; T2 hyperintensity in globus pallidus and putamen
	Dystonia	
	Jerky tremor	
	'Cock walk'	

Table 11.4 Selected causes of late-onset parkinsonism

Cause	Typical features	Investigations
Neurodegenerative		
PD, DLB, PSP, AD	As above	MRI: unremarkable
PAGF	Difficulty in initiating gait	
	Freezing of gait or speech	
	Minimal limb rigidity and tremor	
	No sustained levodopa response	
	No dementia or ophthalmoplegia within the first 5 years	
Secondary		
Vascular parkinsonism	Freezing and falls	MRI: deep subcortical infarcts
	'Lower body parkinsonism'	
	Pyramidal signs	
	Early cognitive involvement	
	Tremor not a main feature	
	Less responsive to levodopa than PD	
Gait disturbance		
NPH	Cognitive decline	MRI: ventriculomegaly without significant cortical atrophy
	Urinary incontinence	Clinical improvement post large volume CSF removal
	Gait disturbance	
	Good response to shunting	
	Can have a good levodopa response	

Table 11.5 Practical steps in approaching parkinsonian patient in the clinic

1. Age of onset	Does this patient present as a
	Juvenile/early onset
	Midlife
	Late onset
	Parkinsonian patient?
2. Disease course	Does the tempo fit with a
	Progressive degenerative syndrome
	Vascular/toxic disorder?
3. Red flags	If the process is a degenerative akinetic-rigid syndrome, does the patient have 'red flags' for atypical parkinsonism?
4. Tremor	Is this most likely to be
	PD tremor
	Dystonic tremor
	Essential tremor/another disorder?
5. Gait	Are the gait, posture and associated features consistent with PD?
6. Initial investigation	Consider structural/nuclear medicine imaging and specialist tests
7. Follow-up	Clinical follow-up is vital
	Assess response to levodopa medication
	Rapidity of progression
	Be vigilant for the appearance of additional/emerging clinical features

Conclusions

Diagnosing PD is a process, which includes initial assessment, investigation and careful follow-up including the clinical course and response to treatment (Table 11.5). Age at onset is an important feature, which helps to stratify the differential diagnosis, and close attention should be paid to the age at onset together with disease progression. Some investigations may be helpful, particularly when there are 'red flags' suggesting alternative diagnoses. Some causes such as drug-induced parkinsonism or Wilson's disease need urgent assessment and treatment. In our opinion the most important aspect of the diagnosis is follow-up in the first year or so after the initiation of treatment when response to treatment and emergence of new clinical features can help to point towards alternative diagnoses.

References

1. Gibb WR, Lees AJ. The relevance of the Lewy body to the pathogenesis of idiopathic Parkinson's disease. J Neurol Neurosurg Psychiatry. 1988;51(6):745–52.
2. Hughes AJ, et al. Accuracy of clinical diagnosis of idiopathic Parkinson's disease: a clinico-pathological study of 100 cases. J Neurol Neurosurg Psychiatry. 1992;55(3):181–4.
3. Goedert M, et al. 100 years of Lewy pathology. Nat Rev Neurol. 2013;9(1):13–24.
4. Cummings JL. Intellectual impairment in Parkinson's disease: clinical, pathologic, and biochemical correlates. J Geriatr Psychiatry Neurol. 1988;1(1):24–36.
5. Hughes TA, et al. A 10-year study of the incidence of and factors predicting dementia in Parkinson's disease. Neurology. 2000;54(8):1596–602.
6. Aarsland D, et al. Prevalence and characteristics of dementia in Parkinson disease: an 8-year prospective study. Arch Neurol. 2003;60(3):387–92.
7. Aarsland D, et al. The effect of age of onset of PD on risk of dementia. J Neurol. 2007;254(1):38–45.
8. Williams-Gray CH, et al. Evolution of cognitive dysfunction in an incident Parkinson's disease cohort. Brain. 2007;130(Pt 7):1787–98.
9. Burn DJ, et al. Motor subtype and cognitive decline in Parkinson's disease, Parkinson's disease with dementia, and dementia with Lewy bodies. J Neurol Neurosurg Psychiatry. 2006;77(5):585–9.
10. Alves G, et al. Changes in motor subtype and risk for incident dementia in Parkinson's disease. Mov Disord. 2006;21(8):1123–30.
11. Braak H, et al. Staging of brain pathology related to sporadic Parkinson's disease. Neurobiol Aging. 2003;24(2):197–211.
12. Ben-Shlomo Y. The epidemiology of Parkinson's disease. Baillieres Clin Neurol. 1997;6(1):55–68.
13. Polymeropoulos MH, et al. Mutation in the alpha-synuclein gene identified in families with Parkinson's disease. Science. 1997;276(5321):2045–7.
14. Simon-Sanchez J, et al. Genome-wide association study reveals genetic risk underlying Parkinson's disease. Nat Genet. 2009;41(12):1308–12.
15. Zimprich A, et al. The PARK8 locus in autosomal dominant parkinsonism: confirmation of linkage and further delineation of the disease-containing interval. Am J Hum Genet. 2004;74(1):11–9.
16. de Lau LM, Breteler MM. Epidemiology of Parkinson's disease. Lancet Neurol. 2006;5(6):525–35.
17. de Rijk MC, et al. Prevalence of parkinsonism and Parkinson's disease in Europe: the EUROPARKINSON Collaborative Study. European Community Concerted Action on the Epidemiology of Parkinson's disease. J Neurol Neurosurg Psychiatry. 1997;62(1):10–5.

18. Tolosa E, et al. Diagnosis and the premotor phase of Parkinson disease. Neurology. 2009;72(7 Suppl):S12–20.
19. Savica R, Rocca WA, Ahlskog JE. When does Parkinson disease start? Arch Neurol. 2010;67(7):798–801.
20. Inose T, et al. Clinical and neuropathological study of a familial case of juvenile parkinsonism. Jpn J Psychiatry Neurol. 1988;42(2):265–76.
21. Ahlskog JE. Parkin and PINK1 parkinsonism may represent nigral mitochondrial cytopathies distinct from Lewy body Parkinson's disease. Parkinsonism Relat Disord. 2009;15(10):721–7.
22. Poulopoulos M, Levy OA, Alcalay RN. The neuropathology of genetic Parkinson's disease. Mov Disord. 2012;27(7):831–42.
23. Doherty KM, et al. Parkin disease: a clinicopathologic entity? JAMA Neurol. 2013;70(5):571–9.
24. Paisan-Ruiz C, et al. Early-onset L-dopa-responsive parkinsonism with pyramidal signs due to ATP13A2, PLA2G6, FBXO7 and spatacsin mutations. Mov Disord. 2010;25(12):1791–800.
25. Lohmann E, et al. A multidisciplinary study of patients with early-onset PD with and without parkin mutations. Neurology. 2009;72(2):110–6.
26. Wickremaratchi MM, et al. The motor phenotype of Parkinson's disease in relation to age at onset. Mov Disord. 2011;26(3):457–63.
27. Kilarski LL, et al. Systematic review and UK-based study of PARK2 (parkin), PINK1, PARK7 (DJ-1) and LRRK2 in early-onset Parkinson's disease. Mov Disord. 2012;27(12):1522–9.
28. Louis ED, et al. Diagnostic criteria for essential tremor: a population perspective. Arch Neurol. 1998;55(6):823–8.
29. Louis ED, et al. Clinical characteristics of essential tremor: data from a community-based study. Mov Disord. 1998;13(5):803–8.
30. Fahn S. Secondary parkinsonism. In Scientific approaches to clinical neurology. Philadelphia: Lea and Febiger; 1977. p. 1159–89.
31. McKeith IG, et al. Diagnosis and management of dementia with Lewy bodies: third report of the DLB Consortium. Neurology. 2005;65(12):1863–72.
32. Quinn N. Multiple system atrophy – the nature of the beast. J Neurol Neurosurg Psychiatry. 1989;52(Suppl):78–89.
33. Litvan I, et al. Clinical research criteria for the diagnosis of progressive supranuclear palsy (Steele-Richardson-Olszewski syndrome): report of the NINDS-SPSP international workshop. Neurology. 1996;47(1):1–9.
34. Williams DR, et al. Characteristics of two distinct clinical phenotypes in pathologically proven progressive supranuclear palsy: Richardson's syndrome and PSP-parkinsonism. Brain. 2005;128(Pt 6):1247–58.
35. Williams DR, et al. Pure akinesia with gait freezing: a third clinical phenotype of progressive supranuclear palsy. Mov Disord. 2007;22(15):2235–41.
36. Bower JH, et al. Incidence of progressive supranuclear palsy and multiple system atrophy in Olmsted County, Minnesota, 1976 to 1990. Neurology. 1997;49(5):1284–8.
37. Gilman S, et al. Second consensus statement on the diagnosis of multiple system atrophy. Neurology. 2008;71(9):670–6.
38. Wenning GK, et al. The natural history of multiple system atrophy: a prospective European cohort study. Lancet Neurol. 2013;12(3):264–74.
39. Wenning GK, et al. Natural history and survival of 14 patients with corticobasal degeneration confirmed at postmortem examination. J Neurol Neurosurg Psychiatry. 1998;64(2):184–9.
40. Brait K, Fahn S, Schwarz GA. Sporadic and familial parkinsonism and motor neuron disease. Neurology. 1973;23(9):990–1002.
41. Bocola V, et al. Neuroleptic induced parkinsonism: MRI findings in relation to clinical course after withdrawal of neuroleptic drugs. J Neurol Neurosurg Psychiatry. 1996;60(2):213–6.
42. Bateman DN, Rawlins MD, Simpson JM. Extrapyramidal reactions with metoclopramide. Br Med J (Clin Res Ed). 1985;291(6500):930–2.
43. Lee MS, Marsden CD. Neurological sequelae following carbon monoxide poisoning clinical course and outcome according to the clinical types and brain computed tomography scan findings. Mov Disord. 1994;9(5):550–8.
44. Grandas F, Artieda J, Obeso JA. Clinical and CT scan findings in a case of cyanide intoxication. Mov Disord. 1989;4(2):188–93.
45. Yamada M, et al. Chronic manganese poisoning: a neuropathological study with determination of manganese distribution in the brain. Acta Neuropathol. 1986;70(3–4):273–8.
46. Karki P, Lee E, Aschner M. Manganese neurotoxicity: a focus on glutamate transporters. Ann Occup Environ Med. 2013;25(1):4.
47. Calne DB, Lees AJ. Late progression of post-encephalitic Parkinson's syndrome. Can J Neurol Sci. 1988;15(2):135–8.
48. Duvoisin RC, Lobo-Antunes J, Yahr MD. Response of patients with postencephalitic Parkinsonism to levodopa. J Neurol Neurosurg Psychiatry. 1972;35(4):487–95.
49. Tse W, et al. Movement disorders and AIDS: a review. Parkinsonism Relat Disord. 2004;10(6):323–34.
50. Zijlmans JC, et al. Clinicopathological investigation of vascular parkinsonism, including clinical criteria for diagnosis. Mov Disord. 2004;19(6):630–40.
51. Bergsneider M, et al. Surgical management of idiopathic normal-pressure hydrocephalus. Neurosurgery. 2005;57(3 Suppl):S29–39. discussion ii–v.
52. Magdalinou NK, et al. Normal pressure hydrocephalus or progressive supranuclear palsy? A clinicopathological case series. J Neurol. 2013;260(4):1009–13.
53. Tang CC, et al. Differential diagnosis of parkinsonism: a metabolic imaging study using pattern analysis. Lancet Neurol. 2010;9(2):149–58.

54. Walter U, et al. Brain parenchyma sonography discriminates Parkinson's disease and atypical parkinsonian syndromes. Neurology. 2003;60(1):74–7.
55. Schrag A, et al. Differentiation of atypical parkinsonian syndromes with routine MRI. Neurology. 2000;54(3):697–702.
56. Massey LA, et al. The midbrain to pons ratio: a simple and specific MRI sign of progressive supranuclear palsy. Neurology. 2013;80(20):1856–61.
57. Brooks DJ. Imaging approaches to Parkinson disease. J Nucl Med. 2010;51(4):596–609.
58. Parkinson Study Group. A multicenter assessment of dopamine transporter imaging with DOPASCAN/SPECT in parkinsonism. Neurology. 2000;50(10):1540–7.

12 The Non-motor Parkinson's Disease

Anna Sauerbier, L. Klingelhoefer, M.A. Qamar, H. Carr, and K. Ray Chaudhuri

12.1 Introduction

Parkinson's disease (PD) is the second commonest neurodegenerative condition, and non-motor symptoms (NMS) are integral to the condition [63]. PD is as much a non-motor disorder as a motor disorder presenting with classical symptoms of rigidity, resting tremor, bradykinesia and postural instability. Indeed, the range and burden of NMS often has a greater impact on the patient's as well as carer's quality of life (QoL), and NMS are the biggest challenge to clinicians and healthcare professionals dealing with PD [16, 58, 85, 89]. Tables 12.1 and 12.2 summarise evidence that NMS play a key role in PD. Irrespective of the disease duration, the motor stage and the cultural background, studies have reported that a typical PD patient reports around ten different NMS [17]. An international survey in 2010 revealed that up to two thirds of PD patients being seen in the clinics, do not mention their NMS. There might be several explanations for this, one might be that the patients feel embarrassed, or the patients simply do not link their NMS to their underlying condition [20]. This highlights how crucial it is to address NMS during clinical consultations to offer the best possible clinical care and as a consequence to improve the QoL [58].

12.2 The Spectrum of Non-motor Problems Occurring in Parkinson's Disease

Originally, James Parkinson described several NMS such as sleep disturbance, constipation, sialorrhoea, urinary incontinence, and "at the last, constant sleepiness with slight delirium" in his essay, "The shaking palsy" published almost 200 years ago [62, 69]. We now know that the NMS of PD can range from autonomic, psychiatric and sleep disorders which reflect the multipeptide involvement of both the central and peripheral nervous system [64]. NMS occur throughout the progression of the disease with some leading the preclinical phase, others the early and untreated phase of PD, while some are present particularly at later advanced stages [43, 98].

A. Sauerbier (✉) • L. Klingelhoefer • M.A. Qamar
H. Carr • K. Ray Chaudhuri
National Parkinson Foundation International Centre of Excellence, King's College Hospital NHS Foundation Trust,
9th Floor Ruskin Wing, Denmark Hill, London SE5 9RS, UK

King's College London, London, UK
e-mail: annasauerbier@nhs.net

C. Falup-Pecurariu et al. (eds.), *Movement Disorders Curricula*,
DOI 10.1007/978-3-7091-1628-9_12

Table 12.1 The importance of non-motor symptoms

A. Historical
James Parkinson outlined several non-motor issues such as sleepiness, cognitive problems, and autonomic dysfunction in his original essay describing PD. This was then reflected in description of PD symptoms by others such as Gowers (Garcia-Ruiz et al. [34])
Frederick Lewy described Lewy bodies in the dorsal motor vagal nucleus, indicating key involvement of a non-motor area. Selective and sometimes a larger degree of non-dopaminergic neuronal involvement have also been recorded in PD for many years (Forno et al. [32])
B. PD has been considered by some to be a neuropsychiatric or a non-motor disorder
C. NMS are now known to present as a preclinical feature
Some NMS can predate motor symptoms by up to 20 years (such as late-onset idiopathic hyposmia and REM sleep behaviour disorder) (Tolosa et al. [88])
D. The burden of NMS
The burden of NMS (as opposed to individual NMS) appears to be the key determinant of quality of life of people with Parkinson's (Martinez-Martin et al. [58])
E. Reports by carers and patients
Patients consistently rate NMS as "most bothersome" using validated self-declarations tools such as the NMS Questionnaire (Politis et al. [65]; Breen and Druyte [13])
F. Relevant NMS-related neuropathy of PD
Heterogeneity of neuropathology includes degeneration of non-dopaminergic nuclei and pathways including serotonergic, cholinergic, and noradrenergic, from the onset of illness and sometimes differentially more affected than dopaminergic nuclei (Forno et al. [32]; Halliday et al. [40]; Hirsch et al. [45]; Iwanaga et al. [45]; Jellinger et al. [50]; Wakabayashi et al. [91]
The Lewy body deposition sites in the brain differ in early onset versus late-onset PD (Halliday et al. [38])

Adapted from Sauerbier and Chaudhuri [75]
PD Parkinson's disease, *NMS* non-motor symptoms, *REM* rapid eye movements

Table 12.2 Reported preclinical non-motor problems in Parkinson's disease

Relationship described	Proposed link
Olfactory dysfunction (Jennings et al. [52])	Urinary dysfunction (Winge et al. [94])
Sleep dysfunction (Postuma et al. [69]; Gao et al. [35]; Abbott et al. [2])	Sexual dysfunction (Gao et al. [36])
Gastrointestinal dysfunction (Cersosimo et al. [15]; Abbott et al. [1])	Cardiovascular problems (Bonuccelli et al. [9]; Jain et al. [49])
Mood disorders (Jacob et al. [48]; Weisskof et al. [93]; Bower et al [10]; Fang et al. [30])	Personality problems (Pont-Sunyer et al. [67])
	Fatigue (Kang et al. [53])
	Pain (Lin et al. [55])
	Weight loss (Chen et al. [23])
	Colour vision (Bertrand et al. [7]; Diederich et al. [26])

Adapted from Sauerbier and Chaudhuri [75]

The validation of holistic NMS tools such as NMS scale (NMSS) or NMSQuest allows conducting holistic studies addressing NMS prevalence [17, 18]. In addition, recent instruments such as the Movement Disorder Society (MDS) revised version of the Unified Parkinson's Disease Rating Scale (UPDRS) now contains a specific non-motor domain [34].

A large single-centre study (DeNoPA) study analysed the non-motor profile of drug naïve patients with PD and reported significantly more NMS compared to healthy controls in the untreated motor phase [59]. Another study by Zis et al. [97] has confirmed these observations that over 45 % of PD patients may have severe to very severe burden of NMS even in the early untreated motor stage. Furthermore, Erro et al. [28] has suggested that most of the NMS occurring at an early stage have the tendency to remain stable during the initial 2 years of the disease.

Politis et al. [65] reported that in general symptoms such as pain, sleep disorders, and anxiety are rated as "most bothersome" ahead of motor symptoms by patients at an early (within 6 years) as well as advanced stage of PD [38, 65]. Additionally, more evidence is indicating that NMS have a close and inverse correlation with the patient's QoL [4, 13, 31, 58].

12.3 Pathophysiology

PD is not a single neurotransmitter (dopaminergic) mediated disorder but a progressive multiorgan disease caused by deficits in numerous neurotransmitter pathway, which also include the cholinergic, noradrenergic, and serotonergic systems [41, 51, 54]. There is growing evidence that the enteric nervous system plays a key role in the pathology of PD, as well as the central and other extra-central nervous systems [42].

The description of Lewy bodies in the dorsal motor vagal nucleus indicates a non-dopaminergic onset of PD. Subsequently, Braak has proposed a theory for the pathogenesis of PD, whereby a six stage process based on Lewy body formation occurs with a "bottom-up" approach as follows [11, 12]:

Stage 1 = degeneration of the olfactory bulb, and the anterior olfactory nucleus, and the lower medulla

Stage 2 = pathological process affecting the lower brainstem with involvement of serotonergic (median raphe), and noradrenergic (locus coeruleus) nuclei in the brainstem, and pons (leading to clinical presentation of NMS such as late-onset hyposmia (olfactory bulb and nucleus) and rapid eye movement behaviour disorder (RBD) (lower brainstem))

Stages 3–6 = correlates with the motor impairment of PD and the onset of further NMS including cognitive and autonomic dysfunction

12.4 The Use of Animal Models to Study Non-motor Problems in PD

Animal models have been essential for the understanding of the pathophysiology of motor PD. Several animal models have been described to address specific NMS including 6-OHDA-lesioned rodents [27], α-synuclein overexpressor (ASO = Thy1-aSYN) mice [24], MPTP-treated primates [27], mouse models of intragastric rotenone administration [61] and Göttingen minipigs (Ellegaard Minipigs ApS) [56, 87]. However, animal models that address the wide range of NMS in PD remain an unmet need.

12.5 Preclinical Non-motor Problems in Parkinson's Disease

We now know that a preclinical phase before the actual onset of motor symptoms (often time of diagnosis) which is dominated by several NMS exists. Hyposmia, RBD, constipation and depression seem to be the most robust markers of the preclinical phase of PD [5, 8, 46, 79]. This is supported by studies reporting an increased risk that patients with idiopathic RBD or idiopathic hyposmia might develop a synucleinopathy [52, 68, 74]. Additionally, REM sleep behavioural events (RBE) have also been described to be associated with an increased risk of developing PD [6, 83].

12.6 Non-motor Subtyping Within Parkinson's Disease

Recent concepts have also driven the emergence of non-motor subtyping within PD. Subtyping within PD has been attempted in the past and broadly, this has concentrated on clinical expression of motor symptoms including akinesia-dominant, tremor-dominant, or postural instability gait difficulty (PIGD)-dominant phenotypes. However, recent evidence suggests that these phenotypes may well be unstable, and over a five-year follow-up period many of the tremor-dominant or akinesia-dominant phenotypes might actually migrate to other variants. Non-motor-dominant phenotypes have been suggested on the basis of several cluster analyses of untreated PD patient's samples and more recently by clinically driven phenotyping concepts [57, 77]. Non-motor phenotyping is based on clinical data collection using validated tools and can be broadly divided into clinical symptoms of Parkinson's expressing a cognitive-dominant phenotype or non-cognitive non-motor-dominant phenotype [77]. They suggest a terminology of Park (see Table 12.3) and further clarified the emergence of these clinical phenotypes with various subtype-specific biomarkers. For example, Park-fatigue group seems to have a selective deficiency of limbic serotonergic binding as shown in DASB-PET imaging, while Park-sleep variant expressing excessive daytime somnolence (EDS) may well have a serotonergic deficiency but in the raphe system of the brain. The latter might express itself as a narcoleptic phenotype with a very specific sensitivity to dopamine D3 agonist, which may precipitate or lead to sleep attacks, suggestive of narcoleptic events.

Further work on clarification of natural history of the various non-motor subtypes and also subtype-specific treatments is currently underway.

Table 12.3 Seven suggested non-motor-dominant subtypes within Parkinson's disease

Park – Cognition
Park – Apathy
Park – Depression/anxiety
Park – Sleep
Park – Pain
Park – Fatigue
Park – Autonomic

Adapted from Sauerbier et al. [76]

12.7 The Possible Impact of Ethnicity on Non-motor Problems in Parkinson's Disease

The impact of ethnicity on different motor and, in particular, NMS occurring in PD is currently underexplored and poorly understood. Previous studies have reported that the non-motor profiles in patients with PD might differ between various ethnic groups [4, 17, 25, 58, 71, 76]. Clustering atypical Parkinsonism has been described from different parts of the world, most recently from northern France [14]. However, possible underlying causes for these differences are still unclear, and the limited access to PD drugs, the varied sociocultural approaches and dietary variations (e.g. foods of Annonaceae family) in different ethnic groups might play an important role [25, 71]. However, evidence-based data are still lacking, and further research addressing this issue as part of a prospective multicentre study led in the UK is currently under way [76].

12.8 Non-motor Fluctuations

Motor fluctuations are common after levodopa therapy is commenced and typically start with "wearing off" of levodopa motor response and thereafter developing into typical "on"–"off" states and development of dyskinesias [29]. In recent years, fluctuations of NMS have also been recognised and classified, with attempts to quantify this phenomenon [86]. Studies have reported a wide range of prevalences, between 17 and 100 % of non-motor fluctuations (NMF) in PD patients [19, 39, 44, 84]. These large differences in prevalence can be attributed to different study populations and different measuring tools used for detecting NMF, e.g. assessed just by "a single open question" or multiple question-based questionnaires. NMF can be associated with motor fluctuations similar to the "on" and "off" phenomena dependent on dopamine replacement therapy (DRT), and the current view is that NMF accompany virtually all forms of motor fluctuations. However, there is also some evidence to suggest that some NMF may also occur independent of motor state and motor fluctuations [19, 44, 72, 95]. NMS combined with NMF can be more troublesome and disabling than motor disturbances alone ([3, 39, 86, 95]). It has been shown that patients with both non-motor and motor fluctuations exhibited more severe motor symptoms, higher NMS burden and a higher levodopa daily dose [81]. NMF is treatable if recognised by similar approaches that would address motor fluctuations; however, in many situations, a focused therapeutic approach is required. The most frequent NMF are listed in Table 12.4.

The NoMoFlu study (non-motor fluctuations in PD) was performed across Germany and the UK to evaluate the frequency and severity of NMS in PD and to correlate these with motor function in patients with fluctuating PD. The authors concluded that patterns of NMF are heterogeneous and complex, but psychiatric NMS fluctuate more frequently and severely. Demographic parameters and motor function do not correlate with NMS or NMF severities in fluctuating PD. Neuropsychiatric NMS, such as anxiety, depression and fatigue, as well as pain, had negative impacts on health-related QoL independent of their occurrence with respect to the motor state. Interestingly, fluctuations of all these NMS but not of fatigue deteriorated QoL. Thus, only the presence but not fluctuations of fatigue as a frequent and highly fluctuating NMS seem to worsen QoL. These discrepancies might be related to differential translation of NMS occurrence into QoL impairment between both motor states. In addition, NMS with high frequencies in "off" state and thus fluctuations might be experienced not only as negative but also as a positive event, providing some relief from these NMS in "on" state. This mixture of experiencing NMF together with potential insensitivity of the PDQ-8 in determining QoL change in fluctuating PD might also explain the relatively mild effects of NMF on QoL.

Table 12.4 A list of the most frequent non-motor fluctuations in "on" and "off" state rated by clinical examination

Non-motor symptoms	Frequency during "off" state [%]	Frequency during "on" state [%]	Reference
Anxiety	88 32.5	10	Witjas et al. [95] Storch et al. [86]
Drenching sweats	59		Witjas et al. [95]
Slowness of thinking	83		Witjas et al. [95]
Fatigue	75 82.5	30	Witjas et al. [95] Storch et al. [86]
Akathisia	63		Witjas et al. [95]
Hallucinations	25		Witjas et al. [95]
Dysphagia	17.5	25	Storch et al. [86]
Depression	55	27.5	Storch et al. [86]
Excessive sweating	25	27.5	Storch et al. [86]
Inner restlessness	50	30	Storch et al. [86]
Pain	45	32.5	Storch et al. [86]
Concentration/attention	62.5	27.5	Storch et al. [86]
Dizziness	35	20	Storch et al. [86]
Bladder urgency	35	27.5	Storch et al. [86]

12.9 Non-motor Symptoms Related to Treatment Complications

In clinical practice, various NMS might be partly treatment related. The most important ones include behavioural problems (impulse control disorders (ICD) and dopamine dysregulation syndromes), a so-called dopamine agonist withdrawal syndrome (DAWS), and drug interactions (e.g. autonomic symptoms of serotonin syndrome) [90]. In the current literature, the estimated prevalence of ICD, due to therapy with dopamine agonists (DA), is reported as being 4.9–19 % [73, 92]. The sudden withdrawal of DA should be avoided as it can lead to DAWS which presents with a wide range of symptoms including panic attacks, anxiety, social phobia, depression, vomiting, and symptomatic orthostatic hypotension [22, 66, 70].

12.10 Validated Tools to Address the Non-motor Symptoms Burden in Clinical Practice

Since 2006, holistic validated tools for patient and health professional completed assessments of the multi-morbid PD patient are available and allow NMS to be effectively detected in clinical practice. The measurement and self-reporting of NMS have been included by several initiatives such as the SCOPA scales (Scales for Outcomes in PD), the NMSQuest, NMSS and a new version of the MDS-UPDRS [21, 37, 60]. The patient completed NMSQuest includes 30 questions covering 10 different domains ranging from gastrointestinal to miscellaneous (Fig. 12.1).

12.11 Treatment of Non-motor Symptoms

Symptomatic NMS in PD may be treated with various options which have been recently discussed by the American Academy of Neurology (2010) and reviewed by the MDS [82, 96]. To address the wide range of symptomatic NMS effectively, dopaminergic as well as non-dopaminergic treatment strategies need to be considered. However, a recent review has concluded that there is only little or no evidence for treatment of many NMS. Prospective-controlled clinical trials addressing these are currently lacking [80]. In order to improve the outcome, future clinical trial populations would be enriched by relevant non-motor subtyping to deliver robust endpoints. Table 12.5 gives a summary of the range of NMS in PD that might be responsive to dopaminergic treatment.

PD NMS QUESTIONNAIRE

Name: .... Date: .... Age: ....

Centre ID: Male ☐ Female ☐

NON-MOVEMENT PROBLEMS IN PARKINSON'S

The movement symptoms of Parkinson's are well known. However, other problems can sometimes occur as part of the condition or its treatment. It is important that the doctor knows about these, particularly if they are troublesome for you.

A range of problems is listed below. Please tick the box 'Yes' if you have experienced it <u>during the past month</u>. The doctor or nurse may ask you some questions to help decide. If you have not experienced the problem in the past month tick the 'No' box. You should answer 'No' even if you have had the problem in the past but not in the past month.

Have you experienced any of the following in the last month?

	Yes	No
1. Dribbling of saliva during the daytime	☐	☐
2. Loss or change in your ability to taste or smell	☐	☐
3. Difficulty swallowing food or drink or problems with choking	☐	☐
4. Vomiting or feelings of sickness (nausea)	☐	☐
5. Constipation (less than 3 bowel movements a week) or having to strain to pass a stool (faeces)	☐	☐
6. Bowel (fecal) incontinence	☐	☐
7. Feeling that your bowel emptying is incomplete after having been to the toilet	☐	☐
8. A sense of urgency to pass urine makes you rush to the toilet	☐	☐
9. Getting up regularly at night to pass urine	☐	☐
10. Unexplained pains (not due to known conditions such as arthritis)	☐	☐
11. Unexplained change in weight (not due to change in diet)	☐	☐
12. Problems remembering things that have happened recently or forgetting to do things	☐	☐
13. Loss of interest in what is happening around you or doing things	☐	☐
14. Seeing or hearing things that you know or are told are not there	☐	☐
15. Difficulty concentrating or staying focussed	☐	☐
16. Feeling sad, 'low' or 'blue'	☐	☐
17. Feeling anxious, frightened or panicky	☐	☐
18. Feeling less interested in sex or more interested in sex	☐	☐
19. Finding it difficult to have sex when you try	☐	☐
20. Feeling light headed, dizzy or weak standing from sitting or lying	☐	☐
21. Falling	☐	☐
22. Finding it difficult to stay awake during activities such as working, driving or eating	☐	☐
23. Difficulty getting to sleep at night or staying asleep at night	☐	☐
24. Intense, vivid dreams or frightening dreams	☐	☐
25. Talking or moving about in your sleep as if you are 'acting' out a dream	☐	☐
26. Unpleasant sensations in your legs at night or while resting, and a feeling that you need to move	☐	☐
27. Swelling of your legs	☐	☐
28. Excessive sweating	☐	☐
29. Double vision	☐	☐
30. Believing things are happening to you that other people say are not true	☐	☐

All the information you supply through this form will be treated with confidence and will only be used for the purpose for which it has been collected. Information supplied will be used for monitoring purposes. Your personal data will be processed and held in accordance with the Data Protection Act 1998.

Fig. 12.1 The Non-motor symptoms Questionnaire (NMSQuest)

Table 12.5 The range of non-motor symptoms in Parkinson's disease that may respond to dopaminergic therapy categorised by strong and weak evidence

Strong evidence	Weak evidence
Depression	Anxiety
Primary PD-related pain (central pain)	Aspects of cognitive dysfunction
Panic attacks (when related to "off" period)	Rapid eye movement sleep behaviour disorder (RBD)
Restless leg syndrome and Periodic limb movements	Erectile failure
Urinary urgency ("off" related)	Nocturia
Urinary frequency ("off" related)	Constipation ("off" related)
Fluctuation-related pain (wearing "off", dyskinesias)	Unsatisfactory voiding of bowel
	Fatigue + Colour vision

Adapted from Chaudhuri and Schapira [18]
PD Parkinson's disease

Conclusions

The evidence of NMS-dominant subtype in PD is evolving and marks a new concept in the landscape of PD. In the future, NMS subtype-specific treatments would be required, as it currently remains under-explored.

Acknowledgements EUROPAR and IPMDS non-motor study group for data collection of studies reported. This paper presents independent research funded by the National Institute for Health Research (NIHR) Mental Health Biomedical Research Centre and Dementia Unit at South London and Maudsley NHS Foundation Trust and King's College London. We acknowledge the help and support of the international Parkinson's non-motor group and in particular Professor Pablo Martinez-Martin and his team in the Institute of Neuroepidemiology, Madrid, for co-leading all studies related to NMSQuest and NMSS described in this paper.

References

1. Abbott RD, Petrovitch H, White LR, et al. Frequency of bowel movements and the future risk of Parkinson's disease. Neurology. 2001;57:456–62.
2. Abbott RD, Ross GW, White LR, et al. Excessive daytime sleepiness and subsequent development of Parkinson disease. Neurology. 2005;65:1442–6.
3. Bayulkem K, Lopez G. Clinical approach to nonmotor sensory fluctuations in Parkinson's disease. J Neurol Sci. 2011;310:82–5.
4. Barone P, Antonini A, Colosimo C, et al. The PRIAMO study: a multicenter assessment of nonmotor symptoms and their impact on quality of life in Parkinson's disease. Mov Disord. 2009;24:1641–9.
5. Berendse HW, Ponsen MM. Detection of preclinical Parkinson's disease along the olfactory trac(t). J Neural Transm Suppl. 2006;70:321–5.
6. Berg D, Postuma RB, Bloem B, et al. Time to redefine PD? Introductory statement of the MDS Task Force on the definition of Parkinson's disease. Mov Disord. 2014;29:454–62.
7. Bertrand JA, Bedetti C, Postuma RB, et al. Color discrimination deficits in Parkinson's disease are related to cognitive impairment and white-matter alterations. Mov Disord. 2012;27:1781–8.
8. Boeve BF, Silber MH, Ferman TJ, et al. Association of REM sleep behavior disorder and neurodegenerative disease may reflect an underlying synucleinopathy. Mov Disord. 2001;16:622–30.
9. Bonuccelli U, Lucetti C, Del Dotto P, et al. Orthostatic hypotension in de novo Parkinson disease. Arch Neurol. 2003;60:1400–4.
10. Bower JH, Grossardt BR, Maraganore DM, et al. Anxious personality predicts an increased risk of Parkinson's disease. Mov Disord. 2010;25:2105–13.
11. Braak H, Del Tredici K, Rueb U, et al. Staging of brain pathology related to sporadic Parkinson's disease. Neurobio Aging. 2003;24:197–210.
12. Braak H, Ghebremedhin E, Rüb U, et al. Stages in the development of Parkinson's disease-related pathology. Cell Tissue Res. 2004;318:121–34.
13. Breen K, Drutyte G. Non motor symptoms of PD disease: the patients perspective. J Neural Transm. 2013;120:531–5.
14. Caparros-Lefebvre D, Golbe LI, Deramecourt V, et al. A geographical cluster of progressive supranuclear palsy in northern France. Neurology. 2015;85:1293–300.
15. Cersosimo MG, Raina GB, Pecci C, et al. Gastrointestinal manifestations in Parkinson's Disease: prevalence and occurrence before motor symptoms. J Neurol. 2013;260:1332–8.
16. Chaudhuri KR, Healy D, Schapira AHV. The non motor symptoms of PD disease. Diagnosis and management. Lancet Neurol. 2006;5:235–45.
17. Chaudhuri KR, Martinez Martin P, Schapira AHV, et al. An international multicenter pilot study of the first comprehensive self-completed non-motor symptoms questionnaire for Parkinson's disease: the NMSQuest study. Mov Disord. 2006;21(7):916–23.
18. Chaudhuri KR, Martinez-Martin P, Brown RG. The metric properties of a novel non-motor symptoms scale for Parkinson's disease: results from an international pilot study. Mov Disord. 2007
19. Chaudhuri KR, Schapira AH. Non-motor symptoms of Parkinson's disease: dopaminergic pathophysiology and treatment. Lancet Neurol. 2009;8:464–74.

20. Chaudhuri KR, Prieto-Jurcynska C, Naidu Y, et al. The nondeclaration of nonmotor symptoms of Parkinson's disease to health care professionals: an international study using the nonmotor symptoms questionnaire. Mov Disord. 2010;25:704–9.
21. Chaudhuri KR, Rojo JM, Schapira AHV, et al. A proposal for a comprehensive gradation of Parkinson's disease severity combining motor and non motor assessments: meeting the unmet need. PLoS One. 2013;8:e57221.
22. Chaudhuri K Ray, Todorova A, Nirenberg MJ, et al. A pilot prospective, multicenter observational study of dopamine withdrawal syndrome in Parkinson's disease. Mov Disord Clin Prac. 2015;2:170–174.
23. Chen H, Zhang SM, Hernan MA, et al. Weight loss in Parkinson's disease. Ann Neurol. 2003;53:676–9.
24. Chesselet MF, Richter F, Zhu C, et al. A progressive mouse model of Parkinson's disease: the Thy1-aSyn ("Line 61") mice. Neurotherapeutics. 2012;9:297–314.
25. Cubo E, Doumbe J, Martinez-Martin P, et al. Comparison of the clinical profile of Parkinson's disease between Spanish and Cameroonian cohorts. J Neurol Sci. 2014;336:122–6.
26. Diederich NJ, Pieri V, Hipp G, et al. Discriminative power of different nonmotor signs in early Parkinson's disease. A case–control study. Mov Disord. 2010;25:882–7.
27. Duty S, Jenner P. Animal models of Parkinson's disease: a source of novel treatments and clues to the cause of the disease. Br J Pharmacol. 2011;164:1357–91.
28. Erro R, Picillo M, Vitale C, et al. Non-motor symptoms in early Parkinson's disease: a 2-year follow-up study on previously untreated patients. J Neurol Neurosurg Psychiatry. 2013;84:14–7.
29. Fahn S. A new look at levodopa based on the ELLDOPA study. J Neural Transm Suppl. 2006;70:419–26.
30. Fang F, Xu Q, Park Y, et al. Depression and the subsequent risk of Parkinson's disease in the NIH-AARP Diet and Health Study. Mov Disord. 2010;25:1157–62.
31. Findley L. The economic impact of Parkinson's disease. Parkinsonism Relat Disord. 2007;13:S8e12.
32. Forno LS. Neuropathology of Parkinson's disease. J Neuropathol Exp Neurol. 1996;55:259–72.
33. Gallagher DA, Goetz CG, Stebbins G, et al. Validation of the MDS-UPDRS part 1 for nonmotor symptoms in Parkinson's disease. Mov Disord. 2012;27(1):79–83.
34. Garcia-Ruiz PJ, Chaudhuri KR, Martinez-Martin P. Non-motor symptoms of Parkinson's disease A review.from the past. J Neurol Sci. 2014;338:30–3.
35. Geo J, Huang X, Park Y, et al. Daytime napping, nighttime sleeping, and Parkinson disease. Am J Epidemiol. 2011;173:1032–8.
36. Gao X, Chen H, Schwarzschild MA, et al. Erectile function and risk of Parkinson's disease. Am J Epidemiol. 2007;166:1446–50.
37. Goetz CG, Fahn S, Martinez-Martin P, et al. Movement Disorder Society sponsored revision of the Unified Parkinson's Disease Rating Sacle (MDS-UPDRS): process, format and clinimetric testing plan. Mov Dosord. 2007;22:41–7.
38. Gulati A, Forbes A, Stegie F, et al. A clinical observational study of the pattern and occurrence of non-motor symptoms in PD disease ranging from early to advanced disease. Mov Disord. 2004;19:S406.
39. Gunal DI, Nurichalichi K, Tuncer N, et al. The clinical profile of nonmotor fluctuations in Parkinson's disease patients. Can J Neurol Sci. 2002;29:61–4.
40. Halliday GM, Blumbergs PC, Cotton RGH, et al. Loss of brainstem serotonin- and substance P-containing neurons in Parkinson's disease. Brain Res. 1990;510:104–7.
41. Halliday G, Lees A, Stern M. Milestones in Parkinson's disease-clinical and pathological features. Mov Disord. 2011;26:1015–21.
42. Hawkes CH, Del Tredici K, Braak H. Parkinson's disease: a dual-hit hypothesis. Neuropathol Appl Neurobiol. 2007;33:599–614.
43. Hawkes CH, Del Tredici K, Braak H. A timeline for Parkinson's disease. Parkinsonism Relat Disord. 2010;16:79e84.
44. Hillen ME, Sage JI. Nonmotor fluctuations in patients with Parkinson's disease. Neurology. 1996;47:1180–3.
45. Hirsch EC, Graybiel AM, Duyckaerts C, et al. Neuronal loss in the pedunculopontine tegmental nucleus in Parkinson's disease and in progressive supranuclear palsy. Proc Natl Acad Sci U S A. 1987;84:5976–80.
46. Iranzo A. Parkinson disease and sleep: sleep-wake changes in the premotor stage of Parkinson disease; impaired olfaction and other prodromal features. Curr Neurol Neurosci Rep. 2013;13:373.
47. Iwanaga K, Wakabayashi K, Yoshimoto M, et al. Lewy body-type degeneration in cardiac plexus in Parkinson's and incidental Lewy body diseases. Neurology. 1999;52:1269–71.
48. Jacob EL, Gatto NM, Thompson A, et al. Occurrence of depression and anxiety prior to Parkinson's disease. Parkinsonism Relat Disord. 2010;16:576–81.
49. Jain S, Ton TG, Perera S, et al. Cardiovascular physiology in premotor Parkinson's disease: a neuroepidemiologic study. Mov Disord. 2012;27:988–95.
50. Jellinger K. Overview of morphological changes in Parkinson's disease. Adv Neurol. 1987;45:1–18.
51. Jellinger KA. Neuropathology of sporadic PD disease: evaluation and change of concepts. Mov Disord. 2012;27:8–30.
52. Jennings D, Siderowf A, Stern M, et al. Evaluating phenoconversion to PD in the PARS prodromal cohort. Mov Disord. 2013;28:S59–60.
53. Kang SY, Ma HI, Lim YM, et al. Fatigue in drug-naïve Parkinson's disease. Eur Neurol. 2013;70:59–64.
54. Kingsbury AE, Bandopadhay R, Silveira-Moriyama L, et al. Brain stem pathology in PD disease: an evaluation of the Braak staging model. Mov Disord. 2010;25:2508–15.
55. Lin CH, Wu RM, Chang HY, et al. Preceding pain symptoms and Parkinson's disease: a nationwide

population-based cohort study. Eur J Neurol. 2013;20:1398–404.
56. Lind NM, Moustgaard A, Jelsing J, et al. The use of pigs in neuroscience: modeling brain disorders. Neurosci Biobehav Rev. 2007;31:728–51.
57. Marras C, Chaudhuri KR. Non motor features of Parkinson's disease subtypes. Mov Disord. 2016;1–8.
58. Martinez-Martin P, Rodriguez-Blazquez C, Kurtis MM, et al. The impact of non motor symptoms on health-related quality of life of patients with Parkinson's disease. Mov Disord. 2011;26:399–406.
59. Mollenhauer B, Trautmann E, Sixel-Döring F, et al. Nonmotor and diagnostic findings in subjects with de novo Parkinson disease of the DeNoPa cohort. Neurology. 2013;81:1226–34.
60. Movement Disorder Society Task Force on Rating Scales for Parkinson's Disease. The Unified Parkinson's Disease Rating Scale (UPDRS): status and recommendations. Mov Disord. 2003;18:738–50.
61. Pan-Montojo F, Anichtchik O, Dening Y, et al. Progression of Parkinson's disease pathology is reproduced by intragastric administration of Rotenone in mice. PLoS One. 2010;5:e8762.
62. Parkinson J. An essay on the shaking palsy. 1817. J Neuropsychiatry Clin Neurosci. 2002;14:223–36.
63. Parkinson's UK. Parkinson's prevalence in the United Kingdom-2009. 2012. http://www.parkinsons.org.uk/pdf/ParkinsonsprevalenceUK.pdf. Accessed 10 July 2013.
64. Perez-Lloret S, Barrantes FJ. Deficits in cholinergic neurotransmission and their clinical correlates in Parkinson's disease. NPJ Parkinson's Dis. 2016;2:1–12.
65. Politis M, Wu K, Molloys S, et al. Parkinson's disease symptoms: the patient's perspectives. Mov Disord. 2010;25:1646–51.
66. Pondal M, Marras C, Miyasaki J, et al. Clinical features of dopamine agonist withdrawal syndrome in a movement disorders clinic. J Neurol Neurosurg Psychiatry. 2013;84:130–5.
67. Pont-Sunyer C, Hotter A, Gaig C, et al. The onset of nonmotor symptoms in Parkinson's disease (the ONSET PD study). Mov Disord. 2015;30:229–37.
68. Postuma RB, Gagnon JF, Montplaisir JY. REM sleep behavior disorder and prodromal neurodegeneration—where are we headed? Tremor Other Hyperkinet Mov. 2013;3. http://tremorjournal.org/article/view/134.
69. Ray Chaudhuri K, Quinn N. What are the non-motor symptoms of Parkinson's disease. In: Ray Chaudhuri K, Tolosa E, Schapira A, Poewe W, editors. Non-motor symptoms of Parkinson's disease. Oxford: Oxford university press; 2009. p. 1–6.
70. Rabinak CA, Nirenberg MJ. Dopamine agonist withdrawal syndrome in Parkinson disease. Arch Neurol. 2010;67:58e63.
71. Rana AQ, Athar A, Owlia A, et al. Impact of ethnicity on non-motor symptoms of Parkinson's disease. J Parkinsons Dis. 2012;2:281–5.
72. Richard IH, Frank S, McDermott MP, et al. The ups and downs of Parkinson disease: a prospective study of mood and anxiety fluctuations. Cogn Behav Neurol. 2004;17:201–7.
73. Rizos A, Sauerbier A, Antonini A, et al. A European multicentre survey of impulse control behaviours in Parkinson's disease patients treated with short- and long-acting dopamine agonists. Eur J Neurol. 2016;1–7.
74. Sakakibara R, Tateno F, Kishi M, Tsuyusaki Y, Terada H, Inaoka T. MIBG myocardial scintigraphy in premotor Parkinson's disease: a review. Parkinsonism Relat Disord. 2014;20:267–73.
75. Sauerbier A, Ray Chaudhuri K. Non-motor symptoms: the core of multi-morbid Parkinson's disease. Br J Hosp Med (Lond). 2014;75:18–24.
76. Sauerbier A, Barretto M, Singhal B, et al. Non motor symptoms profile in black and south Asian minority ethnic subjects compared to white Caucasians with Parkinson's disease: A prospective multicentre comparative study between London South and India [abstract]. Mov Disord. 2014;29:1060.
77. Sauerbier A, Jenner P, Todorova A, et al. Non motor subtypes and Parkinson's disease. Parkinsonism Relat Disord. 2016;22:41–6.
78. Saper CB, Sorrentino DM, German DC, et al. Medullary catecholaminergic neurons in the normal human brain and Parkinson's disease. Ann Neurol. 1991;29:577–84.
79. Schenck CH, Boeve BF, Mahowald MW. Delayed emergence of a parkinsonian disorder or dementia in 81% of older men initially diagnosed with idiopathic rapid eye movement sleep behavior disorder: a 16-year update on a previously reported series. Sleep Med. 2013;14:744–8.
80. Schrag A, Sauerbier A, Chaudhuri KR, et al. New clinical trials for non-motor manifestations of Parkinson's disease. Mov Disord. 2015;30:11490–504.
81. Seki M, Takahashi K, Uematsu D, et al. Clinical features and varieties of non-motor fluctuations in Parkinson's disease: a Japanese multicenter study. Parkinsonism Relat Disord. 2013;19:104–8.
82. Seppi K, Weintraub D, Coelho M, et al. The Movement Disorder Society Evidence-Based Medicine Review Update: Treatments for the non-motor symptoms of Parkinson's disease. Mov Disord. 2011;26:S42–80.
83. Sixel-Döring F, Trautmann E, Mollenhauer B, Trenkwalder C. Rapid eye movement sleep behavioral events: a new marker for neurodegeneration in early Parkinson Disease? Sleep. 2014;37:431–8.
84. Stacy MA, Murck H, Kroenke K. Responsiveness of motor and nonmotor symptoms of Parkinson disease to dopaminergic therapy. Prog Neuropsychopharmacol Biol Psychiatry. 2010;34:57–61.
85. Stern MB, Lang A, Poewe W. Toward a redefinition of Parkinson's disease. Mov Disord . 2012;27:54–60.

86. Storch A, Schneider CB, Wolz M, et al. Nonmotor fluctuations in Parkinson disease: severity and correlation with motor complications. Neurology. 2013;80:800–9.
87. Todorova A, Jenner P, Ray CK. Non-motor Parkinson's: integral to motor Parkinson's, yet often neglected. Pract Neurol. 2014;14:310–22.
88. Tolosa E, Pont-Sunyer C. Progress in defining the premotor phase of Parkinson's disease. J Neurol Sci. 2011;310:4–8.
89. Van der Marck MA, Munneke M, Mulleners W, et al. Integrated multidisciplinary care in Parkinson's disease: a non-randomised, controlled trial (IMPACT). Lancet Neurol. 2013;12:947–56.
90. Voon V, Fox SH. Medication-related impulse control and repetitive behaviors in Parkinson disease. Arch Neurol. 2007;64:1089–96.
91. Wakabayashi K, Takahashi H. The intermediolateral nucleus and Clarke's column in Parkinson's disease. Acta Neuropathol(Berl). 1997;94:287–9.
92. Weintraub D, Koester J, Potenza MN, et al. Impulse control disorders in Parkinson disease: a cross-sectional study of 3090 patients. Arch Neurol. 2010;67:589–95.
93. Weisskoft MG, Chen H, Schwarzschild MA, et al. Prospective study of phobic anxiety and risk of Parkinson's disease. Mov Disord. 2003;18:646–51.
94. Winge K, Fowler CJ. Bladder dysfunction in Parkinsonism: mechanisms, prevalence, symptoms, and management. Mov Disord. 2006;21:737–45.
95. Witjas T, Kaphan E, Azulay JP, et al. Nonmotor fluctuations in Parkinson's disease: frequent and disabling. Neurology. 2002;59:408–13.
96. Zesiewicz TA, Sullivan KL, Arnulf I, et al. Practice parameter: treatment of nonmotor symptoms of Parkinson disease. Report of the quality standards subcommittee of the American academy of neurology. Neurology. 2010;74:924e31.
97. Zis P, Rizos A, Martinez-Martin P. Non-Motor Symptoms profile and burden in drug naïve versus long-term Parkinson's disease patients. J Parkinsons Dis. 2014;4:541–7.
98. Zis P, Erro R, Walton CC, et al. The range and nature of non-motor symptoms in drug-naive Parkinson's disease patients: a state-of-the-art systematic review. NPJ Parkinson's Dis. 2015;1:1–8.

The Natural History of Parkinson's Disease

13

Miguel Coelho and Joaquim J. Ferreira

13.1 Introduction

Parkinson's disease (PD) is a neurodegenerative disorder associated with neuronal loss of the dopaminergic neurons of the substantia nigra (SN) pars compacta [1], but extranigral pathology of the cholinergic, noradrenergic and serotonergic systems have also been well documented [1–3]. At the onset of motor signs in PD, it has been estimated that about two-thirds of cell loss in the lateral ventral tier of the SN pars compacta (SNc) has already occurred [4], and the occurrence of a presymptomatic phase of 5 years is also suggested according to the curve of cell loss in the SN [4, 5]. Clinically, cardinal manifestations of PD are characterised by the presence of asymmetric or even unilateral bradykinesia, rest tremor and rigidity, and postural instability later in the disease course [6, 7]. Classically, the natural history of PD has been regarded as the progression in severity of motor symptoms and the emergence of levodopa-induced motor complications (MC) [6]; however, non-motor symptoms (NMS) of PD, such as dementia, depression, psychosis or dysautonomia, are now well accepted as important features of PD, and they have changed the way we regard the natural history of PD [8–10].

Some of these NMS, notably hyposmia, REM sleep behaviour disorder (RBD), constipation or depression, may manifest before the onset of motor symptoms, sometimes even for decades [11]. Several studies have shown that their presence in individuals without parkinsonism increase the odds for PD, which is in accordance with pathological data [1, 12–19]. This has heralded the emergence of a new nomenclature, such as prodromal and premotor PD, which will be discussed below, and the need for a new definition of PD [20]. On the opposite extreme of the disease course, studies have found that NMS increase in frequency and severity with disease progression and that NMS together with axial motor symptoms are the ones that most impact on the disability of patients and are strong predictors of both institutionalisation and death [21].

In the last decade, major breakthroughs have been made in understanding the genetic causes of

M. Coelho, MD (✉)
Neurology Service, Department of Neurosciences and Clinical Pharmacology Unit, Instituto de Medicina Molecular, Hospital de Santa Maria, Avenida Professor Egas Moniz, 1649-028 Lisbon, Portugal
e-mail: migcoelho2002@yahoo.es

J.J. Ferreira, MD, PhD
Neurology Service, Department of Neurosciences and Clinical Pharmacology Unit, Instituto de Medicina Molecular, Hospital de Santa Maria, Avenida Professor Egas Moniz, 1649-028 Lisbon, Portugal

Laboratório de Farmacologia Clínica e Terapêutica, Faculdade de Medicina de Lisboa, Av. Prof. Egas Moniz, Lisboa 1649-028, Portugal
e-mail: joaquimjfereira@gmail.com

C. Falup-Pecurariu et al. (eds.), *Movement Disorders Curricula*,
DOI 10.1007/978-3-7091-1628-9_13

PD [22, 23], questioning the use of the terminology *idiopathic* PD. Some forms of monogenic PD have distinct clinical features and disease progression, and the same heterogeneity is found in the different subtypes of sporadic PD, which might make it difficult and misleading to describe a one-size-fits-all model for the natural history of PD [24, 25].

On the other hand, in the post-levodopa era, it is almost impossible to disentangle the history of PD from its pharmacological treatment with levodopa (L-dopa) [26]. The development of levodopa-induced MC is a distinctive marker of PD [27], making it no longer accurate to talk about a *natural* history of PD but instead a mixed *natural plus pharmacological* history of PD.

13.2 Prodromal Parkinson's Disease

Substantial and fast increasing data, either epidemiological, clinical, imagiological, genetic or pathological, show that biological changes that are specific to PD occur before the onset of motor symptoms of PD [28]. These individuals cannot be diagnosed with PD according to current clinical criteria because they (still) lack the traditional motor signs of PD [28, 29]. Different designations have been used to name these individuals. An expert meeting held in 2011 tried to put order on this growing field of research [28]. Individuals with prodromal or premotor PD (the time before the onset of clinical apparent classical motor symptoms of PD) can be divided into different stages according to the presence of certain clinical, imagiological, physiological and pathological features as well as risk markers for PD [30]. A hierarchical pyramid classifying these individuals without clinical PD has been suggested and is termed *Parkinson's disease at risk syndrome* (PARS) [30–32]: prodromal PD is divided into four stages that consist of (1) pre-diagnostic phase, (2) premotor phase, (3) preclinical phase and (4) pre-physiological phase.

In the pre-diagnostic phase, patients manifest the classic features of PD, but they do not fulfil the clinical criteria for PD yet; these individuals manifest mild motor signs of parkinsonism [30]. In the next premotor phase, individuals do not show the classic motor signs of PD, but they manifest NMS that have been shown to antedate the motor features of PD, such as RBD or hyposmia [30]. These NMS have distinct predictive values for the future development of PD [30]. In the preclinical phase, individuals are asymptomatic regarding either motor or non-motor features of PD; nevertheless, they show biological changes with a certain specificity for PD which can be detected using biomarkers techniques [30]. These techniques can be functional imaging of the brain to detect depletion of dopamine (DAT SPECT or [18f]-fluorodopa PET), functional imaging of the heart to detect sympathetic denervation ((metaiodobenzylguanidine (MIBG) SPECT)), structural imaging of the brainstem to detect an increased area of echogenicity in the SN (transcranial ultrasound of the midbrain) or pathology of peripheral tissue such as autonomic enteric nervous system to detect Lewy pathology (biopsy of peripheral tissue) [30]. In the pre-physiological phase, individuals have no signs of disease, neither clinically nor biologically detectable; instead, they have traits such as genetic mutations or environmental exposures that increase the odds of developing PD in the future [30].

In prodromal PD, the NMS that have been most robustly associated with PD are the presence of RBD, hyposmia, constipation and depression [12–19]. The presence of RBD is the strongest clinical predictor of developing an alpha-synucleinopathy such as PD, dementia with Lewy bodies (DLB) or multiple system atrophy (MSA) [15, 33]. The risk of conversion from idiopathic RBD to a neurodegenerative disease is between 40 and 65 % at 10 years, with one-half developing parkinsonism and the other half dementia [33]. The specificity of RBD in diagnosing prodromal PD is high, although sensitivity is low as only 50 % of PD patients have RBD [34]. On the contrary, olfactory defect has the highest sensitivity, being present in >80 % of PD patients, but its specificity is low [35, 36]. Similarly, constipation has a moderate-high sensitivity to detect PD, although its specificity is also low [18, 37]. A longitudinal study found an odds ratio (OR) of 2.3 for PD in those individuals reporting <1 bowel movement per day compared to those with ≥1 bowel movements per day [18]. Depression is present in 30–40 % of PD patients but is also present in 30 % of the general population, yielding a low sensitivity and specificity, although one study showed an OR of 2.4 for the association of PD with premorbid depression [38]. These NMS have distinct time profiles of manifestation before the onset of motor symptoms PD, some reports dating back their onset even for decades before motor symptoms [11].

Likewise clinical symptoms, pathological and imaging studies have also found evidence for PD-specific changes starting before the onset of motor parkinsonism [39, 40]. In a recent observational study from the PARS cohort, DAT imaging using [^{123}I]β-CIT SPECT found a significant deficit in 11 % of hyposmic healthy individuals compared to 1 % of normosmic subjects [41]. Combining hyposmia to male sex and the presence of constipation increased the frequency of dopaminergic deficit to more than 40 % in hyposmic subjects [41]. Asymptomatic individuals may display compensatory mechanisms to this dopamine deficit, as suggested by the finding that *LRRK2* asymptomatic mutation carriers have increased grey matter volume of the cuneus compared to healthy controls [42]. In this study, *LRRK2* asymptomatic mutation carriers also had hyperechogenicity of the SN using transcranial sonography, adding evidence to the presence of morphological PD-specific changes in the premotor stages of the disease [42]. In a cohort of healthy subjects 50 years or above, the PRIPS study found that SN hyperechogenicity at baseline had 82.4 % sensitivity and 82.5 % specificity for the diagnosis of PD at 5 years follow-up [43]. Premotor changes in the central and peripheral nervous system have also been documented in post-mortem studies [39, 44]. Autopsy findings of Lewy body pathology (LP) in individuals without clinical manifest parkinsonism suggest that these incidental Lewy bodies\neurites are markers of prodromal PD [39]. The term incidental Lewy body disease (ILBD) refers to the presence of LP in the same type of neurons and in the same areas of the nervous system as those usually encountered in patients with clinically manifest PD [1, 45]. The significance of ILBD as premotor markers of PD is stronger when found in the autopsy of individuals without motor parkinsonism but already manifesting premotor symptoms, as recently reported [44]. Iranzo et al. reported a patient with RBD who developed depression, mild cognitive impairment, constipation, hyposmia and dopamine deficit in DAT imaging for a 10-year period but in whom parkinsonism was always absent; in autopsy, neuronal loss and LP were found in the peripheral autonomic nervous system and in various brain regions, including the CNS [44].

13.3 Early and Intermediate Parkinson's Disease

PD is an heterogeneous disorder, namely in its presenting motor syndrome [46–48]. Age at disease onset is a strong determinant of the presenting clinical features and disease course [46–48]. Younger onset PD patients, regardless their genetic status, have more dystonia at onset and during treatment, have less tremor and gait difficulties at onset, have a better response to L-dopa and develop more levodopa-induced dyskinesias and seem to have a lower rate of dementia and disease progression [25, 46–50]. Depending on the dominant motor features, different phenotypic subtypes of PD have been identified [25, 51–53]. Nomenclatures vary between reports, but the usual described motor phenotypes are tremor-dominant, akinetic-rigid and mixed phenotypes or tremor-dominant versus postural instability and gait disorder phenotype (PIGD), with better outcomes being associated with the tremor-dominant phenotype [25, 50, 52, 53]. In the early and intermediate phases of PD, the presence of NMS has been well documented, even in recently diagnosed cases, and they affect all domains of NMS [21, 54–57].

Despite clinical heterogeneity at presentation, clinical criteria for the diagnosis of PD has been developed and validated, the most widely used being the Queen Square Brain Bank Criteria [58]. The presence of unequivocal bradykinesia is mandatory for the diagnosis, defined as slowness of the initiation of voluntary movement with progressive reduction in speed and amplitude in repetitive actions [59]. Although various tremor types exist in PD, the most typical is a slow pill-rolling rest tremor of the hands (4–6 Hz) [59]. Other component of parkinsonism is rigidity, which is a resistance felt when moving the patient's relaxed limb, classically described as "lead pipe." The typical parkinsonian gait consists of small shuffling steps, usually with associated reduced arm swing, whereas postural instability tends to occur later in the disease course and results in falls in many instances. The onset of PD is gradual and asymmetrical or even unilateral, and patients have a good and sustained response to L-dopa [59]. Functional neuroimaging using [^{123}I]β-CIT SPECT depicts reduced striatal uptake of the dopamine transporter radioligand, usually asymmetrical. However, about 10 % of patients enrolled in clinical trials and diagnosed with early PD were found to have normal DAT scans (SWEDDS – scans without evidence of dopaminergic deficit), some of whom might have been misdiagnosed with dystonic tremor [60, 61].

The progression of PD is non-linear, with a more pronounced rate of deterioration of motor scores in patients with shorter disease duration and lower motor impairment at baseline, although considerable variability exists between individuals [62, 63]. Annual decline of motor scores in patients randomised to the placebo arm in several clinical trials is between 8–11 and 5–7 points in the UPDRS total and motor section, respectively [63]. The progression of PD is also characterised by the development of levodopa-induced MC in a substantial number of patients. The presence of MC has been widely regarded as heralding the onset of the advanced stage of PD.

13.4 Advanced Parkinson's Disease

Although not consensual, the definition of *advanced stage* PD is usually anchored on the severity of motor symptoms, the presence of postural instability or the emergence of levodopa-induced MC [6, 64, 65]. According to the Hoehn and Yahr scale (HY), which staged parkinsonism into five stages depending on the severity of motor impairment and the presence of postural instability, advanced PD is usually defined as stages 4 and 5 (loss of physical independence) [6]. However, reaching HY stage 3 (loss of balance) is of critical importance, as it has been associated with a poorer prognosis, namely, a higher risk of dementia and mortality [66]. The emergence of levodopa-induced MC, or at least troublesome MC, is an alternative definition for *advanced PD* [64]. The majority of PD patients will develop levodopa-induced MC after an initial phase of sustained and smooth response to dopaminergic drugs [64, 67, 68]. The frequency of MC vary considerably depending on the instrument used to capture the event, the type of PD patients, the design of the study, the length of follow-up and the drugs used to treat parkinsonism. Nevertheless, Ahlskog and Muenter have found an overall frequency of MC of about 40 % after 4–6 years of L-dopa treatment [67]. L-dopa substantially increases the risk of MC compared to other antiparkinsonian agents; however, this difference and its clinical importance might dilute over time [69, 70]. The frequency of MC also increases with disease duration and severity, and they are a major source of disability for patients and caregivers, and they negatively impact on the quality of life (QoL) and the independence for performing the activities of daily living (ADL) [64, 71]. Additionally, the treatment of MC adds complexity to the drug regimen of PD patients, causing an extra burden for patients, caregivers and treating physicians. In fact, MC are the major indication for advanced therapies in the management of PD, such as functional surgery and apomorphine and levodopa/carbidopa intestinal gel pumps. MC consist of motor fluctuations (MF) and dyskinesias; MF are characterised by a shortage of the clinical response to each L-dopa dose, leading the patients to alternate between periods of good motor function (on period) and others of bad motor function (off period) [72]. MF manifest as different phenomena, such as the predictable waning of the effect of L-dopa after a certain amount of time (wearing off), the increase in time to the start of L-dopa effect (delayed-on) or the sudden and unpredictable loss of L-dopa action (sudden off) [72]. On the other hand, dyskinesias refer to the presence of abnormal involuntary movements, which may happen at the peak of L-dopa effect (peak dose dyskinesias), during the onset or offset of L-dopa action (respectively, begin of dose and end of dose dyskinesias, or diphasic if both present) or during the off period (off-period dystonia) [68, 72]. In a similar way to motor symptoms, NMS may fluctuate with levodopa response. Non-motor fluctuations (NMF) are frequent and disabling in patients with levodopa-induced MF, and most NMS seem worse in off compared to on [73–76]. The most frequent NMF are neuropsychiatric, especially anxiety, autonomic and fatigue [73–76], and one study found that the overall number of NMF correlated with motor disability [74]. More recently, Tolosa and Katzenschlager [77] defined *advanced stage* as those patients manifesting the cardinal motor symptoms of PD, associated with motor and non-motor complications, either disease related (e.g. freezing) or drug induced (e.g. fluctuations or hallucinations).

Besides MC, PD patients in advanced stage also manifest several NMS and axial motor features resistant to L-dopa such as postural instability, falls and dysphagia, which increase in frequency and severity with longer disease duration [21, 55, 69, 73, 78, 79]. L-dopa-resistant symptoms, either axial motor or NMS, become the dominant features of PD in advanced stage, having a stronger impact on disability and QoL compared with L-dopa-responsive motor symptoms or MC, emerging as the strongest independent predictors of nursing home placement and death [6, 73, 80–83]. Even when comparing the disability caused by levodopa-induced fluctuations, NMF are rated by 17.5–30 % of patients as more disabling than MF [74, 75]. Regarding the relative frequency of NMS, both longitudinal and cross-sectional studies give largely a similar hierarchic order. With slight differences between studies, the most frequent reported NMS are anxiety, depression, fatigue, urinary dysfunction, attention and memory deficit, hallucinations, excessive daytime sleepiness, postural hypotension, constipation, pain and apathy [8, 9, 21, 73]. NMS tend to progress together with axial symptoms [84, 85], and it has been shown that the association of cognitive impairment, psychosis, depression, daytime sleepiness, autonomic dysfunction and axial symptoms is strongly correlated with PD progression [21, 86]. Indeed, Kempster et al. found that four major events, visual hallucinations, falls, dementia and institutionalisation, which the authors designated by disability milestones, clustered together in the later phase of PD, preceding death by 5 years on average [81, 82]. Indeed, axial motor symptoms has been identified as an independent risk factors for the occurrence of major NMS in advanced PD, such as psychosis, dementia and dysautonomia [87, 88]. Similarly, some NMS are risk factors for the emergence of other NMS, such as fatigue increasing the risk for depression, anxiety, apathy and sleep disorders, and psychosis or apathy increasing the risk for dementia [88–91]. The sequence of events reported by Kempster et al. is independent of age of PD onset, disease duration or age at death [81, 82]. On the other hand, deep brain stimulation (DBS) has been a major step forward in the treatment of levodopa-induced MC, and overall its benefit is maintained in the long term [92–94]. However, even though DBS is also effective in treating NMS, it does not avoid the emergence of these disability milestones that ultimately determine the health status of patients in later stages [75, 80, 94].

The subset of patients progressing to this later phase of PD is highly disabled due to motor symptoms or NMS that are resistant to L-dopa and thus do not fulfil the usual definition of *advanced stage* (disabling levodopa-induced MC), although generally classified under the umbrella of *advanced stage PD* [10, 73, 80, 95, 96]. They present with a distinct phenotype, and we have recently proposed the term late-stage PD to refer to these patients who are highly dependent on caregivers for ADL owing to motor symptoms or NMS that are resistant to L-dopa, in whom MC are no longer the most disabling symptom [10].

Most data indicates that PD is associated with increased mortality (mortality ratios 0.9–3.8 compared with matched control populations), although considerable heterogeneity exists between studies [97, 98]. If calculation of mortality ratios is restricted to inception cohorts with low heterogeneity, the mortality ratio is 1.41 (95% CI, 1.28–1.55) [97]. A systematic review found a decrease in survival of 5% per year of follow-up, with mean disease duration at death ranging from 6.9 to 14.3 years in post-mortem studies, although heterogeneity between studies precluded performing a meta-analysis [97]. Studies from longer ago and with older age at recruitment predicted shorter survival, while older age at disease onset and dementia were the factors most consistently associated with increased death [97].

Conclusion

Recent data indicates that the natural history of PD starts well before the onset of motor cardinal features. The course of PD after motor onset and initiation of antiparkinsonian therapy is modulated by pharmacological agents and more recently by DBS, but considerable difference in disease progression exists between different subtypes of PD. Mortality is increased about 1.5 times that of control population in inception cohorts, and older age at onset and dementia are consistently associated with increased mortality.

References

1. Braak H, Del Tredici K, Rub U, de Vos RA, Jansen Steur EN, Braak E. Staging of brain pathology related to sporadic Parkinson's disease. Neurobiol Aging. 2003;24(2):197–211.
2. Schapira AH, Bezard E, Brotchie J, Calon F, Collingridge GL, Ferger B, et al. Novel pharmacological targets for the treatment of Parkinson's disease. Nat Rev Drug Discov. 2006;5(10):845–54.
3. Brooks DJ. Imaging non-dopaminergic function in Parkinson's disease. Mol Imaging Biol. 2007;9(4):217–22.
4. Fearnley JM, Lees AJ. Ageing and Parkinson's disease: substantia nigra regional selectivity. Brain. 1991;114(Pt 5):2283–301.
5. Greffard S, Verny M, Bonnet AM, Beinis JY, Gallinari C, Meaume S, et al. Motor score of the Unified Parkinson Disease Rating Scale as a good predictor of Lewy body-associated neuronal loss in the substantia nigra. Arch Neurol. 2006;63(4):584–8.
6. Hoehn MM, Yahr MD. Parkinsonism: onset, progression and mortality. Neurology. 1967;17(5):427–42.
7. Martin WE, Loewenson RB, Resch JA, Baker AB. Parkinson's disease. Clinical analysis of 100 patients. Neurology. 1973;23(8):783–90.
8. Chaudhuri KR, Martinez-Martin P, Schapira AH, Stocchi F, Sethi K, Odin P, et al. International multicenter pilot study of the first comprehensive self-completed nonmotor symptoms questionnaire for Parkinson's disease: the NMSQuest study. Mov Disord. 2006;21(7):916–23.
9. Martinez-Martin P, Schapira AH, Stocchi F, Sethi K, Odin P, MacPhee G, et al. Prevalence of nonmotor symptoms in Parkinson's disease in an international setting; study using nonmotor symptoms questionnaire in 545 patients. Mov Disord. 2007;22(11):1623–9.
10. Coelho M, Ferreira JJ. Late-stage Parkinson disease. Nat Rev Neurol. 2012;8(8):435–42.
11. Claassen DO, Josephs KA, Ahlskog JE, Silber MH, Tippmann-Peikert M, Boeve BF. REM sleep behavior disorder preceding other aspects of synucleinopathies by up to half a century. Neurology. 2010;75(6):494–9.
12. Berg D, Godau J, Seppi K, Behnke S, Liepelt-Scarfone I, Lerche S, et al. The PRIPS study: screening battery for subjects at risk for Parkinson's disease. Eur J Neurol. 2013;20(1):102–8.
13. Diederich NJ, Pieri V, Hipp G, Rufra O, Blyth S, Vaillant M. Discriminative power of different nonmotor signs in early Parkinson's disease. A case-control study. Mov Disord. 2010;25(7):882–7.
14. Iranzo A, Stockner H, Serradell M, Seppi K, Valldeoriola F, Frauscher B, et al. Five-year follow-up of substantia nigra echogenicity in idiopathic REM sleep behavior disorder. Mov Disord. 2014;29(14):1774–80.
15. Iranzo A, Fernandez-Arcos A, Tolosa E, Serradell M, Molinuevo JL, Valldeoriola F, et al. Neurodegenerative disorder risk in idiopathic REM sleep behavior disorder: study in 174 patients. PLoS One. 2014;9(2):e89741.
16. Ross GW, Petrovitch H, Abbott RD, Tanner CM, Popper J, Masaki K, et al. Association of olfactory dysfunction with risk for future Parkinson's disease. Ann Neurol. 2008;63(2):167–73.
17. Abbott RD, Ross GW, White LR, Tanner CM, Masaki KH, Nelson JS, et al. Excessive daytime sleepiness and subsequent development of Parkinson disease. Neurology. 2005;65(9):1442–6.
18. Abbott RD, Petrovitch H, White LR, Masaki KH, Tanner CM, Curb JD, et al. Frequency of bowel movements and the future risk of Parkinson's disease. Neurology. 2001;57(3):456–62.
19. Leentjens AF, Van den Akker M, Metsemakers JF, Lousberg R, Verhey FR. Higher incidence of depression preceding the onset of Parkinson's disease: a register study. Mov Disord. 2003;18(4):414–8.

20. Berg D, Postuma RB, Bloem B, Chan P, Dubois B, Gasser T, et al. Time to redefine PD? Introductory statement of the MDS Task Force on the definition of Parkinson's disease. Mov Disord. 2014;29(4):454–62.
21. Barone P, Antonini A, Colosimo C, Marconi R, Morgante L, Avarello TP, et al. The PRIAMO study: a multicenter assessment of nonmotor symptoms and their impact on quality of life in Parkinson's disease. Mov Disord. 2009;24(11):1641–9.
22. Healy DG, Falchi M, O'Sullivan SS, Bonifati V, Durr A, Bressman S, et al. Phenotype, genotype, and worldwide genetic penetrance of LRRK2-associated Parkinson's disease: a case-control study. Lancet Neurol. 2008;7(7):583–90.
23. Correia Guedes L, Ferreira JJ, Rosa MM, Coelho M, Bonifati V, Sampaio C. Worldwide frequency of G2019S LRRK2 mutation in Parkinson's disease: a systematic review. Parkinsonism Relat Disord. 2010;16(4):237–42.
24. Brock mann K, Srulijes K, Pflederer S, Hauser AK, Schulte C, Maetzler W, et al. GBA-associated Parkinson's disease: reduced survival and more rapid progression in a prospective longitudinal study. Mov Disord. Mov Disord. 2015;30(3):407–11.
25. Thenganatt MA, Jankovic J. Parkinson disease subtypes. JAMA Neurol. 2014;71(4):499–504.
26. Cotzias GC. L-Dopa for Parkinsonism. N Engl J Med. 1968;278(11):630.
27. Marsden CD, Parkes JD. "On-off" effects in patients with Parkinson's disease on chronic levodopa therapy. Lancet. 1976;1(7954):292–6.
28. Berg D, Poewe W. Can we define "pre-motor" Parkinson's disease? Mov Disord. 2012;27(5):595–6.
29. Hughes AJ, Daniel SE, Kilford L, Lees AJ. Accuracy of clinical diagnosis of idiopathic Parkinson's disease: a clinico-pathological study of 100 cases. J Neurol Neurosurg Psychiatry. 1992;55(3):181–4.
30. Siderowf A, Lang AE. Premotor Parkinson's disease: concepts and definitions. Mov Disord. 2012;27(5):608–16.
31. Siderowf A, Stern MB. Preclinical diagnosis of Parkinson's disease: are we there yet? Curr Neurol Neurosci Rep. 2006;6(4):295–301.
32. Stern MB. The preclinical detection of Parkinson's disease: ready for prime time? Ann Neurol. 2004;56(2):169–71.
33. Postuma RB, Gagnon JF, Vendette M, Fantini ML, Massicotte-Marquez J, Montplaisir J. Quantifying the risk of neurodegenerative disease in idiopathic REM sleep behavior disorder. Neurology. 2009;72(15):1296–300.
34. Gagnon JF, Postuma RB, Mazza S, Doyon J, Montplaisir J. Rapid-eye-movement sleep behaviour disorder and neurodegenerative diseases. Lancet Neurol. 2006;5(5):424–32.
35. Doty RL, Stern MB, Pfeiffer C, Gollomp SM, Hurtig HI. Bilateral olfactory dysfunction in early stage treated and untreated idiopathic Parkinson's disease. J Neurol Neurosurg Psychiatry. 1992;55(2):138–42.
36. Hawkes CH, Shephard BC, Daniel SE. Olfactory dysfunction in Parkinson's disease. J Neurol Neurosurg Psychiatry. 1997;62(5):436–46.
37. Savica R, Carlin JM, Grossardt BR, Bower JH, Ahlskog JE, Maraganore DM, et al. Medical records documentation of constipation preceding Parkinson disease: a case-control study. Neurology. 2009;73(21):1752–8.
38. Reijnders JS, Ehrt U, Weber WE, Aarsland D, Leentjens AF. A systematic review of prevalence studies of depression in Parkinson's disease. Mov Disord. 2008;23(2):183–9. quiz 313.
39. Dickson DW, Fujishiro H, DelleDonne A, Menke J, Ahmed Z, Klos KJ, et al. Evidence that incidental Lewy body disease is pre-symptomatic Parkinson's disease. Acta Neuropathol. 2008;115(4):437–44.
40. Marek KL, Seibyl JP, Zoghbi SS, Zea-Ponce Y, Baldwin RM, Fussell B, et al. [123I] beta-CIT/SPECT imaging demonstrates bilateral loss of dopamine transporters in hemi-Parkinson's disease. Neurology. 1996;46(1):231–7.
41. Jennings D, Siderowf A, Stern M, Seibyl J, Eberly S, Oakes D, et al. Imaging prodromal Parkinson disease: the Parkinson Associated Risk Syndrome Study. Neurology. Neurology. 2014;83(19):1739–46.
42. Brockmann K, Groger A, Di Santo A, Liepelt I, Schulte C, Klose U, et al. Clinical and brain imaging characteristics in leucine-rich repeat kinase 2-associated PD and asymptomatic mutation carriers. Mov Disord. 2011;26(13):2335–42.
43. Berg D, Behnke S, Seppi K, Godau J, Lerche S, Mahlknecht P, et al. Enlarged hyperechogenic substantia nigra as a risk marker for Parkinson's disease. Mov Disord. 2013;28(2):216–9.
44. Iranzo A, Gelpi E, Tolosa E, Molinuevo JL, Serradell M, Gaig C, et al. Neuropathology of prodromal Lewy body disease. Mov Disord. 2014;29(3):410–5.
45. Iwanaga K, Wakabayashi K, Yoshimoto M, Tomita I, Satoh H, Takashima H, et al. Lewy body-type degeneration in cardiac plexus in Parkinson's and incidental Lewy body diseases. Neurology. 1999;52(6):1269–71.
46. Lewis SJ, Foltynie T, Blackwell AD, Robbins TW, Owen AM, Barker RA. Heterogeneity of Parkinson's disease in the early clinical stages using a data driven approach. J Neurol Neurosurg Psychiatry. 2005;76(3):343–8.
47. Wickremaratchi MM, Knipe MD, Sastry BS, Morgan E, Jones A, Salmon R, et al. The motor phenotype of Parkinson's disease in relation to age at onset. Mov Disord. 2011;26(3):457–63.
48. Szewczyk-Krolikowski K, Tomlinson P, Nithi K, Wade-Martins R, Talbot K, Ben-Shlomo Y, et al. The influence of age and gender on motor and non-motor features of early Parkinson's disease: initial findings from the Oxford Parkinson Disease Center (OPDC) discovery cohort. Parkinsonism Relat Disord. 2014;20(1):99–105.
49. Foltynie T, Brayne CE, Robbins TW, Barker RA. The cognitive ability of an incident cohort of Parkinson's patients in the UK. The CamPaIGN study. Brain. 2004;127(Pt 3):550–60.

50. Post B, Muslimovic D, van Geloven N, Speelman JD, Schmand B, de Haan RJ. Progression and prognostic factors of motor impairment, disability and quality of life in newly diagnosed Parkinson's disease. Mov Disord. 2011;26(3):449–56.
51. van Rooden SM, Colas F, Martinez-Martin P, Visser M, Verbaan D, Marinus J, et al. Clinical subtypes of Parkinson's disease. Mov Disord. 2011;26(1):51–8.
52. Jankovic J, McDermott M, Carter J, Gauthier S, Goetz C, Golbe L, et al. Variable expression of Parkinson's disease: a base-line analysis of the DATATOP cohort. The Parkinson Study Group. Neurology. 1990;40(10):1529–34.
53. Marras C, Lang A. Parkinson's disease subtypes: lost in translation? J Neurol Neurosurg Psychiatry. 2013;84(4):409–15.
54. Williams-Gray CH, Evans JR, Goris A, Foltynie T, Ban M, Robbins TW, et al. The distinct cognitive syndromes of Parkinson's disease: 5 year follow-up of the CamPaIGN cohort. Brain. 2009;132(Pt 11):2958–69.
55. Riedel O, Klotsche J, Spottke A, Deuschl G, Forstl H, Henn F, et al. Frequency of dementia, depression, and other neuropsychiatric symptoms in 1,449 outpatients with Parkinson's disease. J Neurol. 2010;257(7):1073–82.
56. Aarsland D, Bronnick K, Alves G, Tysnes OB, Pedersen KF, Ehrt U, et al. The spectrum of neuropsychiatric symptoms in patients with early untreated Parkinson's disease. J Neurol Neurosurg Psychiatry. 2009;80(8):928–30.
57. O'Sullivan SS, Williams DR, Gallagher DA, Massey LA, Silveira-Moriyama L, Lees AJ. Nonmotor symptoms as presenting complaints in Parkinson's disease: a clinicopathological study. Mov Disord. 2008;23(1):101–6.
58. Hughes AJ, Ben-Shlomo Y, Daniel SE, Lees AJ. What features improve the accuracy of clinical diagnosis in Parkinson's disease: a clinicopathologic study. 1992. Neurology. 2001;57(10 Suppl 3):S34–8.
59. Lees AJ, Hardy J, Revesz T. Parkinson's disease. Lancet. 2009;373(9680):2055–66.
60. Scherfler C, Schwarz J, Antonini A, Grosset D, Valldeoriola F, Marek K, et al. Role of DAT-SPECT in the diagnostic work up of parkinsonism. Mov Disord. 2007;22(9):1229–38.
61. Schneider SA, Edwards MJ, Mir P, Cordivari C, Hooker J, Dickson J, et al. Patients with adult-onset dystonic tremor resembling parkinsonian tremor have scans without evidence of dopaminergic deficit (SWEDDs). Mov Disord. 2007;22(15):2210–5.
62. Schrag A, Dodel R, Spottke A, Bornschein B, Siebert U, Quinn NP. Rate of clinical progression in Parkinson's disease. A prospective study. Mov Disord. 2007;22(7):938–45.
63. Poewe W, Mahlknecht P. The clinical progression of Parkinson's disease. Parkinsonism Relat Disord. 2009;15 Suppl 4:S28–32.
64. Obeso JA, Rodriguez-Oroz MC, Chana P, Lera G, Rodriguez M, Olanow CW. The evolution and origin of motor complications in Parkinson's disease. Neurology. 2000;55(11 Suppl 4):S13–20. discussion S1–3.
65. Goetz CG, Poewe W, Rascol O, Sampaio C, Stebbins GT, Counsell C, et al. Movement Disorder Society Task Force report on the Hoehn and Yahr staging scale: status and recommendations. Mov Disord. 2004;19(9):1020–8.
66. Roos RA, Jongen JC, van der Velde EA. Clinical course of patients with idiopathic Parkinson's disease. Mov Disord. 1996;11(3):236–42.
67. Ahlskog JE, Muenter MD. Frequency of levodopa-related dyskinesias and motor fluctuations as estimated from the cumulative literature. Mov Disord. 2001;16(3):448–58.
68. Schrag A, Quinn N. Dyskinesias and motor fluctuations in Parkinson's disease. A community-based study. Brain. 2000;123(Pt 11):2297–305.
69. Hely MA, Morris JG, Reid WG, Trafficante R. Sydney Multicenter Study of Parkinson's disease: non-L-dopa-responsive problems dominate at 15 years. Mov Disord. 2005;20(2):190–9.
70. Katzenschlager R, Head J, Schrag A, Ben-Shlomo Y, Evans A, Lees AJ. Fourteen-year final report of the randomized PDRG-UK trial comparing three initial treatments in PD. Neurology. 2008;71(7):474–80.
71. Chapuis S, Ouchchane L, Metz O, Gerbaud L, Durif F. Impact of the motor complications of Parkinson's disease on the quality of life. Mov Disord. 2005;20(2):224–30.
72. Fox SH, Lang AE. Levodopa-related motor complications – phenomenology. Mov Disord. 2008;23 Suppl 3:S509–14.
73. Coelho M, Marti MJ, Tolosa E, Ferreira JJ, Valldeoriola F, Rosa M, et al. Late-stage Parkinson's disease: the Barcelona and Lisbon cohort. J Neurol. 2010;257(9):1524–32.
74. Witjas T, Kaphan E, Azulay JP, Blin O, Ceccaldi M, Pouget J, et al. Nonmotor fluctuations in Parkinson's disease: frequent and disabling. Neurology. 2002; 59(3):408–13.
75. Witjas T, Kaphan E, Regis J, Jouve E, Cherif AA, Peragut JC, et al. Effects of chronic subthalamic stimulation on nonmotor fluctuations in Parkinson's disease. Mov Disord. 2007;22(12):1729–34.
76. Storch A, Schneider CB, Wolz M, Sturwald Y, Nebe A, Odin P, et al. Nonmotor fluctuations in Parkinson disease: severity and correlation with motor complications. Neurology. 2013;80(9):800–9.
77. Eduardo Tolosa RK. Pharmacological management of Parkinson's disease. In: Joseph Jankovic ET, editor. Parkinson's disease & movement disorders. Philadelphia: Lippincott Williams & Wilkins; 2007. p. 110–45.
78. Hely MA, Reid WG, Adena MA, Halliday GM, Morris JG. The Sydney multicenter study of Parkinson's disease: the inevitability of dementia at 20 years. Mov Disord. 2008;23(6):837–44.
79. Williams-Gray CH, Mason SL, Evans JR, Foltynie T, Brayne C, Robbins TW, et al. The CamPaIGN study of Parkinson's disease: 10-year outlook in an

incident population-based cohort. J Neurol Neurosurg Psychiatry. 2013;84(11):1258–64.
80. Coelho M, Marti MJ, Sampaio C, Ferreira JJ, Valldeoriola F, Rosa MM, et al. Dementia and severity of parkinsonism determines the handicap of patients in late-stage Parkinson's disease: the Barcelona-Lisbon cohort. Eur J Neurol. 2015;22(2):305–12.
81. Kempster PA, Williams DR, Selikhova M, Holton J, Revesz T, Lees AJ. Patterns of levodopa response in Parkinson's disease: a clinico-pathological study. Brain. 2007;130(Pt 8):2123–8.
82. Kempster PA, O'Sullivan SS, Holton JL, Revesz T, Lees AJ. Relationships between age and late progression of Parkinson's disease: a clinico-pathological study. Brain. 2010;133(Pt 6):1755–62.
83. Goetz CG, Stebbins GT. Risk factors for nursing home placement in advanced Parkinson's disease. Neurology. 1993;43(11):2227–9.
84. Khoo TK, Yarnall AJ, Duncan GW, Coleman S, O'Brien JT, Brooks DJ, et al. The spectrum of nonmotor symptoms in early Parkinson disease. Neurology. 2013;80(3):276–81.
85. Factor SA, Steenland NK, Higgins DS, Molho ES, Kay DM, Montimurro J, et al. Disease-related and genetic correlates of psychotic symptoms in Parkinson's disease. Mov Disord. 2011;26(12):2190–5.
86. van Rooden SM, Visser M, Verbaan D, Marinus J, van Hilten JJ. Patterns of motor and non-motor features in Parkinson's disease. J Neurol Neurosurg Psychiatry. 2009;80(8):846–50.
87. Alves G, Wentzel-Larsen T, Aarsland D, Larsen JP. Progression of motor impairment and disability in Parkinson disease: a population-based study. Neurology. 2005;65(9):1436–41.
88. Aarsland D, Andersen K, Larsen JP, Perry R, Wentzel-Larsen T, Lolk A, et al. The rate of cognitive decline in Parkinson disease. Arch Neurol. 2004;61(12):1906–11.
89. Metta V, Logishetty K, Martinez-Martin P, Gage HM, Schartau PE, Kaluarachchi TK, et al. The possible clinical predictors of fatigue in Parkinson's disease: a study of 135 patients as part of international nonmotor scale validation project. Park Dis. 2011;2011:125271.
90. Saez-Francas N, Hernandez-Vara J, Corominas Roso M, Alegre Martin J, Casas BM. The association of apathy with central fatigue perception in patients with Parkinson's disease. Behav Neurosci. 2013;127(2):237–44.
91. Forsaa EB, Larsen JP, Wentzel-Larsen T, Goetz CG, Stebbins GT, Aarsland D, et al. A 12-year population-based study of psychosis in Parkinson disease. Arch Neurol. 2010;67(8):996–1001.
92. Krack P, Batir A, Van Blercom N, Chabardes S, Fraix V, Ardouin C, et al. Five-year follow-up of bilateral stimulation of the subthalamic nucleus in advanced Parkinson's disease. N Engl J Med. 2003;349(20):1925–34.
93. Deuschl G, Schade-Brittinger C, Krack P, Volkmann J, Schafer H, Botzel K, et al. A randomized trial of deep-brain stimulation for Parkinson's disease. N Engl J Med. 2006;355(9):896–908.
94. Castrioto A, Lozano AM, Poon YY, Lang AE, Fallis M, Moro E. Ten-year outcome of subthalamic stimulation in Parkinson disease: a blinded evaluation. Arch Neurol. 2011;68(12):1550–6.
95. Weerkamp NJ, Zuidema SU, Tissingh G, Poels PJ, Munneke M, Koopmans RT, et al. Motor profile and drug treatment of nursing home residents with Parkinson's disease. J Am Geriatr Soc. 2012;60(12):2277–82.
96. Weerkamp NJ, Tissingh G, Poels PJ, Zuidema SU, Munneke M, Koopmans RT, et al. Nonmotor symptoms in nursing home residents with Parkinson's disease: prevalence and effect on quality of life. J Am Geriatr Soc. 2013;61(10):1714–21.
97. Macleod AD, Taylor KS, Counsell CE. Mortality in Parkinson's disease: a systematic review and meta-analysis. Mov Disord. 2014;29(13):1615–22.
98. Pinter B, Diem-Zangerl A, Wenning GK, Scherfler C, Oberaigner W, Seppi K, et al. Mortality in Parkinson's disease: a 38-year follow-up study. Mov Disord. Mov Disord. 2015;30(2):266–9.

Medical Treatment of Parkinson's Disease

14

Anabela Valadas and Joaquim J. Ferreira

14.1 Introduction

Parkinson's disease (PD) is a neurodegenerative progressive disorder. The rate at which the disease progresses to disability varies from one individual to another, with uncertain functional prognosis at the time of diagnosis [1–6]. Nonmotor symptoms have been identified and may precede the motor manifestations of PD by decades. Nevertheless, clinical diagnosis continues to be based on the identification of the cardinal motor signs: bradykinesia, resting tremor, rigidity and postural instability [7]. Generally, in the early stages symptoms are usually mild, with minimal or no disability, and anti-PD medications provide an efficacious and constant control of motor symptoms and signs throughout the day [1–6, 8]. However, after this period, most patients experience a loss of effectiveness of anti-PD medications, as expressed by shorter duration of symptomatic effect or insufficient control of motor signs of the disease. Usually at this stage motor complications arise, characterized by motor fluctuations and dyskinesia, forcing a new treatment strategy to be implemented [8–19]. In general, 10–12 years after treatment onset, patients experience a worsening of axial signs, translated by imbalance and falls, often followed by cognitive decline and dementia [20–22]. The management of individual patients is complex, requiring careful consideration of a number of factors, including age, disease stage, years of disease duration, degree of functional disability, level of physical activity, and productivity. Currently, there are several therapeutic approaches in PD: pharmacological, nonpharmacological, and surgical therapies. This chapter will address the medical treatment of PD.

14.2 The Medical Treatment of Motor Signs in PD

Compared with other neurodegenerative disorders, the array of pharmacological agents for managing motor symptoms in PD is broad and includes levodopa (combined with a peripheral decarboxylase inhibitor, carbidopa or benserazide), dopamine agonists (DAs), monoamine oxidase B (MAO-B) inhibitors, anticholinergic drugs, amantadine, and catechol-O-methyltransferase (COMT) inhibitors. The symptomatic effect is significantly different between drug classes, with some controlling par-

A. Valadas (✉)
Hospital de São Bernardo,
Centro Hospitalar de Setúbal,
Rua Camilo Castelo Branco,
2910-446 Setubal, Portugal
e-mail: fanavaladas@sapo.pt

J.J. Ferreira
Faculdade de Medicina de Lisboa, Laboratório de Farmacologia Clínica e Terapêutica,
Av. Prof. Egas Moniz, 1649-028 Lisboa, Portugal
e-mail: joaquimjferreira@gmail.com

C. Falup-Pecurariu et al. (eds.), *Movement Disorders Curricula*,
DOI 10.1007/978-3-7091-1628-9_14

kinsonism better than others. Levodopa is the most efficacious drug for the treatment of motor symptoms of PD followed by DAs [23, 24]. MAO-B inhibitors, and amantadine, although effective are less potent than DAs [23, 24]. Anticholinergic drugs have been used for controlling tremor with modest effect on the other cardinal signs [23, 24]. The COMT inhibitors are only effective when combined with levodopa [23, 24] (Table. 14.1). In addition to the efficacy of medications, other considerations must be taken into account in the management of PD patients, including but not limited to the disease stage, i.e., early vs. complicated disease with motor fluctuations.

Table 14.1 Characteristics of pharmacological groups used in symptomatic treatment of PD

Pharmacological group	Doses	Titration	Efficacy in controlling parkinsonism	Adverse events
Levodopa (plus peripheral decarboxylase inhibitor, carbidopa or benserazide)	Avoid until possible the use of >400 mg/day; rarely >1 g/day	Yes	+++	Nausea, vomiting, somnolence, orthostatic hypotension, motor fluctuations, dyskinesia, psychiatric symptoms
				Dopaminergic dysregulation syndrome especially if in conjunction with DAs
Dopamine agonists (DAs)[a]		Yes	++	Nausea, vomiting, somnolence, orthostatic hypotension, peripheral edema, psychiatric symptoms, dopamine dysregulation syndrome, impulse control disorders
Ropinirole	Max. 24 mg/day			Skin reactions with transdermal rotigotine. Valvular heart disease is not a concern with newer DAs
Pramipexole	Max. 3.3 mg/day			
Rotigotine	2–6 mg/24 h			
Apomorphine	2–6 mg (pen administration)			Side effects are more often limiting than with levodopa
MAO-B inhibitors			+	Nausea, headache Amphetamine metabolites of selegiline can cause insomnia and often causes confusion in the elderly
Selegiline	5 mg, bid	No		
Rasagiline	1 mg, id	No		
Safinamide	50–100 mg/day	Yes		Insomnia, dyskinesia, somnolence, dizziness, headache, cataracts, orthostatic hypotension
COMT inhibitors		No	With levodopa	Elevation of liver enzymes with tolcapone, orange discoloration of the urine with entacapone, dyskinesia, insomnia, dizziness, psychosis
Tolcapone	100 mg, 3id			
Entacapone	200 mg with each dose of levodopa (max. 8 tablets/day)			
Opicapone	50 mg, id			
Glutamate receptor antagonist		Yes	+	Livedo reticularis, ankle edema, confusion, hallucinations
Amantadine	100 mg, bid-qid			
Anticholinergics	Depends on the drug used	Yes	+	Dry mouth, blurred vision, constipation, nausea, urinary retention, and tachycardia. Caution use in patients with prostatic hypertrophy or closed-angle glaucoma. Memory impairment, confusion, and hallucinations especially in elderly and cognitively impaired patients are often limiting

[a]Only nonergot derivatives were considered

Table 14.2 Hoehn and Yahr scale

Stage	Description
1	Unilateral involvement only usually with minimal or no functional disability
2	Bilateral or midline involvement without impairment of balance
3	Bilateral disease: mild to moderate disability with impaired postural reflexes; physically independent
4	Severely disabling disease; still able to walk or stand unassisted
5	Confinement to bed or wheelchair unless aided

14.2.1 Treatment of Early PD

Early PD is characterized by mild uni- or bilateral motor signs without impairment of balance and no motor fluctuations. These patients correspond to Hoehn and Yahr stages 1 and 2, respectively (Table. 14.2) [1]. Usually, at this stage the degree of disability is mild or nonexistent. The initial management of early PD, beyond pharmacological treatment, must also take into account proper diagnosis, educating patients and their families regarding symptoms and signs, future complications, and the long-term prognosis of the disease [8]. At the present time, the unique clinical criterion that supports the decision of when medical treatment should be initiated is provided by the patient's degree of disability and takes into account age, level of physical activity, and professional productivity [8]. Currently, the discussion around medical treatment of early PD includes neuroprotection and symptomatic effect.

14.2.1.1 Neuroprotective Therapy for PD

Neuroprotective therapy for PD is based on the concept that dopaminergic neurons in human *substantia nigra* may in some way be protected from the complex degenerative process that causes premature cell death characteristic of PD. Functional imaging studies ([18F]-dopa PET) have shown that striatum cell loss is more pronounced in the early years of the disease and, therefore, neuroprotective drugs would be more effective in patients with minimal clinical signs or potentially in asymptomatic individuals with a genetic risk [25–28]. Several drugs have shown some promise as disease-modifying agents in animal models and humans [29]. Almost all pharmacological classes currently used in PD were at some point involved in the field of neuroprotection [29–31]. However, in recent years the agents that have solicited the most attention are the MAO-B inhibitors, selegiline and rasagiline, and the complex I mitochondrial fortifier coenzyme Q10 (CoQ10) [29, 32]. In 1989, the results of a large study with early PD patients never exposed to levodopa, the DATATOP study, showed that patients treated with selegiline 10 mg/day reached clinical disability and needed levodopa later than patients treated with placebo, presumably due to the disease-modifying effect of selegiline [18]. However, subsequent data showed that this outcome was not sustained over time, selegiline had symptomatic effects in PD, and the cohort of patients originally randomized to selegiline showed the same degree of long-term disability as the placebo group [15–17]. In an attempt to bypass the problem of the symptomatic effect of drugs in neuroprotection trials, and in order to distinguish between disease-modifying and symptomatic effects, a new trial design, called delayed start design, was performed with rasagiline in the TEMPO and ADAGIO studies [33, 34]. While the small sample size and short duration of the TEMPO study had led to underpowered results, interpreting the results of ADAGIO proved to be quite complex [35, 37]. The latter study showed that all predetermined endpoints for a possible disease-modifying effect were met with 1 mg daily dose of rasagiline. The 2 mg daily dose failed the test, thus postponing the issue of neuroprotection [35–37]. Currently, rasagiline is only approved as symptomatic therapy for early PD, and in patients with motor complications [23, 24]. More definitive results on neuroprotection have recently been published with CoQ10. Despite the promising results of an exploratory study which reported that patients treated with CoQ10 for 14 months scored less on the UPDRS rating scale without evidence of underlying symptomatic effect, a more recent CoQ10 high-dosage randomized clinical trial in early PD excluded a neuroprotective effect

[38–41]. Similar results were found with vitamin E after the early published data from the DATATOP study [18]. Despite the growing interest devoted to the issue of neuroprotection, several other treatments are still under investigation (i.e., active and passive immunization against α-synuclein, neurotrophic factors, caffeine, etc.); currently, there are no licensed disease-modifying agents for PD [42–44].

14.2.1.2 Symptomatic Therapy for PD

Since the original data from Cotzias's studies, levodopa has been established as the most efficacious treatment for PD [45, 46]. However, the in vitro toxicity of levodopa to dopamine neurons, together with concern of the motor complications, has been the reason to delay the use of this standard therapy in early PD [47–49]. In recent years, an increasing body of evidence has been contradicting these assumptions. The clinical data from the original ELLDOPA trial, the first levodopa dose-response study conducted in early PD patients, showed that all dosages of levodopa (37.5–150, 150–300, and 300–600 mg/day) provided clinical benefit compared to placebo as measured by the UPDRS scores throughout the study [50]. The study also showed that the risk of developing motor complications was dose dependent, increasing in frequency with higher doses of levodopa [50]. Supporting these data, the STRIDE-PD study showed that the strongest risk factors for developing motor complications are early age at disease onset and high doses of levodopa intake (>400 mg/day) [51]. Thus, these clinical data seem to support the concept that levodopa does not hasten disease progression. Likewise, against the assumption that motor fluctuations could be delayed with continuous dopamine stimulation in the striatum since the beginning of treatment, the results of the CR FIRST using the sustained-release formulation of levodopa, and the STRIDE-PD using the COMT inhibitor, entacapone, did not show less motor complications, especially dyskinesia, in patients with early PD [51, 52]. DAs are synthetic agents that directly stimulate postsynaptic dopamine receptors not depending on metabolic conversion, amino acid transport, or neuronal uptake. While the early DAs (bromocriptine, pergolide, and cabergoline) were ergot derivatives with the risk of inducing fibrosis, especially cardiac valvulopathy, the newer agents (pramipexole, ropinirole, and rotigotine) are nonergot compounds and are not associated with such a risk [53]. So far, none of the DAs has proved to be significantly better than another, and recommendations are based solely on the safety profile (better with nonergot DAs) [12, 54–60]. Clinical trials comparing levodopa against DAs have shown that levodopa is more efficacious for treating PD motor signs, but the onset of treatment with DAs delays the beginning of motor complications during the first 2–5 years of treatment [12, 61–63]. However, they have also established that other important side effects are increased with DA therapy (Table. 14.1) [12, 61–63]. Recently, extended-release formulations have been introduced: ropinirole prolonged release and pramipexole extended released. They are effective as monotherapies and noninferior to immediate-release formulations [64, 65]. The more recent DA is rotigotine, a transdermal release formulation. In clinical trials, rotigotine has been shown to be effective in early PD and noninferior to pramipexole [66]. The benefit of a transdermal formulation appears to be related to improving patients' compliance through its convenience, and rotigotine transdermal patch may be better tolerated even in the elderly [67]. Thus, while levodopa-induced motor complications are age dependent, elderly and demented patients are more susceptible to psychiatric side effects from DAs (see Table 14.1). DAs are currently most frequently used as monotherapy for early PD, especially in patients younger than 65 years [23, 24]. However, the long-term usefulness of this strategy remains a matter of debate due to the fact that motor complications inevitably emerge once levodopa is combined with DAs. Regarding motor symptom control in early PD, the MAO-B inhibitors rasagiline and selegiline are both approved [23, 24]. These agents are not involved in the genesis of motor complications but clinical benefits are relatively mild compared with levodopa [23, 24]. Still, the unresolved question of rasagiline's neuroprotection should be taken into account when therapeutic options are discussed with early

PD patients [23, 24]. Amantadine is an antiviral agent with mild effects in early PD. Currently it is mainly used to suppress levodopa-induced dyskinesia in more advanced PD [23, 24]. Anticholinergic drugs are especially used in patients with the tremor-dominant phenotype; however, the available data suggest a very modest therapeutic effect on all motor manifestations of PD [23, 24]. Moreover, given the unfavorable safety profile, its clinical use is currently limited to sporadic cases or in those countries where for economic reasons the access to other anti-PD treatment is limited [23, 24].

14.2.2 Treatment of Motor Complications in PD

PD motor complications comprise motor fluctuations and dyskinesia and are considered late adverse reactions to levodopa treatment. Nevertheless, in the ELLDOPA trial, the onset of motor fluctuations and dyskinesia occurred as quickly as 5–6 months up to 2 years, depending on the daily dose of levodopa [50]. Data from the STRIDE-PD study demonstrated that the strongest risk factors for developing motor complications were young age at disease onset and higher levodopa doses [51]. Motor complications may be of particular concern in patients with PD onset before the age of 50 [51]. The underlying pathophysiology of levodopa-induced motor complications is unknown. The general opinion is that increasing degeneration makes striatal dopamine receptors more sensitive to the discontinuous stimulation as opposed to the continuous supply of dopamine in healthy individuals [68, 69]. Motor complications are not easy to manage, and there are no clinical trials to prove that one therapeutic regimen is superior to another.

14.2.2.1 Management of Motor Fluctuations

Motor fluctuations are defined as alternating periods between "on" when the patient has a good response to treatment and "off" when the signs and symptoms of the underlying PD arise. Motor fluctuations can present as an "end-of-dose" wearing-"off" phenomenon sometimes with even unpredictable "off" episodes. In addition, a "delayed-on" or "no-on" response after medication intake may occur. Theoretically, motor fluctuations could be managed with prolonged D2 dopaminergic stimulation. This can be undertaken by increasing the daily dose of levodopa or by dividing the daily dose shortening the intervals between smaller doses. However, with the progression of the disease the "therapeutic window" becomes increasingly dependent on the pharmacodynamics of drugs, and the risk of dyskinesia and worsening of parkinsonism makes these approaches sustainable only for a short period of time. Thus, new treatment strategies are essential in the management of these patients [49, 69]. A new oral extended-release capsule of carbidopa-levodopa, IPX066, containing combined immediate- and sustained-release pellets is now available for fluctuating PD patients. In the ADVANCE-PD study, IPX06 reduced daily "off" time by 1.17 h compared to placebo, and in the ASCEND-PD study, IPX06 proved to be superior to carbidopa-levodopa-entacapone in terms of "off" time reduction [70, 71]. However, as a new formulation, impact on daily practice remains to be established. DAs, initially developed as add-on therapy to levodopa, are commonly used to reduce the amount of "off" time in patients with advanced PD, about 1.1–1.5 h per day, and may even allow the dose of levodopa to be reduced [56, 72–81]. The DA apomorphine, with a short half-life of about 45 min via pen administration, can be used as a rescue therapy when patients suddenly turn "off" [82]. COMT inhibitors, such as tolcapone and entacapone, increase the half-life of levodopa enhancing the effect of each tablet in about 30% [83–86]. Although tolcapone has a greater ability of COMT inhibition (central and peripheral acting agent) due to cases of severe liver toxicity (three deaths recorded), regular blood examination is required [87]. In a systematic review, entacapone reduced the mean daily "off" time by about 41 min/day when given with each levodopa dosage [88]. Recently, the COMT inhibitor opicapone was approved. In a randomized controlled trial, a 50 mg daily dose proved to be effective in reducing the "off" time, increasing the "on" time without troublesome dyskinesia in PD patients. It is not inferior to entacapone, and its major advantages seem related to the absence of liver toxicity and the possibility of a more simplified dosing regimen in fluctuating PD patients [89]. The MAO-B inhibitors have also a role in this stage of the disease. The LARGO trial evaluated 687 PD patents with motor complications. Patients were randomly assigned to receive daily either rasagiline 1 mg, entacapone 200 mg with every levodopa dose, or placebo. Both rasagiline and entacapone reduced mean daily "off" time by about 1 h compared with placebo, and both increased daily "on" time without troublesome dyskinesia compared with placebo. The beneficial effect of rasagiline was independent of age and of adjunct with DAs [90]. For selegiline, the clinical benefit is less robust [23, 24]. The reversible MAO-B inhibitor, safinamide, which also has a role in the modulation of the excessive release of glutamate, was recently approved by the European Medicines Agency (EMA) as add-on therapy to levodopa alone or in combination with other PD treatments in the mid-to-late stage of fluctuating PD patients. Safinamide was compared to placebo in two main studies involving 1,218 fluctuating patients. In both studies, 6-month treatment increased the "on" time by 30–60 min when compared to placebo. Another study showed maintenance of benefit for 24 months. Currently, in early PD patients without fluctuations, safinamide has not shown a clear benefit [91, 92]. The anticholinergic drugs and amantadine are not very effective in the management of wearing-"off" phenomena and are rarely indicated for this purpose [23, 24]. In addition, at this stage of the disease the competition of levodopa with neutral amino acids for transport across the gut and the brain may be responsible for "off" periods after meals, and protein redistribution in a patient's diet may be required to control these symptoms [93–95]. Also, it has been proposed that the delayed gastric motility which results in inadequate levodopa plasma concentrations has been implicated in delayed-"off" episodes. Prokinetic agents, cisapride and domperidone, could be helpful. Cisapride was discontinued due to major drug interactions and fatal cardiac arrhythmias. Domperidone, a selective peripheral D2 blocker, does not cross the blood-brain barrier and therefore does not cause central nervous system effects. Animal studies suggest that domperidone could predispose to cardiac arrhythmias, but it seems to be safe at doses up to 60 mg/day [96–98].

14.2.2.2 Management of Dyskinesia

Dyskinesia consists of abnormal involuntary movements that are usually choreic or dystonic but when severe may be ballistic in nature. Dyskinesia occurs in about 30–40 % of PD patients after 5 years of treatment with levodopa, and almost 60 % of patients have dyskinesia after 10 years [99]. But not all dyskinesia have to be treated. A retrospective analysis suggests that dyskinesia requiring therapy adjustments at 5 and 10 years after levodopa is 17 % and 43 %, respectively [99]. Peak-dose dyskinesia is usually choreiform, typically starting 60–90 min after levodopa intake. In theory it can be managed with lowering the medication dosage or reducing adjunctive drugs. However, in more advanced disease it may result in a complete failure to turn "on." In these situations, and depending on the patient's characteristics, the dosage of DAs could be increased and the dosage of levodopa reduced. Less frequently there a pattern of dysphasic dyskinesia occurs when patients turn "on" and then when they turn "off." This pattern of dyskinesia is usually unrecognized and extremely difficult to manage and usually requires more frequent levodopa dosing to prevent wearing "off" and the reemergent of "off" dystonia prior to each dose [99]. Amantadine may be useful in treating dyskinesia in PD. In randomized controlled trials, amantadine decreased the incidence of dyskinesia in 24–60 % of patients in the short period of the trial [100, 101]. In a 1-year trial, amantadine appeared to maintain the effect in 56 % of patients [101]. Low-dose clozapine, an antipsychotic drug, reduced dyskinesia in several open-label trials; these results were replicated in a randomized trial [102–104]. The usefulness of clozapine is limited by its potential of inducing bone marrow suppression, thereby requiring white blood cell and absolute neutrophil count at baseline and weekly thereafter during the first 6 months of treatment. Olanzapine has been reported to have similar effects to clozapine in a randomized controlled trial but was associated with unacceptable increases in parkinsonism and "off" time [105]. Dystonia can appear at peak levodopa plasma concentrations but usually reflects "off" periods indicating the low valley of dopaminergic stimulation occurring usually in the early morning. "Off" dystonia that occurs early in the morning is usually managed with sustained-release levodopa before bedtime or by taking levodopa or DAs during the night or in the morning before rising [106].

Finally, if motor complications cannot be satisfactorily controlled by orally delivered medications, other therapeutic strategies must be considered [107]. Besides surgical treatments, continuous dopaminergic drug delivery can be achieved by continuous subcutaneous apomorphine infusions or duodenal infusions of levodopa (Duodopa) via portable minipumps. Both drugs are effective in the treatment of advanced PD [108, 109]. Unlike for surgery, age and cognitive status are less limiting factors [110, 111]. Both require adjustments by the patient or caregiver and regular office visits. Adverse effects are usually associated with infusion systems and can be potentially serious [112, 113].

Although a strong rationale exists for the development of nondopaminergic drugs to treat the motor complications in PD, so far, the available results are disappointing [114].

14.3 Treatment of Frequent Nonmotor Manifestations in PD

PD, in addition to the motor signs, is associated with nonmotor manifestations, many of which arise years before the development of parkinsonism. These manifestations may be attributed to the pathological process of the disease itself, and some may be aggravated by the drugs used during the course of the disease.

14.3.1 Management of the Neuropsychiatric Symptoms in PD

14.3.1.1 Cognitive Decline and Dementia

Cognitive decline and dementia are frequent in PD [115]. A systematic review of prevalence studies of dementia in PD suggests that 24–31 % of PD patients have dementia and that 3–4 % of the dementia in the population could be due to PD with dementia (PDD) [20, 116]. Early signs of cognitive decline include executive dysfunction and visuospatial and verbal memory impairments [117, 118]. The main risk factors associated with dementia are older age, age at disease onset, duration, and severity of parkinsonism [117, 119]. In the management of PDD patients, the gradual withdrawal of drugs implicated in the worsening of cognitive decline, particularly anticholinergics, should be considered. Symptomatic pharmacological strategies include the acetylcholinesterase inhibitors (ACI) (rivastigmine, donepezil, and galantamine). Rivastigmine is the best studied ACI in PDD. Since a 24-week, double-blind, placebo-controlled study in mild to moderate PDD, which showed a 2.1 point improvement in the Alzheimer's Disease Assessment Scale-Cognitive subscale (ADAS-Cog), rivastigmine is considered efficacious for the treatment of PDD [120]. Although donepezil appears to be beneficial for treating dementia associated with PD, studies have failed to show benefit on all proposed primary endpoints [121–123]. To date, there are insufficient data to consider galantamine useful in the treatment of PDD [124]. Side effects such as worsening of tremor, nausea, and vomiting have been reported with ACI and should be taking into account at the time of prescription [120–124]. The benefit of the other antidemential drug memantine (an antagonist to glutamate NMDA receptor) approved for Alzheimer's disease, although well tolerated in some studies, has not been established in PDD patients [125–127].

14.3.1.2 Psychosis and Hallucinations

Psychosis is a frequent complication in PD, mainly characterized by hallucinations and delusions, often paranoid in nature [128, 129]. Hallucinations are the most frequent manifestation and affect up to 40 % of PD patients, particularly those demented and in advanced stages of disease [130]. When hallucinations are intermittent and patients remain critical about the episodes, pharmacological intervention may not be required. In PDD patients with hallucinations, a potential benefit with ACI has been reported [120, 131]. The management of psychosis includes therapeutics review with discontinuation of non-antiparkinsonian medications with anticholinergic action. In patients with more disabling symptoms, it is sometimes necessary to reduce the anti-PD medication in the reverse order of efficacy: anticholinergics, amantadine, MAO-B inhibitors, COMT inhibitors, DAs. Additionally, atypical antipsychotic agents may be helpful in low doses. Clozapine is effective in treating PD-associated psychosis without worsening parkinsonism [132–134]. However, the need for weekly hematological monitoring during the first 6 months of treatment due to the risk of agranulocytosis makes its use troublesome in clinical practice [132–135]. Quetiapine is an alternative option. It seems to be effective without the need for regular monitoring of side effects and no significant worsening of parkinsonian signs [136–139]. Other atypical antipsychotics, such as risperidone and olanzapine, and typical neuroleptic drugs due to unacceptable deterioration of motor symptoms should not be considered [140–143]. Pimavanserin seems to be a promising antipsychotic agent in PD. One randomized placebo-controlled study reported pimavanserin to be effective, well tolerated, and not associated with worsening of motor signs or other significant side effects [144].

14.3.1.3 Depression

Depression is one of the most frequent nonmotor symptom in PD found in up to 40 % of patients and may occur years before the onset of motor signs [145, 146]. There is no consensus regarding the treatment of depression in PD patients [146]. Some data suggest that tricyclic antidepressants (TCAs) are effective in the treatment of depressive symptoms in patients with PD; however, the anticholinergic side effects of TCAs, including cognitive impairment and orthostatic hypotension, may be particularly troublesome in these patients [147–149]. Despite conflicting data on the efficacy of selective serotonin reuptake inhibitors (SSRIs), these are usually considered a first choice in the treatment of PD-associated depression when the potential benefits are weighed against the potential side effects of TCAs [147, 150, 151]. Regarding safety concerns, revised data show that SSRIs aggravate tremor in only 4–5 % of patients and occasionally the parkinsonism. The serotonin syndrome was found in only 0.24 % of patients with PD treated with selegiline [152–154]. Data on the serotonin-norepinephrine reuptake inhibitor (SNRI), venlafaxine, are suggestive of benefit in PD-associated depression [150]. There is a larger body of evidence reporting DAs, mainly pramipexole, are beneficial in the treatment of depressive symptoms in PD [155].

14.3.2 Management of Autonomic Dysfunction

Autonomic dysfunction is a common disorder in PD patients. Orthostatic hypotension, urinary disturbance, gastrointestinal motility disorders, and sialorrhea are frequent and disabling problems.

14.3.2.1 Orthostatic Hypotension

Orthostatic hypotension (OH) is defined as a fall in systolic blood pressure above 20 mmHg and/or in diastolic blood pressure greater than 10 mmHg in the first 3 min of being in a standing position. Although the clinical benefits of nonpharmacological measures have not been extensively studied in the treatment of PD-associated OH, these include wearing waist-high elastic stockings and/or abdominal binders; increasing the intake of salt; head-up tilt of the bed at night (30–40°); avoiding large meals, alcohol, and caffeine at night; avoiding exposure to a hot environment; and preventing volume depletion [156]. Although medications known to cause or worsen OH should be avoided, some of them, including levodopa, DAs, and atypical antipsychotics, are difficult to withdraw or even reduce in this setting. Midodrine and fludrocortisone are agents used in the treatment of neurogenic OH. Although specific data in PD-associated OH are scarce, midodrine, an alpha-adrenergic agonist, has shown a significant increase in standing blood pressure but only during a few hours in PD patients. The main side effects include supine hypertension, paresthesias, and chills [157, 158]. Fludrocortisone enhances sodium reabsorption and potassium excretion in the kidney. Only small studies have been conducted with PD patients showing a trend to increase systolic blood pressure upon standing [159]. In a study including 17 patients with PD, fludrocortisone and domperidone showed improvement in OH, although four dropouts were reported [156]. Hypertension, hypokalemia, and ankle edema are the main side effects of fludrocortisone [160]. At least 4–5 days of treatment are necessary to start the therapeutic response to fludrocortisone, and full benefit requires high dietary salt and adequate fluid intake. Droxidopa is a synthetic catechol-amino acid that is converted to norepinephrine after oral administration. On average, droxidopa elevates standing systolic blood pressure by 10 mmHg. Lying systolic blood pressure is also elevated, and thus supine hypertension is a possible side effect of this drug. Indicated in neurogenic OH, it can be used over the short term in PD patients with OH. However, the long-term efficacy has not been proved [161].

14.3.2.2 Urinary Dysfunction

Urinary disturbance occurs in up to 71 % of patients with PD [162]. The management of urinary dysfunction depends on the type of subjacent problem and implicates the identification of other medical problems or other reversible causes, such as urinary tract infections and diabetes mellitus. In nocturia, a reduction in liquid intake after the late afternoon as well as a head-up tilt of the bed at night could help reduce urine production. Intranasal desmopressin spray has shown some response in PD patients [163]. In general, neurogenic bladder problems with an overactive bladder improve with anticholinergics. Oxybutynin, which controls the hyperactivity of the detrusor muscle, and tolterodine and trospium chloride, which decrease urinary frequency and incontinence episodes, may be considered in patients with PD [164, 165]. However, in PD patients it is important to balance the therapeutic benefits and side effects of these drugs. Apomorphine injections may be beneficial if outflow obstruction is the dominant problem [166].

14.3.2.3 Gastrointestinal Motility Problems

Gastrointestinal motility dysfunction is a complaint in PD patients, with constipation being the most frequent problem [167]. Increased intake of fluids and dietary fibers are recommended. When possible, anticholinergics that worse constipation should be reduced or even withdrawn. Data from a small placebo-controlled trial showed that macrogol is effective in chronic PD-associated constipation [168]. Also, tagaserod, a 5-HT 4 partial agonist, has proven to be efficacious and a safe therapy in a small trial with 15 PD patients [169]. Domperidone has been reported to accelerate gastric emptying and reduces dopaminergic drug-related gastrointestinal symptoms in PD patients [96]. Metoclopramide use, a peripheral and central dopamine-blocking agent, is considered unaccepted by the risk of worsening parkinsonian signs [170, 171].

14.3.2.4 Sialorrhea

Sialorrhea and drooling are common symptoms in PD. Glycopyrrolate, an anticholinergic agent with limited ability to cross the blood-brain barrier, was effective in short-term studies [172]. In patients with less disability, other anticholinergics could be considered (oral amitriptyline and hyoscyamine, sublingual ipratropium bromide, and atropine ophthalmic solution) [173, 174]. An increasing body of evidence suggests that botulinum toxin injections (type A and B) into salivary glands are effective and safe in controlling drooling [175–178].

14.3.3 Management of Sleep Disorders

Significant sleep disorders are common in PD. It is estimated that 60–90 % of patients complain of difficulties associated with sleep, including nocturnal sleep and daytime sleepiness manifestations [179]. REM sleep behavior disorder (RBD), a parasomnia of REM sleep, is one of the most frequent sleep-associated disorders in PD, present in 25–50 % of patients [180]. Small case series have concluded that clonazepam, in small doses, is effective for RBD treatment. However, daytime sedation and exacerbation of obstructive breathing symptoms are common side effects [181, 182]. Contradictory data from small open-label studies have emerged on the efficacy of pramipexole in RBD [183–185]. It should be kept in mind that many antidepressants, especially SSRIs and mirtazapine, may carry a risk of worsening RBD, restless legs syndrome, and periodic leg movements of sleep [186]. Daytime somnolence assessed by the Epworth Sleepiness Scale (ESS) and episodes of sudden-onset sleep episodes (sleep attacks) reach frequencies of about 33 % and between 3.8 % and 20.8 %, respectively, in patients with PD [187–194]. Management recommendations for daytime sleepiness include the assessment of nocturnal sleep disturbances, reduction or discontinuation of sedative drugs, and a decrease of dopaminergic drugs, especially DAs. Driving should be discouraged. Although the data on treatment of daytime sleepiness are sparse and conflicting in PD, the judicious use of modafinil or methylphenidate during the day may be offered [195–198].

Conclusions

- PD is a progressive neurodegenerative disorder with uncertain prognosis at the time of diagnosis.
- Treatment should be individualized, taking into account patients' age at disease onset, disease stage, and functional status.
- Currently there are no disease-modifying therapies for PD.
- In early PD, it is usually simple to control motor symptoms in a relatively satisfactory manner for patients.
- Levodopa and DAs are the most efficacious agents in early PD.
- The choice between DAs and levodopa in early PD should mainly take into account patients' age at disease onset and the degree of functional impairment.
- Motor complications can be delayed in the first 2–5 years of disease onset with DAs, but these effects are not sustained over the long term.
- Motor fluctuations are best managed with DAs, MAO-B inhibitors, and COMT inhibitors with no evidence of superiority of one agent over another; choice should be based on the individual patient's profile.
- Amantadine is the most effective agents for the treatment of peak-dose dyskinesia.
- Early-morning "off" dystonia is best managed with extended-release levodopa formulations at bedtime or extra dosages of immediate-release levodopa or DAs overnight.
- When all these oral treatments fail to control advanced PD motor symptoms, more invasive therapies should be considered. In addition to surgery, apomorphine and duodenal infusion of levodopa can be considered.
- PD nonmotor manifestations are frequent and potentially very disturbing to patients and their relatives.
- General recommendations for managing nonmotor symptoms in PD include a review of therapeutic and even the reduction or withdrawal of possible offensive current drug treatment.
- Pharmacological strategies in PDD include ACI, mainly rivastigmine.
- Management of psychosis and hallucinations in PD includes atypical neuroleptics, clozapine and quetiapine. Regular hematological monitoring is required with clozapine. ACIs have shown some positive results in PDD patients with hallucinations.
- Pharmacological treatment of depression in PD is conflicting. SSRIs are often the first treatment option due to the side-effect profile of TCAs.
- In PD-associated OH, beside nonpharmacological measures, midodrine, fludrocortisone, domperidone, and droxidopa may be considered.

- Management of bladder dysfunction depends on the specific urinary dysfunction. In PD patients, oxybutynin, tolterodine, and trospium chloride can be used for an overactive bladder. Apomorphine is useful if flow obstruction is the dominant problem.
- Macrogol and tagaserod are effective in PD-associated constipation.
- Sialorrhea can be managed with oral anticholinergics, mainly glycopyrrolate. Botulinum toxin (type A and B) injections into salivary glands are effective and safe in the treatment of sialorrhea associated with PD.
- Clonazepam is effective in RBD treatment, but daytime sleepiness and exacerbation of obstructive breathing problems should be considered.
- Patients with daytime somnolence and sleep attacks should not drive. A review of dopaminergic therapy, especially DAs, is recommended. Modafinil and methylphenidate may be considered.

References

1. Hoehn MM, Yahr MD. Parkinsonism: onset, progression and mortality. Neurology. 1967;17(5):427–42.
2. Hoehn MM. Parkinsonism treated with levodopa: progression and mortality. J Neurol Transm Suppl. 1983; 19:253–64.
3. Marttila RJ, Rinne UK. Disability and progression in Parkinson's disease. Acta Neurol Scand. 1977;56(2): 159–69.
4. Hoehn MM. The natural history of Parkinson's disease in the pre-levodopa and post-levodopa eras. Neurol Clin. 1992;10(2):331–9.
5. Tetrud JW, Langston JW. The effect of deprenyl (selegiline) on the natural history of Parkinson's disease. Science. 1989;245(4917):519–22.
6. Stern PH, McDowell F, Miller JM, Robinson MB. Levodopa therapy effects on natural history of Parkinsonism. Arch Neurol. 1972;27(6):481–5.
7. Hughes AJ, Daniel SE, Kilford L, Lees AJ. Accuracy of clinical diagnosis of idiopathic Parkinson's disease. A clinico-pathological study of 100 cases. JNNP. 1992;55:181–4.
8. Olanow CW, Watts RL, Koller WC. An algorithm (decision tree) for the management of Parkinson's disease (2001): treatment guidelines. Neurology. 2001; 56(11 Suppl 5):S9–29.
9. Rajput AH, Stern W, Laverty WH. Chronic low-dose levodopa therapy in Parkinson's disease: an argument for delaying levodopa therapy. Neurology. 1984;34(8):991–6.
10. Poewe WH, Wenning GK. The natural history of Parkinson's disease. Ann Neurol. 1998;44(3 Suppl 1): S1–9.
11. Hely MA, Morris JG, Reid WG, O'Sullivan DJ, Williamson PM, Rail D, Broe GA, Margrie S. The Sydney Multicentre Study of Parkinson's disease: a randomised, prospective five year study comparing low dose bromocriptine with low dose levodopa-carbidopa. J Neurol Neurosurg Psychiatry. 1994;57(8):903–10.
12. Montastruc JL, Rascol O, Senard JM, Rascol A. A randomised controlled study comparing bromocriptine to which levodopa was later added, with levodopa alone in previously untreated patients with Parkinson's disease: a five year follow up. J Neurol Neurosurg Psychiatry. 1994;57(9):1034–8.
13. Dupont E, Andersen A, Boas J, Boisen E, Borgmann R, Helgetveit AC, Kjaer MO, Kristensen TN, Mikkelsen B, Pakkenberg H, Presthus J, Stien R, Worm-Petersen J, Buch D. Sustained-release Madopar HBS compared with standard Madopar in the long-term treatment of de novo parkinsonian patients. Acta Neurol Scand. 1996;93(1):14–20.
14. Parkinson Study Group. Pramipexole vs levodopa as initial treatment for Parkinson disease: a randomized controlled trial. Parkinson Study Group. JAMA. 2000;284(15):1931–8.
15. Parkinson Study Group. Mortality in DATATOP: a multicenter trial in early Parkinson's disease. Ann Neurol. 1998;43(3):318–25.
16. Parkinson Study Group. Impact of deprenyl and tocopherol treatment on Parkinson's disease in DATATOP patients requiring levodopa. Parkinson Study Group. Ann Neurol. 1996;39(1):37–45.
17. Parkinson Study Group. Effects of tocopherol and deprenyl on the progression of disability in early Parkinson's disease. N Engl J Med. 1993;328(3):176–83.
18. Parkinson Study Group. DATATOP: a multicenter controlled clinical trial in early Parkinson's disease. Arch Neurol. 1989;46(10):1052–60.
19. Koller WC, Hutton JT, Tolosa E, Capilldeo R. Immediate-release and controlled-release carbidopa/levodopa in PD: a 5-year randomized multicenter study. Carbidopa/Levodopa Study Group. Neurology. 1999;53(5):1012–9.
20. Aarsland D, Andersen K, Larsen JP, Lolk A, Kragh-Sorensen P. Prevalence and characteristic of dementia in Parkinson disease: an 8-years prospective study. Arch Neurol. 2003;60(3):387–92.
21. Biggins CA, Boyd JL, Harrop FM, Madeley P, Mindham RH, Randall JL, Spokes EG. A controlled, longitudinal study of dementia in Parkinson's disease. J Neurol Neurosurg Psychiatry. 1992;55:566–71.
22. Levy G, Schupf N, Tang MX, Cote L, Alfaro B, Mejia H, Tern Y, Marder K. Combined effect of age and severity on the risk of dementia in Parkinson's disease. Ann Neurol. 2002;51(6):722–9.

23. Fox SH, Katzenschlager R, Lim SY, Ravina B, Seppi K, Coelho M, Poewe W, Rascol O, Goetz CG, Sampaio C. The movement disorder society evidence-based medicine review update: treatments for the motor symptoms of Parkinson's disease. Mov Disord. 2011;26 Suppl 3:S2–41.
24. Ferreira JJ, Katzenschlager R, Bloem BR, Bonuccelli U, Burn D, Deuschl G, Dietrichs E, Fabbrini G, Friedman A, Kanovsky P, Kostic V, Nieuwboer A, Odin P, Poewe W, Rascol O, Sampaio C, Schüpbach M, Tolosa E, Trenkwalder C, Schapira A, Berardelli A, Oertel WH. Summary of the recommendations of the EFNS/MDS-ES review on therapeutic management of Parkinson's disease. Eur J Neurol. 2013;20(1):5–15.
25. Hilker R, Schweitzer K, Coburger S, Ghaemi M, Weisenbach S, Jacobs AH, Rudolf J, Herholz K, Heiss WD. Nonlinear progression of Parkinson disease as determined by serial positron emission tomographic imaging of striatal fluorodopa F 18 activity. Arch Neurol. 2005;62(3):38–82.
26. Nurmi E, Ruottinen H, Kaasinen V, Bergman J, Haaparanta M, Solin O, Rinne JO. Progression in Parkinson's disease: a positron emission tomography study with a dopamine transporter ligand [18F] CTF. Ann Neurol. 2000;47:804–8.
27. Morrish PK, Rakshi JS, Bailey DL, Sawle GV, Brooks DJ. Measuring the rate of progression and estimating the preclinical period of Parkinson's disease with [18F]dopa PET. J Neurol Neurosurg Psychiatry. 1998;64(3):314–9.
28. Vingerhoets FJG, Snow BJ, Lee CS, Schulzer M, Mak E, Calne DB. Longitudinal fluorodopa positron emission tomographic studies of the evolution of idiopathic Parkinsonism. Ann Neurol. 1994;36:759–64.
29. Ravina BM, Fagan SC, Hart RG, Hovinga CA, Murphy DD, Dawson TM, Marler JR. Neuroprotective agents for clinical trials in Parkinson's disease: a systematic assessment. Neurology. 2003;60(8):1234–40.
30. Schapira AH, Olanow CW. Neuroprotection in Parkinson disease: mysteries, myths, and misconceptions. JAMA. 2004;291(3):358–64.
31. LeWitt PA. Clinical trials of neuroprotection for Parkinson's disease. Neurology. 2004;63(7 Suppl 2): S23–31.
32. Hart RG, Pearce LA, Ravina BM, Yaltho TC, Marler JR. Neuroprotection trials in Parkinson's disease: systematic review. Mov Disord. 2009;24(5):647–54.
33. Jenner P. Preclinical evidence for neuroprotection with monoamine oxidase-B inhibitors in Parkinson's disease. Neurology. 2004;63(7 Suppl 2):S13–22.
34. Parkinson Study Group. A controlled, randomized, delayed-start study of rasagiline in early Parkinson disease. Arch Neurol. 2004;61(4):561–6.
35. Olanow CW, Rascol O, Hauser R, Feigin PD, Jankovic J, Lang A, Langston W, Melamed E, Poewe W, Stocchi F, Tolosa E, ADAGIO Study Investigators. A double-blind, delayed-start trial of rasagiline in Parkinson's disease. N Engl J Med. 2009;361(13): 1268–78.
36. Ahlskog JE, Uitti RJ. Rasagiline, Parkinson neuroprotection, and delayed-start trials: still no satisfaction? Neurology. 2010;74(14):1143–8.
37. Lewitt PA. MAO-B inhibitor know-how: back to the pharm. Neurology. 2009;72(15):1352–7.
38. Rascol O, Fitzer-Attas CJ, Hauser R, Jankovic J, Lang A, Langston JW, Melamed E, Poewe W, Stocchi F, Tolosa E, Eyal E, Weiss YM, Olanow CW. A double-blind, delayed-start trial of rasagiline in Parkinson's disease (the ADAGIO study): prespecified and post-hoc analyses of the need for additional therapies, changes in UPDRS scores, and non-motor outcomes. Lancet Neurol. 2011;10(5):415–23.
39. Shults CW, Oakes D, Kieburtz K, Beal MF, Haas R, Plumb S, Juncos JL, Nutt J, Shoulson I, Carter J, Kompoliti K, Perlmutter JS, Reich S, Stern M, Watts RL, Kurlan R, Molho E, Harrison M, Lew M, Parkinson Study Group. Effects of coenzyme Q10 in early Parkinson disease: evidence of slowing of the functional decline. Arch Neurol. 2002;59(10):1541–50.
40. Horstink MW, van Engelen BG. The effect of coenzyme Q10 therapy in Parkinson disease could be symptomatic. Arch Neurol. 2003;60(8):1170–2.
41. Storch A, Jost WH, Vieregge P, Spiegel J, Greulich W, Durner J, Müller T, Kupsch A, Henningsen H, Oertel WH, Fuchs G, Kuhn W, Niklowitz P, Koch R, Herting B, Reichmann H, German Coenzyme Q(10) Study Group. Randomized, double-blind, placebo-controlled trial on symptomatic effects of coenzyme Q(10) in Parkinson disease. Arch Neurol. 2007;64(7):938–44.
42. Beal MF, Oakes D, Shoulson I, Parkinson Study Group QE3 Investigators. A randomized clinical trial of high-dosage coenzyme Q10 in early Parkinson disease: no evidence of benefit. JAMA Neurol. 2014;71:543–52.
43. Visanji NP, Brooks PL, Hazrati L-N, Lange AE. The prion hypothesis in Parkinson's disease: Braak to the future. Acta Neuropathol Commun. 2013;1:2.
44. Postuma RB, Lang AE, Munhoz RP, Charland K, Pelletier A, Moscovich M, Filla L, Zanatta D, Rios Romenets S, Altman R, Shah B. Caffeine for treatment of Parkinson disease: a randomized controlled trial. Neurology. 2012;79:651–8.
45. Lang AE, Gill S, Patel NK, Lozano A, Nutt JG, Penn R, Brooks DJ, Hotton G, Moro E, Heywood P, Brodsky MA, Burchiel K, Kelly P, Dalvi A, Scott B, Stacy M, Turner D, Wooten VG, Elias WJ, Laws ER, Dhawan V, Stoessl AJ, Matcham J, Coffey RJ, Traub M. Randomized controlled trial of intraputamenal glial cell line-derived neurotrophic factor infusion in Parkinson disease. Ann Neurol. 2016;59:459–66.
46. Cotzias GC, Van Woert MH, Schiffer LM. Aromatic amino acids and modification of parkinsonism. N Engl J Med. 1967;276:374–9.
47. Cotzias GC, Papavasiliou PS, Gellene R. Modification of parkinsonism-chronic treatment with L-dopa. N Engl J Med. 1969;280:337–45.
48. Tanaka M, Sotomatsu A, Kanai H, Hirai S. Dopa and dopamine cause cultured neuronal death in the presence of iron. J Neurol Sci. 1991;101(2):198–203.

49. Olanow CW, Agid Y, Mizuno Y, Albanese A, Bonuccelli U, Damier P, De Yebenes J, Gershanik O, Guttman M, Grandas F, Hallett M, Hornykiewicz O, Jenner P, Katzenschlager R, Langston WJ, LeWitt P, Melamed E, Mena MA, Michel PP, Mytilineou C, Obeso JA, Poewe W, Quinn N, Raisman-Vozari R, Rajput AH, Rascol O, Sampaio C, Stocchi F. Levodopa in the treatment of Parkinson's disease: current controversies. Mov Disord. 2004;19(9):997–1005.
50. Mouradian MM, Heuser IJ, Baronti F, Fabbrini G, Juncos JL, Chase TN. Pathogenesis of dyskinesias in Parkinson's disease. Ann Neurol. 1989;25(5):523–6.
51. Fahn S, Oakes D, Shoulson I, Kieburtz K, Rudolph A, Lang A, Olanow CW, Tanner C, Marek K, Parkinson Study Group. Levodopa and the progression of Parkinson's disease. N Engl J Med. 2004;351(24): 2498–508.
52. Stocchi F, Rascol O, Kieburtz K, Poewe W, Jankovic J, Tolosa E, Barone P, Lang AE, Olanow CW. Initiating levodopa/carbidopa therapy with and without entacapone in early Parkinson disease: the STRIDE-PD study. Ann Neurol. 2010;68(1):18–27.
53. Capildeo R. Implications of the 5-year CR FIRST trial. Sinemet CR Five-Year International Response Fluctuation Study. Neurology. 1998;50(6 Suppl 6):S15–7. discussion S44–S48.
54. Zanettini R, Antonini A, Gatto G, Gentile R, Tesei S, Pezzoli G. Valvular heart disease and the use of dopamine agonists for Parkinson's disease. N Engl J Med. 2007;356(1):39–46.
55. Korczyn AD, Brunt ER, Larsen JP, Nagy Z, Poewe WH, Ruggieri S. A 3-year randomized trial of ropinirole and bromocriptine in early Parkinson's disease. The 053 Study Group. Neurology. 1999;53:364–70.
56. LeWitt PA, Ward CD, Larsen TA, Raphaelson MI, Newman RP, Foster N, Dambrosia JM, Calne DB. Comparison of pergolide and bromocriptine therapy in parkinsonism. Neurology. 1983;33:1009–14.
57. Pezzoli G, Martignoni E, Pacchetti C, Angeleri VA, Lamberti P, Muratorio A, De Mari M, Foschi N, Cossutta E, et al. Pergolide compared with bromocriptine in Parkinson's disease: a multicenter, crossover, controlled study. Mov Disord. 1994;9:431–6.
58. Korczyn AD, Brooks DJ, Brunt ER, Poewe WH, Rascol O, Stocchi F. Ropinirole versus bromocriptine in the treatment of early Parkinson's disease: a 6-month interim report of a 3-year study. 053 Study Group. Mov Disord. 1998;13:46–8.
59. Barone P, Bravi D, Bermejo-Pareja F, Marconi R, Kulisevsky J, Malagù S, Weiser R, Rost N. Pergolide monotherapy in the treatment of early PD: a randomized, controlled study. Pergolide Monotherapy Study Group. Neurology. 1999;53:573.
60. Hubble JP, Koller WC, Cutler NR, Sramek JJ, Friedman J, Goetz C, Ranhosky A, Korts D, Elvin A. Pramipexole in patients with early Parkinson's disease. Clin Neuropharmacol. 1995;18:338–47.
61. Adler CH, Sethi KD, Hauser RA, Davis TL, Hammerstad JP, Bertoni J, Taylor RL, Sanchez-Ramos J, O'Brien CF. Ropinirole for the treatment of early Parkinson's disease. The Ropinirole Study Group. Neurology. 1997;49:393–9.
62. Stowe RL, Ives NJ, Clarke C, van Hilten J, Ferreira J, Hawker RJ, Shah L, Wheatley K, Gray R. Dopamine agonist therapy in early Parkinson's disease. Cochrane Database Syst Rev. 2008;2:CD006564.
63. Rascol O, Brooks DJ, Korczyn AD, De Deyn PP, Clarke CE, Lang AE. A five-year study of the incidence of dyskinesia in patients with early Parkinson's disease who were treated with ropinirole or levodopa. 056 Study Group. N Engl J Med. 2000;342:1484–91.
64. Holloway RG, Shoulson I, Fahn S, Kieburtz K, Lang A, Marek K, McDermott M, Seibyl J, Weiner W, Parkinson Study Group, et al. Pramipexole vs levodopa as initial treatment for Parkinson disease: a 4-year randomized controlled trial. Arch Neurol. 2004;61:1044–53.
65. Stocchi F, Hersh BP, Scott BL, Nausieda PA, Giorgi L, Ease-PD Monotherapy Study Investigators. Ropinirole 24-hour prolonged release and ropinirole immediate release in early Parkinson's disease: a randomized, double-blind, non-inferiority crossover study. Curr Med Res Opin. 2008;24(10):2883–95.
66. Poewe W, Rascol O, Barone P, Hauser RA, Mizuno Y, Haaksma M, Salin L, Juhel N, Schapira AH, Pramipexole ER Studies Group. Extended-release pramipexole in early Parkinson disease: a 33-week randomized controlled trial. Neurology. 2011;77(8): 759–66.
67. Watts RL, Jankovic J, Waters C, Rajput A, Boroojerdi B, Rao J. Randomized, blind, controlled trial of transdermal rotigotine in early Parkinson disease. Neurology. 2007;68(4):272–6.
68. Pellicano C, Benincasa D, Fanciulli A, Latino P, Giovannelli M, Pontieri FE. The impact of extended release dopamine agonists on prescribing patterns for therapy of early Parkinson's disease: an observational study. Eur J Med Res. 2013;18(1):60–5.
69. Olanow CW, Obeso JA, Stocchi F. Continuous dopamine-receptor treatment of Parkinson's disease: scientific rationale and clinical implications. Lancet Neurol. 2006;5(8):677–87.
70. Ossig C, Reichmann H. Treatment of Parkinson's disease in the advanced stage. J Neural Transm. 2013;120:523–9.
71. Hauser RA, Hsu A, Kell S, Espay AJ, Sethi K, Stacy M, Ondo W, O'Connell M, Gupta S, IPX066 ADVANCE-PD Investigators. Extended-release carbidopa-levodopa (IPX066) compared with immediate-release carbidopa-levodopa in patients with Parkinson's disease and motor fluctuations: a phase 3 randomised, double-blind trial. Lancet Neurol. 2013;12(4):346–56.
72. Stocchi F, Hsu A, Kell S, Ellenbogen A, Mahler A, Liang G, Dillmann U, Rubens R, Kell S, Gupta S. Comparison of IPX066 with carbidopa-levodopa plus entacapone in advanced PD patients. Parkinsonism Relat Disord. 2014;20:1335–40.
73. Olanow CW, Fanh S, Muenter M, Klawans H, Hurtig H, Stern M, Shoulson I, Kurlan R, Grimes

JD, Jankovic, et al. A multicenter double-blinde placebo-controlled trial of pergolide as an adjunct to Sinemet in Parkinson's disease. Mov Disord. 1994;9(1):40–7.
74. Rascol O, Lees AJ, Senard JM, Pirtosek Z, Montastruc JL, Fuell D. Ropinirole in the treatment of levodopa-induced motor fluctuations in patients with Parkinson's disease. Clin Neuropharmacol. 1996;19(3):234–45.
75. Lieberman A, Ranhosky A, Korts D. Clinical evaluation of pramipexole in advanced Parkinson's disease: results of a double-blind, placebo-controlled, parallel-group study. Neurology. 1997;49(1):162–8.
76. Lieberman A, Olanow CW, Sethi K, Swanson P, Waters CH, Fahn S, Hurtig H, Yahr M. A multicenter trial of ropinirole as adjunct treatment for Parkinson's disease. Ropinirole Study Group. Neurology. 1998; 51(4):1057–62.
77. Pahwa R, Stacy MA, Factor SA, Lyons KE, Stocchi F, Hersh BP, Elmer LW, Truong DD, Earl NL, EASE-PD Adjunct Study Investigators. Ropinirole 24-hour prolonged release: randomized, controlled study in advanced Parkinson disease. Neurology. 2007;68(14): 1108–15.
78. LeWitt PA, Lyons KE, Pahwa R, SP 650 Study Group. Advanced Parkinson disease treated with rotigotine transdermal system: PREFER Study. Neurology. 2007;68(16):1262–7.
79. Schapira AH, Barone P, Hauser RA, Mizuno Y, Rascol O, Busse M, Salin N, Poewe W, Pramipexole ER Studies Group. Extended-release pramipexole in advanced Parkinson disease: a randomized controlled trial. Neurology. 2011;77(8):767–74.
80. Guttman M. Double-blind comparison of pramipexole and bromocriptine treatment with placebo in advanced Parkinson's disease. International Pramipexole-Bromocriptine Study Group. Neurology. 1997;49(4):1060–5.
81. Clarke CE, Deane KD. Cabergoline versus bromocriptine for levodopa-induced complications in Parkinson's disease. Cochrane Database Syst Rev. 2001;1:CD001519. Poewe WH, Rascol O, Quinn N, Tolosa E, Oertel WH, Martignoni E, Rupp M, Boroojerdi B; SP 515 Investigators. Efficacy of pramipexole and transdermal rotigotine in advanced Parkinson's disease: a double-blind, double-dummy, randomised controlled trial. Lancet Neurol. 2007; 6(6):513–20.
82. Dewey Jr RB, Hutton JT, LeWitt PA, Factor SA. A randomized, double-blind, placebo-controlled trial of subcutaneously injected apomorphine for parkinsonian off-state events. Arch Neurol. 2001;58:1385–92.
83. Nutt JG. Catechol-O-methyltransferase inhibitors for treatment of Parkinson's disease. Lancet. 1998; 351(9111):1221–2.
84. Rajput AH, Martin W, Saint-Hilaire MH, Dorflinger E, Pedder S. Tolcapone improves motor function in parkinsonian patients with the "wearing-off" phenomenon: a double-blind, placebo-controlled, multicenter trial. Neurology. 1997;49(4):1066–71.
85. Baas H, Beiske AG, Ghika J, Jackson M, Oertel WH, Poewe W, Ransmayer G. Catechol-O-methyltransferase inhibition with tolcapone reduces the "wearing off" phenomenon and levodopa requirements in fluctuating parkinsonian patients. J Neurol Neurosurg Psychiatry. 1997;63(4):421–8.
86. Parkinson Study Group. Entacapone improves motor fluctuations in levodopa-treated Parkinson's disease patients. Ann Neurol. 1997;42(5):747–55.
87. Watkins P. COMT inhibitors and liver toxicity. Neurology. 2000;55(11 Suppl 4):S51–2.
88. Deane KH, Spieker S, Clarke CE. Catechol-O-methyltransferase inhibitors for levodopa-induced complications in Parkinson's disease. Cochrane Database Syst Rev. 2004;4:CD004554.
89. Ferreira JJ, Lees A, Rocha JF, Poewe W, Rascol O, Soares-da-Silva P; Bi-Park 1 Investigators. Opicapone as an adjunct to levodopa in patients with Parkinson's disease and end-of-dose motor fluctuations: a randomised, double-blind, controlled trial. Lancet Neurol. 2015 Dec 22. pii: S1474-4422(15)00336-1.
90. Rascol O, Brooks DJ, Melamed E, Oertel W, Poewe W, Stocchi F, Tolosa E, LARGO Study Group. Rasagiline as an adjunct to levodopa in patients with Parkinson's disease and motor fluctuations (LARGO, Lasting effect in Adjunct therapy with Rasagiline Given Once daily, study): a randomized, double-blind, parallel-group trial. Lancet. 2005;365(9463): 947–54.
91. Borgohain R, Szasz J, Stanzione P, Meshram C, Bhatt M, Chirilineau D, Stocchi F, Lucini V, Giuliani R, Forrest E, Rice P, Anand R, Study 016 Investigators. Randomized trial of safinamide add-on to levodopa in Parkinson's disease with motor fluctuations. Mov Disord. 2014;29:229–37.
92. Borgohain R, Szasz J, Stanzione P, Meshram C, Bhatt M, Chirilineau D, Stocchi F, Lucini V, Giuliani R, Forrest E, Rice P, Anand R, Study 018 Investigators. Two-year, randomized, controlled study of safinamide as add-on to levodopa in mid to late Parkinson's disease. Mov Disord. 2014;29:1273–80.
93. Nutt JG, Woodward WR, Hammerstad JP, Carter JH, Anderson JL. The "on-off" phenomenon in Parkinson's disease. Relation to levodopa absorption and transport. N Engl J Med. 1984;310:483–8.
94. Karstaedt PJ, Pincus JH. Protein redistribution diet remains effective in patients with fluctuating parkinsonism. Arch Neurol. 1992;49:149–51.
95. Riley D, Lang AE. Practical application of a low-protein diet for Parkinson's disease. Neurology. 1988;38:1026–31.
96. SoyKan I, Sarosiek I, Shifflett J, Wooten GF, McCallum RW. Effect of chronic oral domperidone therapy on gastrointestinal symptoms and gastric emptying in patients with Parkinson's disease. Mov Disord. 1997;12(6):952–7.
97. Jost WH. Gastrointestinal motility problems in patients with Parkinson's disease. Effects of antiparkinsonian treatment and guidelines for management. Drugs Aging. 1997;10(4):249–58.

98. Drolet B, Rousseau G, Daleau P, Cardinal R, Turgeon J. Domperidone should not be considered a no-risk alternative to cisapride in the treatment of gastrointestinal motility disorders. Circulation. 2000;102(16):1883–5.
99. Ahlskog JE, Muenter MD. Frequency of levodopa-related dyskinesias and motor fluctuations as estimated from the cumulative literature. Mov Disord. 2001;16(3):448–58.
100. Snow BJ, Macdonald L, Mcauley D, Wallis W. The effect of amantadine on L-dopa-induced dyskinesias in Parkinson's disease: a double-blind, placebo-controlled study. Clin Neuropharmacol. 2000;23(2):82–5.
101. Metman LV, Del Dotto P, LePoole K, Konitsiotis S, Fang J, Chase TN. Amantadine for levodopa-induced dyskinesias: a 1-year follow-up study. Arch Neurol. 1999;56(11):1383–6.
102. Durif F, Vidailhet M, Assal F, Roche C, Bonnet AM, Agid Y. Low-dose clozapine improves dyskinesias in Parkinson's disease. Neurology. 1997;48(3):658–62.
103. Bennet JP, Landow ER, Schuh LA. Suppression of dyskinesias in advanced Parkinso's disease. II. Increasing daily clozapine doses suppress dyskinesias and improve parkinsonism symptoms. Neurology. 1993;43(8):1551–5.
104. Durif F, Debilly B, Galitzky M, Morand D, Viallet F, Borg M, Thobois S, Broussolle E, Rascol O. Clozapine improves dyskinesias in Parkinson's disease: a double-blind, placebo-controlled study. Neurology. 2004;62(3):381–8.
105. Manson AJ, Schrag A, Lees AJ. Low-dose olanzapine for levodopa induced dyskinesias. Neurology. 2000;55(6):795–9.
106. Jankovic J, Poewe W. Therapies in Parkinson's disease. Curr Opin Neurol. 2012;25(4):433–47.
107. Hilker R, Antonini A, Odin P. What is the best treatment for fluctuating Parkinson's disease: continuous drug delivery or deep brain stimulation of the subthalamic nucleus? J Neural Transm. 2011;118(6):907–14.
108. Neef C, van Laar T. Pharmacokinetic-pharmacodynamic relationships of apomorphine in patients with Parkinson's disease. Clin Pharmacokinet. 1999;37(3):257–71.
109. Honig H, Antonini A, Martinez-Martin P, Forgacs I, Faye GC, Fox T, Fox K, Mancini F, Canesi M, Odin P, Chaudhuri KR. Intrajejunal levodopa infusion in Parkinson's disease: a pilot multicenter study of effects on nonmotor symptoms and quality of life. Mov Disord. 2009:24(10):1468–74.
110. Antonini A, Mancini F, Canesi M, Zangaglia R, Isaias IU, Manfredi L, Pacchetti C, Zibetti M, Natuzzi F, Lopiano L, Nappi G, Pezzoli G. Duodenal levodopa infusion improves quality of live in advanced Parkinson's disease. Neurodegener Dis. 2008;5(3–4):244–6.
111. Morgante L, Basile G, Epifanio A, Spina E, Antonini A, Stocchi F, Di Rosa AE. Continuous apomorphine infusion (CAI) and neuropsychiatric disorders in patients with advanced Parkinson 's disease: a follow-up of two years. Arch Gerontol Geriatr Suppl. 2004;9:291–6.
112. Bowron A. Practical considerations in the use of apomorphine injectable. Neurology. 2004;62(6 Suppl 4):S32–6.
113. Eggert K, Schrader C, Hahn M, Stamelou M, Russmann A, Dengler R, Oertel W, Odin P. Continuous jejunal levodopa infusion in patients with advanced Parkinson disease: practical aspects and outcome of motor of motor and non-motor complications. Clin Neuropharmacol. 2008;31(3): 151–66.
114. Rascol O, Perez-Lloret S, Ferreira JJ. New treatments for levodopa-induced motor complications. Mov Disord. 2015;30:1451–60.
115. Svenningsson P, Westman E, Ballard C, Aarsland D. Cognitive impairment in patients with Parkinson's disease: diagnosis, biomarkers, and treatment. Lancet Neurol. 2012;11:697–707.
116. Aarsland D, Zaccai J, Brayne C. A systematic review of prevalence studies of dementia in Parkinson's disease. Mov Discord. 2005;20:1255–63.
117. Muslimovic D, Post B, Speelman JD, Schmand B. Cognitive profile of patients with newly diagnosed Parkinson disease. Neurology. 2005;65:1239–45.
118. Levin BE, Llabre MM, Reisman S, Weiner WJ, Sanchez-Ramos J, Singer C, Brown MC. Visual impairment in Parkinson's disease. Neurology. 1991;41:365–9.
119. Butter TC, van der Hout A, Mattheus FE, Larsen JP, Brayne C, Aarsland D. Dementia and survival in Parkinson's disease: a 12-year population study. Neurology. 2008;70:1017–22.
120. Emre M, Aarsland D, Albanese A, Byrne EJ, Deuschl G, De Deyn PP, Durif F, Kulisevsky J, van Laar T, Lees A, Poewe W, Robillard A, Rosa MM, Wolters E, Quarg P, Tekin S, Lane R. Rivastigmine for dementia associated with Parkinson's disease. N Engl J Med. 2004;351:2509–18.
121. Aarsland D, Laake K, Larsen J, Javin C. Donepezil for cognitive impairment in Parkinson's disease: a randomised controlled study. J Neurol Neurosurg Psychiatry. 2002;68:708–12.
122. Ravina B, Putt M, Siderowf A, Farrar JT, Gillespie M, Crawley A, Fernandez HH, Trieschmann MM, Reichwein S, Simuni T. Donepezil for dementia in Parkinson's disease: a randomised, double blind, placebo controlled, crossover study. J Neurol Neurosurg Psychiatry. 2005;76:934–9.
123. Leroi I, Brandt J, Reich SG, Lyketsos CG, Grill S, Thompson R, Marsh L. Randomized placebo-controlled trial of donepezil in cognitive impairment in Parkinson's disease. Int J Geriatr Psychiatry. 2004;19:1–8.
124. Litvinenko I, Odinak M, Mogil'naya V, Emelin A. Efficacy and safety of galantamine (reminyl) for dementia in patients with Parkinson's disease (an open controlled trial). Neurosci Behav Physiol. 2008;38:937–45.

125. Aarsland D, Ballard C, Walker Z, Bostrom F, Alves G, Kossakowski K, Leroi I, Pozo-Rodriguez F, Minthon L, Londos E. Memantine in patients with Parkinson's disease dementia or dementia with Lewy bodies: a double-blind, placebo-controlled, multicentre trial. Lancet Neurol. 2009;8:613–8.
126. Emre M, Tsolaki M, Bonuccelli U, Destée A, Tolosa E, Kutzelnigg A, Ceballos-Baumann A, Zdravkovic S, Bladström A, Jones R, 11018 Study Investigators. Memantine for patients with Parkinson's disease dementia or dementia with Lewy bodies: a randomized double-blind, placebo-controlled trial. Lancet Neurol. 2010;9:969–77.
127. Leroi I, Overshott R, Byrne EJ, Daniel E, Burns A. Randomized controlled trial of memantine in dementia associated with Parkinson's disease. Mov Disord. 2009;24:1217–21.
128. Friedman JH. Parkinson's disease psychosis 2010: a review article. Parkinsonism Relat Disord. 2010;16(9):553–60.
129. Forsaa EB, Larsen JP, Wentzel-Larsen T, Goetz CG, Stebbins GT, Aarsland D, Alves G. A 12-year population-based study of psychosis in Parkinson disease. Arch Neurol. 2010;67(8):996–1001.
130. Zahodne LB, Fernandez HH. Pathophysiology and treatment of psychosis in Parkinson's disease: a review. Drugs Aging. 2008;25(8):665–82.
131. Burn D, Emre M, McKeith I, De Deyn PP, Aarsland D, Hsu C, Lane R. Effects of rivastigmine in patients with and without visual hallucinations in dementia associated with Parkinson's disease. Mov Disord. 2006;21(11):1899–907.
132. Parkinson Study Group. Low-dose clozapine for the treatment of drug-induced psychosis in Parkinson's disease. N Engl J Med. 1999;340:757–63.
133. Factor SA, Friedman JH, Lannon MC, Oakes D, Bourgeois K, Parkinson Study Group. Clozapine for the treatment of drug-induced psychosis in Parkinson's disease: results of the 12 week open label extension in the PSYCLOPS trial. Mov Disord. 2001;16:135–9.
134. Pollak P, Tison F, Rascol O, Destée A, Péré JJ, Senard JM, Durif F, Bourdeix I. Clozapine in drug induced psychosis in Parkinson's disease: a randomised, placebo controlled study with open follow up. J Neurol Neurosurg Psychiatry. 2004;75:689–95.
135. Schulte P. Risk of clozapine-associated agranulocytosis and mandatory white blood cell monitoring. Ann Pharmacother. 2006;40:683–8.
136. Fernandez HH, Friedman JH, Jacques C, Rosenfeld M. Quetiapine for the treatment of drug-induced psychosis in Parkinson's disease. Mov Disord. 1999;14:484–7.
137. Morgante L, Epifanio A, Spina E, Di Rosa AE, Zappia M, Basile G, La Spina P, Quattrone A. Quetiapine versus clozapine: a preliminary report of comparative effects on dopaminergic psychosis in patients with Parkinson's disease. Neurol Sci. 2002;23(Supl 2):S89–90.
138. Juncos JL, Roberts VJ, Evatt ML, Jewart RD, Wood CD, Potter LS, Jou HC, Yeung PP. Quetiapine improves psychotic symptoms and cognition in Parkinson's disease. Mov Disord. 2004;19:29–35.
139. Shotbolt P, Samuel M, David A. Quetiapine in the treatment of psychosis in Parkinson's disease. Ther Adv Neurol Disord. 2010;3:339–50.
140. Breier A, Sutton VK, Feldman PD, Kadam DL, Ferchland I, Wright P, Friedman JH. Olanzapine in the treatment of dopamimetic-induced psychosis in patients with Parkinson's disease. Biol Psychiatry. 2002;52:438–45.
141. Goetz C, Blasucci L, Leurgans S, Pappert E. Olanzapine and clozapine: comparative effects on motor function in hallucinating PD patients. Neurology. 2000;55(6):789–94.
142. Mohr E, Mendis T, Hildebrand K, De Deyn PP. Risperidone in the treatment of dopamine-induced psychosis in Parkinson's disease: an open pilot trial. Mov Disord. 2000;15(6):1230–7.
143. Meco G, Alessandria A, Bonifati V, Giustini P. Risperidone for hallucinations in levodopa-treated in Parkinson's disease patients. Lancet. 1994;343(8909):1370–1.
144. Cummings J, Isaacson S, Mills R, Williams H, Chi-Burris K, Corbett A, Dhall R, Ballard C. Pimavanserin for patients with Parkinson's disease psychosis: a randomised, placebo-controlled phase 3 trial. Lancet. 2014;383(9916):533–40.
145. Cummings JL. Depression and Parkinson's disease: a review. Am J Psychiatry. 1992;149(4):443–54.
146. Burn DJ. Beyond the iron mask: towards better recognition and treatment of depression associated with Parkinson's disease. Mov Disord. 2002;17(3):445–54.
147. Miyasaki JM, Shannon K, Voon V, Ravina B, Kleiner-Fisman G, Anderson K, Shulman LM, Gronseth G, Weiner WJ, Quality Standards Subcommittee of the American Academy of Neurology. Practice parameter: evaluation and treatment of depression, psychosis, and dementia in Parkinson's disease (an evidence-based review): report of the Quality Standards Subcommittee of the American Academy of Neurology. Neurology. 2006;66(7):996–1002.
148. Andersen J, Aabro E, Gulmann N, Hjelmsted A, Pedersen HE. Antidepressive treatment in Parkinson's disease: a controlled trial of the effect of nortriptyline in patients with Parkinson's disease treated with L-dopa. Acta Neurol Scand. 1980;62:210–9.
149. Menza M, Dobkin RD, Marin H, Mark MH, Gara M, Buyske S, Bienfait K, Dicke A. A controlled trial of antidepressants in patients with Parkinson disease and depression. Neurology. 2009;72(10):886–92.
150. Richard IH, McDermott MP, Kurlan R, Lyness JM, Como PG, Pearson N, Factor SA, Juncos J, Serrano Ramos C, Brodsky M, Manning C, Marsh L, Shulman L, Fernandez HH, Black KJ, Panisset M, Christine CW, Jiang W, Singer C, Horn S, Pfeiffer R, Rottenberg D, Slevin J, Elmer L, Press D, Hyson HC, McDonald W, SAD-PD Study Group. A randomized, double-blind, placebo-controlled trial of

antidepressants in Parkinson disease. Neurology. 2012;78(16):1229–36.

151. Leentjens AF, Vreeling FW, Luijeckx GJ, Verhey FR. SSRIs in the treatment of depression in Parkinson's disease. Int J Geriatr Psychiatry. 2003;18(6):552–4.
152. Ceravolo R, Nuti A, Piccinni A, Dell'Agnello G, Bellini G, Gambaccini G, Dell'Osso L, Murri L, Bonuccelli U. Paroxetine in Parkinson's disease: effects on motor and depressive symptoms. Neurology. 2000;55(8):1216–8.
153. Leo RJ. Movement disorders associated with the serotonin selective reuptake inhibitors. J Clin Psychiatry. 1996;57(10):449–54.
154. Richard IH, Kurlan R, Tanner C, Factor S, Hubble J, Suchowersky O, Waters C. Serotonin syndrome and the combined use of deprenyl and an antidepressant in Parkinson's disease. Parkinson Study Group. Neurology. 1997;48(4):1070–7.
155. Barone P, Poewe W, Albrecht S, Debieuvre C, Massey D, Rascol O, Tolosa E, Weintraub D. Pramipexole for the treatment of depressive symptoms in patients with Parkinson's disease: a randomised, double-blind, placebo-controlled trial. Lancet Neurol. 2010;9(6):573–80.
156. Scoffer KL, Henderson RD, O'Maley K, O'Sullivan JD. Nonpharmacological treatment, fludrocortisone, and domperidone for orthostatic hypotension in Parkinson's disease. Mov Disord. 2007;22(11):1543–9.
157. Jankovic J, Gilden JL, Hiner BC, Kaufmann H, Brown DC, Coghlan CH, Rubin M, Fouad-Tarazi FM. Neurogenic orthostatic hypotension: a double-blind placebo-controlled study with midodrine. Am J Med. 1993;95:38–48.
158. Low PA, Gilden FL, Freeman R, Sheng KN, McElligott MA. Efficacy of midodrine vs placebo in neurogenic orthostatic hypotension. A randomized double-blind multicenter study. Midodrine study group. JAMA. 1997;277:1046 51.
159. Hoehn MM. Levodopa induced postural hypotension. Treatment with fludrocortisone. Arch Neurol. 1975;32:50–1.
160. Riley DE. Orthostatic hypotension in multiple system atrophy. Curr Treat Options Neurol. 2000;2:225–30.
161. Fox SH, Marras C. Orthostatic hypotension in Parkinsonism: what is it and how can we treat it? Mov Disord. 2015;5:601–3.
162. Singer C, Weiner W, Sanchez-Ramos J. Autonomic dysfunction in men with Parkinson's disease. Eur Neurol. 1992;32:134–40.
163. Suchowersky O, Furtado S, Rohs G. Beneficial effect of intranasal desmopressin for nocturnal polyuria in Parkinson's disease. Mov Disord. 1995;10:337–40.
164. Yarker YE, Goa KL, Fitton A. Oxybutynin: a review of its pharmacokinetic properties and its therapeutic use in detrusor instability. Drugs Aging. 1995;6(3):243–62.
165. Appell RA. Clinical efficacy and safety of tolterodine in the treatment of overactive bladder: a pooled analysis. Urology. 1997;50:90–6.
166. Christmas TJ, Kempster PA, Chapple CR, Frankel JP, Lees AJ, Stern GM, Milroy EJ. Role of subcutaneous apomorphine in parkinsonian voiding dysfunction. Lancet. 1988;2:1451–3.
167. Byrne C, Pfeiffer R, Quigley EM. Gastrointestinal dysfunction in Parkinson's disease: a report of clinical experience at a single center. J Clin Gastroenterol. 1994;19:11–6.
168. Zangaglia R, Martignoni E, Glorioso M, Ossola M, Riboldazzi G, Calandrella D, Brunetti G, Pacchetti C. Macrogol for the treatment of constipation in Parkinson's disease. A randomized placebo-controlled study. Mov Disord. 2007;22(9):1239–44.
169. Sullivan KL, Staffetti JF, Hauser RA, Dunne PB, Zesiewicz TA. Tegaserod (Zelnorm) for the treatment of constipation in Parkinson's disease. Mov Disord. 2006;21(1):115–6.
170. Miller LG, Jankovic J. Metoclopramide-induced movement disorders. Clinical findings with a review of the literature. Arch Intern Med. 1989;149(11):2486–92.
171. Ganzini L, Casey DE, Hoffman WF, McCall AL. The prevalence of metoclopramide-induced tardive dyskinesia and acute extrapyramidal movement disorders. Arch Intern Med. 1993;153(12):1469–75.
172. Arbouw ME, Movig KL, Koopmann M, Poels PJ, Guchelaar HJ, Egberts TC, Neef C, van Vugt JP. Glycopyrrolate for sialorrhea in Parkinson's disease: a randomized, double-blind, crossover trial. Neurology. 2010;74(15):1203–7.
173. Hyson HC, Johnson AM, Jog MS. Sublingual atropine for sialorrhea secondary to parkinsonism: a pilot study. Mov Disord. 2002;17(6):1318–20.
174. Thomsen TR, Galpern WR, Asante A, Arenovich T, Fox SH. Ipratropium bromide spray as treatment for sialorrhea in Parkinson's disease. Mov Disord. 2007;22:2268–73.
175. Chinnapongse R, Gullo K, Nemeth P, Zhang Y, Griggs L. Safety and efficacy of botulinum toxin type B for treatment of sialorrhea in Parkinson's disease: a prospective double-blind trial. Mov Disord. 2012;27(2):219–26.
176. Ondo WG, Hunter C, Moore W. A double-blind placebo-controlled trial of botulinum toxin B for sialorrhea in Parkinson's disease. Neurology. 2004;62(1):37–40.
177. Lagalla G, Millevolte M, Capecci M, Provinciali L, Ceravolo MG. Long-lasting benefits of botulinum toxin type B in Parkinson's disease-related drooling. J Neurol. 2009;256(4):563–7.
178. Lagalla G, Millevolte M, Capecci M, Provinciali L, Ceravolo MG. Botulinum toxin type A for drooling in Parkinson's disease: a double-blind, randomized, placebo-controlled study. Mov Disord. 2006;21(5):704–7.
179. Factor SA, McAlarney T, Sanchez-Ramos JR, Weiner WJ. Sleep disorders and sleep effect in Parkinson's disease. Mov Disord. 1990;5(4):280–5.
180. Iranzo A, Milonuevo JL, Santamaria J, Serradell M, Martí MJ, Valldeoriola F, Tolosa E. Rapid-

eye-movement sleep behavior disorder as an early marker for a neurodegenerative disorder: a descriptive study. Lancet Neurol. 2006;5(7):572–7.
181. Iranzo A, Santamaría J, Rye DB, Valldeoriola F, Martí MJ, Muñoz E, Vilaseca I, Tolosa E. Characteristics of idiopathic REM sleep behavior disorder and that associated with MSA and PD. Neurology. 2005;65(2):247–52.
182. Olson EJ, Boeve BF, Silber MH. Rapid eye movement sleep behavior disorder: demographic, clinical, and laboratory findings in 93 cases. Brain. 2000;123:331–9.
183. Fantini ML, Gagnon JF, Filipini D, Montplaisir J. The effects of pramipexole in REM sleep behavior disorder. Neurology. 2003;61(10):1418–20.
184. Schmidt MH, Koshal VB, Schmidt HS. Use of pramipexole in REM sleep behavior disorder: results from a case series. Sleep Med. 2006;7(5):418–23.
185. Kumru H, Iranzo A, Carrasco E, Valldeoriola F, Marti MJ, Santamaria J, Tolosa E. Lack of effects of pramipexole on REM sleep behavior disorder in Parkinson's disease. Sleep. 2008;31:1418–21.
186. Winkelman JW, James L. Serotoninergic antidepressants are associated with REM sleep without atonia. Sleep. 2004;27(2):317–21.
187. Tan EK, Lum SY, Fook-Chong SM, Teoh ML, Yih Y, Tan L, Tan A, Wong MC. Evaluation of somnolence in Parkinson's disease: comparison with age- and sex-matched controls. Neurology. 2002;58(3):465–8.
188. Högl B, Rothdach A, Wetter TC, Trenkwalder C. The effect of cabergoline on sleep, periodic leg movements in sleep, and early morning function in patients with Parkinson's disease. Neuropsychopharmacology. 2003;28:866–70.
189. Ferreira JJ, Desboeuf K, Galitzky M, Thalamas C, Brefel-Courbon C, Fabre N, Senard JM, Montastruc JL, Sampaio C, Rascol O. Sleep disruption, daytime somnolence and 'sleep attacks' in Parkinson's disease: a clinical survey in PD patients and age matched healthy volunteers. Eur J Neurol. 2006;13(3):209–14.
190. Montastruc JL, Brefel-Courbon C, Senard JM, Bagheri H, Ferreira J, Rascol O, Lapeyre-Mestre M. Sleep attacks and antiparkinsonian drugs: a pilot prospective pharmacoepidemiologic study. Neuropharmacology. 2001;24(3):181–3.
191. Hosborn DE, Lang AE, Martin WR, Razmy A, Rivest J, Fleming J. Excessive daytime sleepiness and sudden-onset sleep in Parkinson's disease: a survey by the Canadian Movement Disorders Group. JAMA. 2002;287(4):455–63.
192. Paus S, Brecht HM, Koster J, Seeger G, Klockgether T, Wullner U. Sleep attacks, daytime sleepiness, and dopamine agonists in Parkinson's disease. Mov Disord. 2003;18(6):659–67.
193. Brodsky MA, Godbold J, Roth T, Olanow CW. Sleepiness in Parkinson's disease: a controlled study. Mov Disord. 2003;18(6):668–72.
194. Körner Y, Meindorfner C, Möller JC, Stiasny-Kolster K, Haja D, Cassel W, Oertel WH, Krüger HP. Predictors of sudden onset sleep in Parkinson's disease. Mov Disord. 2004;19(11):298–305.
195. Högl B, Saletu M, Brandauer E, Glatzl S, Frauscher B, Seppi K, Ulmer H, Wenning G, Poewe W. Modafinil for the treatment of daytime sleepiness in Parkinson's disease: a double-blind, randomized, crossover, placebo-controlled polygraphic trial. Sleep. 2002;25(8):905–9.
196. Adler CH, Caviness JN, Hentz JG, Lind M, Tiede J. Randomized trial of modafinil for treating subjective daytime sleepiness in patients with Parkinson's disease. Mov Disord. 2003;18(3):287–93.
197. Ondo WG, Fayle R, Atassi F, JanKovic J. Modafinil for daytime somnolence in Parkinson's disease: double blind, placebo controlled parallel trial. J Neurol Neurosurg Psychiatry. 2005;76(12):1636–9.
198. Mendonça DA, Menezes K, Jog MS. Methylphenidate improves fatigue scores in Parkinson's disease: a randomized controlled trail. Mov Disord. 2007;22(14):2070–6.

Surgical Treatment of Parkinson's Disease, Transplantations and Restorative Therapies for Parkinson's Diseases

15

Lisa Klingelhoefer, Ismail Ughratdar, Michael Samuel, K. Ray Chaudhuri, and Keyoumars Ashkan

Abbreviations

ADL	Activities of daily living
DBS	Deep brain stimulation
DRT	Dopamine replacement therapy
GPi	Globus pallidus internus
HRQoL	Health-related quality of life
ICD	Impulse control disorder
IPG	Implantable pulse generator
LED	Levodopa equivalent dose
MPTP	1-methyl-4-phenyl-1,2,3,6-tetrahydropyridine
MRI	Magnetic resonance imaging
NMS	Non-motor symptom
NMSS	Non-motor symptom scale
PD	Parkinson's disease
STN	Subthalamic nucleus
UPDRS	Unified Parkinson's disease rating scale
VIM	Thalamic ventralis intermedius

L. Klingelhoefer, MD (✉)
Department of Neurology, Technical University Dresden, Fetscherstraße 74, Dresden, Germany

National Parkinson Foundation International Centre of Excellence, Department of Neurology, King's College Hospital and King's College, SE5 9RS, Denmark Hill, London, UK
e-mail: lisa.klingelhoefer@nhs.net

I. Ughratdar, FRCS • K. Ashkan, MD, FRCP, FRCS
Department of Neurosurgery, King's College Hospital, Denmark Hill, London, UK
e-mail: k.ashkan@nhs.net

M. Samuel, MD • K. Ray Chaudhuri, MD, FRCP
National Parkinson Foundation International Centre of Excellence, Department of Neurology, King's College Hospital and King's College, SE5 9RS, Denmark Hill, London, UK

15.1 Surgical Treatment of Parkinson's Disease

Contemporary neurosurgical techniques for Parkinson's disease (PD) trace their origins to Dr. Irving Cooper when he inadvertently ligated the anterior choroidal artery in a patient resulting in serendipitous improvement in tremor and rigidity. This was largely superseded by thalamotomy which conferred beneficial results. However, concerns about irreversibility and complications associated with bilateral ablation has resulted in high-frequency deep brain stimulation (DBS) becoming the gold standard surgical procedure in PD and other movement disorders such as essential tremor or dystonia.

DBS involves identification of basal ganglia target nuclei utilising high-resolution imaging, especially MRI, and subsequent implantation of electrode leads using stereotactic techniques. The procedure is usually performed under local anaesthetic to allow

C. Falup-Pecurariu et al. (eds.), *Movement Disorders Curricula*,
DOI 10.1007/978-3-7091-1628-9_15

for neurophysiological and clinical confirmation of optimal electrode placement. The leads are then connected subcutaneously via extension wires to an implantable pulse generator (IPG) which is implanted in the chest wall. The IPG serves both as a battery and programming device able to alter the electrical output from the leads.

15.1.1 Intracranial Target

The intracranial target for DBS is dependent upon the predominant symptoms of the patient (Table 15.1). The subthalamic nucleus (STN) is the standard target in majority of PD patients and confers significant improvement in all three cardinal PD motor symptoms as well as control of motor fluctuations and dyskinesias following the reduction of dopamine replacement therapies (DRT). The globus pallidus internus (GPi) allows a comparable control of motor symptoms with a possible advantage of less neuropsychiatric complications compared with STN stimulation. However, DRT cannot be significantly reduced. GPi stimulation may expend the battery more rapidly due to the need of higher stimulation parameters [1–3]. In older patients where tremor is the predominant symptom, thalamic ventralis intermedius (VIM) for tremor control may be considered [4].

15.1.2 Complications

In general, rate of major complications such as haemorrhage or infection with DBS is low (0.4–3 %) [5, 6]. Neuropsychological and psychiatric side effects occur most often in the immediate postoperative period after DBS, possibly related to the changes in DRT or the surgery itself [7–9]. Stimulation-induced side effects such as paraesthesia, dysarthria, ataxia, dystonia or brain steam effects such as flashing lights in the visual fields are dependent of the electrode position, primarily transient and may be treated by change of stimulation parameters.

Table 15.1 Comparison of stimulation on different DBS targets in PD

PD symptoms	STN	GPi	VIM
Tremor	++	+	+++
Akinesia	+++	++	–
Rigidity	+++	+++	–
Dyskinesia	++	++	–
Off dystonia	+++	++	–
Reduction of DRT	+++	–/+	–
Battery consumption	Low	High	Low

– no, + slight, ++ good, +++ excellent control

15.1.3 Patient Selection

The key challenge with DBS remains patient selection and is facilitated by multidisciplinary assessment. The ideal candidate has a diagnosis of idiopathic PD based on the UK Brain Bank criteria with significant off symptoms resulting in disability in activities of daily living (ADL), continued levodopa responsiveness with a levodopa challenge test >30 % improvement of PD symptoms (exception in tremor dominant PD) and motor complications such as fluctuations or dyskinesia.

Exclusion criteria and surgical risk factors include:

- Imaging (e.g. severe brain atrophy, brain lesions causing anatomical changes).
- Neuropsychiatric and neuropsychological (active psychiatric disease, e.g. psychosis, personality disorder or substance abuse, major depression with suicidal ideation, dementia) – thus a psychiatric assessment with cognitive testing should be performed preoperatively.
- General medical (e.g. cardiovascular co-morbidities, coagulopathy).

15.1.4 Motor Outcomes

There is good long-term evidence on effectiveness of DBS to improve motor symptoms in advanced PD with significant benefits in tremor, rigidity and bradykinesia [10–15]. Recently it has been shown that DBS implantation performed earlier in the course of the disease confers significant benefits on motor symptoms and health-related quality of life (HRQoL) [11].

Typically improvements in general motor state as measured by UPDRS III of 50 %, reduction in off periods during the day by 70 % and prolongation of periods with good mobility of approximately 20 % are expected [11, 12, 16, 17]. Overall, tremor and rigidity show better long-term improvement than bradykinesia. Axial symptoms that respond to the levodopa usually also improve with STN DBS. Furthermore, complications like motor fluctuations and dyskinesias decrease by 60–70 % after STN DBS [11, 12, 17]. Despite these benefits, the natural neurodegenerative course of PD does not appear to be altered by DBS and, thus in the long term, worsening of axial symptoms and akinesia should be expected. Cognitive decline is also unchanged reflecting the natural course of the disease. Nevertheless, a consistent marked motor improvement especially of tremor, rigidity, motor fluctuations and dyskinesias without worsening has been reported in studies after 5 and up to 10 years after STN DBS [14, 18].

Levodopa equivalent dose (LED) of Parkinsonian daily medications can be reduced by 40–60 % which is maintained after 5 years.

Recently, it has been shown that motor improvements after STN DBS is not limited to patients with advanced PD. The randomised, prospective multicentre EARLYSTIM trial [11] hypothesised that DBS would be beneficial at an earlier stage of disease. Patients in an earlier stage of PD, mainly defined by younger age (52 years), shorter duration of PD symptoms (7.5 years) and shorter existence of motor fluctuations and dyskinesias (1.6 years) were randomised to best medical therapy ($n = 127$) or bilateral STN DBS ($n = 120$) [11]. The primary outcome assessing quality of life using the PDQ-39 score showed a 26 % improvement in the neurostimulation group opposed to a 1 % worsening in the medical therapy group which was sustained at 24-months follow-up, and this improvement in the neurostimulation group is as good as it was found in PD patients in advanced stage (25 %) [11, 12]. UPDRS III motor scores off medication improved 53 % in the DBS group. Additionally, DBS was superior to medical therapy with respect to ADLs ($p < 0.001$), levodopa-induced motor complications ($p < 0.001$) and time with good mobility and no dyskinesia ($p = 0.01$). Cognitive change did not differ between groups; however, mood and overall psychiatric morbidity were more favourable in the neurostimulation group. Given these results, especially when applied before the onset of disabling motor symptoms, DBS has been advocated at an earlier stage in the disease process than the current practice. However, long-term outcome in this cohort is awaited.

15.1.5 Non-motor Outcomes

Non-motor symptoms (NMS) are common in PD patients and can have a huge impact on patients' HRQoL [19, 20]. They are more frequent and severe in advanced PD [21] but are also present in early stages of PD and even before dopaminergic medication has been initiated [22]. Therefore, therapies instigated in patients with PD, independent of disease stage, must address motor and non-motor symptoms to provide optimal quality of life, health status and individual well-being [23]. Though DBS literature has primarily focused on motor symptoms, evidence indicates that STN DBS can improve NMS in selected patients [24]. Given the relative paucity of literature on non-motor outcome following DBS, we aim to provide a detailed review here.

Mean improvement of 36 % on non-motor symptom scale (NMSS) [25] and a significant decrease in the number and the severity of most NMS after STN DBS [26] with associated improved QoL and ADLs [27] have been reported. However, not all NMS improve and indeed some may deteriorate both transiently and permanently [7, 28]. The underlying mechanism for changes in NMS following DBS may be related to the alterations in the dopamine replacement therapy (DRT) that follows DBS, the surgery itself (e.g. oedema along the tract and micro-lesion effect at the target) or the electrical stimulation at the active electrode contact [23].

The effect of STN DBS on mood disorders like depression, mania and anxiety is variable. These can improve [9, 26], remain unchanged

[29] or worsen [30] compared to the preoperative state. Both postoperative DRT changes and DBS may be responsible. Direct postoperative changes in mood such as mania have been described by the anatomical localisation of the electrodes and current spread to, e.g. ventral-medial limbic portion of the STN or the limbic circuits [31, 32]. Pre-existing drug-induced psychotic symptoms like hallucinations disappear after STN DBS in nearly all PD patients following reduction of DRT [33]. On the other hand, transient psychotic symptoms such as delirium may be seen in the immediate postoperative period as the direct result of surgery, possibly related to peri-electrode oedema [23].

Similarly behavioural disorders may occur and should be carefully monitored following DBS. Impulse control disorders (ICD), mainly caused by dopaminergic medication, can improve markedly or disappear after STN DBS [7, 34]. This effect may be due to decreased stimulation of non-motor dopaminergic circuits by reduction of dopaminergic medication, a less pulsatile and non-suprathreshold stimulation of the mesolimbic dopamine receptors or direct modulation by DBS of the reward-seeking brain circuitry [35]. However, there are also reports of occurrence or worsening of ICDs after STN DBS [36, 37]. The time period between DBS and the development of ICD varied, but most of the ICDs were transient and resolved within a year of their development. Thus, vigilance is required for patients with a previous history of ICD or compulsive medication use. Although there are no absolute rules, in general, for PD patients with DRT-induced ICD, STN DBS may be of benefit, whilst for PD patients with ICD independent of DRT, DBS may lead to worsening of the ICD.

Though small, the mortality in the first year following STN DBS has been reported at 0.4 %, and suicide, especially in these patients, is an important risk [38]. It is postulated whether the decision to undergo DBS may self-select a subgroup of patients willing to take higher risks than the general population leading to a higher risk for suicidal behaviour afterwards [11]. Therefore, it may be that the DBS as a procedure is not associated with a higher risk of suicide but that the personality trait of PD patients' deciding for DBS is.

Postoperative apathy may be caused primarily by the withdrawal of DRT as many patients recover completely after treatment with dopaminergic therapy [39, 40]. As apathy is not reversed in all PD patients following DRT, STN DBS in itself may be an additional cause of apathy in a proportion of patients [41]. Given the diversity of the literature on the association between STN DBS and apathy, we hypothesise that different types of apathy, such as transient direct postoperative apathy or apathy in association with depression and/or cognitive deficits, might be caused by different mechanisms [23].

Multiple studies and meta-analysis have consistently shown that STN DBS does not impair overall cognition over short- and long-term follow-up in carefully selected patients, although there may be a selective decrease in the frontal cognitive function with impairment of phonemic and semantic verbal fluency and executive function [29, 42, 43]. These changes do not affect the improvements in QoL which accompanies STN DBS [2] and in fact in self-assessed questionnaire studies showing overall improvement in cognition after STN DBS [11].

Impairment of sleep is one of the most frequent NMS in PD patients. An objective improvement in sleep following STN DBS has been shown with studies using polysomnography through an increase in sleep efficiency and quality, increase in continuous sleep time, decrease in the arousal index, decrease in nocturnal and early morning dystonia and improvement of nocturnal mobility [44]. Furthermore, this objective improvement led to a subjective enhancement in sleep in PD patients after STN DBS measured by NMSS, NMSQuest and PSQI [45]. DBS seems to have a direct effect on sleep regulatory centres without changing the relative percentage of sleep stages [46]. Additional benefits on sleep may be indirectly achieved by reduction in DRT or improvement of mobility and daytime somnolence [47].

Pain and sensory symptoms seem to be improved after STN DBS, especially when they are associated with "off" motor conditions or dystonia in PD patients [48]. This positive effect persisted on a long-term follow-up of 24 months, even when new, mainly musculoskeletal, pain developed [49].

The effect of STN DBS on autonomic dysfunction is rarely investigated and has only been described in a small number of studies. An improvement of sweating and/or bladder and bowel function after STN DBS in PD patients has been reported in small case series [26, 27, 50]. A positive direct effect of STN DBS is suggested by a significant correlation between bladder state, using urodynamic measures, and increased cerebral blood flow (rCBF) in the lateral frontal cortex measured by PET in patients with STN DBS. The improvement in bladder dysfunction after STN DBS is thought to be partly due to a delay in the first desire to void due to an increase in bladder capacity and modulation of bladder control [51, 52].

Furthermore STN DBS appears to have a positive effect on cardiovascular dysautonomia in PD patients [53, 54].

15.2 Transplantations and Restorative Therapies for Parkinson's Disease

Transplantations and restorative therapies for PD have a long history, dating to 1970s, but are still only in use as part of clinical trials. In a randomised study of 40 patients with severe PD receiving either a transplant of human embryonic dopamine neurons or a sham surgery, it was shown that the transplanted cells survived and resulted in some clinical benefit in younger but not older patients [55]. Furthermore, clinical benefit and graft viability were sustained up to 4 years after transplantation, and the imaging changes reliably correlated with clinical outcome over the entire post-transplantation time course [56]. In contrast, in another prospective 24-month double-blind placebo-controlled trial of foetal nigral transplantation in 34 patients with advanced PD, a slight treatment effect in patients with milder disease was observed. Fifty-six percent of the transplanted patients, however, developed off-phase dyskinesia [57]. These dyskinesias were also described by other groups and can persist up to 11 years [58, 59]. Striatal fluorodopa uptake was significantly increased after transplantation, and robust survival of dopamine neurons was observed at post-mortem examination [57]. Thus, currently neural transplantation remains as an experimental therapy. Further studies are necessary to obtain objective evidence of benefit, define target patient population and determine the optimal cells for transplant and the exact brain target area for transplantation [60].

15.3 Optogenetics

Recent advances in optogenetics have allowed for precise modulation of targeted neurons using light. The technique involves developing a genetic construct using a light-activated protein (opsin) which is delivered into brain using viruses. Opsin is expressed in the target neurons, and when laser light of a specific wavelength is shone via an optrode, this induces ion channels in the neuron to open leading to physiological effects. In vivo experiments in Parkinsonian rodents have shown improvement of disease symptoms by preferentially activating neurons that link to the subthalamic nucleus region of the brain [61].

15.4 Near-Infrared Light Therapy

Exposure to near-infrared light treatment, also referred to as photobiomodulation, has been shown to protect dopaminergic cells from degeneration both in vitro and in vivo 1-methyl-4-phenyl-1,2,3,6-tetrahydropyridine (MPTP)-treated animals [62–64]. A recent study has involved implantation of an optical fibre linked to a LED or laser device into the lateral ventricle of MPTP rodents and has confirmed neuroprotection without toxic side effects [65].

These less invasive methods show good promise to be included in the armamentarium for PD treatment, but further translational work in humans is still required.

References

1. Rodriguez-Oroz MC, Obeso JA, Lang AE, Houeto JL, Pollak P, Rehncrona S, et al. Bilateral deep brain stimulation in Parkinson's disease: a multicentre study with 4 years follow-up. Brain. 2005;128(Pt 10):2240–9.
2. Follett KA, Weaver FM, Stern M, Hur K, Harris CL, Luo P, et al. Pallidal versus subthalamic deep-brain stimulation for Parkinson's disease. N Engl J Med. 2010;362(22):2077–91.
3. Follett KA, Torres-Russotto D. Deep brain stimulation of globus pallidus interna, subthalamic nucleus, and pedunculopontine nucleus for Parkinson's disease: which target? Parkinsonism Relat Disord. 2012;18 Suppl 1:S165–7.
4. Hariz MI, Krack P, Alesch F, Augustinsson LE, Bosch A, Ekberg R, et al. Multicentre European study of thalamic stimulation for parkinsonian tremor: a 6 year follow-up. J Neurol Neurosurg Psychiatry. 2008;79(6):694–9.
5. Voges J, Krauss JK. Neurological and technical aspects of deep brain stimulation. Nervenarzt. 2010;81(6):702–10.
6. Voges J, Hilker R, Botzel K, Kiening KL, Kloss M, Kupsch A, et al. Thirty days complication rate following surgery performed for deep-brain-stimulation. Mov Disord. 2007;22(10):1486–9.
7. Lim SY, O'Sullivan SS, Kotschet K, Gallagher DA, Lacey C, Lawrence AD, et al. Dopamine dysregulation syndrome, impulse control disorders and punding after deep brain stimulation surgery for Parkinson's disease. J Clin Neurosci. 2009;16(9):1148–52.
8. Frank MJ, Samanta J, Moustafa AA, Sherman SJ. Hold your horses: impulsivity, deep brain stimulation, and medication in parkinsonism. Science. 2007;318(5854):1309–12.
9. Volkmann J, Daniels C, Witt K. Neuropsychiatric effects of subthalamic neurostimulation in Parkinson disease. Nat Rev Neurol. 2010;6(9):487–98.
10. Benabid AL, Pollak P, Gross C, Hoffmann D, Benazzouz A, Gao DM, et al. Acute and long-term effects of subthalamic nucleus stimulation in Parkinson's disease. Stereotact Funct Neurosurg. 1994;62(1–4):76–84.
11. Schuepbach WM, Rau J, Knudsen K, Volkmann J, Krack P, Timmermann L, et al. Neurostimulation for Parkinson's disease with early motor complications. N Engl J Med. 2013;368(7):610–22.
12. Deuschl G, Schade-Brittinger C, Krack P, Volkmann J, Schafer H, Botzel K, et al. A randomized trial of deep-brain stimulation for Parkinson's disease. N Engl J Med. 2006;355(9):896–908.
13. Ashkan K, Wallace B, Bell BA, Benabid AL. Deep brain stimulation of the subthalamic nucleus in Parkinson's disease 1993–2003: where are we 10 years on? Br J Neurosurg. 2004;18(1):19–34.
14. Krack P, Batir A, Van Blercom N, Chabardes S, Fraix V, Ardouin C, et al. Five-year follow-up of bilateral stimulation of the subthalamic nucleus in advanced Parkinson's disease. N Engl J Med. 2003;349(20):1925–34.
15. Williams A, Gill S, Varma T, Jenkinson C, Quinn N, Mitchell R, et al. Deep brain stimulation plus best medical therapy versus best medical therapy alone for advanced Parkinson's disease (PD SURG trial): a randomised, open-label trial. Lancet Neurol. 2010;9(6):581–91.
16. Kuopio AM, Marttila RJ, Helenius H, Toivonen M, Rinne UK. The quality of life in Parkinson's disease. Mov Disord. 2000;15(2):216–23.
17. Kleiner-Fisman G, Herzog J, Fisman DN, Tamma F, Lyons KE, Pahwa R, et al. Subthalamic nucleus deep brain stimulation: summary and meta-analysis of outcomes. Mov Disord. 2006;21 Suppl 14:S290–304.
18. Rodriguez-Oroz MC, Moro E, Krack P. Long-term outcomes of surgical therapies for Parkinson's disease. Mov Disord. 2012;27(14):1718–28.
19. Chaudhuri KR, Schapira AH. Non-motor symptoms of Parkinson's disease: dopaminergic pathophysiology and treatment. Lancet Neurol. 2009;8(5):464–74.
20. Martinez-Martin P, Rodriguez-Blazquez C, Kurtis MM, Chaudhuri KR. The impact of non-motor symptoms on health-related quality of life of patients with Parkinson's disease. Mov Disord. 2011;26(3):399–406.
21. Leonardi M, Raggi A, Pagani M, Carella F, Soliveri P, Albanese A, et al. Relationships between disability, quality of life and prevalence of nonmotor symptoms in Parkinson's disease. Parkinsonism Relat Disord. 2012;18(1):35–9.
22. Muller B, Assmus J, Herlofson K, Larsen JP, Tysnes OB. Importance of motor vs. non-motor symptoms for health-related quality of life in early Parkinson's disease. Parkinsonism Relat Disord. 2013;19(11):1027–32.
23. Klingelhoefer L, Samuel M, Chaudhuri KR, Ashkan K. An update of the impact of deep brain stimulation on non motor symptoms in Parkinson's disease. J Parkinsons Dis. 2014;4(2):289–300.
24. Witt K, Daniels C, Reiff J, Krack P, Volkmann J, Pinsker MO, et al. Neuropsychological and psychiatric changes after deep brain stimulation for Parkinson's disease: a randomised, multicentre study. Lancet Neurol. 2008;7(7):605–14.
25. Reich MM, Chaudhuri KR, Ashkan K, Hulse N, Costello A, Moriarty J, et al. Changes in the non-motor symptom scale in Parkinson's disease after deep brain stimulation. Basal Ganglia. 2011;1(3):131–3.
26. Wolz M, Hauschild J, Fauser M, Klingelhofer L, Reichmann H, Storch A. Immediate effects of deep brain stimulation of the subthalamic nucleus on non-motor symptoms in Parkinson's disease. Parkinsonism Relat Disord. 2012;18(8):994–7.
27. Nazzaro JM, Pahwa R, Lyons KE. The impact of bilateral subthalamic stimulation on non-motor symptoms of Parkinson's disease. Parkinsonism Relat Disord. 2011;17(8):606–9.

28. Fasano A, Daniele A, Albanese A. Treatment of motor and non-motor features of Parkinson's disease with deep brain stimulation. Lancet Neurol. 2012; 11(5):429–42.
29. Fasano A, Romito LM, Daniele A, Piano C, Zinno M, Bentivoglio AR, et al. Motor and cognitive outcome in patients with Parkinson's disease 8 years after subthalamic implants. Brain. 2010;133(9):2664–76.
30. Pinsker M, Amtage F, Berger M, Nikkhah G, van Elst LT. Psychiatric side-effects of bilateral deep brain stimulation for movement disorders. Acta Neurochir Suppl. 2013;117:47–51.
31. Ulla M, Thobois S, Llorca PM, Derost P, Lemaire JJ, Chereau-Boudet I, et al. Contact dependent reproducible hypomania induced by deep brain stimulation in Parkinson's disease: clinical, anatomical and functional imaging study. J Neurol Neurosurg Psychiatry. 2011;82(6):607–14.
32. Bejjani BP, Damier P, Arnulf I, Thivard L, Bonnet AM, Dormont D, et al. Transient acute depression induced by high-frequency deep-brain stimulation. N Engl J Med. 1999;340(19):1476–80.
33. Umemura A, Oka Y, Okita K, Matsukawa N, Yamada K. Subthalamic nucleus stimulation for Parkinson disease with severe medication-induced hallucinations or delusions. J Neurosurg. 2011;114(6):1701–5.
34. Shotbolt P, Moriarty J, Costello A, Jha A, David A, Ashkan K, et al. Relationships between deep brain stimulation and impulse control disorders in Parkinson's disease, with a literature review. Parkinsonism Relat Disord. 2012;18(1):10–6.
35. Weintraub D, Potenza MN. Impulse control disorders in Parkinson's disease. Curr Neurol Neurosci Rep. 2006;6(4):302–6.
36. Kim YE, Kim HJ, Lee JY, Yun JY, Kim JY, Paek SH, et al. Impulse control and related behaviors after bilateral subthalamic stimulation in patients with Parkinson's disease. J Clin Neurosci. 2013;20(7): 964–9.
37. Demetriades P, Rickards H, Cavanna AE. Impulse control disorders following deep brain stimulation of the subthalamic nucleus in Parkinson's disease: clinical aspects. Parkinsons Dis. 2011;2011:658415.
38. Voon V, Krack P, Lang AE, Lozano AM, Dujardin K, Schupbach M, et al. A multicentre study on suicide outcomes following subthalamic stimulation for Parkinson's disease. Brain. 2008;131(Pt 10):2720–8.
39. Thobois S, Ardouin C, Lhommee E, Klinger H, Lagrange C, Xie J, et al. Non-motor dopamine withdrawal syndrome after surgery for Parkinson's disease: predictors and underlying mesolimbic denervation. Brain. 2010;133(Pt 4):1111–27.
40. Thobois S, Lhommee E, Klinger H, Ardouin C, Schmitt E, Bichon A, et al. Parkinsonian apathy responds to dopaminergic stimulation of D2/D3 receptors with piribedil. Brain. 2013;136(Pt 5): 1568–77.
41. Kirsch-Darrow L, Zahodne LB, Marsiske M, Okun MS, Foote KD, Bowers D. The trajectory of apathy after deep brain stimulation: from pre-surgery to 6 months post-surgery in Parkinson's disease. Parkinsonism Relat Disord. 2011;17(3):182–8.
42. Yaguez L, Costello A, Moriarty J, Hulse N, Selway R, Clough C, et al. Cognitive predictors of cognitive change following bilateral subthalamic nucleus deep brain stimulation in Parkinson's disease. J Clin Neurosci. 2014;21(3):445–50.
43. Wu B, Han L, Sun BM, Hu XW, Wang XP. Influence of deep brain stimulation of the subthalamic nucleus on cognitive function in patients with Parkinson's disease. Neurosci Bull. 2013;30(1):153–61.
44. Iranzo A, Valldeoriola F, Santamaria J, Tolosa E, Rumia J. Sleep symptoms and polysomnographic architecture in advanced Parkinson's disease after chronic bilateral subthalamic stimulation. J Neurol Neurosurg Psychiatry. 2002;72(5):661–4.
45. Amara AW, Standaert DG, Guthrie S, Cutter G, Watts RL, Walker HC. Unilateral subthalamic nucleus deep brain stimulation improves sleep quality in Parkinson's disease. Parkinsonism Relat Disord. 2012;18(1): 63–8.
46. Monaca C, Ozsancak C, Jacquesson JM, Poirot I, Blond S, Destee A, et al. Effects of bilateral subthalamic stimulation on sleep in Parkinson's disease. J Neurol. 2004;251(2):214–8.
47. Lyons KE, Pahwa R. Effects of bilateral subthalamic nucleus stimulation on sleep, daytime sleepiness, and early morning dystonia in patients with Parkinson disease. J Neurosurg. 2006;104(4):502–5.
48. Kim HJ, Paek SH, Kim JY, Lee JY, Lim YH, Kim MR, et al. Chronic subthalamic deep brain stimulation improves pain in Parkinson disease. J Neurol. 2008;255(12):1889–94.
49. Kim HJ, Jeon BS, Lee JY, Paek SH, Kim DG. The benefit of subthalamic deep brain stimulation for pain in Parkinson disease: a 2-year follow-up study. Neurosurgery. 2012;70(1):18–23. discussion 23–4.
50. Halim A, Baumgartner L, Binder DK. Effect of deep brain stimulation on autonomic dysfunction in patients with Parkinson's disease. J Clin Neurosci. 2011;18(6):804–6.
51. Herzog J, Weiss PH, Assmus A, Wefer B, Seif C, Braun PM, et al. Improved sensory gating of urinary bladder afferents in Parkinson's disease following subthalamic stimulation. Brain. 2008;131(Pt 1): 132–45.
52. Herzog J, Weiss PH, Assmus A, Wefer B, Seif C, Braun PM, et al. Subthalamic stimulation modulates cortical control of urinary bladder in Parkinson's disease. Brain. 2006;129(Pt 12):3366–75.
53. Stemper B, Beric A, Welsch G, Haendl T, Sterio D, Hilz MJ. Deep brain stimulation improves orthostatic regulation of patients with Parkinson disease. Neurology. 2006;67(10):1781–5.
54. Liu KD, Shan DE, Kuo TB, Yang CC. The effects of bilateral stimulation of the subthalamic nucleus on heart rate variability in patients with Parkinson's disease. J Neurol. 2013;260(7):1714–23.
55. Freed CR, Greene PE, Breeze RE, Tsai WY, DuMouchel W, Kao R, et al. Transplantation of

embryonic dopamine neurons for severe Parkinson's disease. N Engl J Med. 2001;344(10):710–9.
56. Ma Y, Tang C, Chaly T, Greene P, Breeze R, Fahn S, et al. Dopamine cell implantation in Parkinson's disease: long-term clinical and (18)F-FDOPA PET outcomes. J Nucl Med. 2010;51(1):7–15.
57. Olanow CW, Goetz CG, Kordower JH, Stoessl AJ, Sossi V, Brin MF, et al. A double-blind controlled trial of bilateral fetal nigral transplantation in Parkinson's disease. Ann Neurol. 2003;54(3):403–14.
58. Hagell P, Piccini P, Bjorklund A, Brundin P, Rehncrona S, Widner H, et al. Dyskinesias following neural transplantation in Parkinson's disease. Nat Neurosci. 2002;5(7):627–8.
59. Hagell P, Cenci MA. Dyskinesias and dopamine cell replacement in Parkinson's disease: a clinical perspective. Brain Res Bull. 2005;68(1–2):4–15.
60. Hyun I, Lindvall O, Ahrlund-Richter L, Cattaneo E, Cavazzana-Calvo M, Cossu G, et al. New ISSCR guidelines underscore major principles for responsible translational stem cell research. Cell Stem Cell. 2008;3(6):607–9.
61. Gradinaru V, Mogri M, Thompson KR, Henderson JM, Deisseroth K. Optical deconstruction of parkinsonian neural circuitry. Science. 2009;324(5925):354–9.
62. Peoples C, Spana S, Ashkan K, Benabid AL, Stone J, Baker GE, et al. Photobiomodulation enhances nigral dopaminergic cell survival in a chronic MPTP mouse model of Parkinson's disease. Parkinsonism Relat Disord. 2012;18(5):469–76.
63. Shaw VE, Peoples C, Spana S, Ashkan K, Benabid AL, Stone J, et al. Patterns of cell activity in the subthalamic region associated with the neuroprotective action of near-infrared light treatment in MPTP-Treated Mice. Parkinsons Dis. 2012;2012:296875.
64. Shaw VE, Spana S, Ashkan K, Benabid AL, Stone J, Baker GE, et al. Neuroprotection of midbrain dopaminergic cells in MPTP-treated mice after near-infrared light treatment. J Comp Neurol. 2010;518(1):25–40.
65. Moro C, Massri NE, Torres N, Ratel D, De Jaeger X, Chabrol C, et al. Photobiomodulation inside the brain: a novel method of applying near-infrared light intracranially and its impact on dopaminergic cell survival in MPTP-treated mice. J Neurosurg. 2014;120(3):670–83.

Quality of Life in Parkinson's Disease

16

Maria João Forjaz, Carmen Rodriguez-Blazquez, and Pablo Martinez-Martin

Abbreviations

15D-QoL	15-dimensional quality of life instrument
COMT	Catechol-O-methyltransferase
EQ-5D-3L	EQ-5D questionnaire with 3 levels of severity
EQ-5D-5L	EQ-5D questionnaire with 5 levels of severity
MDS	Movement Disorders Society
NHP	Nottingham health profile
NMS	Non-motor symptoms
PD	Parkinson's disease
PDQ-8	8-item Parkinson's disease questionnaire
PDQ-39	39-item Parkinson's disease questionnaire
PDQL	Parkinson's disease quality of life questionnaire
PIMS	Parkinson's impact scale
PRO	Patient-reported outcome
QoL	Quality of life
SCOPA-PS	Scales for outcomes in Parkinson's disease-psychosocial
SF-36	36-item short-form health survey
SIP	Sickness impact profile

M.J. Forjaz (✉)
National School of Public Health, Carlos III Institute of Health and REDISSEC,
C/ Monforte de Lemos 5, 28029 Madrid, Spain
e-mail: jforjaz@isciii.es

C. Rodriguez-Blazquez • P. Martinez-Martin
National Center of Epidemiology, Carlos III Institute of Health and CIBERNED,
C/ Monforte de Lemos 5, 28029 Madrid, Spain
e-mail: crodb@isciii.es; pmartinez@isciii.es

16.1 Measuring Quality of Life

According to the World Health Organization, quality of life (QoL) is defined as "the individuals' perception of their position in life in the context of the culture and value systems in which they live, and their relation to their goals, expectations, standards and concerns" [1]. This definition refers to global QoL, a construct formed by several dimensions including physical health, psychological and social aspects, and relationship with important aspects of the environment. Health-related QoL is a more restricted construct, focused on the QoL aspects related with health: health status, assistance, and social support.

Usually, generic health-related QoL measures include dimensions such as physical and functional state, psychological (both emotional and cognitive aspects), and social aspects (role, relationships, support). Also, health perception and overall QoL are frequently considered [2]. QoL measures designed for a specific health condition (specific QoL measures) include items related to characteristic disease symptoms and consequences.

C. Falup-Pecurariu et al. (eds.), *Movement Disorders Curricula*,
DOI 10.1007/978-3-7091-1628-9_16

Measuring health results from the patient's perspective is generally referred as patient-reported outcome measures (PROs). Besides QoL, other PROs include well-being, general health perceptions and health status, functioning and disability, satisfaction with health care, and symptoms. All PROs are obtained from the patient's perspective, either directly through self-report (the preferred way) or interview focused on the patient's views. They are developed as measures through standardized procedures and provide valid and reliable data, important to complement the clinical information. PROs are frequently used in research, including epidemiological studies and clinical trials. They also provide clinical information at the individual level, which can be used to best tailor the treatment and clinical interventions to the patient's needs.

16.2 Instruments Applied for Assessment of QoL in Parkinson's Disease

There are several validated questionnaires available to assess QoL in Parkinson's disease (PD). In 2011, a Movement Disorders Society (MDS) task force critically reviewed the QoL scales in PD [3], recommending the use of four generic and five specific scales (Table 16.1), all with sound psychometric properties and widely used in studies on PD populations.

The main advantage of using generic scales is that they allow the comparison between PD patients and general population subjects or patients with other health conditions. However, generic scales are less responsive as they fail to capture the impact of some symptoms that are specific to PD. Thus, the use of specific questionnaires provides more focused and detailed information.

16.2.1 Generic Measures of QoL Recommended for Use in PD

The EQ-5D is a health status questionnaire with econometric applications [4]. Its five dimensions can be combined into a single index value for health status ranging from −1 to 1, in which higher scores represent better health status. It also contains a visual analogue scale that assesses the current health status from 0 (worst) to 100 (best health state). The EQ-5D is accessible in many languages and general population norms are available. It may be administered as a self-rated measure or by proxy, as well as interview or web-based forms. Recently, the 3-point response scale of original version (EQ-5D-3L) was extended to 5 points (EQ-5D-5L) [5]. The EQ-5D-5L shows adequate psychometric properties in Parkinson's disease [6, 7].

The Nottingham Health Profile (NHP) is formed by two parts, though the second one is optional [8]. Domain scores are based on item weights and are expressed in a scale from 0 (good subjective health status) to 100 (poor subjective health status). The NHP total score is calculated by averaging the six domain scores.

The 36-item short-form health survey (SF-36) is a measure of health status and health-related QoL [9]. Total scores are expressed in a 0 (lowest level of functioning) to 100 (highest level of functioning) scale. Population norms are available. There are short versions, the SF-12 [10] or the SF-8 with one item representing each dimension [11].

The sickness impact profile (SIP) measures changes in behavior as a consequence of illness [12]. Scores can be obtained for the total scale, the two dimensions or for each category, by summing the corresponding endorsed items and expressing them in a 0 (lowest) to 100 (greatest dysfunction) scale. There is a shorter version of the SIP with 68 items [13].

16.2.2 Specific QoL Measures for PD

The 39-item Parkinson's disease questionnaire (PDQ-39) is probably the most widely used QoL instrument in PD, with extensively tested and well-established psychometric properties [14]. Time frame is the last month. Dimension scores are expressed as a percentage over the maximum dimension score. A summary index can also be calculating by averaging the dimension scores.

Table 16.1 Generic and PD-specific QoL questionnaires recommended by the MDS task force [3]

Scale [reference]	Number of items	Dimensions	Response scale	Time frame	Time to complete
Generic scales					
EQ-5D [4]	5 dimensions + visual analogue scale	5 dimensions: mobility, self-care, usual activities, pain/discomfort and anxiety/depression	3 (EQ-5D-3L) or 5 (EQ-5D-5L) levels of severity, from no problems to severe problems	"Today"	5–10 min
NHP [8]	Part I: 38 items Part II: 7 items about the limitations caused by health problems in functional areas of activities of daily living	6 domains in part I: pain, energy, sleep, mobility, emotional reaction, and social isolation	Yes/no	"At the moment"	5–10 min
SF-36 [9]	36	8 dimensions grouped into 2 components (physical and mental): physical functioning, role limitations due to physical health, role limitations due to emotional problems, energy/fatigue, emotional well-being, social functioning, pain, and general health	Likert-type scales with 5–6 points or with 2–3 points	Previous month (standard) or week (acute version)	SF-36, 10 min or less; SF-8, 2 min or less
SIP [12]	136	12 categories grouped into 2 dimensions Physical dimension: ambulation, mobility, and body care and movement Psychosocial dimension: social interaction, alertness behavior, emotional behavior, and communication Independent categories: sleep and rest, eating, work, home management, and recreation and pastimes	Subjects check the items that apply to them	Current day	68-item version: 15–20 min to administer [13] 136-item version: 20–30 min
PD-specific scales					
PDQ-39 [14]	39	8 dimensions: mobility, activities of daily living, emotional well-being, stigma, social support cognition, communication, and bodily pain	0 (no problem) to 4 (continuous problems or unable to do it)	Past month	10–20 min

(continued)

Table 16.1 (continued)

Scale [reference]	Number of items	Dimensions	Response scale	Time frame	Time to complete
PDQL [16]	37	4 dimensions: parkinsonian and systemic symptoms, and social and emotional function	1 (all the time) to 5 (never)	Past 3 months	20 min [125]
PIMS [18, 19]	10	4 factors: subjective physical aspects of the disease, psychological dimension, social aspects, and sexuality	0 (no change) to 4 (severe)	Unspecified	Less than 10 min [18]
SCOPA-PS [20]	11	There are no dimensions, just a total score	0 (not at all) to 3 (very much)	Previous month	5–10 min (estimated)

NHP Nottingham health profile, *SF-36* 36-item short-form health survey, *SIP* sickness impact profile, *PDQ-39* 39-item Parkinson's disease questionnaire, *PDQL* Parkinson's disease quality of life questionnaire, *PIMS* Parkinson's impact scale, *SCOPA-PS* scales for outcomes in Parkinson's disease-psychosocial

There is a short version, the PDQ-8 [15]. Both instruments have been used in many studies and clinical trials and translated and validated into many languages.

The Parkinson's disease quality of life questionnaire (PDQL) is formed by 37 items grouped into four dimensions: parkinsonian and systemic symptoms, and social and emotional function [16]. Higher values on the total sum score represent worse QoL. The scale may be self-completed or as an interview [17].

The Parkinson's impact scale (PIMS) measures nonphysical aspects of PD [18, 19]. The total score is obtained by adding weighted item scores. This scale may be rated by the patient or a caregiver. The PIMS has sound psychometric properties, but its use may be limited by the lack of questions on physical and mental aspects of PD.

The scales for outcomes in Parkinson's disease-psychosocial (SCOPA-PS) assesses the social or emotional consequences of PD [20]. The SCOPA-PS has been validated in several cultural contexts. The SCOPA-PS includes one item that addresses sexual problems, which leads to a high percentage of missing values.

16.3 Quality of Life in PD

PD is expressed through a wide range of different manifestations that deteriorate the patient's QoL. Knowledge about factors that influence QoL is important to develop interventions that will have an impact on the patient's live. Both, mental (for example, depression and cognitive impairment) and physical aspects (for example, postural instability and disability) are significant aspects associated to QoL in PD in cross-sectional studies [21].

Throughout the disease course, PD affects many areas of the patient's life which contribute to a gradual decrease of his/her QoL. Longitudinal studies report significant deterioration in QoL components over time [22–24]. Most influential factors on QoL deterioration are functional limitations and dependence, postural instability, depression, and cognitive dysfunction [24, 25]. Changes in QoL over 1 year were of small to moderate magnitude, probably buffered by adaptation of patients to their condition [22, 23]. To adequately capture change over time, specific QoL measures are preferred [26]. Nonetheless, as generic measures provide information on important aspects of global health, the combined use of specific and generic scales is recommended.

The effects of motor symptoms on QoL have been well documented. Studies showed that motor impairment expressed as limitations for mobility, gait disorder and falls, and disability are consistent determinants of QoL [24–27]. Motor complications, especially biphasic dyskinesias and nocturnal akinesia, also worsen importantly patients' QoL [28].

Non-motor symptoms (NMS) have even a greater impact on QoL than motor symptoms [18, 25, 26, 29, 30]. The most frequent NMS were nocturia, fatigue, and dribbling saliva, measured as per the NMS scale (NMSS) [31, 32], and the domains that had a highest impact on QoL were mood/apathy, sleep/fatigue, and miscellaneous [25, 26, 29, 30, 33]. Patients with NMS also had a significantly lower QoL than patients without symptoms. NMS influence negatively not only patients' but also caregivers' QoL [34].

16.4 The Impact of Treatment Approaches on QoL in PD

A 2007 review of the impact of treatment options on QoL showed that the following drug therapies were efficacious in the improvement of QoL in PD: conversion from levodopa to standard controlled-release levodopa formulation, tolcapone when given as an add-on to levodopa, and rasagiline [35]. Results were inconclusive about the effects of cabergoline, entacapone, and pramipexole on QoL. Other works also review the impact of treatments on QoL in PD [36–39].

16.4.1 Levodopa as Mono or Adjuvant Therapy

Levodopa is considered to be the most effective treatment in PD [40]. Its efficacy was confirmed in a review of the impact of several treatment options in the improvement of QoL in PD [35] and also in more recent trials offering a high level of evidence [41–43]. One of the main concerns about its long-term use is the development of dyskinesias [44]. However, the number of patients who developed severe dyskinesias was relatively low, and QoL scores were similar for patients treated with levodopa or dopaminergic agonists [35].

Tolcapone, a catechol-O-methyltransferase (COMT) inhibitor, when given as an add-on to levodopa was also beneficial and efficacious in improving the QoL of PD patients [35]. Patients with wearing-off fluctuations taking tolcapone showed a significantly larger increase in their QoL than patients on pergolide [45]. Clinical trials measuring the effect of adjunctive tolcapone to levodopa on QoL of patients with advanced motor fluctuations provided contradictory results [46–49]. The use of tolcapone is restricted and requires a strict monitoring of liver function due to its hepatotoxicity [36].

Entacapone is a COMT inhibitor taken in conjunction with levodopa. The benefits of entacapone on QoL are different according to PD stage, with studies providing mixed results, but it significantly improves patient's QoL as a whole [50, 51, 53].

16.4.2 Dopamine Agonists

Dopamine agonists have a longer half-life than levodopa, which might contribute to delay the onset of levodopa-induced motor complications [37, 54]. They are used as initial monotherapy or as adjuvant therapy. There are several dopamine agonists available for the treatment for PD, such as rotigotine, pramipexole, cabergoline, ropinirole, pergolide, piribedil, and bromocriptine.

Rotigotine is a dopamine agonist delivered continuously through transdermal patches. A study reported no significant improvement in the EQ-5D questionnaire for the rotigotine group at 6-months follow-up [55]. According to a large randomized, double-blind double-dummy trial, transdermal rotigotine was as beneficial for QoL as pramipexole when used as adjunct therapies for patients with wearing-off fluctuations [56]. In a double-blind, placebo-control trial, after treatment with rotigotine patients with bad control of early morning symptoms showed a significant greater benefit on PDQ-8 items than controls [57, 58]. Another study documented a beneficial effect on QoL, but not on non-motor symptoms [59]. Rotigotine was considered to be efficacious [54] and safe treatment for patients in early states of PD or as adjuvant therapy in more advanced stages [60].

Pramipexole is an oral, non-ergotamine-derived dopamine agonist. When used as initial treatment and in comparison to a group on levodopa, QoL ratings improved on both groups at 6 months, with a decrease to baseline at 48 months [61, 62]. This decline was more accentuated in the levodopa group than for patients on pramipexole [63]. When taken as an adjuvant to levodopa, pramipexole was efficacious in improving QoL at 3-month follow-up in a group of depressed patients and with no fluctuations or dyskinesias [64]. In two studies, QoL results favored the treatment groups, and QoL scores of patients on pramimexole were not significantly different for those on rotigotine [56] or bromocriptine [65].

Cabergoline in conjunction with levodopa improved the QoL of patients with wearing off [52]. However, the magnitude of change was higher for patients on cabergoline than for those on entacapone. Other studies confirmed the QoL benefits of cabergoline as an adjunct therapy [66–68]. No added effect on QoL was observed in patients who switched from standard to extended-release pramipexole [69].

When comparing the effect of *ropinirole* and levodopa as initial treatment, there were no significant QoL differences [70]. In a large randomized, double-blind trial in advanced PD patients with wearing off, prolonged-release ropinirole taken as an adjunct to levodopa demonstrated an improvement in QoL dimensions of emotional well-being, stigma, and communication [71].

Piribedil had a positive effect on QoL after 12 weeks of treatment in a small, randomized, double-blind trial with PD patients that had undergone DBS and complained of apathy symptoms [72]. Furthermore, piribedil as monotherapy in early PD disease [73], or taken as add-on to levodopa, resulted in improvement in motor function and ability to carry on activities of daily living [74–76].

There are very few studies about the effect of *bromocriptine* or *pergolide* in QoL. After a 14-year follow-up, patients on levodopa reported a better QoL than those on bromocriptine [77, 78]. In addition, another study did not find significant differences with the EQ-5D between the group of patients on bromocriptine and placebo controls, but QoL improvement comparable to pramipexole with other measure [65]. Pergolide as an add-on to levodopa had a significant effect on QoL for patients with wearing off, but its benefit was smaller than the one found for tolcapone [45].

16.4.3 Monoamine Oxidase Inhibitors

16.4.3.1 Selegiline

The first selective monoamine oxidase B (MAO-B) inhibitor developed for PD treatment was selegiline. One study showed improvement in QoL, although small in magnitude [79]. Two other studies, where patients changed over from selegiline to rasagiline, indicate lead to inconsistent results [80, 81]. However, these three trials were open label. In a study comparing the effect of monotherapy against levodopa combined with rasagiline or selegiline, results favored combined therapy [82].

16.4.3.2 Rasagiline

Rasagiline is an irreversible, selective MAO-B inhibitor. When used as monotherapy, beneficial effects of QoL were found after 6 months of treatment [83]. An open-label trial analyzed a group of 30 patients on a stable drug therapy, who switched from selegiline to rasagiline [81]. The changeover to rasagiline resulted in an amelioration of PD symptoms, with no change in QoL scores. According to a cost-effectiveness study, comparing rasagiline with pramipexole, rasagiline was advantageous in terms of quality-adjusted life-years over 5 years [84]. However, in another study also comparing these two drugs, QoL scores remained stable in the rasagiline group [85]. A 2015 review concluded that rasagiline has a beneficial effect on QoL and non-motor symptoms such as fatigue [86].

16.4.3.3 Safinamide

It is a benzylamino derivative, developed for the PD treatment. A large sample trial, using a randomized, placebo-controlled design, showed significant QoL improvement at 6 and 24 months [87, 88]. Despite having a good safety profile, there is a lack of studies in de novo patients [89].

16.4.4 Other Drugs

Rivastigmine is a cholinesterase inhibitor that showed a positive effect on activities of daily living of PD patients with apathy and no depression or dementia. In a double-blind, placebo-controlled study, no significant QoL improvement was observed [90]. However, another study reported a trend effect for QoL benefit in PD patients with mild-cognitive impairment [91].

16.4.5 Treatment for Advanced PD: Surgery, Duodopa, and Apomorphine

16.4.5.1 Surgical Procedures

Concerning the surgical options for advanced-stage PD patients, pallidotomy and deep brain stimulation (DBS) were considered efficacious for improving patient's QoL in a 2007 review about the effect of treatment options on QoL [35]. Studies performed since then confirm the beneficial results of DBS on QoL [92–96]. The effect of subthalamic nucleus DBS was more pronounced in women than in men [95]. When comparing DBS of the globus pallidus interna or subthalamic nucleus, results were similar and showed an initial QoL benefit gradually decreasing at 36 months [94].

The pharmaceutical treatment options for advanced patients include continuous intestinal infusion of levodopa/carbidopa gel (duodopa) and subcutaneous infusion of apomorphine, which are especially useful to address severe dyskinesias and motor fluctuations that cannot be controlled with oral combination therapy [97].

16.4.5.2 Duodopa

A literature review shows that 23 studies included QoL as an outcome measure of the effect of duodopa on PD since 2007 [98] (Table 16.2). The relative change in PDQ-39 summary index or PDQ-8 showed a great variability, between 14 % [99] and 69 % [100], which is probably due to sample characteristics rather than to the length of the follow-up.

The DIREQT is a randomized, open-label, crossover trial which included a group of 12 patients on conventional therapy for 3 weeks, crossing over with duodopa as monotherapy for other 3 weeks, and another group that received treatment in the opposite order [101–103]. At the end of the trial, QoL instruments favored the duodopa treatment arm [101]. Patients on duodopa, at the 6-month follow-up, showed a relative change of 27 % [103]. The DIREQT trial included a subset of four patients in the comparator arm who used apomorphine, showing that duodopa treatment led to a better QoL than apomorphine [102].

Another study compared seven duodopa-naïve patients with eight previous users, after a 6-month follow-up [100]. QoL improvement on the PDQ-8 was significant for the drug-naïve patients, with a relative change of 69 %. The study by Devos et al. comprises the largest sample of advanced PD patients on duodopa, with 71 patients [104]. After a follow-up of 18 months, 92 % of them reported subjective improvement on QoL.

Long-term follow-up, up to a maximum of 42 months, was recorded on a small sample of seven to nine patients on duodopa [105–107]. QoL improvement was 46 % at 6 months, and 37 % at the end of the follow-up period, which indicates that duodopa QoL benefits are long lasting. Another study documented a 24 % increase in QoL ratings after a 3-year follow-up period [108].

16.4.5.3 Apomorphine

There are few trials that qualify the effect of treatment with apomorphine, a dopamine agonist, on QoL [102, 109–112] (Table 16.3). QoL improvement was reported by all studies, although in one of them, QoL improvement was only observed in 50 % of the sample [109].

A study compared patients on apomorphine with a control on conventional therapy [110]. While the group on apomorphine significantly improved its QoL by 45 %, the control group showed worsening (25 %). However, in a trial with four patients that compared the effect of apomorphine-duodopa combination therapy with duodopa alone [102], better results on QoL were observed for the duodopa alone arm [102]. Another study comparing apomorphine with levodopa infusion found that QoL results, after a 6-month follow-up, were similar for both treatment arms [112].

Table 16.2 Studies providing data about effect of continuous intestinal infusion of levodopa/carbidopa (duodopa) on quality of life

Reference	Type of study	Control (yes/no)	Sample size (n)	Follow-up (months)	QoL measure	QoL improvement
Nyholm et al. [101]	DIREQT trial: randomized, open label, crossover	Yes: conventional treatment	12+12	1.5	PDQ-36, 15D-QoL	Better for treatment with duodenal levodopa infusion. 28 % for PDQ-36; 8 % for 15D-QoL (based on medians)
Antonini et al. [98]	Open label	No	9 (7 to follow-up)	12	PDQ-39	Improvement on 4/8 subscales
Antonini et al. [126]	Open label	No	22 (17 to follow-up)	24	PDQ-39	12 months, 21 %; 24 months, 17 %
Isacson et al. [103]	DIREQT trial: randomized, open label, crossover	Yes (conventional treatment)	12 out of 18	6	PDQ-39	26–33 %
Annic et al. [127]	Open label	No	7	6	PDQ-39	No QoL change
Devos [104]	Open label	No	102, 71 with QoL data	18	3-point QoL scale	92 % report improvement
Honig [128]	Open label	No	22	6	PDQ-8	56 %
Nyholm et al. [102]	DIREQT trial: randomized, open label, crossover	Yes. Monotherapy with duodopa vs. combination therapy with apomorphine	4	3+3 weeks	PDQ-36, 15D-QoL	Greater benefit for duodopa. PDQ-36 change: 3–31. 15D-QoL change: 0.06–0.13
Puente et al. [129]	Open label	No	9	18	PDQ-39	38 %
Santos-Garcia et al. [106]	Open label	No	9 out of 11	Mean: 18.2 (range: 4.5–31)	PDQ-39	48 %
Meppelink et al. [100]	Open label	Yes: drug-naïve vs. previous users	15	6	PDQ-8	62–69 %, nonsignificant
Fasano et al. 2012	Open label	No	14	24	PDQ-8	No significant differences for total group. QoL improvement for subgroup of patients with improvement in motor function and functionality
Palhagen et al. [99]	Open label	No	25 out of 36	12	PDQ-39	14 %, nonsignificant
Reddy et al. [130]	Open label	Yes	17+9	6	PDQ-8	Significant improvement in treated group (effect size = 1.12)

Table 16.2 (continued)

Reference	Type of study	Control (yes/no)	Sample size (n)	Follow-up (months)	QoL measure	QoL improvement
Santos-Garcia et al. [107]	Open label	No	9 out of 11	6-month evaluation, median follow-up: 25 months	PDQ-39	46 % at 6 months; 37 % at the end of follow-up
Santos-Garcia et al. [105]	Open label	No	7	31.4±7.9 (range: 23–42)	PDQ-39	37 % at the end of follow-up
Foltynie et al. [131]	Open label	No	12 (11 on follow-up)	3–12 months	PDQ-39	3 months, 28 %; latest follow-up, 22 %
Zibetti et al. [108]	Open label	No	17/25	Mean: 36.2±11.5	PDQ-39	27 %
Caceres-Redondo et al. [132]	Open label	No	29	24 months	PDQ-39 and EQ-5D	13.3 % (PDQ-39)
Martinez-Martin et al. [112]	Open label	No	43	6 months	PDQ-8	34.2 %
Olanow et al. [43]	Placebo controlled	Yes	37	12 weeks	PDQ-39	31.0 %
Sensi et al. [133]	Open label	No	17	24 months	PDQ-8	30.9 %
Antonini et al. [134]	Open label	No	375	12 months	PDQ-8, EQ-5D	17.7 %

QoL quality of life, *PDQ-39* 39-item Parkinson's disease questionnaire, *PDQ-8* 8-item Parkinson's disease questionnaire, *15D-QoL* 15-dimensional quality of life instrument, *DIREQT* duodopa infusion: randomized efficacy and quality of life study trial

The largest trial was conducted in France and 142 patients were followed for 6 months [113]. Similarly to the previous studies, significant QoL improvement was registered. There is a lack of randomized controlled trials testing the QoL effect of apomorphine.

IPEX066 (RYTARY) is an extended-release oral formulation of carbidopa-levodopa in the form of microbeads that dissolve at different rates, thus combining the effects of quick abortion and sustained release for extended periods [114]. A review of its clinical efficacy showed that IPEX066 improves QoL as well as function, morbidity, and mortality [115].

16.4.6 Nonsurgical, Non-pharmacological Therapies

A recent review of multidisciplinary interventions to improve QoL in PD found inconclusive evidence [38]. Most interventions had an educational component (78 %), and two thirds included a rehabilitation program. However, pooled results from the nine reviewed studied did not show significant differences between treatment and control groups. These results are consistent with another review that focused on the effect of physiotherapy on PD: although small short-term benefits were found across studies for velocity, balance, and disability, there was no statistically significant difference between groups on QoL outcomes [116]. More recent studies provided mixed results, with three studies reporting a beneficial effect on QoL [117–119] and one study finding no effect [120]. A recent systematic review of 14 studies about physical exercise based rehabilitation programs concluded that the following program characteristics are associated with benefits on QoL: two to four times a week, 1-h sessions, 6–12-week program duration [121].

A smartphone intervention that provided feedback on gait performance leads to better QoL results than conventional gait training at home

Table 16.3 Studies providing data about effect of apomorphine on quality of life

Reference	Drug treatment	Type of study	Control (yes/no)	Sample size (n)	Follow-up (months)	QoL measure	QoL improvement
Manson et al. [111]	Intravenous apomorphine	Open label	No	6	Mean: 7 (range: 0.5–18)	Subjective improvement on QoL	"Marked improvement on QoL"
Castaño et al. [109]	Apomorphine (CSAI)	Open label	No	7	6	PDQ-39	Improvement in 3 patients
Nyholm et al. [102]	Apomorphine (CSAI), duodopa (intraduodenal levodopa/carbidopa infusion)	DIREQT trial: open, crossover, randomized	Yes: monotherapy with duodopa vs. combination therapy with apomorphine	4	3 + 3 weeks	PDQ-39, 15D-QoL	Greater benefit for duodopa. PDQ-36 change in the duodopa arm: −3 to −31. 15D-QoL change: 0.06–0.13
Martinez-Martin et al. [110]	Apomorphine (CSAI)	Open label	Yes: 17 patients on conventional therapy	17	12.5 ± 11.5	PDQ-8	42 % improvement for the apomorphine group; 25 % worsening for the control group
Martinez-Martin et al. [112]	Apomorphine (CSAI) vs. levodopa infusion	Open label	No	43	6 months	PDQ-8	29.75 % (apomorphine)
Drapier et al. [113]	Apomorphine (CSAI)	Open label	No	142	6 months	PDQ-39	13.3 %

QoL quality of life, *CSAI* continuous subcutaneous infusion of apomorphine, *PDQ-39* 39-item Parkinson's disease questionnaire, *PDQ-8* 8-item Parkinson's disease questionnaire, *15D-QoL* 15-dimensional quality of life instrument, *DIREQT* duodopa infusion: randomized efficacy and quality of life study trial

[122]. Music-based movement therapy improved walking velocity, with no effects on QoL [123]. According to another study, a group singing intervention, for 8 weeks, showed a positive effect on the QoL of 27 PD participants [124].

Conclusions

Quality of life is as important PRO, and it should be used as an additional endpoint in clinical practice, research studies, and clinical trials. There are several general and PD-specific QoL measures recommended to assess QoL in PD. Motor and NMS have a great impact on patients' QoL, and the contribution of the latter could outweigh the former. Previous studies have documented the positive effect of surgical and pharmaceutical treatment options on QoL. There is inconclusive evidence about the effect of non-pharmacological therapies in QoL. Concerning pharmacological options for advanced PD, several studies provide evidence for the positive effect of duodopa on PD patient's QoL. However, there is a need for randomized controlled trials that assess the effect of apomorphine on QoL.

References

1. World Health Organization Division of Mental Health and Prevention of Substance. WHOQOL : measuring quality of life [Internet]. 1997. http://apps.who.int/iris/handle/10665/63482.
2. Ware JEJ. The status of health assessment 1994. Annu Rev Public Health. 1995;16:327–54.
3. Martinez-Martin P, Jeukens-Visser M, Lyons KE, Rodriguez-Blazquez C, Selai C, Siderowf A, et al. Health-related quality-of-life scales in Parkinson's disease: critique and recommendations. Mov Disord. 2011;26(13):2371–80.
4. EuroQol Group. EuroQol – a new facility for the measurement of health-related quality of life. Health Policy. 1990;16(3):199–208.
5. Herdman M, Gudex C, Lloyd A, Janssen M, Kind P, Parkin D, et al. Development and preliminary testing of the new five-level version of EQ-5D (EQ-5D-5L). Qual Life Res. 2011;20(10):1727–36.
6. Alvarado-Bolaños A, Cervantes-Arriaga A, Rodríguez-Violante M, Llorens-Arenas R, Calderón-Fajardo H, Millán-Cepeda R, et al. Convergent validation of EQ-5D-5L in patients with Parkinson's disease. J Neurol Sci. 2015;358(1–2):53–7.
7. García-Gordillo MÁ, del Pozo-Cruz B, Adsuar JC, Sánchez-Martínez FI, Abellán-Perpiñán JM. Validation and comparison of 15-D and EQ-5D-5L instruments in a Spanish Parkinson's disease population sample. Qual Life Res. 2014;23(4):1315–26.
8. Hunt SM, McEwen J, McKenna SP. Measuring health status: a new tool for clinicians and epidemiologists. J R Coll Gen Pract. 1985;35(273):185–8.
9. Ware JEJ, Sherbourne CD. The MOS 36-item short-form health survey (SF-36). I. Conceptual framework and item selection. Med Care. 1992;30(6):473–83.
10. Ware JJ, Kosinski M, Keller SD. A 12-item short-form health survey: construction of scales and preliminary tests of reliability and validity. Med Care. 1996;34(3):220–33.
11. Turner-Bowker DM, Bayliss MS, Ware JEJ, Kosinski M. Usefulness of the SF-8 Health Survey for comparing the impact of migraine and other conditions. Qual Life Res. 2003;12(8):1003–12.
12. Bergner M, Bobbitt RA, Carter WB, Gilson BS. The sickness impact profile: development and final revision of a health status measure. Med Care. 1981;19(8):787–805.
13. Post MW, Gerritsen J, Diederikst JP, DeWittet LP. Measuring health status of people who are wheelchair-dependent: validity of the Sickness Impact Profile 68 and the Nottingham Health Profile. Disabil Rehabil. 2001;23(6):245–53.
14. Peto V, Jenkinson C, Fitzpatrick R, Greenhall R. The development and validation of a short measure of functioning and well being for individuals with Parkinson's disease. Qual Life Res. 1995;4(3):241–8.
15. Jenkinson C, Fitzpatrick R, Peto V, Greenhall R, Hyman N. The PDQ-8: development and validation of a short-form Parkinson's disease Questionnaire. Psychol Health. 1997;12(6):805–14.
16. de Boer AG, Wijker W, Speelman JD, de Haes JC. Quality of life in patients with Parkinson's disease: development of a questionnaire. J Neurol Neurosurg Psychiatry. 1996;61(1):70–4.
17. Damiano AM, Snyder C, Strausser B, Willian MK. A review of health-related quality-of-life concepts and measures for Parkinson's disease. Qual Life Res. 1999;8(3):235–43.
18. Calne S, Schulzer M, Mak E, Guyette C, Rohs G, Hatchard S, et al. Validating a quality of life rating scale for idiopathic parkinsonism: Parkinson's Impact Scale (PIMS). Parkinsonism Relat Disord. 1996;2(2):55–61.
19. Schulzer M, Mak E, Calne SM. The psychometric properties of the Parkinson's Impact Scale (PIMS) as a measure of quality of life in Parkinson's disease. Parkinsonism Relat Disord. 2003;9(5):291–4.
20. Marinus J, Visser M, Martínez-Martín P, van Hilten JJ, Stiggelbout AM. A short psychosocial questionnaire for patients with Parkinson's disease: the SCOPA-PS. J Clin Epidemiol. 2003;56(1):61–7.
21. Schrag A, Jahanshahi M, Quinn N. What contributes to quality of life in patients with Parkinson's disease? J Neurol Neurosurg Psychiatry. 2000;69(3):308–12.

22. Martínez-Martin P, Carod-Artal FJ, da Silveira Ribeiro L, Ziomkowski S, Vargas AP, Kummer W, et al. Longitudinal psychometric attributes, responsiveness, and importance of change: an approach using the SCOPA-psychosocial questionnaire. Mov Disord. 2008;23(11):1516–23.
23. Schrag A, Spottke A, Quinn NP, Dodel R. Comparative responsiveness of Parkinson's disease scales to change over time. Mov Disord. 2009;24(6):813–8.
24. Karlsen KH, Tandberg E, Arsland D, Larsen JP. Health related quality of life in Parkinson's disease: a prospective longitudinal study. J Neurol Neurosurg Psychiatry. 2000;69(5):584–9.
25. Marras C, McDermott MP, Rochon PA, Tanner CM, Naglie G, Lang AE. Predictors of deterioration in health-related quality of life in Parkinson's disease: results from the DATATOP trial. Mov Disord. 2008;23(5):653–9; quiz 776.
26. Reuther M, Spottke EA, Klotsche J, Riedel O, Peter H, Berger K, et al. Assessing health-related quality of life in patients with Parkinson's disease in a prospective longitudinal study. Parkinsonism Relat Disord. 2007;13(2):108–14.
27. Chapuis S, Ouchchane L, Metz O, Gerbaud L, Durif F. Impact of the motor complications of Parkinson's disease on the quality of life. Mov Disord. 2005;20(2):224–30.
28. Rahman S, Griffin HJ, Quinn NP, Jahanshahi M. Quality of life in Parkinson's disease: the relative importance of the symptoms. Mov Disord. 2008;23(10):1428–34.
29. Barone P, Antonini A, Colosimo C, Marconi R, Morgante L, Avarello TP, et al. The PRIAMO study: a multicenter assessment of nonmotor symptoms and their impact on quality of life in Parkinson's disease. Mov Disord. 2009;24(11):1641–9.
30. Leonardi M, Raggi A, Pagani M, Carella F, Soliveri P, Albanese A, et al. Relationships between disability, quality of life and prevalence of nonmotor symptoms in Parkinson's disease. Parkinsonism Relat Disord. 2012;18(1):35–9.
31. Chaudhuri KR, Martinez-Martin P, Brown RG, Sethi K, Stocchi F, Odin P, et al. The metric properties of a novel non-motor symptoms scale for Parkinson's disease: results from an international pilot study. Mov Disord. 2007;22(13):1901–11.
32. Martinez-Martin P, Rodriguez-Blazquez C, Abe K, Bhattacharyya KB, Bloem BR, Carod-Artal FJ, et al. International study on the psychometric attributes of the non-motor symptoms scale in Parkinson disease. Neurology. 2009;73(19):1584–91.
33. Martinez-Martin P, Rodriguez-Blazquez C, Kurtis MM, Chaudhuri KR. The impact of non-motor symptoms on health-related quality of life of patients with Parkinson's disease. Mov Disord. 2011;26(3):399–406.
34. Martinez-Martin P, Rodriguez-Blazquez C, Forjaz MJ. Quality of life and burden in caregivers for patients with Parkinson's disease: concepts, assessment and related factors. Expert Rev Pharmacoecon Outcomes Res. 2012;12(2):221–30.
35. Martinez-Martin P, Deuschl G. Effect of medical and surgical interventions on health-related quality of life in Parkinson's disease. Mov Disord. 2007;22(6):757–65.
36. Gallagher DA, Schrag A. Impact of newer pharmacological treatments on quality of life in patients with Parkinson's disease. CNS Drugs. 2008;22(7):563–86.
37. Iaconi AI, Zimmerman MA, Kulkarni AS, Balkrishnan R. Outcomes associated with pharmacologic treatments in Parkinson's disease: a review of recent literature. Expert Opin Pharmacother. 2008;9(2):163–74.
38. Tan SB, Williams AF, Kelly D. Effectiveness of multidisciplinary interventions to improve the quality of life for people with Parkinson's disease: a systematic review. Int J Nurs Stud. 2014;51(1):166–74.
39. Martinez-Martin P, Rodriguez-Blazquez C, Forjaz MJ, Kurtis MM. Impact of pharmacotherapy on quality of life in patients with Parkinson's disease. CNS Drugs. 2015;29(5):397–413.
40. Luquin MR, García-Ruiz PJ, Martí MJ, Rojo A, Vela L, Grandas FJ, et al. Levodopa in the treatment of Parkinson's disease: myths and realties. Rev Neurol. 2012;55(11):669–88.
41. Hauser RA, Hsu A, Kell S, Espay AJ, Sethi K, Stacy M, et al. Extended-release carbidopa-levodopa (IPX066) compared with immediate-release carbidopa-levodopa in patients with Parkinson's disease and motor fluctuations: a phase 3 randomised, double-blind trial. Lancet Neurol. 2013;12(4):346–56.
42. Pahwa R, Lyons KE, Hauser RA, Fahn S, Jankovic J, Pourcher E, et al. Randomized trial of IPX066, carbidopa/levodopa extended release, in early Parkinson's disease. Parkinsonism Relat Disord. 2014;20(2):142–8.
43. Olanow CW, Kieburtz K, Odin P, Espay AJ, Standaert DG, Fernandez HH, et al. Continuous intrajejunal infusion of levodopa-carbidopa intestinal gel for patients with advanced Parkinson's disease: a randomised, controlled, double-blind, double-dummy study. Lancet Neurol. 2014;13(2):141–9.
44. Encarnacion EV, Hauser RA. Levodopa-induced dyskinesias in Parkinson's disease: etiology, impact on quality of life, and treatments. Eur Neurol. 2008;60(2):57–66.
45. Koller W, Lees A, Doder M, Hely M, Tolcapone/Pergolide Study Group. Randomized trial of tolcapone versus pergolide as add-on to levodopa therapy in Parkinson's disease patients with motor fluctuations. Mov Disord. 2001;16(5):858–66.
46. Rajput AH, Martin W, Saint-Hilaire MH, Dorflinger E, Pedder S. Tolcapone improves motor function in parkinsonian patients with the «wearing-off» phenomenon: a double-blind, placebo-controlled, multicenter trial. Neurology. 1997;49(4):1066–71.

47. Baas H, Beiske AG, Ghika J, Jackson M, Oertel WH, Poewe W, et al. Catechol-O-methyltransferase inhibition with tolcapone reduces the «wearing off» phenomenon and levodopa requirements in fluctuating parkinsonian patients. J Neurol Neurosurg Psychiatry. 1997;63(4):421–8.
48. Adler CH, Singer C, O'Brien C, Hauser RA, Lew MF, Marek KL, et al. Randomized, placebo-controlled study of tolcapone in patients with fluctuating Parkinson disease treated with levodopa-carbidopa. Tolcapone Fluctuator Study Group III. Arch Neurol. 1998;55(8):1089–95.
49. Welsh MD, Dorflinger E, Chernik D, Waters C. Illness impact and adjustment to Parkinson's disease: before and after treatment with tolcapone. Mov Disord. 2000;15(3):497–502.
50. Grandas F, Hernández B, PRACTICOMT Study Group. Long-term effectiveness and quality of life improvement in entacapone-treated Parkinson's disease patients: the effects of an early therapeutic intervention. Eur J Neurol. 2007;14(3):282–9.
51. Reichmann H, Boas J, Macmahon D, Myllyla V, Hakala A, Reinikainen K, et al. Efficacy of combining levodopa with entacapone on quality of life and activities of daily living in patients experiencing wearing-off type fluctuations. Acta Neurol Scand. 2005;111(1):21–8.
52. Deuschl G, Vaitkus A, Fox G-C, Roscher T, Schremmer D, Gordin A, et al. Efficacy and tolerability of Entacapone versus Cabergoline in parkinsonian patients suffering from wearing-off. Mov Disord. 2007;22(11):1550–5.
53. Tolosa E, Hernández B, Linazasoro G, López-Lozano JJ, Mir P, Marey J, et al. Efficacy of levodopa/carbidopa/entacapone versus levodopa/carbidopa in patients with early Parkinson's disease experiencing mild wearing-off: a randomised, double-blind trial. J Neural Transm. 2014;121(4):357–66.
54. Martinez-Martin P, Kurtis MM. Systematic review of the effect of dopamine receptor agonists on patient health-related quality of life. Parkinsonism Relat Disord. 2009;15 Suppl 4:S58–64.
55. Jankovic J, Watts RL, Martin W, Boroojerdi B, SP 512 Rotigotine Transdermal System Clinical Study Group. Transdermal rotigotine: double-blind, placebo-controlled trial in Parkinson disease. Arch Neurol. 2007;64(5):676–82.
56. Poewe WH, Rascol O, Quinn N, Tolosa E, Oertel WH, Martignoni E, et al. Efficacy of pramipexole and transdermal rotigotine in advanced Parkinson's disease: a double-blind, double-dummy, randomised controlled trial. Lancet Neurol. 2007;6(6):513–20.
57. Ghys L, Surmann E, Whitesides J, Boroojerdi B. Effect of rotigotine on sleep and quality of life in Parkinson's disease patients: post hoc analysis of RECOVER patients who were symptomatic at baseline. Expert Opin Pharmacother. 2011;12(13): 1985–98.
58. Trenkwalder C, Kies B, Rudzinska M, Fine J, Nikl J, Honczarenko K, et al. Rotigotine effects on early morning motor function and sleep in Parkinson's disease: a double-blind, randomized, placebo-controlled study (RECOVER). Mov Disord. 2011;26(1):90–9.
59. Antonini A, Bauer L, Dohin E, Oertel WH, Rascol O, Reichmann H, et al. Effects of rotigotine transdermal patch in patients with Parkinson's disease presenting with non-motor symptoms – results of a double-blind, randomized, placebo-controlled trial. Eur J Neurol. 2015;22(10):1400–7.
60. Lyons KE, Pahwa R. Outcomes of rotigotine clinical trials: effects on motor and nonmotor symptoms of Parkinson's disease. Neurol Clin. 2013;31(3 Suppl):S51–9.
61. Parkinson Study Group. Pramipexole vs levodopa as initial treatment for Parkinson disease: a randomized controlled trial. Parkinson Study Group. JAMA. 2000;284(15):1931–8.
62. Holloway RG, Shoulson I, Fahn S, Kieburtz K, Lang A, Marek K, et al. Pramipexole vs levodopa as initial treatment for Parkinson disease: a 4-year randomized controlled trial. Arch Neurol. 2004;61(7):1044–53.
63. Noyes K, Dick AW, Holloway RG, Parkinson Study Group. Pramipexole versus levodopa in patients with early Parkinson's disease: effect on generic and disease-specific quality of life. Value Health. 2006;9(1):28–38.
64. Barone P, Scarzella L, Marconi R, Antonini A, Morgante L, Bracco F, et al. Pramipexole versus sertraline in the treatment of depression in Parkinson's disease: a national multicenter parallel-group randomized study. J Neurol. 2006;253(5):601–7.
65. Guttman M. Double-blind comparison of pramipexole and bromocriptine treatment with placebo in advanced Parkinson's disease. International Pramipexole-Bromocriptine Study Group. Neurology. 1997;49(4):1060–5.
66. Linazasoro G, Spanish Dopamine Agonists Study Group. Conversion from dopamine agonists to cabergoline: an open-label trial in 128 patients with advanced Parkinson disease. Clin Neuropharmacol. 2008;31(1):19–24.
67. Baas HK, Schueler P. Efficacy of cabergoline in long-term use: results of three observational studies in 1,500 patients with Parkinson's disease. Eur Neurol. 2001;46 Suppl 1:18–23.
68. Odin P, Oehlwein C, Storch A, Polzer U, Werner G, Renner R, et al. Efficacy and safety of high-dose cabergoline in Parkinson's disease. Acta Neurol Scand. 2006;113(1):18–24.
69. Takanashi M, Shimo Y, Hatano T, Oyama G, Hattori N. Efficacy and safety of a once-daily extended-release formulation of pramipexole switched from an immediate-release formulation in patients with advanced Parkinson's disease: results from an open-label study. Drug Res (Stuttg). 2013;63(12):639–43.

70. Hauser RA, Rascol O, Korczyn AD, Jon Stoessl A, Watts RL, Poewe W, et al. Ten-year follow-up of Parkinson's disease patients randomized to initial therapy with ropinirole or levodopa. Mov Disord. 2007;22(16):2409–17.
71. Pahwa R, Stacy MA, Factor SA, Lyons KE, Stocchi F, Hersh BP, et al. Ropinirole 24-hour prolonged release: randomized, controlled study in advanced Parkinson disease. Neurology. 2007;68(14):1108–15.
72. Thobois S, Lhommée E, Klinger H, Ardouin C, Schmitt E, Bichon A, et al. Parkinsonian apathy responds to dopaminergic stimulation of D2/D3 receptors with piribedil. Brain. 2013;136(5):1568–77.
73. Rascol O, Dubois B, Caldas AC, Senn S, Del Signore S, Lees A, et al. Early piribedil monotherapy of Parkinson's disease: a planned seven-month report of the REGAIN study. Mov Disord. 2006;21(12):2110–5.
74. Salazar Tortolero G, Wix Ramos R, Salazar Aladrén P, Jiménez León JC. The effectiveness and tolerance of piribedil as adjunct therapy to levodopa in patients with Parkinson's disease: a nine month follow up. Rev Neurol. 2004;38(8):715–9.
75. Evidente VGH, Esteban RP, Domingo FM, Carbajal LO, Parazo MA. Piribedil as an adjunct to levodopa in advanced Parkinson's disease: the Asian experience. Parkinsonism Relat Disord. 2003;10(2):117–21.
76. Suwantamee J, Nidhinandana S, Srisuwananukorn S, Laptikultham S, Pisarnpong A, Chankrachang S, et al. Efficacy and safety of piribedil in early combination with L-dopa in the treatment of Parkinson's disease: a 6-month open study. J Med Assoc Thai. 2004;87(11):1293–300.
77. Katzenschlager R, Head J, Schrag A, Ben-Shlomo Y, Evans A, Lees AJ, et al. Fourteen-year final report of the randomized PDRG-UK trial comparing three initial treatments in PD. Neurology. 2008;71(7):474–80.
78. Shannon KM. Long-term outcome in Parkinson disease: no advantage to initiating therapy with dopamine agonists. Nat Clin Pract Neurol. 2008; 4(11):590–1.
79. Reichmann H, Jost WH. Efficacy and tolerability of rasagiline in daily clinical use – a post-marketing observational study in patients with Parkinson's disease. Eur J Neurol. 2010;17(9):1164–71.
80. Jost WH, Klasser M, Reichmann H. Rasagiline in daily clinical use. Results of a treatment study of Parkinson patients with a combination treatment. Fortschr Neurol Psychiatr. 2008;76(10):594–9.
81. Müller T, Hoffmann JA, Dimpfel W, Oehlwein C. Switch from selegiline to rasagiline is beneficial in patients with Parkinson's disease. J Neural Transm. 2013;120(5):761–5.
82. Krishna R, Ali M, Moustafa AA. Effects of combined MAO-B inhibitors and levodopa vs. monotherapy in Parkinson's disease. Front Aging Neurosci. 2014;6:180.
83. Biglan KM, Schwid S, Eberly S, Blindauer K, Fahn S, Goren T, et al. Rasagiline improves quality of life in patients with early Parkinson's disease. Mov Disord. 2006;21(5):616–23.
84. Haycox A, Armand C, Murteira S, Cochran J, François C. Cost effectiveness of rasagiline and pramipexole as treatment strategies in early Parkinson's disease in the UK setting: an economic Markov model evaluation. Drugs Aging. 2009;26(9):791–801.
85. Viallet F, Pitel S, Lancrenon S, Blin O. Evaluation of the safety and tolerability of rasagiline in the treatment of the early stages of Parkinson's disease. Curr Med Res Opin. 2013;29(1):23–31.
86. Stocchi F, Fossati C, Torti M. Rasagiline for the treatment of Parkinson's disease: an update. Expert Opin Pharmacother. 2015;16(14):2231–41.
87. Kandadai RM, Jabeen SA, Kanikannan MA, Borgohain R. Safinamide for the treatment of Parkinson's disease. Expert Rev Clin Pharmacol. 2014;7(6):747–59.
88. Borgohain R, Szasz J, Stanzione P, Meshram C, Bhatt M, Chirilineau D, et al. Randomized trial of safinamide add-on to levodopa in Parkinson's disease with motor fluctuations. Mov Disord. 2014;29(2):229–37.
89. Stocchi F, Torti M. Adjuvant therapies for Parkinson's disease: critical evaluation of safinamide. Drug Des Devel Ther. 2016;10:609–18.
90. Devos D, Moreau C, Maltête D, Lefaucheur R, Kreisler A, Eusebio A, et al. Rivastigmine in apathetic but dementia and depression-free patients with Parkinson's disease: a double-blind, placebo-controlled, randomised clinical trial. J Neurol Neurosurg Psychiatry. 2014;85(6):668–74.
91. Mamikonyan E, Xie SX, Melvin E, Weintraub D. Rivastigmine for mild cognitive impairment in Parkinson disease: a placebo-controlled study. Mov Disord. 2015;30(7):912–8.
92. Witt K, Daniels C, Reiff J, Krack P, Volkmann J, Pinsker MO, et al. Neuropsychological and psychiatric changes after deep brain stimulation for Parkinson's disease: a randomised, multicentre study. Lancet Neurol. 2008;7(7):605–14.
93. Montel S, Bonnet A-M, Bungener C. Quality of life in relation to mood, coping strategies, and dyskinesia in Parkinson's disease. J Geriatr Psychiatry Neurol. 2009;22(2):95–102.
94. Weaver FM, Follett KA, Stern M, Luo P, Harris CL, Hur K, et al. Randomized trial of deep brain stimulation for Parkinson disease: thirty-six-month outcomes. Neurology. 2012;79(1):55–65.
95. Hariz G-M, Limousin P, Zrinzo L, Tripoliti E, Aviles-Olmos I, Jahanshahi M, et al. Gender differences in quality of life following subthalamic stimulation for Parkinson's disease. Acta Neurol Scand. 2013;128(4):281–5.
96. Baláž M, Bočková M, Rektor I. DBS amplitude setting can improve aspects of quality of life in patients with Parkinson's disease. J Neural Transm. 2013;120(4):643–8.

97. Clarke CE. Neuroprotection and pharmacotherapy for motor symptoms in Parkinson's disease. Lancet Neurol. 2004;3(8):466–74.
98. Antonini A, Isaias IU, Canesi M, Zibetti M, Mancini F, Manfredi L, et al. Duodenal levodopa infusion for advanced Parkinson's disease: 12-month treatment outcome. Mov Disord. 2007;22(8):1145–9.
99. Pålhagen SE, Dizdar N, Hauge T, Holmberg B, Jansson R, Linder J, et al. Interim analysis of long-term intraduodenal levodopa infusion in advanced Parkinson disease. Acta Neurol Scand. 2012;126(6):e29–33.
100. Meppelink AM, Nyman R, van Laar T, Drent M, Prins T, Leenders KL. Transcutaneous port for continuous duodenal levodopa/carbidopa administration in Parkinson's disease. Mov Disord. 2011;26(2):331–4.
101. Nyholm D, Nilsson Remahl AIM, Dizdar N, Constantinescu R, Holmberg B, Jansson R, et al. Duodenal levodopa infusion monotherapy vs oral polypharmacy in advanced Parkinson disease. Neurology. 2005;64(2):216–23.
102. Nyholm D, Constantinescu R, Holmberg B, Dizdar N, Askmark H. Comparison of apomorphine and levodopa infusions in four patients with Parkinson's disease with symptom fluctuations. Acta Neurol Scand. 2009;119(5):345–8.
103. Isacson D, Bingefors K, Kristiansen IS, Nyholm D. Fluctuating functions related to quality of life in advanced Parkinson disease: effects of duodenal levodopa infusion. Acta Neurol Scand. 2008;118(6):379–86.
104. Devos D. Patient profile, indications, efficacy and safety of duodenal levodopa infusion in advanced Parkinson's disease. Mov Disord. 2009;24(7):993–1000.
105. Santos-García D, Añón MJ, Fuster-Sanjurjo L, de la Fuente-Fernández R. Duodenal levodopa/carbidopa infusion therapy in patients with advanced Parkinson's disease leads to improvement in caregivers' stress and burden. Eur J Neurol. 2012;19(9):1261–5.
106. Santos-García D, Macías M, Llaneza M, Fuster-Sanjurjo L, Echarri-Piudo A, Belmonte S, et al. Experience with continuous levodopa enteral infusion (Duodopa(®)) in patients with advanced Parkinson's disease in a secondary level hospital. Neurologia. 2010;25(9):536–43.
107. Santos-García D, Sanjurjo LF, Macías M, Llaneza M, Carpintero P, de la Fuente-Fernández R. Long-term exposure to duodenal levodopa/carbidopa infusion therapy improves quality of life in relation especially to mobility, activities of daily living, and emotional well-being. Acta Neurol Scand. 2012;125(3):187–91.
108. Zibetti M, Merola A, Ricchi V, Marchisio A, Artusi CA, Rizzi L, et al. Long-term duodenal levodopa infusion in Parkinson's disease: a 3-year motor and cognitive follow-up study. J Neurol. 2013;260(1):105–14.
109. Castaño B, Mateo D, Giménez-Roldán S. Shifting to subcutaneous infusion of apomorphine in advanced Parkinson's disease patients on an out-patient basis: experience and recommendations. Neurologia. 2007;22(3):133–7.
110. Martinez-Martin P, Reddy P, Antonini A, Henriksen T, Katzenschlager R, Odin P, et al. Chronic subcutaneous infusion therapy with apomorphine in advanced Parkinson's disease compared to conventional therapy: a real life study of non motor effect. J Parkinsons Dis. 2011;1(2):197–203.
111. Manson AJ, Hanagasi H, Turner K, Patsalos PN, Carey P, Ratnaraj N, et al. Intravenous apomorphine therapy in Parkinson's disease clinical and pharmacokinetic observations. Brain. 2001;124(2):331–40.
112. Martinez-Martin P, Reddy P, Katzenschlager R, Antonini A, Todorova A, Odin P, et al. EuroInf: a multicenter comparative observational study of apomorphine and levodopa infusion in Parkinson's disease. Mov Disord. 2015;30(4):510–6.
113. Drapier S, Eusebio A, Degos B, Vérin M, Durif F, Azulay JP, et al. Quality of life in Parkinson's disease improved by apomorphine pump: the OPTIPUMP cohort study. J Neurol. 2016;263(6):1111–9.
114. Hauser RA. IPX066: a novel carbidopa-levodopa extended-release formulation. Expert Rev Neurother. 2012;12(2):133–40.
115. Dhall R, Kreitzman DL. Advances in levodopa therapy for Parkinson disease: review of RYTARY (carbidopa and levodopa) clinical efficacy and safety. Neurology. 2016;86(14 Suppl 1):S13–24.
116. Tomlinson CL, Patel S, Meek C, Herd CP, Clarke CE, Stowe R, et al. Physiotherapy intervention in Parkinson's disease: systematic review and meta-analysis. BMJ. 2012;345:e5004.
117. Rose MH, Løkkegaard A, Sonne-Holm S, Jensen BR. Improved clinical status, quality of life, and walking capacity in Parkinson's disease after body weight-supported high-intensity locomotor training. Arch Phys Med Rehabil. 2013;94(4):687–92.
118. Tickle-Degnen L, Ellis T, Saint-Hilaire MH, Thomas CA, Wagenaar RC. Self-management rehabilitation and health-related quality of life in Parkinson's disease: a randomized controlled trial. Mov Disord. 2010;25(2):194–204.
119. Yousefi B, Tadibi V, Khoei AF, Montazeri A. Exercise therapy, quality of life, and activities of daily living in patients with Parkinson disease: a small scale quasi-randomised trial. Trials. 2009;10:67.
120. Lauhoff P, Murphy N, Doherty C, Horgan NF. A controlled clinical trial investigating the effects of cycle ergometry training on exercise tolerance, balance and quality of life in patients with Parkinson's disease. Disabil Rehabil. 2013;35(5):382–7.
121. da Silva FC, Iop Rda R, Dos Santos PD, Bezerra LM, Gutierres PJ, da Silva R. Effects of physical exercise based rehabilitation programs on quality of life in Parkinson's disease patients: a systematic review of randomized controlled trials. J Aging Phys Act. 2016. [Epub ahead of print].

122. Ginis P, Nieuwboer A, Dorfman M, Ferrari A, Gazit E, Canning CG, et al. Feasibility and effects of home-based smartphone-delivered automated feedback training for gait in people with Parkinson's disease: a pilot randomized controlled trial. Parkinsonism Relat Disord. 2016;22:28–34.
123. de Dreu MJ, van der Wilk ASD, Poppe E, Kwakkel G, van Wegen EEH. Rehabilitation, exercise therapy and music in patients with Parkinson's disease: a meta-analysis of the effects of music-based movement therapy on walking ability, balance and quality of life. Parkinsonism Relat Disord. 2012;18 Suppl 1:S114–9.
124. Stegemöller EL, Radig H, Hibbing P, Wingate J, Sapienza C. Effects of singing on voice, respiratory control and quality of life in persons with Parkinson's disease. Disabil Rehabil. 2016:1–7. doi:10.3109/09638288.2016.1152610.
125. Serrano-Dueñas M, Serrano S. Psychometric characteristics of PIMS – compared to PDQ-39 and PDQL – to evaluate quality of life in Parkinson's disease patients: validation in Spanish (Ecuadorian style). Parkinsonism Relat Disord. 2008;14(2):126–32.
126. Antonini A, Mancini F, Canesi M, Zangaglia R, Isaias IU, Manfredi L, et al. Duodenal levodopa infusion improves quality of life in advanced Parkinson's disease. Neurodegener Dis. 2008;5(3–4):244–6.
127. Annic A, Devos D, Seguy D, Dujardin K, Destée A, Defebvre L. Continuous dopaminergic stimulation by Duodopa in advanced Parkinson's disease: efficacy and safety. Rev Neurol (Paris). 2009;165(8–9):718–27.
128. Honig H, Antonini A, Martinez-Martin P, Forgacs I, Faye GC, Fox T, et al. Intrajejunal levodopa infusion in Parkinson's disease: a pilot multicenter study of effects on nonmotor symptoms and quality of life. Mov Disord. 2009;24(10):1468–74.
129. Puente V, De Fabregues O, Oliveras C, Ribera G, Pont-Sunyer C, Vivanco R, et al. Eighteen month study of continuous intraduodenal levodopa infusion in patients with advanced Parkinson's disease: impact on control of fluctuations and quality of life. Parkinsonism Relat Disord. 2010;16(3):218–21.
130. Reddy P, Martinez-Martin P, Rizos A, Martin A, Faye GC, Forgacs I, et al. Intrajejunal levodopa versus conventional therapy in Parkinson disease: motor and nonmotor effects. Clin Neuropharmacol. 2012;35(5):205–7.
131. Foltynie T, Magee C, James C, Webster GJM, Lees AJ, Limousin P. Impact of duodopa on quality of life in advanced Parkinson's disease: a UK case series. Parkinson's Disease [Internet]. 2013. http://www.hindawi.com/journals/pd/2013/362908/abs/.
132. Cáceres-Redondo MT, Carrillo F, Lama MJ, Huertas-Fernández I, Vargas-González L, Carballo M, et al. Long-term levodopa/carbidopa intestinal gel in advanced Parkinson's disease. J Neurol. 2014;261(3):561–9.
133. Sensi M, Preda F, Trevisani L, Contini E, Gragnaniello D, Capone JG, et al. Emerging issues on selection criteria of levodopa carbidopa infusion therapy: considerations on outcome of 28 consecutive patients. J Neural Transm. 2014;121(6):633–42.
134. Antonini A, Yegin A, Preda C, Bergmann L, Poewe W, GLORIA Study Investigators and Coordinators. Global long-term study on motor and non-motor symptoms and safety of levodopa-carbidopa intestinal gel in routine care of advanced Parkinson's disease patients; 12-month interim outcomes. Parkinsonism Relat Disord. 2015;21(3):231–5.

Part III

Other Movement Disorders

Multiple System Atrophy

17

Johannes Levin, Sylvia Maaß,
Madeleine Schuberth, and Günter Höglinger

Abbreviations

CPAP	Continuous positive airway pressure
FDG-PET	Fluorodeoxyglucose positron emission tomography
GCIs	Glial cytoplasmic inclusions
GNIs	Glial nuclear inclusions
GWAS	Genome-wide association studies
LBD	Dementia with Lewy bodies
L-threo-DOPS	L-threodihydroxy-phenylserine
MSA	Multiple system atrophy
MSA-C	MSA of the cerebellar type
MSA-P	MSA of the parkinsonian type
MSCs	Mesenchymal stem cells
NCIs	Neuronal cytoplasmic inclusions
NNIs	Neuronal nuclear inclusions
OH	Orthostatic hypotension
PD	Parkinson's disease
PSP	Progressive supranuclear palsy
rhGH	Recombinant human growth hormone
SNCA	α-Synuclein gene

J. Levin (✉) • M. Schuberth
Neurologische Klinik, Ludwig-Maximilians-Universität München, Klinikum der Universität – Großhadern, Marchioninistraße 15, 81377 Munich, Germany
e-mail: Johannes.Levin@med.uni-muenchen.de; Madeleine.Schuberth@med.uni-muenchen.de

S. Maaß • G. Höglinger
Deutsches Zentrum für Neurodegenerative Erkrankungen (DZNE) & Klinik für Neurologie, Klinikum rechts der Isar, Technische Universität München, Feodor-Lynen Str. 17, 81377 Munich, Germany
e-mail: Sylvia.Maass@dzne.de; Guenter.Hoeglinger@dzne.de

17.1 Epidemiology

MSA is considered a rare disease. MSA has an estimated prevalence of 1.9–4.9 per 100.000 [8, 65]. An annual incidence of approximately 0.6 in 100,000 was reported in the USA [8]. This incidence seems to be quite stable across distinct populations. For example, in Iceland and Great Britain, similar incidences were observed [7, 48]. The incidence of MSA increases with age, which is illustrated by the increase in the US American population above the age of 50 years [8]. A French study reported an increase to 12 per 100,000 in the population above the age of 70 years [11]. The mean age at onset was reported consistently in European and Asian populations within the age of 50–70 years [30, 68]. The disease affects men and women alike and does not show a gender-specific course [4]. In Europe about 60 % of MSA patients present with a parkinsonian phenotype (MSA-P) [32, 67], whereas in Japan cerebellar (MSA-C) and mixed phenotypes are more common [70].

C. Falup-Pecurariu et al. (eds.), *Movement Disorders Curricula*,
DOI 10.1007/978-3-7091-1628-9_17

17.2 Neuropathology

In this section, you will find a summary of the neuropathology of MSA. MSA has been broadly divided into subtypes with predominant affection of the striatonigral system and the olivopontocerebellar system. However, in most cases, changes in both systems can be observed even if these changes are usually more pronounced in one of these systems [28]. The affection of the anatomical systems that are vulnerable to the disease process can be observed macroscopically by their atrophy ([1, 13]). MSA cases with *primary affection of the striatonigral system* show atrophy and dark discoloration of the putamen, which is more pronounced in the posterior part and which can reach to the caudate nucleus. Like in Parkinson's disease, pallor of the substantia nigra and locus coeruleus can be observed. Furthermore, mild cortical atrophy in the frontal lobes has been described [60]. In MSA cases with *primary affection of the olivopontocerebellar system*, the cerebellum is reduced in size. Cortical atrophy of the cerebellum, narrowing of the folia, and a change in color and decreased size of the cerebellar white matter can be observed. Often severe atrophy of the pontine base and middle cerebellar peduncle is present. Furthermore, in these cases also pallor of the substantia nigra and locus coeruleus has been described, however, often less severe than in MSA cases with primary affection of the striatonigral system. MSA belongs to the group of α-synucleinopathies, characterized by intracellular proteinaceous inclusions containing α-synuclein [53]. In contrast to other α-synucleinopathies, e.g., Parkinson's disease and dementia with Lewy bodies, α-synuclein inclusions in MSA are not primarily found in neurons but mainly in *oligodendroglia* [53]. These so-called glial cytoplasmic inclusions (*GCIs*) or Papp-Lantos bodies are pathognomonic for MSA [28]. The neuropathology working group on MSA recommends: "A definite neuropathological diagnosis of MSA is established when there is evidence of widespread and abundant CNS α-synuclein-positive GCIs in association with neurodegenerative changes in striatonigral or olivopontocerebellar structures" [59].

17.3 Etiology/Pathogenesis

In recent years, efforts in genetics, epidemiology, histopathology, and cell biology have contributed to an increased insight in the complex processes leading to the development of MSA. Available genetic evidence suggests that α-synuclein, neuroinflammation, as well as mitochondrial dysfunction and oxidative stress may be involved in disease development [6, 17]. However, MSA pathogenesis is only partially understood so far. An interaction of genetic vulnerability and environmental factors is probable. In general, MSA is considered a sporadic disease. However, cases have been reported within families suggestive for autosomal dominant and recessive patterns of inheritance [18]. Recently, homozygous and compound heterozygous mutations in the *COQ2* gene, which codes for the parahydroxybenzoate-polyprenyl transferase, have been described in familial MSA in Japanese patients [42]. However, one of these mutations, the p.V343A variant, is relatively common among the Japanese population. This suggests that *COQ2* mutations are likely to represent a risk factor for MSA. In a European population, this finding could not be confirmed [51]. These findings are relevant as they foster the link between mitochondrial dysfunction and the etiology of MSA. Despite substantial efforts, no other disease-associated mutations have been identified in these families so far [52, 69]. Other approaches to detect possible genetic factors in the pathogenesis of MSA were screening for candidate genes as well as genome-wide association studies (GWAS). An obvious candidate gene was the α-synuclein gene (*SNCA*). Initial findings using sequencing and gene expression analysis in studies of small size did not reveal changes in the SNCA gene or the RNA level in oligodendrocytes of pathology proven MSA [40]. In a test of candidate single nucleotide polymorphisms, a significant association for two SNCA variants was found associated with MSA [47], but not confirmed.

17.4 Clinical Characteristics

17.4.1 Symptoms

17.4.1.1 MSA with Predominant Parkinsonism (MSA-P)

MSA-P is characterized by a hypokinetic-rigid syndrome in combination with postural instability early in the disease course. Due to the loss of postural reflexes, falls occur early in the disease course, but usually not within the first year after disease onset [32]. Irregular, jerky postural tremor can occur as well, whereas the characteristic pill-rolling tremor of Parkinson's disease is rare [63]. L-Dopa responsiveness can be observed initially in 83 % of the patients [32, 63]. However, the effect is usually transient; in a large multicenter cohort, only 31 % showed a response to levodopa that continued for a mean period of 3.5 years [67]. In some of these patients, motor fluctuations with wearing-off phenomena and off-bound dystonia were detected [67].

17.4.1.2 MSA of the Cerebellar Type (MSA-C)

In MSA-C, the most frequent sign is broad-based gait ataxia [5, 32, 56, 67], but affected patients can also develop limb ataxia, cerebellar oculomotor disturbances (e.g., sustained spontaneous, gaze-evoked, or downbeat nystagmus), scanning dysarthria, and intention tremor.

17.4.1.3 Autonomic Symptoms

Autonomic failure characteristically accompanies motor dysfunction in both MSA-P and MSA-C. "Pure autonomic dysfunction" [71] is rare, but can precede motor dysfunction in MSA. Dysautonomia in MSA typically involves urogenital, orthostatic, and sometimes gastrointestinal dysfunction. Early erectile dysfunction in men and urinary incontinence or incomplete bladder emptying may be the initial feature in 5–30 % of MSA patients [5]. Orthostatic hypotension can be symptomatic or asymptomatic. Typically, orthostatic hypotension occurs after the onset of genitourinary symptoms [31]. Gastrointestinal dysfunction appears as chronic constipation in one-third of the patients [32].

17.4.1.4 Additional Symptoms/Red Flags

Additional characteristic symptoms observed in MSA, the so-called red flags, should be used as a clue to consider the diagnosis. Nine to 69 % of the patients suffer from an inspiratory stridor, commonly associated with an advanced stage of the disease and constituting a poor prognostic predictor [27]. Pyramidal signs are reported in 30–50 % [32] and could help to distinguish between MSA-P and PD. Pyramidal signs can be found more frequently in MSA-C-patients than in MSA-P-patients. Other red flags would include rapid progression, early postural instability, emotional incontinence (inappropriate laughing or crying), and bulbar dysfunction (including severe dysphonia/dysarthria and dysphagia). Furthermore, respiratory dysfunction (diurnal and nocturnal inspiratory stridor as mentioned above and/or inspiratory sighs) and abnormal postures like Pisa syndrome, disproportionate antecollis, and contractures of the hands or feet are also considered red flags for the disease. Köllensperger et al. [32] propose a combination of two out of six red flag categories as suggestive for probable MSA-P.

17.4.2 Technical Investigations

17.4.2.1 MRI

Routine 1.5 tesla MRI should be performed in all patients with suspected MSA to rule out other symptomatic causes for the clinical presentation. In several large cohort studies performing MRI in MSA patients, a significant atrophy was detected in the following brain regions: putamen, middle cerebellar peduncles, and brainstem regions (pons, medulla oblongata, midbrain) [10, 34]. Also signal abnormalities on T2-weighted images are reported, most characteristically the so-called "hot-cross bun" sign, indicating a characteristic cruciform hypointensity in the pons [49] and the "putaminal slit" sign that marks a marginal hyperintensity lateral from the bilateral putamina [46]. In the recent consensus criteria [21], those features have not been included, but brain atrophy detected by MRI has been included as an additional feature for possible MSA-P and for possible MSA-C.

17.4.2.2 PET

18-Fluorodeoxyglucose positron emission tomography (FDG-PET) can distinguish patients with MSA-P from those with PD by showing a different pattern of decreased glucose metabolism. In MSA, but not PD, the brainstem, cerebellum, basal ganglia, thalamus, and cerebral cortex are affected [19]. Gilman et al. suggest that in the absence of clinically evident ataxia in a patient with parkinsonian features, demonstration of cerebellar hypometabolism can point to the diagnosis of MSA-P rather than Parkinson's disease: conversely, in the absence of parkinsonian features in a patient with cerebellar ataxia, evidence of nigrostriatal dopaminergic denervation from functional imaging may point to the diagnosis of MSA-C [21]. Assigning patients to MSA on the basis of the characteristic metabolic pattern should be possible with a highly specific positive predictive value of 97 % [55].

17.4.2.3 CSF

α-Synuclein levels have been measured in CSF and plasma of MSA patients at lower CSF concentrations than in healthy controls and patients with other neurological diseases, differentiating on a group level, but with a high overlap of values on the level of individual patients [41], thus yielding low sensitivity and specificity with the methods available so far.

17.4.2.4 Autonomic Function Testing

Cardiovascular function: For the diagnosis of probable MSA, a reduction of systolic blood pressure by at least 30 mmHg or a reduction of diastolic blood pressure by at least 15 mmHg is required to occur in a Schellong test [21].

Bladder function: A standard urine analysis will exclude lower urinary tract infections which often cause urinary symptoms. Ultrasound measurement or transurethral catheterization can determine urine residual volume or incomplete bladder emptying. For differentiation between hypocontractile detrusor function and hyperreflexic sphincter–detrusor dyssynergia, a cystometry can be necessary [65].

For both orthostatic hypotension, urinary incontinence or retention, and erectile dysfunction, symptomatic causes have to be excluded before attributing them to MSA.

17.4.3 Diagnostic Criteria

In 1998 a consensus conference in MSA established widely accepted diagnostic criteria [20]. A second consensus statement was published in 2008 [21], adding new implications from clinical, laboratory, neuropathologic, and imaging studies and simplifying the previous criteria. The new criteria retain the diagnostic categories of MSA with predominant parkinsonism and MSA with predominant cerebellar ataxia to designate the predominant motor features and also retain the designations of definite, probable, and possible MSA.

Definite MSA requires neuropathologic demonstration of CNS α-synuclein-positive GCIs with neurodegenerative changes in striatonigral or olivopontocerebellar structures.

Probable MSA requires a sporadic, progressive adult-onset disorder including rigorously defined autonomic failure and poorly levodopa-responsive parkinsonism or cerebellar ataxia.

Possible MSA requires a sporadic, progressive adult-onset disease including parkinsonism or cerebellar ataxia and at least one feature suggesting autonomic dysfunction plus one other feature that may be a clinical or a neuroimaging abnormality.

17.4.4 Disease Course

Disease progression in MSA is faster than in PD so that after 5 years, more than 40 % of patients are wheelchair bound or severely disabled [61]. The progression of MSA has been reported to occur at a remarkably stable rate in several clinical trials, as assessed by the unified MSA rating scale (UMSARS). In a recent observational study, the first-year progression rate for the UMSARS motor examination subscale was 44.9 % (8.2 points, standard deviation 7.0) relative to baseline. In the second year, a decline of 17.2 % (5.0, 5.4) relative to

12-month scores was observed. Mean survival after the first clinical manifestation ranges between 6 and 10 years [67].

17.5 Differential Diagnoses

Differentiating MSA-P from Parkinson's disease early in the disease course can prove very difficult due to overlapping symptoms. In the early stages, similarities between MSA-P and other atypical parkinsonian syndromes like progressive supranuclear palsy (PSP) or corticobasal syndromes may complicate the establishment of a diagnosis. Furthermore MSA-C must be distinguished from inherited or acquired cerebellar ataxias. To distinguish MSA-P from PSP, oculomotor function testing is vital as a vertical gaze palsy (downward gaze) is highly suggestive for the diagnosis of PSP. Coexisting frontal symptoms such as apathy and reduced verbal fluency can also hint versus PSP [9]. The Luria sequence can be used as a simple bedside test to detect a frontal syndrome and has shown to be one of the best predictors in PSP. To differentiate corticobasal syndromes from MSA, the examiner should look out for coexisting cortical symptoms such as aphasia, apraxia, cortical sensory loss, and alien limb phenomena. An atypical parkinsonian syndrome that additionally shows cognitive fluctuations and optical hallucinations is highly suggestive for dementia with Lewy bodies.

The main differential diagnosis for MSA-C would be other forms of adult-onset cerebellar ataxia. Clinically, the presence of autonomic symptoms and/or parkinsonism can help differentiate MSA-C from other adult-onset cerebellar ataxias. Adult-onset ataxias can be classified into sporadic etiologies, symptomatic forms (including toxins, e.g., alcohol, vitamin E deficiency, tumors, and infections), or genetic disorders. Hereditary ataxias, such as spinocerebellar ataxias, Friedreich's ataxia, and fragile X-associated ataxia syndrome, can present with a phenotype strongly resembling MSA-C and therefore be considered a genocopy of MSA [2]. Moreover, these diseases can present as seemingly sporadic disorders. A complete history of the disease, workup of the family history, and investigations to rule out acquired forms followed by investigations (MRI) can help to narrow the differential diagnosis of MSA-C considerably. The challenge remains to differentiate so-called sporadic degenerative ataxia (including MSA-C) from idiopathic late-onset cerebellar ataxia, a term that is usually used to refer to cases with negative family history, where acquired causes have been ruled out, genetic testing has proved negative and consensus criteria for MSA are not met [37].

17.6 Therapy

17.6.1 Symptomatic Therapy

To date, no effective treatment exists for cerebellar ataxia or pyramidal affection in MSA, but levodopa can improve parkinsonism in about one-third of the patients, yet only transiently [12, 63]. Most authors recommend that symptomatic therapy should focus on autonomic symptoms, as these interfere most with quality of life in MSA patients [50]. Among them, orthostatic hypotension, constipation, genitourinary, and breathing disorders are treatable pharmacologically and by alternative treatment options.

17.6.1.1 Parkinsonism

A poor levodopa response is one of the core features in the consensus criteria for the diagnosis of MSA [21] and helps to differentiate atypical parkinsonian disorders including MSA from Parkinson's disease [62, 64]. However, one-third of all the patients show some form of a transient levodopa response. This effect will be seen mainly in the MSA-P subtype, as would be expected [12]. In some cases, this effect will only be noticed after withdrawal of levodopa. Wenning and colleagues [62] documented a distinct and persisting benefit from a levodopa therapy (as in Parkinson's disease) in 13 % of MSA patients. More recent data from a large European prospective cohort study documented a beneficial levodopa response in 31 % of patients, also preferably in MSA-P patients that lasted for about 3.5 years [67]. These data could also show that a beneficial levodopa response was related to a somewhat slower disease progression.

The management of MSA is largely empirical in the absence of evidence from randomized placebo-controlled drug trials, but most specialists would recommend using levodopa as a first-line medication in daily doses up to 1 g, depending on tolerability and necessity [20, 66]. As a second choice, dopamine agonists can be given in PD titration schemes, even if there are no controlled studies available. Amantadine can be given as a third-line medication (3 × 100–200-mg daily dosage). A short-term add-on treatment with paroxetine 30-mg tid has shown to improve motor symptoms in a double-blind placebo-controlled randomized trial that was performed during 2 weeks with 19 MSA patients [33]. Hence, paroxetine as an add-on therapy is worthwhile.

In addition to pharmacotherapy and physiotherapy, occupational therapy and speech therapy should be an integral part of the therapy of motor features in MSA, both parkinsonian and cerebellar subtype.

17.6.1.2 Dystonia

For dystonia (orofacial and limb, antecollis excluded), local injections of botulinum toxin would be recommended [43]. Note that injections with botulinum toxin for treatment of antecollis into the cervical muscles, especially the usually targeted sternocleidomastoid muscles, can provoke dysphagia or enhance preexisting dysphagic problems, especially when injected in the lower two-thirds of the muscles. Therefore this type of treatment is not currently recommended [57].

17.6.1.3 Cerebellar Ataxia

For cerebellar ataxia there is to date no effective pharmacological treatment available. All therapy is based on physiotherapy as well as occupational and speech therapy.

17.6.1.4 Autonomic Failure

In a large prospective clinical cohort study among autonomic symptoms, urinary dysfunction was more common (83 %) than symptomatic orthostatic dysregulation (75 %) [54]. Since autonomic symptoms can be most inconvenient for the patient and are mostly affecting quality of life in clinical studies [50], therapy should focus on these symptoms.

Orthostatic Hypotension

The first choice for treating orthostatic hypotension should always be nonpharmacological strategies such as wearing elastic support stockings or tights, a high-salt diet, sufficient fluid intake, frequent and small meals a day, head-up tilt of the bed at night, and slowly getting up from a lying position. Constipation can also be addressed by sufficient fluid intake and by ingestion of macrogol water solution [15].

If conservative measures prove insufficient, fludrocortisone (0.1–0.3 mg) at night can be added. As a second-line therapy, midodrine (15–30 mg/day) can be added combined with fludrocortisone. Midodrine showed significant benefit in randomized placebo-controlled trials [26] in patients with orthostatic hypotension.

If these measures prove unsatisfactory, midodrine could be replaced by ephedrine (15–45 mg tid) or the norepinephrine precursor L-threodihydroxy-phenylserine (L-threo-DOPS) (100 mg tid). The latter has been used for this indication in Japan for years; its efficacy has been shown by two double-blind placebo-controlled trials including patients with MSA [29, 39].

Postprandial hypotension can be reduced by avoiding alcohol and excessive single-meal caloric intake or by increasing water and coffee consumption. In severe cases, octreotide 25–50 mg s.c. may have a beneficial effect on postprandial hypotension [16, 36].

Urge Incontinence

Anticholinergic substances like trospium chloride (2–3 × 10–15 mg/day) [23] or tolterodine (2 × 2 mg/day) can be useful for treating detrusor hyperreflexia or sphincter–detrusor dyssynergy. Oxybutinin (2 × 2.5–5 mg/day) can be used as a second-line medication, as it has shown to be less well tolerated, concerning central side effects. Also, the control of postmicturition residue is necessary.

If anticholinergic medication proves unsatisfactory or if side effects are not well tolerated, admission of desmopressin (10–40-μg spray, 100–400-μg tablets) can have a positive effect on nycturia [16].

Incomplete Bladder Emptying

Postmicturition residue of 100 ml is an indication for intermittent self-catheterization. In the advanced stages of MSA, a urethral or suprapubic catheter may become necessary. Surgical therapies for neurogenic bladder problems should be avoided in MSA, because postoperative worsening of bladder control is most likely [3].

Erectile Dysfunction

Sildenafil citrate has been shown effective in a double-blind placebo-controlled randomized trial in patients with PD and MSA [25]. Since it may worsen or exacerbate orthostatic hypotension, measurement of lying and standing blood pressure before prescribing sildenafil to men with parkinsonism is recommended. If necessary, oral yohimbine can be used for erectile dysfunction. Lastly, intracavernosal injection of papaverine or a penis implant can be a possibility in young patients with predominant erectile dysfunction [3].

Inspiratory Stridor

About 30 % of patients suffer from inspiratory stridor. Here ventilation by continuous positive airway pressure (CPAP) may be helpful and in some of these patients even suitable as a long-term therapy [22]. In rare cases, a tracheostomy will have to be performed.

17.6.1.5 Depression

Depression is more prevalent in MSA than in PD [58] and correlates with poor quality of life [50]. Next to psychotherapy, a therapy with selective serotonergic reuptake inhibitors is justified [33] with a less expected risk of inducing orthostatic hypotension than tricyclic drugs, even though to date there are no controlled trials available concerning antidepressant therapy in patients with MSA.

17.6.2 Disease Modification

So far, several compounds have been tested for a disease-modifying effect including riluzole [5], rhGH [24], fluoxetine (Rascol et al. study not yet published, ClinicalTrials.gov Identifier, NCT01146548), rasagiline [44], minocycline [14], and rifampicin [38]. All these compounds did not show a significant effect on disease progression in humans. Also, mesenchymal stem cell transplantation was tested by administering intra-arterial and intravenous infusion of MSC four times total. The results showed that MSC therapy could delay the progression of neurological deficits in patients with MSA-C, suggesting the potential of MSC therapy as a treatment candidate of MSA [35]. Still, these results have to be taken with caution as the rationale for such a trial was comparatively weak as the underlying mechanisms of action remain unclear and need more preclinical explanation [45].

17.7 Perspectives

MSA is considered a rare disorder, however frequent enough and severely affecting the affected patients' lives, to be recognized by treating physicians and researchers. This article demonstrates the present knowledge but also the current limitations with regard to etiology, early diagnosis, and symptomatic treatment options, but foremost preventive or curative options. Thus, further intensification of research into the identification of biological or imaging biomarkers to identify the disease ideally in its preclinical state, as well as therapeutic interventions targeting the core molecular mechanisms of neurodegeneration, is urgently needed.

References

1. Adams RD, Van Bogaert L, Van Der Eecken H. Striato-nigral degeneration. J Neuropathol Exp Neurol. 1964;23:584–608.
2. Ahmed Z, Asi YT, Sailer A, Lees AJ, Houlden H, Revesz T, Holton JL. The neuropathology, pathophysiology and genetics of multiple system atrophy. Neuropathol Appl Neurobiol. 2012;38(1):4–24.

3. Beck RO, Betts CD, Fowler CJ. Genitourinary dysfunction in multiple system atrophy: clinical features and treatment in 62 cases. J Urol. 1994;151(5): 1336–41.
4. Ben-Shlomo Y, Wenning GK, Tison F, Quinn NP. Survival of patients with pathologically proven multiple system atrophy: a meta-analysis. Neurology. 1997;48(2):384–93.
5. Bensimon G, Ludolph A, Agid Y, Vidailhet M, Payan C, Leigh PN, NNIPPS Study Group. Riluzole treatment, survival and diagnostic criteria in Parkinson plus disorders: the NNIPPS study. Brain. 2009;132(Pt 1):156–71.
6. Berg D, Hochstrasser H. Iron metabolism in parkinsonian syndromes. Mov Disord. 2006;21:1299–310.
7. Bjornsdottir A, Gudmundsson G, Blondal H, Olafsson E. Incidence and prevalence of multiple system atrophy: a nationwide study in Iceland. J Neurol Neurosurg Psychiatry. 2013;84(2):136–40.
8. Bower JH, Maraganore DM, McDonnell SK, Rocca WA. Incidence of progressive supranuclear palsy and multiple system atrophy in Olmsted County, Minnesota, 1976 to 1990. Neurology. 1997;49(5):1284–8.
9. Brown RG, Lacomblez L, Landwehrmeyer BG, Bak T, Uttner I, Dubois B, Agid Y, Ludolph A, Bensimon G, Payan C, Leigh NP, NNIPPS Study Group. Cognitive impairment in patients with multiple system atrophy and progressive supranuclear palsy. Brain. 2010;133(Pt 8):2382–93.
10. Bürk K, Bühring U, Schulz JB, Zühlke C, Hellenbroich Y, Dichgans J. Clinical and magnetic resonance imaging characteristics of sporadic cerebellar ataxia. Arch Neurol. 2005;62(6):981–5.
11. Chrysostome V, Tison F, Yekhlef F, Sourgen C, Baldi I, Dartigues JF. Epidemiology of multiple system atrophy: a prevalence and pilot risk factor study in Aquitaine, France. Neuroepidemiology. 2004;23(4):201–8.
12. Constantinescu R, Richard I, Kurlan R. Levodopa responsiveness in disorders with parkinsonism: a review of the literature. Mov Disord. 2007;22(15):2141–8.
13. Déjérine J, Thomas A. L'atrophie olivo pontocerebelleuse. Nouvelle iconographie de la Salpetriere: Clinique des malacies du systeme nerveux. 1900;13:330–70.
14. Dodel R, Spottke A, Gerhard A, Reuss A, Reinecker S, Schimke N, Trenkwalder C, Sixel-Döring F, Herting B, Kamm C, Gasser T, Sawires M, Geser F, Köllensperger M, Seppi K, Kloss M, Krause M, Daniels C, Deuschl G, Böttger S, Naumann M, Lipp A, Gruber D, Kupsch A, Du Y, Turkheimer F, Brooks DJ, Klockgether T, Poewe W, Wenning G, Schade-Brittinger C, Oertel WH, Eggert K. Minocycline 1-year therapy in multiple-system-atrophy: effect on clinical symptoms and [(11)C] (R)-PK11195 PET (MEMSA-trial). Mov Disord. 2010;25(1):97–107.
15. Eichhorn TE, Oertel WH. Macrogol 3350/electrolyte improves constipation in Parkinson's disease and multiple system atrophy. Mov Disord. 2001;16(6):1176–7.
16. Fanciulli A, Wenning GK. Multiple system atrophy. N Engl J Med. 2015;372(3):249–63.
17. Frumkin H. Multiple system atrophy following chronic carbon disulfide exposure. Environ Health Perspect. 1998;106(9):611–3.
18. Fujioka S, Ogaki K, Tacik PM, Uitti RJ, Ross OA, Wszolek ZK. Update on novel familial forms of Parkinson's disease and multiple system atrophy. Parkinsonism Relat Disord. 2014;20 Suppl 1: S29–34.
19. Gilman S. Biochemical changes in multiple system atrophy detected with positron emission tomography. Parkinsonism Relat Disord. 2001;7(3):253–6.
20. Gilman S, Low PA, Quinn N, Albanese A, Ben-Shlomo Y, Fowler CJ, Kaufmann H, Klockgether T, Lang AE, Lantos PL, Litvan I, Mathias CJ, Oliver E, Robertson D, Schatz I, Wenning GK. Consensus statement on the diagnosis of multiple system atrophy. American Autonomic Society and American Academy of Neurology. J Auton Nerv Syst. 1998;74(2–3):189–92.
21. Gilman S, Wenning GK, Low PA, Brooks DJ, Mathias CJ, Trojanowski JQ, Wood NW, Colosimo C, Dürr A, Fowler CJ, Kaufmann H, Klockgether T, Lees A, Poewe W, Quinn N, Revesz T, Robertson D, Sandroni P, Seppi K, Vidailhet M. Second consensus statement on the diagnosis of multiple system atrophy. Neurology. 2008;71(9):670–6.
22. Ghorayeb I, Bioulac B, Tison F. Sleep disorders in multiple system atrophy. J Neural Transm. 2005;112(12):1669–75.
23. Halaska M, Ralph G, Wiedemann A, Primus G, Ballering-Brühl B, Höfner K, Jonas U. Controlled, double-blind, multicentre clinical trial to investigate long-term tolerability and efficacy of trospium chloride in patients with detrusor instability. World J Urol. 2003;20(6):392–9.
24. Holmberg B, Johansson JO, Poewe W, Wenning G, Quinn NP, Mathias C, Tolosa E, Cardozo A, Dizdar N, Rascol O, Slaoui T, Growth-Hormone MSA Study Group, European MSA Study Group. Safety and tolerability of growth hormone therapy in multiple system atrophy: a double-blind, placebo-controlled study. Mov Disord. 2007;22(8):1138–44.
25. Hussain IF, Brady CM, Swinn MJ, Mathias CJ, Fowler CJ. Treatment of erectile dysfunction with sildenafil citrate (Viagra) in parkinsonism due to Parkinson's disease or multiple system atrophy with observations on orthostatic hypotension. J Neurol Neurosurg Psychiatry. 2001;71(3):371–4.
26. Jankovic J, Gilden JL, Hiner BC, Kaufmann H, Brown DC, Coghlan CH, Rubin M, Fouad-Tarazi FM. Neurogenic orthostatic hypotension: a double-blind, placebo-controlled study with midodrine. Am J Med. 1993;95(1):38–48.
27. Jecmenica-Lukic M, Poewe W, Tolosa E, Wenning GK. Premotor signs and symptoms of multiple system atrophy. Lancet Neurol. 2012;11(4):361–8.
28. Jellinger KA, Seppi K, Wenning GK. Grading of neuropathology in multiple system atrophy: proposal for a novel scale. Mov Disord. 2005;20 Suppl 12:S29–36.
29. Kaufmann H, Saadia D, Voustianiouk A, Goldstein DS, Holmes C, Yahr MD, Nardin R, Freeman R.

Norepinephrine precursor therapy in neurogenic orthostatic hypotension. Circulation. 2003;108(6):724–8.
30. Kim HJ, Jeon BS, Lee JY, Yun JY. Survival of Korean patients with multiple system atrophy. Mov Disord. 2011;26(5):909–12.
31. Kirchhof K, Apostolidis AN, Mathias CJ, Fowler CJ. Erectile and urinary dysfunction may be the presenting features in patients with multiple system atrophy: a retrospective study. Int J Impot Res. 2003;15(4):293–8.
32. Köllensperger M, Geser F, Ndayisaba JP, Boesch S, Seppi K, Ostergaard K, Dupont E, Cardozo A, Tolosa E, Abele M, Klockgether T, Yekhlef F, Tison F, Daniels C, Deuschl G, Coelho M, Sampaio C, Bozi M, Quinn N, Schrag A, Mathias CJ, Fowler C, Nilsson CF, Widner H, Schimke N, Oertel W, Del Sorbo F, Albanese A, Pellecchia MT, Barone P, Djaldetti R, Colosimo C, Meco G, Gonzalez-Mandly A, Berciano J, Gurevich T, Giladi N, Galitzky M, Rascol O, Kamm C, Gasser T, Siebert U, Poewe W, Wenning GK. EMSA-SG. Presentation, diagnosis, and management of multiple system atrophy in Europe: final analysis of the European multiple system atrophy registry. Mov Disord. 2010;25(15):2604–12.
33. Friess E, Kuempfel T, Modell S, Winkelmann J, Holsboer F, Ising M, Trenkwalder C. Paroxetine treatment improves motor symptoms in patients with multiple system atrophy. Parkinsonism Relat Disord. 2006;12(7):432–7.
34. Lee EA, Cho HI, Kim SS, Lee WY. Comparison of magnetic resonance imaging in subtypes of multiple system atrophy. Parkinsonism Relat Disord. 2004;10(6):363–8.
35. Lee PH, Lee JE, Kim HS, Song SK, Lee HS, Nam HS, Cheong JW, Jeong Y, Park HJ, Kim DJ, Nam CM, Lee JD, Kim HO, Sohn YH. A randomized trial of mesenchymal stem cells in multiple system atrophy. Ann Neurol. 2012;72(1):32–40.
36. Levin J, Kurz A, Arzberger T, Giese A, Höglinger GU. The differential diagnosis and treatment of atypical Parkinsonism. Dtsch Arztebl Int. 2016;113(5):61 9.
37. Lin DJ, Hermann KL, Schmahmann JD. Multiple system atrophy of the cerebellar type: clinical state of the art. Mov Disord. 2014;29(3):294–304.
38. Low PA, Robertson D, Gilman S, Kaufmann H, Singer W, Biaggioni I, Freeman R, Perlman S, Hauser RA, Cheshire W, Lessig S, Vernino S, Mandrekar J, Dupont WD, Chelimsky T, Galpern WR. Efficacy and safety of rifampicin for multiple system atrophy: a randomised, double-blind, placebo-controlled trial. Lancet Neurol. 2014;13(3):268–75.
39. Mathias CJ, Senard JM, Braune S, Watson L, Aragishi A, Keeling JE, Taylor MD. L-threo-dihydroxyphenylserine (L-threo-DOPS; droxidopa) in the management of neurogenic orthostatic hypotension: a multi-national, multi-center, dose-ranging study in multiple system atrophy and pure autonomic failure. Clin Auton Res. 2001;11(4):235–42.
40. Miller DW, Johnson JM, Solano SM, Hollingsworth ZR, Standaert DG, Young AB. Absence of alpha-synuclein mRNA expression in normal and multiple system atrophy oligodendroglia. J Neural Transm. 2005;112(12):1613–24.
41. Mollenhauer B, Locascio JJ, Schulz-Schaeffer W, Sixel-Döring F, Trenkwalder C, Schlossmacher MG. α-Synuclein and tau concentrations in cerebrospinal fluid of patients presenting with parkinsonism: a cohort study. Lancet Neurol. 2011;10(3):230–40.
42. Mutations in COQ2 in familial and sporadic multiple-system atrophy. Multiple-System Atrophy Research Collaboration. N Engl J Med. 2013;369(3):233–44.
43. Müller J, Wenning GK, Wissel J, Seppi K, Poewe W. Botulinum toxin treatment in atypical parkinsonian disorders associated with disabling focal dystonia. J Neurol. 2002;249(3):300–4.
44. Poewe W, Barone P, Gliadi N, Gilman S, Low PA, Sampaio C, Seppi K, Wenning GK, Rasagiline-for-MSA Investigators. A randomized, placebo-controlled clinical trial to assess the effects of rasagiline in patients with multiple system atrophy of the parkinsonian subtype. Mov Disord. 2012;27(1):S1–523.
45. Quinn N, Barker RA, Wenning GK. Are trials of intravascular infusions of autologous mesenchymal stem cells in patients with multiple system atrophy currently justified, and are they effective? Clin Pharmacol Ther. 2008;83(5):663–5. doi:10.1038/sj.clpt.6100454.
46. Savoiardo M, Strada L, Girotti F, Zimmerman RA, Grisoli M, Testa D, Petrillo R. Olivopontocerebellar atrophy: MR diagnosis and relationship to multisystem atrophy. Radiology. 1990;174(3 Pt 1):693–6.
47. Scholz SW, Houlden H, Schulte C, Sharma M, Li A, Berg D, Melchers A, Paudel R, Gibbs JR, Simon-Sanchez J, Paisan-Ruiz C, Bras J, Ding J, Chen H, Traynor BJ, Arepalli S, Zonozi RR, Revesz T, Holton J, Wood N, Lees A, Oertel W, Wüllner U, Goldwurm S, Pellecchia MT, Illig T, Riess O, Fernandez HH, Rodriguez RL, Okun MS, Poewe W, Wenning GK, Hardy JA, Singleton AB, Del Sorbo F, Schneider S, Bhatia KP, Gasser T. SNCA variants are associated with increased risk for multiple system atrophy. Ann Neurol. 2009;65(5):610–4.
48. Schrag A, Ben-Shlomo Y, Quinn NP. Prevalence of progressive supranuclear palsy and multiple system atrophy: a cross-sectional study. Lancet. 1999;354(9192):1771–5.
49. Schrag A, Good CD, Miszkiel K, Morris HR, Mathias CJ, Lees AJ, Quinn NP. Differentiation of atypical parkinsonian syndromes with routine MRI. Neurology. 2000;54(3):697–702.
50. Schrag A, Geser F, Stampfer-Kountchev M, Seppi K, Sawires M, Köllensperger M, et al. Health-related quality of life in multiple system atrophy. Mov Disord. 2006;21:809–15.
51. Sharma M, Wenning G, Krüger R, European Multiple-System Atrophy Study Group (EMSA-SG). Mutant COQ2 in multiple-system atrophy. N Engl J Med. 2014;371(1):80–1.

52. Soma H, Yabe I, Takei A, Fujiki N, Yanagihara T, Sasaki H. Heredity in multiple system atrophy. J Neurol Sci. 2006;240(1–2):107–10.
53. Spillantini MG, Goedert M. The alpha-synucleinopathies: Parkinson's disease, dementia with Lewy bodies, and multiple system atrophy. Ann N Y Acad Sci. 2000;920:16–27.
54. Stefanova N, Bücke P, Duerr S, Wenning GK. Multiple system atrophy: an update. Lancet Neurol. 2009;8(12):1172–8.
55. Tang CC, Eidelberg D. Abnormal metabolic brain networks in Parkinson's disease from blackboard to bedside. Prog Brain Res. 2010;184:161–76.
56. Testa D, Monza D, Ferrarini M, Soliveri P, Girotti F, Filippini G. Comparison of natural histories of progressive supranuclear palsy and multiple system atrophy. Neurol Sci. 2001;22(3):247–51.
57. Thobois S, Broussolle E, Toureille L, Vial C. Severe dysphagia after botulinum toxin injection for cervical dystonia in multiple system atrophy. Mov Disord. 2001;16:764–5.
58. Tison F, Yekhlef F, Chrysostome V. Depression and self-reported depressive symptoms in multiple system atrophy compared to Parkinson's disease. Mov Disord. 2006;21(7):1056–7.
59. Trojanowski JQ, Revesz T, Neuropathology Working Group on MSA. Proposed neuropathological criteria for the post mortem diagnosis of multiple system atrophy. Neuropathol Appl Neurobiol. 2007; 33(6):615–20.
60. Wakabayashi K, Yoshimoto M, Tsuji S, Takahashi H. Alpha-synuclein immunoreactivity in glial cytoplasmic inclusions in multiple system atrophy. Neurosci Lett. 1998;249(2–3):180–2.
61. Watanabe H, Saito Y, Terao S, Ando T, Kachi T, Mukai E, Aiba I, Abe Y, Tamakoshi A, Doyu M, Hirayama M, Sobue G. Progression and prognosis in multiple system atrophy: an analysis of 230 Japanese patients. Brain. 2002;125(Pt 5):1070–83.
62. Wenning GK, Ben Shlomo Y, Magalhães M, Daniel SE, Quinn NP. Clinical features and natural history of multiple system atrophy. An analysis of 100 cases. Brain. 1994;117(Pt 4):835–45.
63. Wenning GK, Tison F, Ben Shlomo Y, Daniel SE, Quinn NP. Multiple system atrophy: a review of 203 pathologically proven cases. Mov Disord. 1997;12(2):133–47.
64. Wenning GK, Ben-Shlomo Y, Hughes A, Daniel SE, Lees A, Quinn NP. What clinical features are most useful to distinguish definite multiple system atrophy from Parkinson's disease? J Neurol Neurosurg Psychiatry. 2000;68(4):434–40.
65. Wenning GK, Tison F, Seppi K, Sampaio C, Diem A, Yekhlef F, Ghorayeb I, Ory F, Galitzky M, Scaravilli T, Bozi M, Colosimo C, Gilman S, Shults CW, Quinn NP, Rascol O, Poewe W, Multiple System Atrophy Study Group. Development and validation of the Unified Multiple System Atrophy Rating Scale (UMSARS). Mov Disord. 2004;19(12):1391–402.
66. Wenning GK, Stefanova N. Recent developments in multiple system atrophy. J Neurol. 2009; 256(11):1791–808.
67. Wenning GK, Geser F, Krismer F, Seppi K, Duerr S, Boesch S, Köllensperger M, Goebel G, Pfeiffer KP, Barone P, Pellecchia MT, Quinn NP, Koukouni V, Fowler CJ, Schrag A, Mathias CJ, Giladi N, Gurevich T, Dupont E, Ostergaard K, Nilsson CF, Widner H, Oertel W, Eggert KM, Albanese A, del Sorbo F, Tolosa E, Cardozo A, Deuschl G, Hellriegel H, Klockgether T, Dodel R, Sampaio C, Coelho M, Djaldetti R, Melamed E, Gasser T, Kamm C, Meco G, Colosimo C, Rascol O, Meissner WG, Tison F, Poewe W, European Multiple System Atrophy Study Group. The natural history of multiple system atrophy: a prospective European cohort study. Lancet Neurol. 2013;12(3):264–74.
68. Wüllner U, Schmitz-Hübsch T, Abele M, Antony G, Bauer P, Eggert K. Features of probable multiple system atrophy patients identified among 4770 patients with parkinsonism enrolled in the multicentre registry of the German Competence Network on Parkinson's disease. J Neural Transm. 2007; 114(9):1161–5.
69. Wüllner U, Schmitt I, Kammal M, Kretzschmar HA, Neumann M. Definite multiple system atrophy in a German family. J Neurol Neurosurg Psychiatry. 2009;80(4):449–50.
70. Yabe I, Soma H, Takei A, Fujiki N, Yanagihara T, Sasaki H. MSA-C is the predominant clinical phenotype of MSA in Japan: analysis of 142 patients with probable MSA. J Neurol Sci. 2006;249(2):115–21.
71. Bradbury S, Eggleston C. Postural hypotension: A report of three cases. American Heart Journal, St. Louis, 1925;1:73–86.

Progressive Supranuclear Palsy

18

Maria Stamelou and Wolfgang H. Oertel

Abbreviations

CBD	Corticobasal degeneration
DATScan	Dopamine transporter imaging
EIF2AK3	Eukaryotic translation initiation factor 2-α kinase 3
ER	Endoplasmic reticulum
FDG-PET	Fluorodeoxyglucose positron emission tomography
GSK-3	Glycogen synthase kinase 3
GWAS	Genome-wide association study
IBZM	^{123}I-iodobenzamide
MAPT	Microtubule-associated protein tau
MIBG	^{123} I-meta-iodobenzylguanidine
MOBP	Myelin-associated oligodendrocyte basic protein
MRS	Magnetic resonance spectroscopy
MSA	Multiple system atrophy
NFTs	Neurofibrillary tangles
NINDS-SPSP	National Institute of Neurological Disorders and Stroke and Society for Progressive Supranuclear Palsy
PAGF	Pure akinesia with gait freezing
PD	Parkinson's disease
PEG	Percutaneous endoscopic gastrostomy
PSP	Progressive supranuclear palsy
SPECT	Single-photon emission computed tomography
SSRIs	Serotonin reuptake inhibitors
STX6	Syntaxin 6
UPR	Unfolded protein response

M. Stamelou, MD, PhD (✉)
Department of Neurology, University Clinic, Philipps University Marburg, Baldingerstrasse 35039, Germany

Movement Disorders Department, Hygeia Hospital, Erythrou Stavrou 4 & Kifisiaw, Marousi, Athens 15123, Greece

Second Department of Neurology, Kapodistrian University of Athens, Rimini 1, Athens 12462, Greece
e-mail: mariastamelou@gmail.com

W.H. Oertel, MD
Department of Neurology, University Clinic, Philipps University Marburg, Baldingerstrasse 35039, Germany
e-mail: oertelw@med.uni-marburg.de

18.1 Epidemiology

Progressive supranuclear palsy (PSP) or Steele-Richardson-Olszewksi syndrome is considered a rare disease. The mean age at onset is approximately 63 years with a mean survival of 9 years from the onset of symptomatology [1]. The youngest age of onset ever reported is 41 years old [2]. PSP presents a prevalence of 5–6/100,000 and an average annual incidence of 5.3 per 100,000 in the

C. Falup-Pecurariu et al. (eds.), *Movement Disorders Curricula*,
DOI 10.1007/978-3-7091-1628-9_18

age range of 50–99 years [3]. A high prevalence of PSP has been reported in the French Antilles, with a minimum prevalence of 14 per 100,000 on the island of Guadeloupe [4, 5].

18.2 Neuropathology

PSP belongs to a family of diseases called tauopathies and is characterized by neuronal loss, gliosis, and accumulation of tau protein in the involved cerebral areas [6]. Tauopathies comprise more than 20 clinicopathological entities, including Alzheimer's dementia (the most common tauopathy), corticobasal degeneration (CBD), and some frontotemporal dementias. The name "tauopathies" derives from the protein tau, which is the most abundant microtubule-associated protein in the human brain. The gene encoding for tau protein (microtubule-associated protein tau, *MAPT*) is present on chromosome 17q21. The protein exists in six isoforms, differing by the presence or absence of 29-amino-acid or 59-amino-acid inserts located in the amino-terminal end and a 31-amino-acid repeat in the microtubule-binding domain. Depending on the presence or the absence of the latter, the domain harbors either 3-repeat (3R) or 4-repeat (4R) sequences, respectively. In the normal adult brain, there are similar levels of 3R and 4R tau [7–13]. In tauopathies, there is an abnormally hyperphosphorylated tau and an altered ratio between 3R and 4R tau. This leads to formation of tau aggregates called neurofibrillary tangles (NFTs) and ultimately to neuronal cell death [14].

The neuropathological abnormalities involve both cortical and subcortical structures and in particular the subthalamic nuclei, globus pallidus, superior colliculi, other cerebellar regions, pretectal regions, periaqueductal gray matter, substantia nigra, and the whole tegmentum [6, 15]. Tau protein aggregates in neurons as spherical NFTs revealed by silver staining or by immunohistochemistry with specific antibodies against the pathological tau protein (e.g., AD2 antibodies) [15–17] (Fig. 18.1). The distribution and type of pathological hallmarks (NFTs formation and tufted astrocytes in the basal ganglia, brainstem, and motor cortices, absence of neuritic plaques) suggest the diagnosis of PSP and help to differentiate from other tauopathies such as CBD [18, 19].

18.3 Etiology

Although the etiology of PSP remains unknown, our knowledge regarding the contribution of genetic factors, environmental factors, and mitochondrial dysfunction is discussed below.

18.3.1 Genetics

PSP is almost always sporadic. A genome-wide association study (GWAS) has confirmed that the most common risk allele for PSP is the H1 haplotype of the *MAPT* gene [20]. The H1 haplotype of the *MAPT* gene (encoding for tau) is found in over 90 % of the patients. It is

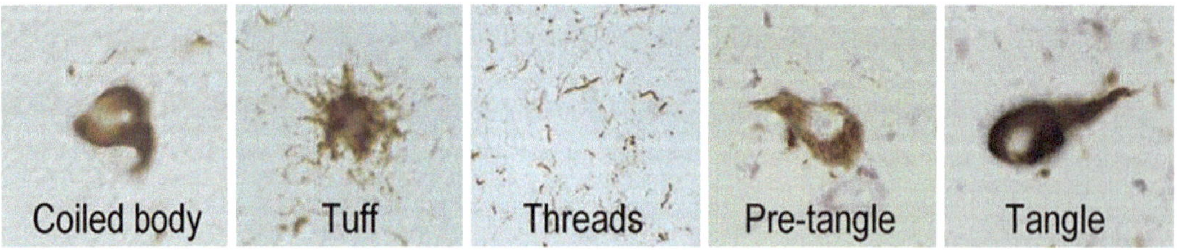

Fig. 18.1 Tau pathology in a postmortem brain of a PSP patient within the basal ganglia. Immunostaining with the AD2 antibody against human tau. Pathological AD2 immunoreaction in cytoplasm of oligodendrocytes (coiled body) and astrocytes (tuff), in neurites (threads), and in neuronal cytoplasm in loose (pre-tangle) and dense aggregation (tangle)

suggested that the presence of the H1 *MAPT* haplotype affects alternative splicing of exon 10 of the *MAPT* gene, which may result in an increased ratio of 4R tau compared with the 3R tau. However, the H1 *MAPT* haplotype did not correlate with age of onset, disease severity, or survival in a study on 63 PSP patients, implying the presence of other modifying factors [21]. Interestingly, Li et al. using genome-wide methylation analysis showed that differential methylation at 17q21.31 correlates with the H1 haplotype in a dose-dependent manner in patients with frontotemporal dementia (FTD) and PSP, pointing for the first time to an epigenetic mediator of neurodegeneration that increases the risk for PSP [22].

Apart from confirming two independent variants in *MAPT* affecting the risk for PSP, the GWAS study identified three significant novel signals associated with PSP risk, which may give some insight in the pathophysiology of the disease: *EIF2AK3* (eukaryotic translation initiation factor 2-α kinase 3), *STX6* (syntaxin 6), and *MOBP* (myelin-associated oligodendrocyte basic protein) [20]. *EIF2AK3* is a gene that encodes PERK, a component of the endoplasmic reticulum (ER) unfolded protein response (UPR). When excess unfolded proteins accumulate in the ER, PERK is activated and protein synthesis is inhibited allowing the ER to clear misfolded proteins. However, tau, which is the primary misfolded protein in PSP, is not expected to traffic through the ER. The second PSP susceptibility gene *STX6* encodes syntaxin 6 (STX6), and genetic variation at STX6 could influence the movement of misfolded proteins from the ER to lysosomes via the endosomal system. Lastly, *MOBP* encodes a protein (MOBP) that is produced by oligodendrocytes and is present in the major dense line of CNS myelin. MOBP is highly expressed in the white matter of the medulla, pons, cerebellum, and midbrain, regions affected in PSP, suggesting that myelin dysfunction or oligodendrocyte misfunction contributes to PSP pathogenesis [20]. Further research is needed to identify the functional links between these risk loci and disease pathophysiology.

18.3.2 Environmental Factors and Mitochondrial Dysfunction

Based on the observation of increased PSP prevalence in Guadeloupe and its association with the consumption of a tropical fruit containing annonacin (a complex I inhibitor) [4, 23, 24], a number of clinical studies and experiments have been conducted [4, 23–28] that identified a possible role of complex I inhibition in tau pathology. Complex I is an enzyme in the mitochondrial respiratory chain, which produces cellular energy. Chronic treatment of rats with the natural complex I inhibitor rotenone induced a pattern of neurodegeneration in the brain that resembled the one seen in PSP [27]. Rotenone-treated rats developed neuronal cytosolic aggregates of hyperphosphorylated tau [23, 27, 28]. Primary cultures of rat striatal neurons treated with annonacin showed a concentration-dependent decrease in adenosine triphosphate (ATP) levels, a redistribution of tau from the axons to the cell body, and cell death [26]. The main consequence of impaired complex I activity is a decrease in oxidative phosphorylation, which results in reduced levels of high-energy phosphates. Indeed, this was confirmed in vivo in PSP patients using phosphorus magnetic resonance spectroscopy [29]. In summary, both experimental and clinical data strengthen the idea that complex I inhibition may be implicated in the etiopathogenesis of PSP.

18.4 Clinical Characteristics

18.4.1 Clinical Features

PSP is typically characterized by symmetric and axial parkinsonism, postural instability with early falls particularly backwards, vertical supranuclear gaze palsy, and a frontal-subcortical dementia. This classical PSP phenotype is now termed Richardson's syndrome. The prognosis is poor, leading to death 6–9 years after disease onset. Postural instability and falls occur also in PD, however, usually later in the disease course. In PSP, the prevailing axial rigidity causes head and trunk hyperextension sometimes with retrocollis (although rarely), unlike the posture in flexion in PD. The typical pill-rolling asymmetric rest tremor typically seen in PD is usually absent [30–33]. Gait may be slightly broad based and does not present typically the short-stepped gait seen in PD. Freezing of gait is common and may lead to diagnostic confusion with multiple system atrophy (MSA).

The characteristic sign of PSP is the supranuclear palsy of vertical gaze followed by abnormalities of horizontal gaze. The ocular motor dysfunction begins with a slowing of vertical saccadic movements, in particular downwards. Markedly reduced blink rate, and closure of eyelids due to eyelid dystonia or "levator inhibition" (also known as "apraxia of eyelid opening"), results in overactivity of the frontalis muscle, in an attempt to keep the eyelids open, leading to a characteristic surprised look. Horizontal saccadic intrusions named "square wave jerks," occurring while staring at an object, are frequently present in PSP patients, while ocular-vestibular reflexes are preserved. Thus, on doll's eye maneuver, the range improves, as vestibulo-ocular reflex is preserved, confirming the supranuclear nature of the gaze palsy [34].

Pseudobulbar palsy with dysarthria and dysphagia is very common and appears earlier in the disease course compared to PD. Subcortical-type dementia is present in PSP patients having dramatically slowed information processing and motor execution as well as difficulty in planning and shifting conceptual sets. Apathy and withdrawal are very common and may initially be confused with depression. Reduced verbal fluency, motor perseveration, which can be detected with the "applause sign," echopraxia, echolalia, and frontal release signs are often present [35]. Patients often display "motor recklessness," e.g., they display no caution in the way they walk, throwing themselves into and out of chairs, taking no account of their lack of balance ("the rocket sign") [36, 37].

18.4.2 The Phenotypic Spectrum of PSP Pathology

The typical PSP phenotype described above is now termed Richardson's syndrome [38]. The second most common phenotype seems to be PSP-parkinsonism which may resemble PD at least at the initial stages, with asymmetric parkinsonism, rest tremor, better levodopa response, and a longer mean survival of 9 years compared to Richardson's syndrome [38]. Further phenotypes include pure akinesia with gait freezing (PAGF), corticobasal syndrome, frontotemporal dementia, progressive nonfluent aphasia, and PSP with cerebellar features [39]. In particular the PAGF phenotype is characterized by severe freezing of gait and speech, and only later in the disease course, the characteristic eye abnormalities may occur [39]. The relative frequency and natural distribution of these phenotypes are not known, and there is currently no clinical sign to accurately predict PSP pathology based on the phenotype. Recently, it has been shown that the phenotypic spectrum of PSP may be even larger than previously thought [2]. Moreover, other diseases such as CBD and frontotemporal dementias may present with the typical Richardson's syndrome phenotype, leading to diagnostic difficulties [40–42].

18.4.3 Diagnostic Criteria

There are several sets of criteria proposed to diagnose PSP, but the most widely used are the NINDS-SPSP (National Institute of Neurological Disorders and Stroke and Society for Progressive Supranuclear Palsy) (Table 18.1) [32]. These criteria have shown high specificity but low sensitivity to diagnose PSP [32, 43]. One possible condition in which these criteria would be expected to have lower sensitivity is when the development of core diagnostic features is delayed [38, 44]. Pathology remains the gold standard for definite diagnosis [32].

18.5 Investigations in PSP

PSP remains largely a clinical diagnosis. However, several abnormalities in magnetic resonance imagining (MRI) have been proposed as possible candidates to differentiate between

Table 18.1 Diagnostic criteria for progressive supranuclear palsy

Diagnostic criteria for possible PSP	Gradually progressive course
	Onset at or after 40 years with
	(a) Vertical supranuclear ophthalmoparesis *or*
	(b) Postural instability with falls since the first year of disease + slowing of saccadic movements, especially vertical saccadic movements
Diagnostic criteria for probable PSP	Gradually progressive course
	Onset at or after 40 years with
	(a) Vertical supranuclear ophthalmoparesis *and*
	(b) Postural instability with falls since the first year of disease
Diagnostic criteria for definitive PSP	Diagnostic criteria for possible and/or probable PSP + histological confirmation
Supportive criteria	Symmetric akinesia or proximal (>distal) rigidity, retrocollis, early dysphagia and dysarthria, poor or absent response of parkinsonism to levodopa therapy, early cognitive disorders, with at least one of the following signs: frontal signs, apathy, abstract thought alterations, language alterations, and imitation or utilization behavior
Mandatory exclusion criteria	Recent history of encephalitis, alien limb syndrome, cortical sensory deficits, focal frontal or temporoparietal atrophy, hallucinations or delusions unrelated to dopaminergic therapy, cortical dementia of Alzheimer type, prominent, early cerebellar symptoms and unexplained dysautonomia, severe asymmetric parkinsonian signs, neuroradiological evidence of relevant structural abnormality, Whipple's disease

atypical parkinsonian syndromes [45]. However, their sensitivity and specificity, assessed retrospectively in pathologically proven cases, were found almost equal to that of clinical diagnosis [45–47]. The most clinically useful MRI abnormalities seen in PSP are signs of midbrain atrophy, superior cerebellar peduncle atrophy, and frontal and parietal cortical atrophy [45–47]. The "morning glory flower sign" and the "humming bird sign" are quite specific but show low sensitivity (50 % and 68.4 %, respectively), in one retrospective study [47].

With regard to functional imaging, dopamine transporter imaging (DATscan) is abnormal in PD and all atypical parkinsonian syndromes are, therefore, not useful in their differential diagnosis. To differentiate with PD, ^{123} meta-iodobenzylguanidine (MIBG) scintigraphy and ^{123}I-iodobenzamide (IBZM) single-photon emission computed tomography (SPECT) may be useful. MIBG is abnormal in PD because of postganglionic sympathetic denervation but is typically normal in PSP. IBZM SPECT assessing the postsynaptic receptors is abnormal in PSP as opposed to PD. However, IBZM SPECT is abnormal in all atypical parkinsonian syndromes (such as MSA and CBD) and therefore cannot differentiate between PSP and other atypical parkinsonian conditions [48, 49]. FDG-PET (fluorodeoxyglucose positron emission tomography) has been shown to help in the differential diagnosis with other atypical parkinsonian syndromes such as MSA and CBD; however, these studies have not been conducted in pathology-proven cases, and it is unknown whether they reflect the phenotype rather than the underlying pathology [50–53].

Novel diagnostic approaches and biomarkers such as proteins in cerebrospinal fluid (a-synuclein, tau, etc.) are still under research [54, 55]. In this regard, neurofilament light chain may be proven useful as a biomarker in the future [56]. Moreover, the development of tau-specific ligands for PET studies is well underway.

18.6 Treatment

18.6.1 Symptomatic Treatment

Currently, there are no effective symptomatic or neuroprotective treatments for PSP [42, 57]. Proposed treatments are based largely on small, uncontrolled studies with no pathological or retrospective confirmation. Supportive treatment, particularly regarding swallowing and prevention of falls, may prolong survival and improve quality of life:

- A trial of levodopa (up to 1 g/day) and amantadine (up to 450 mg/day) is worthwhile.
- Botulinum toxin injections can be used to treat levator inhibition.
- Serotonin reuptake inhibitors (SSRIs) may be used for apathy with no clear benefit.
- Supportive measures such as physiotherapy, walking aids, and percutaneous endoscopic gastrostomy (PEG) for swallowing difficulties may be helpful.

18.6.2 Disease Modification

As in most sporadic neurodegenerative conditions, research has focused in the recent years on the development of disease-modifying treatments [57]. In PSP, the targets of such treatments have been aimed mainly at tau dysfunction [10, 58–60] and in particular at the inhibition of aggregation and/or phosphorylation, reduction of tau levels, and microtubule stabilization [61–64].

Glycogen synthase kinase 3 (GSK-3) is a kinase important in tau hyperphosphorylation [62, 63, 65, 66], and its inhibition has been found to reduce tau phosphorylation in vitro and in vivo [61, 62, 67, 68]. However, tideglusib, a GSK-3b inhibitor, failed to show efficacy on the clinical endpoints in a recent double-blind, randomized, placebo-controlled phase II clinical trial in PSP [67]. However, there were treatment-related differences in progressive brain atrophy in a small subgroup of patients who underwent longitudinal volumetric MRI scans as part of the study [69], suggesting that further studies with kinase inhibitors might be warranted.

Stabilization of microtubules has been proposed as a strategy to compensate for loss of tau function [70]. Recently, davunetide, a peptide derived from the growth factor activity-dependent neurotrophic protein, was reported to promote microtubule stability. However, the compound failed to show efficacy in a 1-year, double-blind, parallel-group, phase II/III, placebo-controlled study with 313 participants [56].

Transcellular spread of altered conformations of tau with prion-like properties has recently emerged as a possible mechanism in sporadic neurodegenerative disorders and offers new therapeutic possibilities for PSP [71–74]. Different strains of pathogenic tau conformations may help to explain the selective vulnerability of different brain networks in the spectrum of tau-related neurodegenerative disease [75]. Therapeutic agents are being developed to reducing tau levels in the extracellular space either by active or passive immunization [76–78], and evidence from animal models is promising [79, 80]. Antisense oligonucleotides have also demonstrated great promise in reducing tau concentrations and their pathogenic consequences in animal models [81] and, when intrathecally delivered, have been shown to be well tolerated in amyotrophic lateral sclerosis, suggesting this approach may be feasible for PSP as well [82, 83]. Lastly, experimental data suggest that small interfering RNAs suppressing human tau expression might be another therapeutic option in the future [84].

Apart from targeting tau, mitochondrial dysfunction has been a therapeutic target of PSP, based on in vitro and in vivo evidence of complex I dysfunction [23, 26–29, 85]. A small, double-blind, placebo-controlled, randomized trial administering coenzyme Q10 for 6 weeks found improved clinical scales as well as improved occipital energy levels in MR spectroscopy [86]; however, a larger, placebo-controlled trial of coenzyme Q10 in 62 PSP patients for 12 months, using clinical scales as primary outcomes, was reported to be negative [87].

18.7 Future Perspectives

Despite the current lack of an effective treatment, new knowledge on the pathophysiology of PSP has contributed to the design of potential new therapies the translation of which into humans is under way. Current limitations for conducting disease-modifying clinical trials include the late diagnosis and the lack of validated biomarkers.

In particular, a well-designed human trial would require validated biomarkers of target engagement to demonstrate that therapies exert their predicted biological effect in humans. Without such biomarkers, the results of negative efficacy trials will be difficult to interpret. Positron emission tomographic imaging using tau-specific ligands and cerebrospinal fluid biomarkers may be proven useful in the near future.

References

1. Litvan I. Update on epidemiological aspects of progressive supranuclear palsy. Mov Disord. 2003;18 Suppl 6:S43–50.
2. Respondek G, Stamelou M, Kurz C, Ferguson LW, Rajput A, Chiu WZ, et al. The phenotypic spectrum of progressive supranuclear palsy: a retrospective multicenter study of 100 definite cases. Mov Disord. 2014;29:1758–66.
3. Nath U, Ben-Shlomo Y, Thomson RG, Lees AJ, Burn DJ. Clinical features and natural history of progressive supranuclear palsy: a clinical cohort study. Neurology. 2003;60:910–6.
4. Caparros-Lefebvre D, Sergeant N, Lees A, Camuzat A, Daniel S, Lannuzel A, et al. Guadeloupean parkinsonism: a cluster of progressive supranuclear palsy-like tauopathy. Brain. 2002;125:801–11.
5. Caparros-Lefebvre D, Elbaz A. Possible relation of atypical parkinsonism in the French West Indies with consumption of tropical plants: a case-control study. Caribbean Parkinsonism Study Group. Lancet. 1999;354:281–6.
6. Daniel SE, de Bruin VM, Lees AJ. The clinical and pathological spectrum of Steele-Richardson-Olszewski syndrome (progressive supranuclear palsy): a reappraisal. Brain. 1995;118(Pt 3):759–70.
7. Bouchard M, Suchowersky O. Tauopathies: one disease or many? Can J Neurol Sci J Can Sci Neurol. 2011;38:547–56.
8. Kouri N, Whitwell JL, Josephs KA, Rademakers R, Dickson DW. Corticobasal degeneration: a pathologically distinct 4R tauopathy. Nat Rev Neurol. 2011;7:263–72.
9. Vandrovcova J, Anaya F, Kay V, Lees A, Hardy J, de Silva R. Disentangling the role of the tau gene locus in sporadic tauopathies. Curr Alzheimers Res. 2010;7:726–34.
10. Gozes I. Tau pathology and future therapeutics. Curr Alzheimers Res. 2010;7:685–96.
11. Sahara N, Maeda S, Takashima A. Tau oligomerization: a role for tau aggregation intermediates linked to neurodegeneration. Curr Alzheimers Res. 2008;5:591–8.
12. Spillantini MG, Goedert M. Tau protein pathology in neurodegenerative diseases. Trends Neurosci. 1998;21:428–33.
13. Spillantini MG, Bird TD, Ghetti B. Frontotemporal dementia and Parkinsonism linked to chromosome 17: a new group of tauopathies. Brain Pathol. 1998;8:387–402.
14. Rampello L, Butta V, Raffaele R, Vecchio I, Battaglia G, Cormaci G, et al. Progressive supranuclear palsy: a systematic review. Neurobiol Dis. 2005;20:179–86.
15. Hauw JJ, Daniel SE, Dickson D, Horoupian DS, Jellinger K, Lantos PL, et al. Preliminary NINDS neuropathologic criteria for Steele-Richardson-Olszewski syndrome (progressive supranuclear palsy). Neurology. 1994;44:2015–9.
16. Duyckaerts C, Verny M, Hauw JJ. Recent neuropathology of parkinsonian syndromes. Rev Neurol. 2003;159:3S11–8.
17. Verny M, Jellinger KA, Hauw JJ, Bancher C, Litvan I, Agid Y. Progressive supranuclear palsy: a clinicopathological study of 21 cases. Acta Neuropathol. 1996;91:427–31.
18. Lee SE, Rabinovici GD, Mayo MC, Wilson SM, Seeley WW, DeArmond SJ, et al. Clinicopathological correlations in corticobasal degeneration. Ann Neurol. 2011;70:327–40.
19. Dickson DW, Ahmed Z, Algom AA, Tsuboi Y, Josephs KA. Neuropathology of variants of progressive supranuclear palsy. Curr Opin Neurol. 2010;23:394–400.
20. Hoglinger GU, Melhem NM, Dickson DW, Sleiman PM, Wang LS, Klei L, et al. Identification of common variants influencing risk of the tauopathy progressive supranuclear palsy. Nat Genet. 2011;43:699–705.
21. Litvan I, Baker M, Hutton M. Tau genotype: no effect on onset, symptom severity, or survival in progressive supranuclear palsy. Neurology. 2001;57:138–40.
22. Li Y, Chen JA, Sears RL, Gao F, Klein ED, Karydas A, et al. An epigenetic signature in peripheral blood associated with the haplotype on 17q21.31, a risk factor for neurodegenerative tauopathy. PLoS Genet. 2014;10, e1004211.
23. Lannuzel A, Michel PP, Hoglinger GU, Champy P, Jousset A, Medja F, et al. The mitochondrial complex I inhibitor annonacin is toxic to mesencephalic dopaminergic neurons by impairment of energy metabolism. Neuroscience. 2003;121:287–96.
24. Lannuzel A, Michel PP, Caparros-Lefebvre D, Abaul J, Hocquemiller R, Ruberg M. Toxicity of Annonaceae for dopaminergic neurons: potential role in atypical parkinsonism in Guadeloupe. Mov Disord. 2002;17:84–90.
25. Lannuzel A, Ruberg M, Michel PP. Atypical parkinsonism in the Caribbean island of Guadeloupe: etiological role of the mitochondrial complex I inhibitor annonacin. Mov Disord. 2008;23:2122–8.
26. Escobar-Khondiker M, Hollerhage M, Muriel MP, Champy P, Bach A, Depienne C, et al. Annonacin, a natural mitochondrial complex I inhibitor, causes tau pathology in cultured neurons. J Neurosci Off J Soc Neurosci. 2007;27:7827–37.
27. Hoglinger GU, Lannuzel A, Khondiker ME, Michel PP, Duyckaerts C, Feger J, et al. The mitochondrial complex I inhibitor rotenone triggers a cerebral tauopathy. J Neurochem. 2005;95:930–9.

28. Champy P, Hoglinger GU, Feger J, Gleye C, Hocquemiller R, Laurens A, et al. Annonacin, a lipophilic inhibitor of mitochondrial complex I, induces nigral and striatal neurodegeneration in rats: possible relevance for atypical parkinsonism in Guadeloupe. J Neurochem. 2004;88:63–9.
29. Stamelou M, Pilatus U, Reuss A, Magerkurth J, Eggert KM, Knake S, et al. In vivo evidence for cerebral depletion in high-energy phosphates in progressive supranuclear palsy. J Cereb Blood Flow Metab: Off J Int Soc Cereb Blood Flow Metab. 2009;29:861–70.
30. Josephs KA, Petersen RC, Knopman DS, Boeve BF, Whitwell JL, Duffy JR, et al. Clinicopathologic analysis of frontotemporal and corticobasal degenerations and PSP. Neurology. 2006;66:41–8.
31. Litvan I, Campbell G, Mangone CA, Verny M, McKee A, Chaudhuri KR, et al. Which clinical features differentiate progressive supranuclear palsy (Steele-Richardson-Olszewski syndrome) from related disorders? A clinicopathological study. Brain. 1997;120(Pt 1):65–74.
32. Litvan I, Mangone CA, McKee A, Verny M, Parsa A, Jellinger K, et al. Natural history of progressive supranuclear palsy (Steele-Richardson-Olszewski syndrome) and clinical predictors of survival: a clinicopathological study. J Neurol Neurosurg Psychiatry. 1996;60:615–20.
33. Osaki Y, Ben-Shlomo Y, Lees AJ, Daniel SE, Colosimo C, Wenning G, et al. Accuracy of clinical diagnosis of progressive supranuclear palsy. Mov Disord. 2004;19:181–9.
34. Marx S, Respondek G, Stamelou M, Dowiasch S, Stoll J, Bremmer F, et al. Validation of mobile eye-tracking as novel and efficient means for differentiating progressive supranuclear palsy from Parkinson's disease. Front Behav Neurosci. 2012;6:88.
35. Dubois B, Slachevsky A, Litvan I, Pillon B. The FAB: a Frontal Assessment Battery at bedside. Neurology. 2000;55:1621–6.
36. Litvan I. Cognitive disturbances in progressive supranuclear palsy. J Neural Transm Suppl. 1994;42:69–78.
37. Paviour DC, Winterburn D, Simmonds S, Burgess G, Wilkinson L, Fox NC, et al. Can the frontal assessment battery (FAB) differentiate bradykinetic rigid syndromes? Relation of the FAB to formal neuropsychological testing. Neurocase. 2005;11:274–82.
38. Williams DR, de Silva R, Paviour DC, Pittman A, Watt HC, Kilford L, et al. Characteristics of two distinct clinical phenotypes in pathologically proven progressive supranuclear palsy: Richardson's syndrome and PSP-parkinsonism. Brain. 2005;128:1247–58.
39. Williams DR, Lees AJ. Progressive supranuclear palsy: clinicopathological concepts and diagnostic challenges. Lancet Neurol. 2009;8:270–9.
40. Stamelou M, Alonso-Canovas A, Bhatia KP. Dystonia in corticobasal degeneration: a review of the literature on 404 pathologically proven cases. Mov Disord. 2012;27:696–702.
41. Stamelou M, Quinn NP, Bhatia KP. "Atypical" atypical parkinsonism: new genetic conditions presenting with features of progressive supranuclear palsy, corticobasal degeneration, or multiple system atrophy-a diagnostic guide. Mov Disord. 2013;28:1184–99.
42. Stamelou M, Bhatia KP. Atypical parkinsonism: diagnosis and treatment. Neurol Clin. 2015;33:39–56.
43. Respondek G, Roeber S, Kretzschmar H, Troakes C, Al-Sarraj S, Gelpi E, et al. Accuracy of the National Institute for Neurological Disorders and Stroke/ Society for Progressive Supranuclear Palsy and neuroprotection and natural history in Parkinson plus syndromes criteria for the diagnosis of progressive supranuclear palsy. Mov Disord. 2013;28:504–9.
44. Williams DR, Holton JL, Strand K, Revesz T, Lees AJ. Pure akinesia with gait freezing: a third clinical phenotype of progressive supranuclear palsy. Mov Disord. 2007;22:2235–41.
45. Stamelou M, Knake S, Oertel WH, Hoglinger GU. Magnetic resonance imaging in progressive supranuclear palsy. J Neurol. 2011;258:549–58.
46. Longoni G, Agosta F, Kostic VS, Stojkovic T, Pagani E, Stosic-Opincal T, et al. MRI measurements of brainstem structures in patients with Richardson's syndrome, progressive supranuclear palsy-parkinsonism, and Parkinson's disease. Mov Disord. 2011;26:247–55.
47. Massey LA, Micallef C, Paviour DC, O'Sullivan SS, Ling H, Williams DR, et al. Conventional magnetic resonance imaging in confirmed progressive supranuclear palsy and multiple system atrophy. Mov Disord. 2012;27:1754–62.
48. Orimo S, Suzuki M, Inaba A, Mizusawa H. 123I-MIBG myocardial scintigraphy for differentiating Parkinson's disease from other neurodegenerative parkinsonism: a systematic review and meta-analysis. Parkinsonism Relat Disord. 2012;18:494–500.
49. Vlaar AM, de Nijs T, Kessels AG, Vreeling FW, Winogrodzka A, Mess WH, et al. Diagnostic value of 123I-ioflupane and 123I-iodobenzamide SPECT scans in 248 patients with parkinsonian syndromes. Eur Neurol. 2008;59:258–66.
50. Tripathi M, Dhawan V, Peng S, Kushwaha S, Batla A, Jaimini A, et al. Differential diagnosis of parkinsonian syndromes using F-18 fluorodeoxyglucose positron emission tomography. Neuroradiology. 2013; 55(4):483–92.
51. Zwergal A, la Fougere C, Lorenzl S, Rominger A, Xiong G, Deutschenbaur L, et al. Functional disturbance of the locomotor network in progressive supranuclear palsy. Neurology. 2013;80:634–41.
52. Hellwig S, Amtage F, Kreft A, Buchert R, Winz OH, Vach W, et al. [(1)(8)F]FDG-PET is superior to [(1)(2)(3)I]IBZM-SPECT for the differential diagnosis of parkinsonism. Neurology. 2012;79:1314–22.
53. Zhao P, Zhang B, Gao S. 18F-FDG PET study on the idiopathic Parkinson's disease from several parkinsonian-plus syndromes. Parkinsonism Relat Disord. 2012;18 Suppl 1:S60–2.
54. Mollenhauer B, Locascio JJ, Schulz-Schaeffer W, Sixel-Doring F, Trenkwalder C, Schlossmacher MG. alpha-Synuclein and tau concentrations in cerebrospinal fluid of patients presenting with parkinsonism: a cohort study. Lancet Neurol. 2011;10:230–40.

55. Stamelou M, Hoeglinger GU. Atypical parkinsonism: an update. Curr Opin Neurol. 2013;26:401–5.
56. Boxer AL, Lang AE, Grossman M, Knopman DS, Miller BL, Schneider LS, et al. Davunetide in patients with progressive supranuclear palsy: a randomised, double-blind, placebo-controlled phase 2/3 trial. Lancet Neurol. 2014;13:676–85.
57. Stamelou M, de Silva R, Arias-Carrion O, Boura E, Hollerhage M, Oertel WH, et al. Rational therapeutic approaches to progressive supranuclear palsy. Brain. 2010;133:1578–90.
58. Gozes I. Microtubules (tau) as an emerging therapeutic target: NAP (davunetide). Curr Pharm Des. 2011;17:3413–7.
59. Schneider A, Mandelkow E. Tau-based treatment strategies in neurodegenerative diseases. Neurother: J Am Soc Exp Neurother. 2008;5:443–57.
60. Goedert M. Tau gene mutations and their effects. Mov Disord. 2005;20 Suppl 12:S45–52.
61. Dominguez JM, Fuertes A, Orozco L, del Monte-Millan M, Delgado E, Medina M. Evidence for irreversible inhibition of glycogen synthase kinase-3beta by tideglusib. J Biol Chem. 2012;287:893–904.
62. Medina M, Garrido JJ, Wandosell FG. Modulation of GSK-3 as a therapeutic strategy on Tau Pathologies. Front Mol Neurosci. 2011;4:24.
63. Ferrer I, Gomez-Isla T, Puig B, Freixes M, Ribe E, Dalfo E, et al. Current advances on different kinases involved in tau phosphorylation, and implications in Alzheimer's disease and tauopathies. Curr Alzheimers Res. 2005;2:3–18.
64. Martinez A, Alonso M, Castro A, Perez C, Moreno FJ. First non-ATP competitive glycogen synthase kinase 3 beta (GSK-3beta) inhibitors: thiadiazolidinones (TDZD) as potential drugs for the treatment of Alzheimer's disease. J Med Chem. 2002;45:1292–9.
65. Hanger DP, Noble W. Functional implications of glycogen synthase kinase-3-mediated tau phosphorylation. Int J Alzheimers Dis. 2011;2011:352805.
66. Meijer L, Flajolet M, Greengard P. Pharmacological inhibitors of glycogen synthase kinase 3. Trends Pharmacol Sci. 2004;25:471–80.
67. Tolosa E, Litvan I, Hoglinger GU, Burn D, Lees A, Andres MV, et al. A phase 2 trial of the GSK-3 inhibitor tideglusib in progressive supranuclear palsy. Mov Disord. 2014;29:470–8.
68. del Ser T, Steinwachs KC, Gertz HJ, Andres MV, Gomez-Carrillo B, Medina M, et al. Treatment of Alzheimer's disease with the GSK-3 inhibitor tideglusib: a pilot study. J Alzheimers Dis. 2013;33:205–15.
69. Hoglinger GU, Huppertz HJ, Wagenpfeil S, Andres MV, Belloch V, Leon T, et al. Tideglusib reduces progression of brain atrophy in progressive supranuclear palsy in a randomized trial. Mov Disord. 2014;29:479–87.
70. Brunden KR, Trojanowski JQ, Smith 3rd AB, Lee VM, Ballatore C. Microtubule-stabilizing agents as potential therapeutics for neurodegenerative disease. Bioorg Med Chem. 2014;22:5040–9.
71. Iba M, Guo JL, McBride JD, Zhang B, Trojanowski JQ, Lee VM. Synthetic tau fibrils mediate transmission of neurofibrillary tangles in a transgenic mouse model of Alzheimer's-like tauopathy. J Neurosci: Off J Soc Neurosci. 2013;33:1024–37.
72. Clavaguera F, Akatsu H, Fraser G, Crowther RA, Frank S, Hench J, et al. Brain homogenates from human tauopathies induce tau inclusions in mouse brain. Proc Natl Acad Sci U S A. 2013;110:9535–40.
73. Clavaguera F, Bolmont T, Crowther RA, Abramowski D, Frank S, Probst A, et al. Transmission and spreading of tauopathy in transgenic mouse brain. Nat Cell Biol. 2009;11:909–13.
74. Yanamandra K, Kfoury N, Jiang H, Mahan TE, Ma S, Maloney SE, et al. Anti-tau antibodies that block tau aggregate seeding in vitro markedly decrease pathology and improve cognition in vivo. Neuron. 2013;80:402–14.
75. Sanders DW, Kaufman SK, DeVos SL, Sharma AM, Mirbaha H, Li A, et al. Distinct tau prion strains propagate in cells and mice and define different tauopathies. Neuron. 2014;82:1271–88.
76. Pride M, Seubert P, Grundman M, Hagen M, Eldridge J, Black RS. Progress in the active immunotherapeutic approach to Alzheimer's disease: clinical investigations into AN1792-associated meningoencephalitis. Neuro-degenerative Dis. 2008;5:194–6.
77. Boutajangout A, Quartermain D, Sigurdsson EM. Immunotherapy targeting pathological tau prevents cognitive decline in a new tangle mouse model. J Neurosci: Off J Soc Neurosci. 2010;30:16559–66.
78. Asuni AA, Boutajangout A, Quartermain D, Sigurdsson EM. Immunotherapy targeting pathological tau conformers in a tangle mouse model reduces brain pathology with associated functional improvements. J Neurosci: Off J Soc Neurosci. 2007;27:9115–29.
79. Chai X, Wu S, Murray TK, Kinley R, Cella CV, Sims H, et al. Passive immunization with anti-Tau antibodies in two transgenic models: reduction of Tau pathology and delay of disease progression. J Biol Chem. 2011;286:34457–67.
80. Boutajangout A, Ingadottir J, Davies P, Sigurdsson EM. Passive immunization targeting pathological phospho-tau protein in a mouse model reduces functional decline and clears tau aggregates from the brain. J Neurochem. 2011;118:658–67.
81. DeVos SL, Goncharoff DK, Chen G, Kebodeaux CS, Yamada K, Stewart FR, et al. Antisense reduction of tau in adult mice protects against seizures. J Neurosci: Off J Soc Neurosci. 2013;33:12887–97.
82. Marc G, Leah R, Ofira E, Oded A, Zohar A, Hanna R. Presymptomatic treatment with acetylcholinesterase antisense oligonucleotides prolongs survival in ALS (G93A-SOD1) mice. BioMed Res Int. 2013;2013:845345.
83. Riboldi G, Zanetta C, Ranieri M, Nizzardo M, Simone C, Magri F, et al. Antisense oligonucleotide therapy for the treatment of C9ORF72 ALS/FTD diseases. Mol Neurobiol. 2014;50(3):721–32.
84. Xu H, Rösler TW, Carlsson T, de Andrade A, Fiala O, Höllerhage M, Oertel WH, Goedert M, et al. Tau silencing by siRNA in the P301S mouse model of tauopathy. Current Gene Therapy 2014;14(5):343–51.

85. Hollerhage M, Matusch A, Champy P, Lombes A, Ruberg M, Oertel WH, et al. Natural lipophilic inhibitors of mitochondrial complex I are candidate toxins for sporadic neurodegenerative tau pathologies. Exp Neurol. 2009;220:133–42.
86. Stamelou M, Reuss A, Pilatus U, Magerkurth J, Niklowitz P, Eggert KM, et al. Short-term effects of coenzyme Q10 in progressive supranuclear palsy: a randomized, placebo-controlled trial. Mov Disord. 2008;23:942–9.
87. Apetauerova DSD, Yacoubian T, Hamill RW, Simon D, Scala S. Effects of coenzyme Q10 in PSP, a multicenter, randomized, placebo-controlled, double-blind study [abstract]. Mov Disord. 2014;29:265.

19 Corticobasal Degeneration

Cristian Falup-Pecurariu and Dafin Fior Mureșanu

Corticobasal degeneration (CBD) was first described by Rebeiz et al. in 1968 [45].

The CBD spectrum is comprised of corticobasal syndrome (CBS), which is based on a clinical diagnosis, and CBD, which is based on a pathologically confirmed diagnosis [13].

19.1 Epidemiology

CBD is a heterogeneous clinical and pathological syndrome; therefore, its incidence and prevalence are difficult to estimate. Reports in the literature describe the low clinical and pathological correlations of CBD [5, 29, 38]. Hughes et al. [29] evaluated 143 patients with parkinsonian syndromes who underwent pathological examinations in a specialized movement disorders center at the National Hospital for Neurology and Neurosurgery in London. Over a 10-year period, three of the patients in this group received a clinical diagnosis of CBD. Pathologically, one case consisted of corticobasal degeneration, one case consisted of frontotemporal dementia, and one case consisted of idiopathic Parkinson's disease. In addition, four patients received a pathological diagnosis of CBD. Only one of these patients was clinically diagnosed with CBD during their lifetime. The other three cases consisted of vascular parkinsonism, progressive supranuclear palsy (PSP), and focal cerebral atrophy with myoclonus, respectively [29].

The low sensitivity of the clinical diagnosis of CBD has also been reported by Litvan et al. [38]. In a series of 105 cases with neuropathological diagnoses, ten patients received CBD diagnoses. In this group, the specificity of the clinical diagnosis of CBD was 99.6 %. The mean sensitivity for the CBD diagnosis increased from 35 % at first visit to 48.3 % at the last visit [38].

Boeve et al. [5] reported that seven of 13 patients with a clinical diagnosis of CBD received neuropathological confirmation. The remaining cases consisted of two cases of Alzheimer's disease; one case each of Pick's disease, PSP, and Creutzfeldt-Jakob disease; and nonspecific degenerative changes in one case [5].

Ling et al. [36] reported the experience of the Queen Square Brain Bank for Neurological Disorders in London; of the 19 patients with neuropathological confirmation of CBD, only five received the diagnosis during their lifetime. The other cases ranged along a broad spectrum that included PSP in eight cases, Parkinson's disease in

C. Falup-Pecurariu, MD, PhD (✉)
Department of Neurology, County Emergency Clinic Hospital, Faculty of Medicine, Transilvania University, Calea Bucuresti 25-27, Brasov 500040, Romania
e-mail: crisfp100@yahoo.co.uk

D.F. Mureşanu, MD, PhD, MBA
Department of Clinical Neurosciences, University of Medicine and Pharmacy "Iuliu Haţieganu", 43 Victor Babes, Cluj-Napoca 400012, Romania

"RoNeuro" Institute for Neurological Research and Diagnostic, Cluj-Napoca 400012, Romania
e-mail: dafinm@ssnn.ro

C. Falup-Pecurariu et al. (eds.), *Movement Disorders Curricula*,
DOI 10.1007/978-3-7091-1628-9_19

two cases, and one case each of frontotemporal lobar degeneration, Pick's disease, Gilles de la Tourette's syndrome, spastic quadriparesis, and myoclonus. Five of the 21 patients with CBS had corticobasal neuropathology. The neuropathological spectrum for these patients was also diverse, consisting of six cases of PSP, five cases of Alzheimer's disease, two cases of Parkinson's disease, and one case of frontotemporal lobar degeneration [36]. The youngest reported case of probable CBD showed onset at 28 years of age [9]. Another report of a young clinical case with onset at 40 years of age has been published [48]. The youngest published case with neuropathological confirmation showed disease onset at 45 years of age [63].

In one report, the mean age of disease onset was 63 ± 7.7 years, and the mean disease duration was 7.9 ± 2.6 years [63].

Regarding gender differences, several reports suggest a slight predominance in women [33, 48, 50, 59].

CBD is typically a sporadic disease. However, a description of a series of neuropathologically confirmed familial cases has been reported [7]. Reports also exist of familial dementia with no specific pathological features presenting with the symptomatology of CBS [8]. In an incidence study in Moscow that involved 1,237,900 participants, Winter et al. [65] reported only one case of CBD. The crude incidence was 0.03 per 100,000 person-years [65].

In their prevalence studies, Schrag et al. [52, 53] did not identify any CBD cases.

From a methodological point of view, the best strategy to identify CBD cases involves utilizing disease registries and case-control studies [60]. CBD and PSP have a similar genetic background; therefore, the same registries and studies can be used to study CBD [10].

19.2 Neuropathology

Rebeiz et al. described the neuropathological findings in three cases of CBD [45]. The main pathological characteristic was neuronal achromasia, consisting of enlarged neurons with swelling of the cell body. The neurons were oval and round shaped, and the main affected areas included the cerebral cortex, substantia nigra (the pigmented portion), and, in two out of three cases, the dentatorubrothalamic system [45]. The nucleus was irregularly shaped or round and pale, and the cytoplasm contained no Nissl substance [45].

Nerve cells with these abnormalities were found mainly in layer V and less in layer VI of the cortex.

Some authors consider swollen neurons a hallmark of CBD [15]. However, recent neuropathological criteria for CBD [11] show that this symptom is nonspecific because cases of CBD patients with no swollen neurons have been reported.

The gross findings of patients demonstrate asymmetric superior frontoparietal and perirolandic cerebral cortical atrophy [11].

Narrowing of cortical gyri is an important feature [11]. Atrophy of the thalamus and caudate, pallor of the substantia nigra, and thinning of the corpus callosum have been reported [11, 58]. In addition, the substantia nigra shows prominent neuronal loss [37].

The gross findings also demonstrate asymmetric cortical atrophy or focal atrophy. In these regions, corresponding neuronal loss and gliosis are present [5]. In addition, status spongiosis has been described, especially in the frontoparietal cortex [5].

Tau-immunopositive neurons are present in CBD patients [61]. Yamada and McGeer [66] defined oligodendroglial microtubule masses as microtubular aggregates in oligodendroglia. Braak and Braak [6] described coiled bodies of silver-stained filaments.

Accumulations of straight filaments appear in the coiled bodies [6]. The white matter changes include coiled bodies and threadlike lesions [11], and astrocytic plaques are present in the white and gray matter [11].

Tau-immunoreactive lesions are present in the putamen and caudate [11], and neurofibrillary tangles have also been described [58].

19.3 Clinical Features

Some symptoms are present at the initial presentation. Over time, these symptoms may worsen or other symptoms may appear [41, 47]. At the initial presentation, the most common feature is a "clumsy, stiff, or jerky arms" [48].

The main characteristic of the arms is that they are rigid and apraxic. One-third of these patients exhibit a fixed, dystonic posture. Postural instability and gait disturbances were reported by one-third of the patients [48], and limb "clumsiness" was described by half of the patients [63]. Falls in the early stages of the disease were described by 21 % of patients. The spectrum of the other symptoms included sensory dysfunction, cognitive and behavioral disturbances, and speech disturbances. In a recent report, Armstrong et al. [1] analyzed 209 neuropathologically proven CBD cases. Limb rigidity was the most common complaint (57 %), followed by bradykinesia or "clumsy limbs." Higher cortical symptoms were also described at the initial presentation including cognitive impairment (52 %), followed by behavioral changes (46 %) and limb apraxia (45 %).

19.3.1 Motor Symptoms

The key feature of CBD is parkinsonism. The most common feature is asymmetrical unilateral parkinsonism that affects one arm [40].

Another key feature is dystonia [18, 20, 33, 56, 62], which affects half of the patients in the first 2 years [56] and another one-third of patients after 4 years from disease onset. Dystonia is sometimes a main symptom in the clinical manifestation of CBD. A recent report showed that dystonia was present in 37.5 % of a large cohort of neuropathologically proven CBD patients [56]. Limb dystonia is usually asymmetric [62].

Vanek and Jankovic [62] reported that half of the patients from their cohort had dystonia. Topographically, the upper limbs were more often affected than the legs (51 % vs. 33 %). One of the most common features of patients is adduction and flexion of the upper limbs, along with extension of interphalangeal joints, in which the fingers flex at the metacarpal-phalangeal joints.

During the course of the disease, other focal dystonias could appear. Cranial (including cervical dystonia and blepharospasm) and trunk dystonias could also be clinical features of the disease. Lower limb dystonia is very rare [28, 36, 50], but different fixed postures with accompanying contractures have been observed [62]. From the onset, dystonia could remain unchanged, spread and become generalized [31], or become hemidystonia [24, 49, 50]. Pain accompanying dystonia was present in 42 % of the patients in one report and was especially strong in the dystonic hand [62].

19.3.2 Cortical Dysfunction

Limb apraxia is one of the most common impairments of CBD [23, 57].

Limb apraxia is typically asymmetric and is often ideomotor. In most cases, patients are typically impaired while using tools and also while performing communicative gestures [64]. CBD patients exhibit different types of apraxia [30, 35, 42]:

1. Limb kinetic apraxia – usually involves fine finger movements and appears less often than ideomotor apraxia [27].
2. Ideational apraxia – many CBD patients are impaired in the use of objects and the performance of symbolic gestures by command or imitation.
3. Truncal apraxia – reported in some cases [42] and involves apraxia of whole body movements, usually appears when the patient is sitting or lying down, and is minimal when standing up.

Apraxia in CBD patients is sometimes bilateral and is difficult to assess due to the combination of dystonia, bradykinesia, and rigidity [40]. Orofacial apraxia is present in many patients, and sequential gestures are also impaired [43].

CBD patients exhibit multifactorial apraxia and an alteration in the organization of motor programming. Ideomotor apraxia (IMA) is characterized by the patient's inability to perform different types of movement when no motor and sensory disturbances are present [51].

A deficit in production and execution is involved in the initial mechanism of apraxia [30].

General semantic memory is affected in some CBD patients. Thus, CBD patients who have more than one deficit involving the use of the objects are more disabled by dyspraxia during activities of daily living [55]. The voluntary movements of the tongue are impaired, and recently, lingual dystonia has been described [19]. Alien limb syndrome is a particular symptom in which the patient perceives one limb as foreign, and this sensation is accompanied by involuntary movements [12]. In this particular syndrome, the patient fails to recognize his/her limbs when visual cues are not available, and the limb movements are perceived to be out of the patient's voluntary control [12, 25].

Alien limb syndrome is one of the main features of CBD [25] and affects many patients. In CBD patients, alien limb symptoms could be one of the first clinical features of the disease or could complicate the disease course. A grasp reflex is commonly associated with this phenomenon [12]. In one study, alien limb symptoms were present in 108 of 150 cases of CBD and were associated with left-sided CBS [21]. One phenotypic variant is the posterior alien limb phenotype, which includes rigidity, apraxia, neglect, sensory disturbances, and alien limb symptoms [12, 16]. Kompoliti et al. [33] reported that 42 % of their cohort of 147 cases exhibited alien limb syndrome.

Other features of these patients include (a) dyspraxia, consisting of intermanual conflict and mirror movements, and (b) frontal lobe reflexes, characterized by a grasping reflex and groping [16]. A case has been reported that involves complex partial seizures with secondary generalization [14].

Cortical reflex myoclonus has been frequently described in CBD patients [40].

19.3.3 Cognition

It was initially thought that cognitive impairment was rare or appeared late during the evolution of the disease [18, 48]; however, reports have suggested that cognitive impairment could appear before the onset of motor symptoms or early in the disease [4, 26, 32, 50].

Some reports have suggested that dementia is an important disease symptom [26]. Cognitive examinations have shown that ideomotor apraxia is significantly more frequent in CBD patients [54]. and Kompoliti et al. [33] reported that dementia occurred in 25 % of their cohort of 147 cases.

Armstrong et al. [1] reported cognitive impairment early during the disease course in 59 of 114 (52 %) cases and during the entire course of the disease in 123 of 175 (70 %) cases.

Impairment of visuospatial skills has been reported [3, 22, 46, 54].

Both episodic and semantic memory is affected by the disease [3, 44]. CBD patients exhibit learning deficits and impairments in motor execution [44]. Using an extensive neuropsychology battery, Pillon et al. [44] compared the performance of a group of patients with CBD ($n = 15$) to that of a group of control subjects ($n = 19$) and groups of patients with PSP and Alzheimer's disease ($n = 15$ in each group). This study suggested that patients with CBD, similar to those with PSP, exhibit dysexecutive syndrome. When the process of praxis was compared between groups, it was noted that CBD patients exhibited impairments in symbolic gesture execution and object utilization tasks. Some lesions that affect anatomical structures such as the premotor and parietal lobes are involved in the asymmetric praxis disorders associated with CBD [44]. CBD patients have impairments in remote memory, but these impairments do not affect recognition or visuospatial memory [3].

19.3.4 Psychiatric Features

The spectrum of psychiatric symptoms in CBD patients is diverse [39]. Litvan et al. [39] evaluated the neuropsychiatric symptoms in 15 patients with CBD using the Neuropsychiatric Inventory (NPI). The spectrum of psychiatric features was dominated by depression (73 %), followed by apathy (40 %) and irritability and agitation (20 %). Irritability was significantly associated with apathy. It has been suggested that frontal-subcortical pathways are not impaired in CBD patients [39].

19.4 Treatment

While the treatment of CBD patients is unsatisfactory overall [2, 40, 58], some reports have shown that treatment produces some benefits.

Motor symptoms respond poorly to dopaminergic medication; however, many CBD patients are included in dopaminergic trials. Kompoliti et al. [33] reported that 92 % of CBD patients received dopaminergic medication.

Levodopa is the first-line medication used to treat motor symptoms, but usually a response is only obtained in a minority of patients (this is also suggested by the diagnostic criteria) [2].

However, the spectrum of medication used to treat CBD patients is diverse [33]; the majority of patients (87 %) receive levodopa and peripheral decarboxylase inhibitors, and 25 % receive bromocriptine or pergolide mesylate; other drugs used include selegiline hydrochloride and amantadine hydrochloride. For dystonic features, injected botulinum toxin has been used in 6 % of CBD patients [33].

When complex treatments were used, no clinical improvement was observed in 71 % of the cases. Some improvements were noted in 24 % of the cases, but 5 % of the patients showed a worsening of symptoms [33]. Levodopa improved the symptoms in 26 % of patients [33]. Ling et al. [36] reported that 56 % of patients showed transient mild-to-moderate symptom improvement.

In addition to CBD patients showing a poor response to levodopa, it can also induce dyskinesia [17]. However, one report [33] suggests that dyskinesia does not occur, even with high doses of dopaminergic drugs.

Ling et al. [36] reported that three of 16 (17 %) patients developed dystonic or choreiform movements of the limbs, which were reversible and dose dependent.

Wening et al. [63] reported that most patients treated with levodopa did not benefit from the treatment. In this study, at the last visit, four of 14 patients received levodopa. Three of the four patients treated with levodopa did not benefit from the treatment. Only one patient showed a moderate response [63].

Vanek [62] reported that 32 patients received levodopa, and 12 were treated with dopamine agonists, with a modest clinical benefit.

Clonazepam was shown to control myoclonus in 23 % of cases. Two of 12 patients showed transient improvements of myoclonus with clonazepam treatment [62]. Kovacs et al. [34] reported that levetiracetam (1,500 mg/day) remarkably improved myoclonus in two patients.

Some improvement of tremor was noted when anticonvulsants and propranolol were used in combination [33].

Antidepressants were not beneficial for the treatment of depression [33].

Of six patients treated with botulinum toxin injections, two showed marked improvement of dystonia and pain and four showed mild-to-moderate improvement [62].

Subthalamic or pallidal deep brain stimulation produced no benefit for CBD patients.

Other potential treatments involve acetylcholinesterase inhibitors and selective serotonin reuptake inhibitors, but there is no data regarding the efficiency of these treatments [2].

Other lines of treatment utilize cognitive therapies, physical therapies to maintain mobility and prevent muscle contractions, occupational therapy to maintain some degree of functional independence, and social work [2, 58]. Speech therapy is very important and has practical applications, including exercises to avoid aspiration due to the swallowing difficulties present in CBD patients.

Depression and obsessive-compulsive symptoms may benefit from selective serotonin reuptake inhibitors. However, clinicians should consider that at higher doses, these medications could induce agitation [58]. Atypical antipsychotics could be used in patients with psychotic behavior and agitation [58]. Sleep problems could be treated with small doses of sedative hypnotics; clonazepam and zolpidem are good options for this type of treatment [58].

Gastrointestinal symptoms in CBD patients include hypersalivation, dysphagia, nausea, and constipation.

Excessive salivation could be treated with small doses of anticholinergics.

Dysphagia should be evaluated by barium swallowing tests or upper gastrointestinal tract endoscopy. Helpful measures include dietary modifications and swallowing maneuvers. When patients become highly disabled, a feeding gastrostomy may be necessary.

References

1. Armstrong MJ, Litvan I, Lang AE, Bak TH, Bhatia KP, Borroni B, Boxer AL, Dickson DW, Grossman M, Hallett M, Josephs KA, Kertesz A, Lee SE, Miller BL, Reich SG, Riley DE, Tolosa E, Tröster AI, Vidailhet M, Weiner WJ. Criteria for the diagnosis of corticobasal degeneration. Neurology. 2013;80(5):496–503.
2. Armstrong MJ, Lang AE. Corticobasal degeneration and corticobasal syndrome. In: Wolters EC, Baumann C, editors. Parkinson disease and other movement disorders. Motor behavioural disorders and behavioural motor disorders. VU University Press, Amsterdem; 2014. p. 411–21.
3. Beatty WW, Scott JG, Wilson DA, Prince JR, Williamson DJ. Memory deficits in a demented patient with probable corticobasal degeneration. J Geriatr Psychiatry Neurol. 1995;8(2):132–6.
4. Bergeron C, Davis A, Lang AE. Corticobasal ganglionic degeneration and progressive supranuclear palsy presenting with cognitive decline. Brain Pathol. 1998;8(2):355–65.
5. Boeve BF, Maraganore DM, Parisi JE, Ahlskog JE, Graff-Radford N, Caselli RJ, Dickson DW, Kokmen E, Petersen RC. Pathologic heterogeneity in clinically diagnosed corticobasal degeneration. Neurology. 1999;53(4):795–800.
6. Braak H, Braak E. Cortical and subcortical argyrophilic grains characterize a disease associated with adult onset dementia. Neuropathol Appl Neurobiol. 1989;15(1):13–26.
7. Brown J, Lantos PL, Roques P, Fidani L, Rossor MN. Familial dementia with swollen achromatic neurons and corticobasal inclusion bodies: a clinical and pathological study. J Neurol Sci. 1996;135(1):21–30.
8. Brown J, Lantos PL, Rossor MN. Familial dementia lacking specific pathological features presenting with clinical features of corticobasal degeneration. J Neurol Neurosurg Psychiatry. 1998;65(4):600–3.
9. DePold HA, Ransom BR, Chun MR, Tröster AI, Samii A. The youngest reported case of corticobasal degeneration. Parkinsonism Relat Disord. 2003;10(1):47–50.
10. Di Maria E, Tabaton M, Vigo T, Abbruzzese G, Bellone E, Donati C, Frasson E, Marchese R, Montagna P, Munoz DG, Pramstaller PP, Zanusso G, Ajmar F, Mandich P. Corticobasal degeneration shares a common genetic background with progressive supranuclear palsy. Ann Neurol. 2000;47(3):374–7.
11. Dickson DW, Bergeron C, Chin SS, Duyckaerts C, Horoupian D, Ikeda K, Jellinger K, Lantos PL, Lippa CF, Mirra SS, Tabaton M, Vonsattel JP, Wakabayashi K, Litvan I, Office of Rare Diseases of the National Institutes of Health. Office of rare diseases neuropathologic criteria for corticobasal degeneration. J Neuropathol Exp Neurol. 2002;61(11):935–46.
12. Doody RS, Jankovic J. The alien hand and related signs. J Neurol Neurosurg Psychiatry. 1992;55(9):806–10.
13. Doran M, du Plessis DG, Enevoldson TP, Fletcher NA, Ghadiali E, Larner AJ. Pathological heterogeneity of clinically diagnosed corticobasal degeneration. J Neurol Sci. 2003;216(1):127–34.
14. Douglas VC, DeArmond SJ, Aminoff MJ, Miller BL, Rabinovici GD. Seizures in corticobasal degeneration: a case report. Neurocase. 2009;15(4):352–6.
15. Feany MB, Dickson DW. Widespread cytoskeletal pathology characterizes corticobasal degeneration. Am J Pathol. 1995;146(6):1388–96.
16. Fisher CM. Alien hand phenomena: a review with the addition of six personal cases. Can J Neurol Sci. 2000;27(3):192–203.
17. Frucht S, Fahn S, Chin S, Dhawan V, Eidelberg D. Levodopa-induced dyskinesias in autopsy-proven cortical-basal ganglionic degeneration. Mov Disord. 2000;15(2):340–3.
18. Gibb WR, Luthert PJ, Marsden CD. Corticobasal degeneration. Brain. 1989;112(Pt 5):1171–92.
19. Giza E, Katsarou Z, Dagklis I, Bostantjopoulou S. Lingual dystonia as a new clinical feature in corticobasal syndrome. J Neurol Sci. 2015;353(1–2):187–8.
20. Godeiro-Junior C, Felício AC, Barsottini OGP, de Carvalho Aguiar PM, Silva SMA, Borges V, Ferraz HB. Clinical features of dystonia in atypical parkinsonism. Arq Neuropsiquiatr. 2008;66(4):800–4.
21. Graff-Radford J, Rubin MN, Jones DT, Aksamit AJ, Ahlskog JE, Knopman DS, Petersen RC, Boeve BF, Josephs KA. The alien limb phenomenon. J Neurol. 2013;260(7):1880–8.
22. Graham NL, Zeman A, Young AW, Patterson K, Hodges JR. Dyspraxia in a patient with corticobasal degeneration: the role of visual and tactile inputs to action. J Neurol Neurosurg Psychiatry. 1999;67(3):334–44.
23. Graham NL, Bak TH, Hodges JR. Corticobasal degeneration as a cognitive disorder. Mov Disord. 2003;18(11):1224–32.
24. Greene PE, Fahn S, Lang AE, Watts RL, Eidelberg D, Powers JM. What is it? Case 1, 1990: progressive unilateral rigidity, bradykinesia, tremulousness, and apraxia, leading to fixed postural deformity of the involved limb. Mov Disord. 1990;5(4):341–51.
25. Grijalvo-Perez AM, Litvan I. Corticobasal degeneration. Semin Neurol. 2014;34(2):160–73.
26. Grimes DA, Lang AE, Bergeron CB. Dementia as the most common presentation of cortical-basal ganglionic degeneration. Neurology. 1999;53(9):1969–74.
27. Heilman KM, Rothi LJG. Apraxia. In: Heilman KM, Valenstein E, editors. Clinical neuropsychology. 3rd ed. Oxford: Oxford University Press; 1993. p. 141–63.

28. Horvath J, Kövari E, Bouras C, Burkhard PR. Neuropathological correlates of lower limb corticobasal degeneration. Neuropathol Appl Neurobiol. 2009;35(6):623–7.
29. Hughes AJ, Daniel SE, Ben-Shlomo Y, Lees AJ. The accuracy of diagnosis of parkinsonian syndromes in a specialist movement disorder service. Brain. 2002;125(Pt 4):861–70.
30. Jacobs DH, Adair JC, Macauley B, Gold M, Gonzalez Rothi LJ, Heilman KM. Apraxia in corticobasal degeneration. Brain Cogn. 1999;40(2):336–54.
31. Jung HH, Bremer J, Streffer J, Virdee K, Spillantini MG, Crowther RA, Brugger P, Van Broeckhoven C, Aguzzi A, Tolnay M. Phenotypic variation of autosomal-dominant corticobasal degeneration. Eur Neurol. 2012;67(3):142–50.
32. Kertesz A, Martinez-Lage P, Davidson W, Munoz DG. The corticobasal degeneration syndrome overlaps progressive aphasia and frontotemporal dementia. Neurology. 2000;55(9):1368–75.
33. Kompoliti K, Goetz CG, Boeve BF, Maraganore DM, Ahlskog JE, Marsden CD, Bhatia KP, Greene PE, Przedborski S, Seal EC, Burns RS, Hauser RA, Gauger LL, Factor SA, Molho ES, Riley DE. Clinical presentation and pharmacological therapy in corticobasal degeneration. Arch Neurol. 1998;55(7):957–61.
34. Kovács T, Farsang M, Vitaszil E, Barsi P, Györke T, Szirmai I, Kamondi A. Levetiracetam reduces myoclonus in corticobasal degeneration: report of two cases. J Neural Transm. 2009;116(12):1631–4.
35. Leiguarda R, Lees AJ, Merello M, Starkstein S, Marsden CD. The nature of apraxia in corticobasal degeneration. J Neurol Neurosurg Psychiatry. 1994;57(4):455–9.
36. Ling H, O'Sullivan SS, Holton JL, Revesz T, Massey LA, Williams DR, Paviour DC, Lees AJ. Does corticobasal degeneration exist? A clinicopathological re-evaluation. Brain. 2010;133(Pt 7):2045–57.
37. Lippa CF, Smith TW, Fontneau N. Corticonigral degeneration with neuronal achromasia. A clinicopathologic study of two cases. J Neurol Sci. 1990;98(2–3):301–10.
38. Litvan I, Agid Y, Goetz C, Jankovic J, Wenning GK, Brandel JP, Lai EC, Verny M, Ray-Chaudhuri K, McKee A, Jellinger K, Pearce RK, Bartko JJ. Accuracy of the clinical diagnosis of corticobasal degeneration: a clinicopathologic study. Neurology. 1997;48(1):119–25.
39. Litvan I, Cummings JL, Mega M. Neuropsychiatric features of corticobasal degeneration. J Neurol Neurosurg Psychiatry. 1998;65(5):717–21.
40. Mahapatra RK, Edwards MJ, Schott JM, Bhatia KP. Corticobasal degeneration. Lancet Neurol. 2004;3(12):736–43.
41. Mastrolilli F, Benvenga A, Di Biase L, Giambattistelli F, Trotta L, Salomone G, Quintiliani L, Landi D, Melgari JM, Vernieri F. An unusual cause of dementia: essential diagnostic elements of corticobasal degeneration – a case report and review of the literature. Int J Alzheimers Dis. 2011;536141:1–6.
42. Okuda B, Tanaka H, Kawabata K, Tachibana H, Sugita M. Truncal and limb apraxia in corticobasal degeneration. Mov Disord. 2001;16(4):760–2.
43. Ozsancak C, Auzou P, Hannequin D. Dysarthria and orofacial apraxia in corticobasal degeneration. Mov Disord. 2000;15(5):905–10.
44. Pillon B, Blin J, Vidailhet M, Deweer B, Sirigu A, Dubois B, Agid Y. The neuropsychological pattern of corticobasal degeneration: comparison with progressive supranuclear palsy and Alzheimer's disease. Neurology. 1995;45(8):1477–83.
45. Rebeiz JJ, Kolodny EH, Richardson Jr EP. Corticodentatonigral degeneration with neuronal achromasia. Arch Neurol. 1968;18(1):20–33.
46. Rey GJ, Tomer R, Levin BE, Sanchez-Ramos J, Bowen B, Bruce JH. Psychiatric symptoms, atypical dementia, and left visual field inattention in corticobasal ganglionic degeneration. Mov Disord. 1995;10(1):106–10.
47. Riley DE, Lang AE, Lewis A, Resch L, Ashby P, Hornykiewicz O, Black S. Cortical-basal ganglionic degeneration. Neurology. 1990;40(8):1203–12.
48. Rinne JO, Lee MS, Thompson PD, Marsden CD. Corticobasal degeneration. A clinical study of 36 cases. Brain. 1994;117(Pt 5):1183–96.
49. Sawle GV, Brooks DJ, Marsden CD, Frackowiak RS. Corticobasal degeneration. A unique pattern of regional cortical oxygen hypometabolism and striatal fluorodopa uptake demonstrated by positron emission tomography. Brain. 1991;114(Pt 1B):541–56.
50. Schneider JA, Watts RL, Gearing M, Brewer RP, Mirra SS. Corticobasal degeneration: neuropathologic and clinical heterogeneity. Neurology. 1997;48(4):959–69.
51. Schnider A, Hanlon RE, Alexander DN, Benson DF. Ideomotor apraxia: behavioral dimensions and neuroanatomical basis. Brain Lang. 1997;58(1):125–36.
52. Schrag A, Ben-Shlomo Y, Quinn NP. Prevalence of progressive supranuclear palsy and multiple system atrophy: a cross-sectional study. Lancet. 1999;354(9192):1771–5.
53. Schrag A, Ben-Shlomo Y, Quinn NP. Cross sectional prevalence survey of idiopathic Parkinson's disease and Parkinsonism in London. BMJ. 2000;321(7252):21–2.
54. Soliveri P, Monza D, Paridi D, Radice D, Grisoli M, Testa D, Savoiardo M, Girotti F. Cognitive and magnetic resonance imaging aspects of corticobasal degeneration and progressive supranuclear palsy. Neurology. 1999;53(3):502–7.
55. Spatt J, Bak T, Bozeat S, Patterson K, Hodges JR. Apraxia, mechanical problem solving and semantic knowledge: contributions to object usage in corticobasal degeneration. J Neurol. 2002;249(5):601–8.
56. Stamelou M, Alonso-Canovas A, Bhatia KP. Dystonia in corticobasal degeneration: a review of the literature on 404 pathologically proven cases. Mov Disord. 2012;27(6):696–702.
57. Stamenova V, Roy EA, Black SE. Limb apraxia in corticobasal syndrome. Cortex. 2011;47(4):460–72.

58. Stover NP, Wainer BH, Watts RL. Corticobasal degeneration. In: Watts RL, Koller WC. Movement disorders, neurologic principles & practice. McGraw-Hill Companies, USA; 2004. p. 763–78.
59. Stover NP, Watts RL. Corticobasal degeneration. Semin Neurol. 2001;21(1):49–58.
60. Tanner CM. Epidemiologic approaches to cortical basal ganglionic degeneration. Mov Disord. 1996;11(3):350.
61. Uchihara T, Mizusawa H, Tsuchiya K, Kondo H, Oda T, Ikeda K. Discrepancy between tau immunoreactivity and argyrophilia by the Bodian method in neocortical neurons of corticobasal degeneration. Acta Neuropathol. 1998;96(6):553–7.
62. Vanek Z, Jankovic J. Dystonia in corticobasal degeneration. Mov Disord. 2001;16(2):252–7.
63. Wenning GK, Litvan I, Jankovic J, Granata R, Mangone CA, McKee A, Poewe W, Jellinger K, Ray Chaudhuri K, D'Olhaberriague L, Pearce RK. Natural history and survival of 14 patients with corticobasal degeneration confirmed at postmortem examination. J Neurol Neurosurg Psychiatry. 1998;64(2):184–9.
64. Wheaton LA, Hallett M. Ideomotor apraxia: a review. J Neurol Sci. 2007;260(1–2):1–10.
65. Winter Y, Bezdolnyy Y, Katunina E, Avakjan G, Reese JP, Klotsche J, Oertel WH, Dodel R, Gusev E. Incidence of Parkinson's disease and atypical parkinsonism: Russian population-based study. Mov Disord. 2010;25(3):349–56.
66. Yamada T, McGeer PL. Oligodendroglial microtubular masses: an abnormality observed in some human neurodegenerative diseases. Neurosci Lett. 1990;120(2):163–6.

The Lewy Body Dementias: Dementia with Lewy Bodies and Related Syndromes

20

Sara Garcia-Ptacek, Alexandra Bernadotte, and Dag Aarsland

20.1 Introduction

The Lewy body dementias comprise disorders characterized by parkinsonism and a dementia syndrome with a predominant attentional, executive and visuospatial component, and with the Lewy body as the core pathological marker. Dementia with Lewy bodies (DLB) and Parkinson's disease with dementia (PDD) are two conditions that meet this definition and are only differentiated by the duration of parkinsonism prior to dementia onset. The standardized clinical criteria for DLB establish an arbitrary 1-year cutoff between symptoms: if dementia begins at the same time or within 1 year of parkinsonism, the patient is presumed to suffer from DLB; if dementia onset occurs more than 1 year after parkinsonism, PDD is assumed. The third report of the DLB consortium [1] highlighted the unresolved boundary issues between DLB and PDD but maintained this arbitrary cut point. The appropriateness of such an artificial cut point for differentiating two similar clinical syndromes has been debated. Indeed, DLB and PDD share many common characteristics and might represent different clinical manifestations of a common underlying process. Even within the PDD group, different cognitive profiles exist [2, 3], and some genetic alterations cause both PDD and DLB within the same family [4]. Thus, it is reasonable to consider these conditions as a continuum of possible symptoms: different patient profiles can be identified but with considerable overlap between groups. For this reason, progressive focus has shifted to defining the early stages of these diseases, where differences may be more apparent or clinically recognizable. In this chapter, we aim to present what is currently known about DLB and PDD, focusing on clinical aspects of diagnosis, treatment, and care as well as a taste of foreseeable developments in the near future.

S. Garcia-Ptacek
Department of Medicine, Universidad Complutense, Madrid, Spain

Division of Clinical Geriatrics, Department of Neurobiology, Care Sciences and Society, Section for Clinical Geriatrics, Karolinska Institutet, Novum plan 5, 141 86 Stockholm, Sweden

A. Bernadotte, MD, PhD
Division of Clinical Geriatrics, Department of Neurobiology, Care Sciences and Society, Section for Clinical Geriatrics, Karolinska Institutet, Novum plan 5, 141 86 Stockholm, Sweden
e-mail: alexandra.bernadotte@gmail.com

D. Aarsland, MD, PhD (✉)
Division of Clinical Geriatrics, Department of Neurobiology, Care Sciences and Society, Section for Clinical Geriatrics, Karolinska Institutet, Novum plan 5, 141 86 Stockholm, Sweden

Centre for Age-Related Medicine, Stavanger University Hospital, Stavanger, Norway

Karolinska University, Stockholm, Sweden
e-mail: daarsland@gmail.com

C. Falup-Pecurariu et al. (eds.), *Movement Disorders Curricula*,
DOI 10.1007/978-3-7091-1628-9_20

20.2 Epidemiology of Cognitive Decline of Presumed Lewy Body Etiology

The prevalence of dementia in cohorts of PD is high, with around 25 % of PD patients affected, which translates to a global prevalence of PDD in the general population over 65 of around 0.5 % [5]. The risk for dementia seems to increase with the duration of the disease, reaching 46 % at 10 years of symptom onset in the CamPaIGN incident cohort [6]. Others have suggested that dementia onset is independent from PD disease duration, occurring around 70 years of age regardless of age of motor symptom onset [7]. However, slight cognitive impairment is already apparent in incident PD cohorts compared to controls, with some describing deficits particularly in verbal memory [8]. Incidentally, vocabulary skills prior to dementia onset distinguished patients who developed dementia in mid-stage PD from those who did so later in the disease process [7].

The rate of cognitive decline in PD is modest in the short term but adds up over time [7]. The trajectory of cognitive decline in PD could be nonlinear, remaining relative stable followed by swift decline after around 13 years of onset [9]. In one study, 18.9 % of incident non-demented untreated PD patients already presented MCI [8], reaching around 26 % of all patients in non-demented prevalent cohorts [10]. The cognitive profile of these patients is varied, with the most frequent being episodic memory deficits (69 %), executive dysfunction (54 %), and language/praxis deficits (50 %) followed by visuospatial/constructional deficits (46 %) and attention/working memory (35 %) deficits [10, 11]. Unsurprisingly, PD patients with MCI are more likely to progress to dementia than cognitively intact PD patients, although a substantial proportion (20 %) revert back to normal [12]. Furthermore, even subtler deficits may be associated with future decline. The concept of subjective cognitive impairment (SCI) – a patient report of cognitive impairment with no significant deficits in formal neuropsychological testing – can also be applied to PD: in one study, patients with the same baseline cognitive performance with and without PD-SCI were followed for 2.5 years. Patients with SCI were more likely to convert to MCI and showed more rapid decline in semantic fluency and visuospatial memory [13]. However, larger studies with longer follow-up are needed to confirm this finding and define the SCI patients who are more likely to present future decline.

Less information exists on the prevalence of DLB, with widely ranging estimates from 0 to 24 % [14]. Underdiagnosis seems to be a widespread problem: whereas DLB is responsible for 4.2 % of all dementias in community-based studies and 7.5 % in clinic-based studies, studies that perform a thorough neurological examination and use the established consensus criteria find that as many as 10–22 % of all dementia cases can be attributable to DLB [15, 16]. As with PDD, there may be a predementia phase in DLB, but identifying patients in this stage is hampered by the lack of criteria for predementia DLB.

20.3 Pathology

The Lewy body (LB), an alpha-synuclein aggregate, is the core pathological marker in both disorders, present in limbic and cortical areas [17–19]. It is unclear whether PDD and LBD present different pathological patterns, although there might be differences in the amount of cortical LB or their distribution [17–20]. Both present with somewhat less cortical atrophy than AD, with abnormal medial temporal lobe structures but less hippocampal atrophy than in AD. The type of pathology and its localization could determine phenotype in both conditions: LB in limbic areas have been linked to earlier onset of hallucinations, while limbic and cortical LB have been associated with visual misperceptions and misidentifications [21].

Amyloid (Aβ) plaques are often found in association to LB and have generally been reported to be higher in DLB than in PDD [18, 22]. It has been suggested that Aβ load might hasten the cognitive decline in DLB relative to PDD [23, 24]. In one study, amyloid burden measured by PiB PET was highest in DLB – where higher amyloid correlated with worse cognition – followed by PDD [23]. Amyloid showed no correlation with motor parkinsonian symptoms. Both

DLB and PDD had significantly higher amyloid than PD. Although less frequent than in AD, neurofibrillary tangles may also be present, influencing the cognitive phenotype in DLB. Indeed, an association between tangle pathology and hallucinations has been described [25].

20.4 Clinical Characteristics

20.4.1 Prodromal Symptoms

Despite their prevalence, the dementias associated with Lewy body pathology present a diagnostic challenge, especially in the early disease stages. The presence of a previous diagnosis of PD may facilitate matters in PDD, but the fluctuating nature of symptoms and overlap with AD complicate matters in DLB. Progressively, prodromal symptoms are being recognized, and the clinician should ask about a previous history of olfactory loss, autonomic dysfunction, and mood and sleep disorders, i.e., REM behavioral disorder (RBD), which can precede memory loss by 1.2–9.3 years [26].

Mild cognitive impairment (MCI) represented a conceptual revolution in AD and served to define a group of patients for early disease characterization and interventional strategies. In PD, cohorts of patients with MCI (PD-MCI) and subjective cognitive complaints (PD-SCI) are progressively being recognized [27]. The search for the DLB-MCI equivalent is underway. Non-demented cases of incidental DLB at autopsy have been examined for symptoms retrospectively, and olfactory dysfunction is a frequent finding [28]. Different types of patients have been proposed to fit this definition, including non-demented patients with autonomic denervation or occipital hypometabolism [26] (see below for a discussion on prodromal DLB).

20.5 Cognitive Profile

The cognitive profile of PDD and DLB includes impaired executive and visuospatial functioning, together with deficits in motivation and attention. Memory deficits are frequent, although deterioration in episodic memory is less pronounced than in AD [29]. Attention deficit and fluctuations in attention are more marked than in AD. PDD and DLB share a similar cognitive profile, although differences exist with some studies finding more pronounced executive dysfunction in DLB than in PD-D [30, 31] or more pronounced auditory attentional disturbances in PDD [32]. It is also likely that different cognitive profiles exist within these cohorts, something that has already been demonstrated in PD and PDD groups [2, 3].

20.6 Visual Disturbances, Hallucinations, and Delusions

A range of visual symptoms can be present, including defects in eye movement, pupillary function, and complex visual functions [33]. Indeed, the occipital cortex is one of the first affected areas in DLB, and visual processing defects might be early markers. Saccadic eye movements are affected to a similar degree in both PDD and DLB and are impaired compared to patients with AD, PD, and controls [34]. Impairment in complex visual function is characteristic of DLB and includes difficulties with object size estimation, identifying overlapping figures, and drawing [33]. The trail-making test, in which the patient is asked to connect dots or numbers, or drawing the Rey-Osterrieth complex figure might reveal some of these difficulties.

Visual hallucinations and delusions are frequent, occurring in around 60–70 % of DLB and PDD cases [35]. Visual hallucinations can be detailed and recurrent, often unpleasant, of short duration, appearing centrally in the visual field and often static, with people or animals being common themes [36]. Although rarer, auditory hallucinations may also be present. Visual hallucinations may also be present in other dementias, but hallucinations within 5 years of dementia onset are suggestive of LBD [21]. Apathy, sleep disturbances, and anxiety are often associated. Compared to DLB, PDD patients may experience more anxiety in relationship to their hallucinations [36]. In one study, patients with DLB with hallucinations were older and had greater deficits in visual attention and executive function, with slightly worse global cognition than patients with the same diagnosis but without hallucinations [37].

Hallucinations may closely be linked to delusions: the themes for these are varied, but delusions of infidelity, theft, and misidentification are frequent. This last term groups a number of delusions characterized by disturbances in recognition or familiarity, which are hypothesized to arise from failures in visual recognition coupled with deficient "fact checking," probably due to frontal lobe dysfunction [38]. The visual processing defects and dysexecutive neuropsychological profile of DLB and PDD make them a fertile ground for delusional misidentification, which can include Capgras syndrome (in which the patient claims that a relative has been substituted by an impostor) and phantom child – or grandchild – syndrome (in which the patient believes in imaginary children or grandchildren, who often "inhabit" the patient's home), among others. One study found delusional misidentification in 16.7 % of PDD patients: patients with delusional misidentification had the same global cognitive function, executive function, and visuospatial abilities as PDD patients without misidentification but demonstrated worse recall in the Rey Auditory Verbal Learning Test (RAVLT), worse performance in tests of semantic fluency, and accompanying visual hallucinations were present in all cases [39].

20.7 Fluctuations in Alertness, Attention, and Cognitive Performance

Fluctuating cognition, particularly attention, is a core feature of DLB but also appears in other neurodegenerative processes such as AD. The first prerequisite of cognitive performance is wakefulness or alertness, with the second being attention. Thus, cognitive fluctuations in LBD have been attributed to one or both of the above [1]. As with other cognitive symptoms, fluctuations are also present in AD albeit with different characteristics. In DLB, fluctuations are more frequent and severe, with greater variance between best and worst performance, and are typically spontaneous, periodic, and transient [40]. This compares to fluctuations in AD, which are typically related to a particular episode of memory failure and can last for longer periods involving one or more days [40]. The spontaneous nature of onset and remission and the absence of identifiable environmental triggers suggest that fluctuations in LBD may be internally generated [40], but their origin remains unclear. In EEG, DLB patients display more variability in attentional and slow electrocortical measures than either AD or controls, and this variability correlates to fluctuation severity [41]. Blood-oxygen-level-dependent (BOLD) resting state network analysis has found an association between fluctuations and reduction in the right hemisphere functional connectivity in DLB patients[42]. The cholinergic system appears to be involved, with cholinergic and dopaminergic changes in thalamic areas [43]. This explanation has been proposed for the improvement in fluctuations and attention observed with cholinesterase inhibitors [44, 45].

The clinical evaluation of fluctuations is complex and often relies on caretaker interviews. The Clinician Assessment of Fluctuation (CAF) is a short scale meant to be administered by a clinician to an informant and, another scale, the Fluctuation Inventory (FI) can also be useful [46]. Changes in choice reaction time (CRT) or in other cognitive tests can also be illustrative [46]. At times, the fluctuations are evident: in an early description of DLB, one patient experienced over 50 % fluctuation in MMSE scores, while another went from mute and unable to stand to capable of sustaining a conversation [47]. In a recent study, DLB patients were assessed for attention using a bedside digit span and for alertness using the Maintenance of Wakefulness Test (MWT) [48], with PD patients without dementia as controls. Compared to the PD patients, DLB patients presented greater differences in best and worse digit span performance, betraying fluctuations in attention, without changes in alertness as measured by the MWT [48]. This supports the use of digit span in the bedside examination of DLB, particularly considering that it is a quick and accessible test.

Fluctuations are also present in some patients with PDD. PDD patients with fluctuations present a cognitive profile with prominent attention and initiation/perseveration dysfunction, making them more similar to DLB patients than PDD patients without fluctuations [49]. Furthermore, patients with PDD with fluctuations and patients with DLB present a similar incidence of visual hallucinations, higher than that observed in nonfluctuating PDD and AD patients [49].

20.8 Depression

Depression is present in 35–50 % of cases [35, 50] and presents worse prognosis [51, 52, 53]. Depression as well as other neuropsychiatric symptoms are more frequent and severe among PD patients with cognitive impairment, Parkinson's disease dementia, and dementia with Lewy bodies [51, 53] and more frequent and severe in DLB than in AD [51].

Of note, depression is usually underdiagnosed and often undertreated in PD patients [54, 55], and this problem likely increases with higher age and in those with dementia.

There are several antidepressant trials in PD, but these have usually excluded people with dementia or substantial cognitive impairment, and thus the positive findings may not generalize to PDD. There is no systematic evidence regarding treatment of depression in DLB. Apathy, characterized by reduced initiative and motivation, is also more frequent than in AD and is often incapacitating and difficult to treat.

20.9 Other Symptoms

Rapid eye movement (REM) sleep behavior disorder (RBD) is another frequent characteristic. This parasomnia is characterized by vivid, frightening dreams accompanied by simple or complex motor behavior and vocalizations while asleep and can lead to injury of the patient or bed partner [56]. RBD can be an early clinical marker of damage to the nigrostriatal pathway: in one cohort, 81 % of patients presenting with RBD eventually presenting with a parkinsonian disorder or dementia [57]. RBD, together with olfactory dysfunction, dysautonomia, and mood disorders seem to precede Lewy body pathology, occur in up to 90 % of cases, and could help identify prodromal cohorts [26].

20.10 Parkinsonism

Most DLB patients develop parkinsonism sooner or later in the disease process. Motor symptoms seem to be less severe than those present in PDD but comparable to PD patients without dementia [58]. However, the progression of motor symptoms seems comparable in PDD and DLB [59]. Symptoms that are not mediated by dopaminergic deficit, such as postural instability and gait, are more severe in DLB patients than in PDD, whereas tremor is more important in PDD [58], where symptoms are also more symmetric [60]. Interestingly, PD patients with prominent gait and postural instability at baseline have a higher dementia risk with follow-up compared to tremor-dominant phenotypes [61].

20.11 Neuroimaging and Other Ancillary Testing

Structural MRI in DLB shows a relatively preserved hippocampus and temporal lobe compared to AD patients, although mild hippocampal atrophy may be present [62, 63]. Unfortunately, there is considerable overlap between AD and DLB, which makes these findings rather unspecific. One study found rates of brain atrophy of 1.4 % for DLB, compared to 0.5–0.7 % for controls and 2.0 % for AD. However, although rates of atrophy differed significantly between controls and dementia, a statistically significant difference was not found between the dementia types [64]. Multivariate MRI protocols might prove more discriminative. A recent study employed a sparse partial least squares (SPLS) classification of cortical thickness and found a pattern of thinning in mid-anterior temporal, occipital, and subgenual cingulate cortex for AD and dorsal cingulate, posterior temporal, and lateral orbitofrontal for

DLB with sensitivity of 78 % and a specificity of 75 % for distinguishing between the two [65].

Diffusion tensor imaging may show increased diffusion and decreased fractional anisotropy (FA) in corpus callosum and pericallosal areas compared to controls and reduced FA in precuneus compared to AD or controls [62], but this is unlikely to be of great use to the clinician evaluating an individual diagnosis. Of greater use are SPECT and PET showing decreased glucose metabolism and perfusion in parietal and occipital areas in DLB, although these regions are also affected in AD [62]. Since severe nigrostriatal dopaminergic degeneration occurs in DLB, brain imaging with ligands that bind dopamine transporter (DAT) are of particular relevance. In this line, SPECT with 123-I-2beta-carbometoxy-3beta-(4-iodophenyl)-N(3-fluoropropyl) nortropane ((123)I-FP-CIT) which binds to DAT has a 77.7 % sensitivity for detecting clinical probable DLB, with 90.4 % specificity for excluding non-DLB dementia [66]. This evaluation was performed blinded for clinical data: in the context of compatible symptoms, low DAT uptake in the basal ganglia as demonstrated by SPECT or PET is highly suggestive of DLB or PDD [66] and should be considered as part of the diagnostic process. However, DAT binding does not distinguish between DLB and PD patients [62]. Amyloid imaging by Pittsburgh compound B (PiB) can be pathological in PDD and DLB, although it is more common and severe in the latter [24, 67].

Thoracic SPECT using 123-I metaiodobenzylguanidine (MIBG) – a marker of postganglionic cardiac sympathetic innervation – shows reduced uptake in DLB and PD and is independent from disease duration and autonomic failure. In one study, all patients with DLB showed decreased MIGB uptake and all patients with AD showed preserved uptake, making this technique uniquely discriminative between the two conditions [68].

20.12 Other Biomarkers

As is already the case with AD, CSF biomarkers in DLB could help define research cohorts and aid clinicians in diagnostically complicated cases. Several such markers have been proposed, with alpha-synuclein being the most logical candidate. Lower CSF alpha-synuclein levels have been observed in patients with synucleinopathies and may be caused by lower levels of neurosin, a cleaving enzyme [69]. In this way, slower degradation would lead to accumulation of insoluble alpha-synuclein. A recent meta-analysis on the published studies dealing with CSF alpha-synuclein found lower mean CSF concentrations in patients with DLB compared to AD, with no difference between DLB and PD, or other neurodegenerative conditions such as multiple systems atrophy (MSA), progressive supranuclear palsy (PSP), frontotemporal dementia (FTD), or vascular dementia [69]. Additionally, no differences were found between mean CSF alpha-synuclein between DLB and controls, although a nonsignificant trend was observed (−0.12 95 % CI −0.29–0.04 $p = 0.13$) [69]. When results were grouped into synucleinopathies and non-synucleinopathies, mean alpha-synuclein CSF was significantly lower in DLB than in non-synucleinopathies, with no difference between DLB and other synucleinopathies. The studies analyzed varied greatly in methodology, with enormous variations in difference means between and within studies [69]. These findings are interesting and warrant future examination, but technical issues around assessment method remain unresolved and cut points are yet to be determined.

A clinician is more likely to have access to CSF amyloid-beta and tau results from dementia work-up from memory clinics where these measures are progressively becoming routine. Alone, these biomarkers cannot distinguish LBD from AD, but they can add interesting information. On average, levels of amyloid-beta in LBD are lower than in PD or controls but not as low as in AD [70, 71]. The relation with cognition is complex, with one study supporting a correlation between AD-like CSF profile with MMSE [72] in DLB but not in PD, while others find that baseline amyloid-beta in PD patients with and without dementia can predict the rate of cognitive decline [73].

Other possible biomarkers such as CSF uric acid [74], transthyretin [74], plasma epidermal growth factor [75], or other species of alpha-synuclein such as oligomeric or phosphorylated forms are receiving progressive attention [76, 77].

20.13 Genetics

Molecular genetic studies suggest an overlap in the genetic causes of AD, PD, PDD, and DLB, and some argue for placing all these diseases in the same continuum [78]. Cohorts of sporadic DLB present mutations associated with the above disorders, such as alpha-synuclein (SNCA)-associated with PD and amyloid precursor protein gene (APP), presenilin 1 gene (PSEN1), and presenilin 2 gene (PSEN2) related to AD [78]. Although most cases of DLB are sporadic, there is clustering of dementia in families with DLB [79]. A number of families have been identified with Mendelian inheritance of DLB, most frequently in an autosomal dominant fashion. These mutations have been described in SNCA, 2p13, and SNCB (beta-synuclein), although in most the mutation was not identified [78]. The first genome-wide linkage study mapped a chromosomal locus for DLB in 2q35-q36 [80], but the mutation associated to this pedigree seems more complex than a simple monogenic disorder [81].

The glucocerebrosidase gene (GBA) may confer some genetic susceptibility, with individuals with parkinsonism presenting heterozygous GBA variants more frequently than controls, while DLBs have a higher mutation rate than PD [82]. Additionally, GBA mutation status is associated with the presence of cortical LBs and the absence of AD-type pathology [82]. Apolipoprotein E (APOE) ε4 is a risk factor for AD and is overrepresented in DLB cohorts [83]. Recently, another allele APO ε 2 has been associated with reduced risk for DLB and later age of onset [84]. The ApoE4 allele may be an independent risk factor for the development of dementia in PD, but its significance is still unclear [85].

At present, routine genetic testing of all patients with PDD or DLB is not warranted, but patients with early-onset parkinsonism or familial occurrence of parkinsonism and dementia deserve further study. Within these families, a range of phenotypes can occur, with some individuals developing only parkinsonism or only cognitive decline. SNCA encodes the alpha-synuclein protein, so mutations in this gene are one possible cause, although they probably account for only a small fraction of all familial cases [4]. Mutations in A53T, A30P, and E46K can cause symptoms ranging from early-onset L-dopa-responsive parkinsonism, early- or late-onset dementia, cortical Lewy body pathology, hypoventilation, postural hypotension, bladder incontinence, and myoclonus [4]. Alterations in the leucine-rich kinase 2 (LRRK2) gene account for 8 % of late-onset PD cases and usually occur without cognitive decline [86]. Paradoxically, they can be associated with DLB cortical pathology [4].

20.14 Treatment

Unfortunately, at the present moment there are no disease-modifying strategies for these dementias, and few large randomized controlled trials have been conducted among DLB [87]. Cholinesterase inhibitors are useful, with rivastigmine having demonstrated improvement in attentional performance and neuropsychiatric symptoms in DLB [44], with an effect comparable to that found in AD [88]. In a placebo-controlled trial with a mean dose of 7 mg of rivastigmine, 63 % of treated DLB patients achieved a 30 % improvement in the Neuropsychiatric Inventory (NPI) scale [44]. Donepezil at doses of 3, 5, or 10 mg has shown a dose-dependent improvement in attention and MMSE, with improvement in neuropsychiatric symptoms as assessed by NPI [89]. Galantamine might also benefit DLB patients, as was shown in an open-label trial with 42 patients [90]. Similar evidence exists for the effect of cholinesterase inhibitors in PDD: rivastigmine has shown improvement in MMSE, attention, and executive function [91], and donepezil might also be effective [92]. An open-label randomized trial with galantamine at a maximum dose of 16 mg/day found benefit of global cognition and neuropsychiatric symptoms [93]. Another open-label trial with galantamine showed improvement in global mental symptoms, hallucinations, and parkinsonism but mild worsening tremor [94]. There are no studies directly comparing the magnitude of benefit between cholinesterase inhibitors and between PDD and DLB, but the magnitude of benefit appears comparable between studies [87]. In both conditions, withdrawal of cholinesterase inhibitors may be poorly tolerated [95].

Additionally, the N-methyl D-aspartate (NMDA) receptor antagonist memantine has also been proposed to target the glutamatergic dysfunction described in LBD. One randomized study suffered from high attrition but showed a benefit in the clinical global impression of change scale with memantine relative to placebo, as well as MMSE [96]. In the 30-week extension of this trial, significant recurrence of symptoms and global deterioration was observed upon withdrawal of memantine in the treatment group [97]. Another study also examining memantine in PDD and DLB found a benefit with memantine in clinical global impression and NPI scales but only in the DLB group [98]. Additionally, memantine decreases symptoms of RBD in both PDD and DLB patients [99].

DLB patients can suffer from severe neuroleptic sensitivity, which includes extrapyramidal features, confusion, autonomic instability, falls, and death [100]. Neuroleptic sensitivity is common to diseases with Lewy body pathology, occurring in 53 % of DLB, 39 % of PDD, and 27 % of PD [101]. However, DLB and PDD patients also present psychotic symptoms that might benefit from neuroleptic treatment. There are few studies on antipsychotic medication in these patients. In one, quetiapine was not more effective than placebo in treating psychosis [102]. Clozapine is an option, and severe neuroleptic sensitivity occurs rarely with clozapine [103, 104], although the risk of agranulocytosis limits its use. For this reason, antipsychotic treatment should be reserved to severe symptoms that cannot be managed otherwise. A novel treatment for psychosis in PD is pimavanserin, a selective serotonin 5-HT2A inverse agonist without dopaminergic, adrenergic, histaminergic, or muscarinic affinity [105]. One double-blind randomized placebo-controlled trial with 40 mg/day of pimavanserin showed efficacy in treating psychotic symptoms in PD, without exacerbation of motor disability [105].

Levodopa may be useful in DLB, although to a lesser extent than in PDD or PD [106, 107]. The drug is well tolerated, although gastrointestinal problems, confusion, sleep disturbances, and hallucinations can occur [106]. However, neuropsychiatric symptoms in PDD did not worsen with L-Dopa [107], and in a study examining sleep disturbances and circadian rhythm inversion in DLB L-Dopa seemed to have no ill effect [108]. Others have described increased psychosis risk with L-Dopa in DLB [109]. In conclusion, despite a potential risk for worsening of cognition and psychiatric symptoms, L-Dopa is a valid option for clinically significant parkinsonian motor symptoms in DLB.

There are very few treatment studies of antidepressants in DLB and PDD, but clinical evidence suggest that depression may respond to conventional treatments. In some cases with severe and treatment-resistant depression, electroconvulsive therapy may be effective and well tolerated in DLB [110]. Delusional misidentification may respond to cholinesterase inhibitors or atypical neuroleptics [39], and cholinesterase inhibitors can improve cognitive fluctuations [44, 98].

The classical treatment for RBD includes modifying the sleep environment to prevent injury [111]. Traditionally, low doses of clonazepam before bedtime or melatonin have been recommended, although improvement with drugs such as pramipexole, donepezil, levodopa, carbamazepine have also been reported [56]. However, both benzodiazepines and dopamine agonists should be used with caution in patients with dementia, and there are questions about the efficacy of L-Dopa and dopamine agonists, with some studies suggesting that these drugs might actually induce or exacerbate RBD [111]. A randomized trial with memantine has been shown to reduce the occurrence of RBD [99]. For this reason, cholinesterase inhibitors and memantine may be the logical choice in patients with RBD and concomitant synucleinopathy [99, 111].

Table 20.1 Treatment options and levels of evidence for DLB and PDD

Treatment	Benefit	Risks	Level of evidence	Dosage used in previous studies
ChEIs	Improvement in cognition, behavior, activities of daily living	Donepezil may be better tolerated than rivastigmine. Tremor more frequent in treated patients	I (Cochrane meta-analysis) [87]	Rivastigmine: 7 mg/day
				Donepezil: 3, 5 or 10 mg/day
				Galantamine 3–16 mg/day)
Memantine	MMSE, CGIC, RBD	Well tolerated	II (several RCT) [96, 98, 99]	10 mg/12 h
Levodopa	Motor symptoms	May increase psychotic symptoms	II and III [107, 109]	Titration to patient needs

ChEIs cholinesterase inhibitors, *MMSE* Mini-Mental State Examination, *CGIC* Clinician Global Impression of Change, *RBD* REM behavioral disorder, *RCT* randomized controlled trial

20.15 Prognosis

Compared to AD, patients with PDD and DLB present with reduced survival [112–116]. Studies comparing DLB and AD usually find worse survival in DLB [112, 113], even after adjusting for cognitive level [114]. Overlapping syndromes fare even worse, with patients diagnosed with DLB or PDD who present AD pathology at autopsy demonstrated reduced survival relative to those with purer LB presentation [117]. Likewise, patients diagnosed with AD who have some Lewy body pathology also have worse disease course [118]. DLB in its turn could be more lethal than PDD [117], which itself presents higher mortality than PD or controls [119]. In a recent study examining mortality risk in SveDem, the Swedish dementia registry, patients with DLB and PDD presented higher mortality risk relative to AD, with HR of 1.64 (95% CI (1.39–1.95) for DLB and 1.47 (95% CI 1.17–1.84) for PDD [120]. In another study, autonomic dysfunction presenting as orthostatic hypotension had poorer prognosis, which was worsened if constipation and urinary incontinence were also present [121].

The rate of cognitive decline seems similar in DLB and AD [122]. One study compared the rate of functional decline, a statistically significant difference was not found between in AD and DLB [123], while another study by the same authors did find greater decline in DLB participants but only in subjects under 81 years of age [124]. Another study found greater risk for DLB relative to AD for hospitalization, institutionalization, and death but not differences in cognitive decline [113] (Table 20.1).

Conclusions

The Lewy body dementias are frequent causes of cognitive decline, but underdiagnosis is a widespread problem. The arbitrary distinction between PDD and DLB and overlapping syndromes with other dementias (particularly AD) complicate matters for the clinician. However, the clinical picture in these dementias is distinctive, and diagnosis can be made confidently, particularly when suggestive symptoms are accompanied by a DAT SCAN revealing nigrostriatal dopamine dysfunction. Despite the absence of disease-modifying treatment strategies, cholinesterase inhibitors have shown efficacy for treating cognitive and neuropsychiatric symptoms, and a range of pharmacological and adjuvant strategies are available. Functional prognosis and mortality is worse in DLB and PDD than in AD, although the rate of cognitive decline appears similar.

References

1. McKeith IG, Dickson DW, Lowe J, Emre M, O'Brien JT, Feldman H, Cummings J, Duda JE, Lippa C, Perry EK, Aarsland D, Arai H, Ballard CG, Boeve B, Burn DJ, Costa D, Del Ser T, Dubois B, Galasko D, Gauthier S, Goetz CG, Gomez-Tortosa E, Halliday G, Hansen LA, Hardy J, Iwatsubo T,

Kalaria RN, Kaufer D, Kenny RA, Korczyn A, Kosaka K, Lee VM, Lees A, Litvan I, Londos E, Lopez OL, Minoshima S, Mizuno Y, Molina JA, Mukaetova-Ladinska EB, Pasquier F, Perry RH, Schulz JB, Trojanowski JQ, Yamada M. Diagnosis and management of dementia with Lewy bodies: third report of the DLB consortium. Neurology. 2005;65:1863–72.
2. Janvin CC, Larsen JP, Aarsland D, Hugdahl K. Subtypes of mild cognitive impairment in Parkinson's disease: progression to dementia. Mov Disord. 2006;21:1343–9.
3. Foltynie T, Brayne CE, Robbins TW, Barker RA. The cognitive ability of an incident cohort of Parkinson's patients in the UK. The campaign study. Brain: J Neurol. 2004;127:550–60.
4. Kurz MW, Schlitter AM, Larsen JP, Ballard C, Aarsland D. Familial occurrence of dementia and parkinsonism: a systematic review. Dement Geriatr Cogn Disord. 2006;22:288–95.
5. Aarsland D, Zaccai J, Brayne C. A systematic review of prevalence studies of dementia in Parkinson's disease. Mov Disord. 2005;20:1255–63.
6. Williams-Gray CH, Mason SL, Evans JR, Foltynie T, Brayne C, Robbins TW, Barker RA. The campaign study of Parkinson's disease: 10-year outlook in an incident population-based cohort. J Neurol Neurosurg Psychiatry. 2013;84:1258–64.
7. Reid WG, Hely MA, Morris JG, Loy C, Halliday GM. Dementia in Parkinson's disease: a 20-year neuropsychological study (Sydney multicentre study). J Neurol Neurosurg Psychiatry. 2011;82:1033–7.
8. Aarsland D, Bronnick K, Larsen JP, Tysnes OB, Alves G. Cognitive impairment in incident, untreated Parkinson disease: the Norwegian parkwest study. Neurology. 2009;72:1121–6.
9. Aarsland D, Muniz G, Matthews F. Nonlinear decline of mini-mental state examination in Parkinson's disease. Mov Disord. 2011;26:334–7.
10. Aarsland D, Bronnick K, Williams-Gray C, Weintraub D, Marder K, Kulisevsky J, Burn D, Barone P, Pagonabarraga J, Allcock L, Santangelo G, Foltynie T, Janvin C, Larsen JP, Barker RA, Emre M. Mild cognitive impairment in Parkinson disease: a multicenter pooled analysis. Neurology. 2010;75:1062–9.
11. Pfeiffer HC, Lokkegaard A, Zoetmulder M, Friberg L, Werdelin L. Cognitive impairment in early-stage non-demented Parkinson's disease patients. Acta Neurol Scand. 2013;129(5):307–18.
12. Pedersen KF, Larsen JP, Tysnes OB, Alves G. Prognosis of mild cognitive impairment in early Parkinson disease: the Norwegian parkwest study. JAMA Neurol. 2013;70:580–6.
13. Hong JY, Sunwoo MK, Chung SJ, Ham JH, Lee JE, Sohn YH, Lee PH. Subjective cognitive decline predicts future deterioration in cognitively normal patients with Parkinson's disease. Neurobiol Aging. 2013;35(7):1739–43.
14. Vann Jones SA, O'Brien JT. The prevalence and incidence of dementia with Lewy bodies: a systematic review of population and clinical studies – erratum. Psychol Med. 2014;44:684.
15. Stevens T, Livingston G, Kitchen G, Manela M, Walker Z, Katona C. Islington study of dementia subtypes in the community. Br J Psychiatr: J Ment Sci. 2002;180:270–6.
16. Rahkonen T, Eloniemi-Sulkava U, Rissanen S, Vatanen A, Viramo P, Sulkava R. Dementia with Lewy bodies according to the consensus criteria in a general population aged 75 years or older. J Neurol Neurosurg Psychiatry. 2003;74:720–4.
17. Aarsland D, Perry R, Brown A, Larsen JP, Ballard C. Neuropathology of dementia in Parkinson's disease: a prospective, community-based study. Ann Neurol. 2005;58:773–6.
18. Harding AJ, Halliday GM. Cortical Lewy body pathology in the diagnosis of dementia. Acta Neuropathol. 2001;102:355–63.
19. Tsuboi Y, Dickson DW. Dementia with Lewy bodies and Parkinson's disease with dementia: are they different? Parkinsonism Relat Disord. 2005;11 Suppl 1:S47–51.
20. Harding AJ, Broe GA, Halliday GM. Visual hallucinations in Lewy body disease relate to Lewy bodies in the temporal lobe. Brain: J Neurol. 2002;125:391–403.
21. Ferman TJ, Arvanitakis Z, Fujishiro H, Duara R, Parfitt F, Purdy M, Waters C, Barker W, Graff-Radford NR, Dickson DW. Pathology and temporal onset of visual hallucinations, misperceptions and family misidentification distinguishes dementia with Lewy bodies from Alzheimer's disease. Parkinsonism Relat Disord. 2013;19:227–31.
22. Edison P, Rowe CC, Rinne JO, Ng S, Ahmed I, Kemppainen N, Villemagne VL, O'Keefe G, Nagren K, Chaudhury KR, Masters CL, Brooks DJ. Amyloid load in Parkinson's disease dementia and Lewy body dementia measured with [11c]pib positron emission tomography. J Neurol Neurosurg Psychiatry. 2008;79:1331–8.
23. Gomperts SN, Locascio JJ, Marquie M, Santarlasci AL, Rentz DM, Maye J, Johnson KA, Growdon JH. Brain amyloid and cognition in Lewy body diseases. Mov Disord. 2012;27:965–73.
24. Gomperts SN, Rentz DM, Moran E, Becker JA, Locascio JJ, Klunk WE, Mathis CA, Elmaleh DR, Shoup T, Fischman AJ, Hyman BT, Growdon JH, Johnson KA. Imaging amyloid deposition in Lewy body diseases. Neurology. 2008;71:903–10.
25. Ballard CG, Jacoby R, Del Ser T, Khan MN, Munoz DG, Holmes C, Nagy Z, Perry EK, Joachim C, Jaros E, O'Brien JT, Perry RH, McKeith IG. Neuropathological substrates of psychiatric symptoms in prospectively studied patients with autopsy-confirmed dementia with Lewy bodies. Am J Psychiatry. 2004;161:843–9.
26. Fujishiro H, Iseki E, Nakamura S, Kasanuki K, Chiba Y, Ota K, Murayama N, Sato K. Dementia with Lewy bodies: early diagnostic challenges. Psychogeriatrics. 2013;13:128–38.

27. Litvan I, Goldman JG, Troster AI, Schmand BA, Weintraub D, Petersen RC, Mollenhauer B, Adler CH, Marder K, Williams-Gray CH, Aarsland D, Kulisevsky J, Rodriguez-Oroz MC, Burn DJ, Barker RA, Emre M. Diagnostic criteria for mild cognitive impairment in Parkinson's disease: movement disorder society task force guidelines. Mov Disord. 2012;27:349–56.
28. Adler CH, Connor DJ, Hentz JG, Sabbagh MN, Caviness JN, Shill HA, Noble B, Beach TG. Incidental Lewy body disease: clinical comparison to a control cohort. Mov Disord. 2010;25:642–6.
29. Emre M. Dementia associated with Parkinson's disease. Lancet Neurol. 2003;2:229–37.
30. Downes JJ, Priestley NM, Doran M, Ferran J, Ghadiali E, Cooper P. Intellectual, mnemonic, and frontal functions in dementia with Lewy bodies: a comparison with early and advanced Parkinson's disease. Behav Neurol. 1998;11:173–83.
31. Aarsland D, Litvan I, Salmon D, Galasko D, Wentzel-Larsen T, Larsen JP. Performance on the dementia rating scale in Parkinson's disease with dementia and dementia with Lewy bodies: comparison with progressive supranuclear palsy and Alzheimer's disease. J Neurol Neurosurg Psychiatry. 2003;74:1215–20.
32. Bronnick KS, Nordby H, Larsen JP, Aarsland D. Disturbance of automatic auditory change detection in dementia associated with Parkinson's disease: a mismatch negativity study. Neurobiol Aging. 2010;31:104–13.
33. Armstrong RA. Visual signs and symptoms of dementia with Lewy bodies. Clin Exp Optom. 2012;95:621–30.
34. Mosimann UP, Muri RM, Burn DJ, Felblinger J, O'Brien JT, McKeith IG. Saccadic eye movement changes in Parkinson's disease dementia and dementia with Lewy bodies. Brain: J Neurol. 2005;128:1267–76.
35. Klatka LA, Louis ED, Schiffer RB. Psychiatric features in diffuse Lewy body disease: a clinicopathologic study using Alzheimer's disease and Parkinson's disease comparison groups. Neurology. 1996;47:1148–52.
36. Mosimann UP, Rowan EN, Partington CE, Collerton D, Littlewood E, O'Brien JT, Burn DJ, McKeith IG. Characteristics of visual hallucinations in Parkinson disease dementia and dementia with Lewy bodies. Am J Geriatr Psychiatr: Off J Am Assoc Geriatr Psychiatr. 2006;14:153–60.
37. Cagnin A, Gnoato F, Jelcic N, Favaretto S, Zarantonello G, Ermani M, Dam M. Clinical and cognitive correlates of visual hallucinations in dementia with Lewy bodies. J Neurol Neurosurg Psychiatry. 2013;84:505–10.
38. Devinsky O. Delusional misidentifications and duplications: right brain lesions, left brain delusions. Neurology. 2009;72:80–7.
39. Pagonabarraga J, Llebaria G, Garcia-Sanchez C, Pascual-Sedano B, Gironell A, Kulisevsky J. A prospective study of delusional misidentification syndromes in Parkinson's disease with dementia. Mov Disord. 2008;23:443–8.
40. Bradshaw J, Saling M, Hopwood M, Anderson V, Brodtmann A. Fluctuating cognition in dementia with Lewy bodies and Alzheimer's disease is qualitatively distinct. J Neurol Neurosurg Psychiatry. 2004;75:382–7.
41. Walker MP, Ayre GA, Perry EK, Wesnes K, McKeith IG, Tovee M, Edwardson JA, Ballard CG. Quantification and characterization of fluctuating cognition in dementia with Lewy bodies and Alzheimer's disease. Dement Geriatr Cogn Disord. 2000;11:327–35.
42. Franciotti R, Falasca NW, Bonanni L, Anzellotti F, Maruotti V, Comani S, Thomas A, Tartaro A, Taylor JP, Onofrj M. Default network is not hypoactive in dementia with fluctuating cognition: an Alzheimer disease/dementia with Lewy bodies comparison. Neurobiol Aging. 2013;34:1148–58.
43. Pimlott SL, Piggott M, Ballard C, McKeith I, Perry R, Kometa S, Owens J, Wyper D, Perry E. Thalamic nicotinic receptors implicated in disturbed consciousness in dementia with Lewy bodies. Neurobiol Dis. 2006;21:50–6.
44. McKeith I, Del Ser T, Spano P, Emre M, Wesnes K, Anand R, Cicin-Sain A, Ferrara R, Spiegel R. Efficacy of rivastigmine in dementia with Lewy bodies: a randomised, double-blind, placebo-controlled international study. Lancet. 2000;356:2031–6.
45. Ikeda M, Mori E, Kosaka K, Iseki E, Hashimoto M, Matsukawa N, Matsuo K, Nakagawa M. Long-term safety and efficacy of donepezil in patients with dementia with Lewy bodies: results from a 52-week, open-label, multicenter extension study. Dement Geriatr Cogn Disord. 2013;36:229–41.
46. Walker MP, Ayre GA, Cummings JL, Wesnes K, McKeith IG, O'Brien JT, Ballard CG. Quantifying fluctuation in dementia with Lewy bodies, Alzheimer's disease, and vascular dementia. Neurology. 2000;54:1616–25.
47. Byrne EJ, Lowe J, Godwin-Austen RB, Arie T, Jones R. Dementia and Parkinson's disease associated with diffuse cortical Lewy bodies. Lancet. 1987;1:501.
48. Bliwise DL, Scullin MK, Trotti LM. Fluctuations in cognition and alertness vary independently in dementia with Lewy bodies. Mov Disord. 2014;29:83–9.
49. Varanese S, Perfetti B, Monaco D, Thomas A, Bonanni L, Tiraboschi P, Onofrj M. Fluctuating cognition and different cognitive and behavioural profiles in Parkinson's disease with dementia: comparison of dementia with Lewy bodies and Alzheimer's disease. J Neurol. 2010;257:1004–11.
50. Yamane Y, Sakai K, Maeda K. Dementia with Lewy bodies is associated with higher scores on the geriatric depression scale than is Alzheimer's disease. Psychogeriatrics. 2011;11:157–65.
51. Fritze F, Ehrt U, Hortobagyi T, Ballard C, Aarsland D. Depressive symptoms in Alzheimer's disease and Lewy body dementia: a one-year follow-up study. Dement Geriatr Cogn Disord. 2011;32:143–9.

52. Aarsland D, Bronnick K, Alves G, Tysnes OB, Pedersen KF, Ehrt U, Larsen JP. The spectrum of neuropsychiatric symptoms in patients with early untreated Parkinson's disease. J Neurol Neurosurg Psychiatry. 2009;80:928–30.
53. Monastero R, Di Fiore P, Ventimiglia GD, Camarda R, Camarda C. The neuropsychiatric profile of Parkinson's disease subjects with and without mild cognitive impairment. J Neural Transm. 2013;120:607–11.
54. Weintraub D, Moberg PJ, Duda JE, Katz IR, Stern MB. Recognition and treatment of depression in Parkinson's disease. J Geriatr Psychiatry Neurol. 2003;16:178–83.
55. Dobkin RD, Rubino JT, Friedman J, Allen LA, Gara MA, Menza M. Barriers to mental health care utilization in Parkinson's disease. J Geriatr Psychiatry Neurol. 2013;26:105–16.
56. Boeve BF, Silber MH, Ferman TJ. REM sleep behavior disorder in Parkinson's disease and dementia with Lewy bodies. J Geriatr Psychiatry Neurol. 2004;17:146–57.
57. Schenck CH, Boeve BF, Mahowald MW. Delayed emergence of a parkinsonian disorder or dementia in 81% of older men initially diagnosed with idiopathic rapid eye movement sleep behavior disorder: a 16-year update on a previously reported series. Sleep Med. 2013;14:744–8.
58. Burn DJ, Rowan EN, Minett T, Sanders J, Myint P, Richardson J, Thomas A, Newby J, Reid J, O'Brien JT, McKeith IG. Extrapyramidal features in Parkinson's disease with and without dementia and dementia with Lewy bodies: a cross-sectional comparative study. Mov Disord. 2003;18:884–9.
59. Ballard C, O'Brien J, Swann A, Neill D, Lantos P, Holmes C, Burn D, Ince P, Perry R, McKeith I. One year follow-up of parkinsonism in dementia with Lewy bodies. Dement Geriatr Cogn Disord. 2000;11:219–22.
60. Gnanalingham KK, Byrne EJ, Thornton A, Sambrook MA, Bannister P. Motor and cognitive function in Lewy body dementia: comparison with Alzheimer's and Parkinson's diseases. J Neurol Neurosurg Psychiatry. 1997;62:243–52.
61. Alves G, Larsen JP, Emre M, Wentzel-Larsen T, Aarsland D. Changes in motor subtype and risk for incident dementia in Parkinson's disease. Mov Disord. 2006;21:1123–30.
62. Hanagasi HA, Bilgic B, Emre M. Neuroimaging, biomarkers, and management of dementia with Lewy bodies. Front Neurol. 2013;4:151.
63. Kantarci K, Ferman TJ, Boeve BF, Weigand SD, Przybelski S, Vemuri P, Murray ME, Senjem ML, Smith GE, Knopman DS, Petersen RC, Jack Jr CR, Parisi JE, Dickson DW. Focal atrophy on MRI and neuropathologic classification of dementia with Lewy bodies. Neurology. 2012;79:553–60.
64. O'Brien JT, Paling S, Barber R, Williams ED, Ballard C, McKeith IG, Gholkar A, Crum WR, Rossor MN, Fox NC. Progressive brain atrophy on serial MRI in dementia with Lewy bodies, ad, and vascular dementia. Neurology. 2001;56:1386–8.
65. Lebedev AV, Westman E, Beyer MK, Kramberger MG, Aguilar C, Pirtosek Z, Aarsland D. Multivariate classification of patients with Alzheimer's and dementia with Lewy bodies using high-dimensional cortical thickness measurements: an MRI surface-based morphometric study. J Neurol. 2013;260:1104–15.
66. McKeith I, O'Brien J, Walker Z, Tatsch K, Booij J, Darcourt J, Padovani A, Giubbini R, Bonuccelli U, Volterrani D, Holmes C, Kemp P, Tabet N, Meyer I, Reininger C. Sensitivity and specificity of dopamine transporter imaging with 123i-fp-cit spect in dementia with Lewy bodies: a phase III, multicentre study. Lancet Neurol. 2007;6:305–13.
67. Maetzler W, Liepelt I, Reimold M, Reischl G, Solbach C, Becker C, Schulte C, Leyhe T, Keller S, Melms A, Gasser T, Berg D. Cortical PIB binding in Lewy body disease is associated with Alzheimer-like characteristics. Neurobiol Dis. 2009;34:107–12.
68. Yoshita M, Taki J, Yamada M. A clinical role for [(123)i]mibg myocardial scintigraphy in the distinction between dementia of the Alzheimer's-type and dementia with Lewy bodies. J Neurol Neurosurg Psychiatry. 2001;71:583–8.
69. Lim X, Yeo JM, Green A, Pal S. The diagnostic utility of cerebrospinal fluid alpha-synuclein analysis in dementia with Lewy bodies – a systematic review and meta-analysis. Parkinsonism Relat Disord. 2013;19:851–8.
70. Mollenhauer B, Locascio JJ, Schulz-Schaeffer W, Sixel-Doring F, Trenkwalder C, Schlossmacher MG. Alpha-synuclein and tau concentrations in cerebrospinal fluid of patients presenting with parkinsonism: a cohort study. Lancet Neurol. 2011;10:230–40.
71. Parnetti L, Tiraboschi P, Lanari A, Peducci M, Padiglioni C, D'Amore C, Pierguidi L, Tambasco N, Rossi A, Calabresi P. Cerebrospinal fluid biomarkers in Parkinson's disease with dementia and dementia with Lewy bodies. Biol Psychiatry. 2008;64:850–5.
72. Andersson M, Zetterberg H, Minthon L, Blennow K, Londos E. The cognitive profile and CSF biomarkers in dementia with Lewy bodies and Parkinson's disease dementia. Int J Geriatr Psychiatr. 2011;26:100–5.
73. Siderowf A, Xie SX, Hurtig H, Weintraub D, Duda J, Chen-Plotkin A, Shaw LM, Van Deerlin V, Trojanowski JQ, Clark C. Csf amyloid {beta} 1-42 predicts cognitive decline in Parkinson disease. Neurology. 2010;75:1055–61.
74. Maetzler W, Stapf AK, Schulte C, Hauser AK, Lerche S, Wurster I, Schleicher E, Melms A, Berg D. Serum and cerebrospinal fluid uric acid levels in Lewy body disorders: associations with disease occurrence and amyloid-beta pathway. J Alzheimers Dis. 2011;27:119–26.
75. Chen-Plotkin AS, Hu WT, Siderowf A, Weintraub D, Goldmann Gross R, Hurtig HI, Xie SX, Arnold SE, Grossman M, Clark CM, Shaw LM, McCluskey

L, Elman L, Van Deerlin VM, Lee VM, Soares H, Trojanowski JQ. Plasma epidermal growth factor levels predict cognitive decline in Parkinson disease. Ann Neurol. 2011;69:655–63.
76. Paleologou KE, Kragh CL, Mann DM, Salem SA, Al-Shami R, Allsop D, Hassan AH, Jensen PH, El-Agnaf OM. Detection of elevated levels of soluble alpha-synuclein oligomers in post-mortem brain extracts from patients with dementia with Lewy bodies. Brain: J Neurol. 2009;132:1093–101.
77. Tokuda T, Qureshi MM, Ardah MT, Varghese S, Shehab SA, Kasai T, Ishigami N, Tamaoka A, Nakagawa M, El-Agnaf OM. Detection of elevated levels of alpha-synuclein oligomers in csf from patients with Parkinson disease. Neurology. 2010;75:1766–72.
78. Meeus B, Theuns J, Van Broeckhoven C. The genetics of dementia with Lewy bodies: what are we missing? Arch Neurol. 2012;69:1113–8.
79. Nervi A, Reitz C, Tang MX, Santana V, Piriz A, Reyes D, Lantigua R, Medrano M, Jimenez-Velazquez IZ, Lee JH, Mayeux R. Familial aggregation of dementia with Lewy bodies. Arch Neurol. 2011;68:90–3.
80. Bogaerts V, Engelborghs S, Kumar-Singh S, Goossens D, Pickut B, van der Zee J, Sleegers K, Peeters K, Martin JJ, Del-Favero J, Gasser T, Dickson DW, Wszolek ZK, De Deyn PP, Theuns J, Van Broeckhoven C. A novel locus for dementia with Lewy bodies: a clinically and genetically heterogeneous disorder. Brain: J Neurol. 2007;130:2277–91.
81. Meeus B, Nuytemans K, Crosiers D, Engelborghs S, Peeters K, Mattheijssens M, Elinck E, Corsmit E, De Deyn PP, Van Broeckhoven C, Theuns J. Comprehensive genetic and mutation analysis of familial dementia with Lewy bodies linked to 2q35-q36. J Alzheimers Dis. 2010;20:197–205.
82. Clark LN, Kartsaklis LA, Wolf Gilbert R, Dorado B, Ross BM, Kisselev S, Verbitsky M, Mejia-Santana H, Cote LJ, Andrews H, Vonsattel JP, Fahn S, Mayeux R, Honig LS, Marder K. Association of glucocerebrosidase mutations with dementia with Lewy bodies. Arch Neurol. 2009;66:578–83.
83. Kobayashi S, Tateno M, Park TW, Utsumi K, Sohma H, Ito YM, Kokai Y, Saito T. Apolipoprotein e4 frequencies in a japanese population with Alzheimer's disease and dementia with Lewy bodies. PLoS One. 2011;6:e18569.
84. Berge G, Sando SB, Rongve A, Aarsland D, White LR. Apolipoprotein e {varepsilon}2 genotype delays onset of dementia with Lewy bodies in a norwegian cohort. J Neurol Neurosurg Psychiatry. 2014;85(11):1227–31.
85. Parsian A, Racette B, Goldsmith LJ, Perlmutter JS. Parkinson's disease and apolipoprotein e: possible association with dementia but not age at onset. Genomics. 2002;79:458–61.
86. Paisan-Ruiz C, Jain S, Evans EW, Gilks WP, Simon J, van der Brug M, Lopez de Munain A, Aparicio S, Gil AM, Khan N, Johnson J, Martinez JR, Nicholl D, Carrera IM, Pena AS, de Silva R, Lees A, Marti-Masso JF, Perez-Tur J, Wood NW, Singleton AB. Cloning of the gene containing mutations that cause park8-linked Parkinson's disease. Neuron. 2004;44:595–600.
87. Rolinski M, Fox C, Maidment I, McShane R. Cholinesterase inhibitors for dementia with lewy bodies, parkinson's disease dementia and cognitive impairment in parkinson's disease. Cochrane Database Syst Rev 2012;(3):CD006504.
88. Rozzini L, Chilovi BV, Bertoletti E, Conti M, Delrio I, Trabucchi M, Padovani A. Cognitive and psychopathologic response to rivastigmine in dementia with Lewy bodies compared to Alzheimer's disease: a case control study. Am J Alzheimers Dis Other Dement. 2007;22:42–7.
89. Mori E, Ikeda M, Kosaka K. Donepezil for dementia with Lewy bodies: a randomized, placebo-controlled trial. Ann Neurol. 2012;72:41–52.
90. Edwards K, Royall D, Hershey L, Lichter D, Hake A, Farlow M, Pasquier F, Johnson S. Efficacy and safety of galantamine in patients with dementia with Lewy bodies: a 24-week open-label study. Dement Geriatr Cogn Disord. 2007;23:401–5.
91. Emre M, Aarsland D, Albanese A, Byrne EJ, Deuschl G, De Deyn PP, Durif F, Kulisevsky J, van Laar T, Lees A, Poewe W, Robillard A, Rosa MM, Wolters E, Quarg P, Tekin S, Lane R. Rivastigmine for dementia associated with Parkinson's disease. N Engl J Med. 2004;351:2509–18.
92. Dubois B, Tolosa E, Katzenschlager R, Emre M, Lees AJ, Schumann G, Pourcher E, Gray J, Thomas G, Swartz J, Hsu T, Moline ML. Donepezil in Parkinson's disease dementia: a randomized, double-blind efficacy and safety study. Mov Disord. 2012;27:1230–8.
93. Litvinenko IV, Odinak MM, Mogil'naya VI, Emelin AY. Efficacy and safety of galantamine (Reminyl) for dementia in patients with Parkinson's disease (an open controlled trial). Neurosci Behav Physiol. 2008;38:937–45.
94. Aarsland D, Hutchinson M, Larsen JP. Cognitive, psychiatric and motor response to galantamine in Parkinson's disease with dementia. Int J Geriatr Psychiatr. 2003;18:937–41.
95. Minett TS, Thomas A, Wilkinson LM, Daniel SL, Sanders J, Richardson J, Littlewood E, Myint P, Newby J, McKeith IG. What happens when donepezil is suddenly withdrawn? An open label trial in dementia with Lewy bodies and Parkinson's disease with dementia. Int J Geriatr Psychiatr. 2003;18:988–93.
96. Aarsland D, Ballard C, Walker Z, Bostrom F, Alves G, Kossakowski K, Leroi I, Pozo-Rodriguez F, Minthon L, Londos E. Memantine in patients with Parkinson's disease dementia or dementia with Lewy bodies: a double-blind, placebo-controlled, multicentre trial. Lancet Neurol. 2009;8:613–8.
97. Johansson C, Ballard C, Hansson O, Palmqvist S, Minthon L, Aarsland D, Londos E. Efficacy of

memantine in PDD and DLB: an extension study including washout and open-label treatment. Int J Geriatr Psychiatr. 2011;26:206–13.
98. Emre M, Tsolaki M, Bonuccelli U, Destee A, Tolosa E, Kutzelnigg A, Ceballos-Baumann A, Zdravkovic S, Bladstrom A, Jones R. Memantine for patients with Parkinson's disease dementia or dementia with Lewy bodies: a randomised, double-blind, placebo-controlled trial. Lancet Neurol. 2010;9:969–77.
99. Larsson V, Aarsland D, Ballard C, Minthon L, Londos E. The effect of memantine on sleep behaviour in dementia with Lewy bodies and Parkinson's disease dementia. Int J Geriatr Psychiatr. 2010;25:1030–8.
100. McKeith I, Fairbairn A, Perry R, Thompson P, Perry E. Neuroleptic sensitivity in patients with senile dementia of Lewy body type. BMJ. 1992;305:673–8.
101. Aarsland D, Perry R, Larsen JP, McKeith IG, O'Brien JT, Perry EK, Burn D, Ballard CG. Neuroleptic sensitivity in Parkinson's disease and parkinsonian dementias. J Clin Psychiatry. 2005;66:633–7.
102. Kurlan R, Cummings J, Raman R, Thal L. Quetiapine for agitation or psychosis in patients with dementia and parkinsonism. Neurology. 2007;68:1356–63.
103. Ballard C, Grace J, McKeith I, Holmes C. Neuroleptic sensitivity in dementia with Lewy bodies and Alzheimer's disease. Lancet. 1998;351:1032–3.
104. Sadek J, Rockwood K. Coma with accidental single dose of an atypical neuroleptic in a patient with Lewy body dementia. Am J Geriatr Psychiatr: Off J Am Assoc Geriatr Psychiatr. 2003;11:112–3.
105. Cummings J, Isaacson S, Mills R, Williams H, Chi-Burris K, Corbett A, Dhall R, Ballard C. Pimavanserin for patients with Parkinson's disease psychosis: a randomised, placebo-controlled phase 3 trial. Lancet. 2014;383:533–40.
106. Molloy S, McKeith IG, O'Brien JT, Burn DJ. The role of levodopa in the management of dementia with Lewy bodies. J Neurol Neurosurg Psychiatry. 2005;76:1200–3.
107. Molloy SA, Rowan EN, O'Brien JT, McKeith IG, Wesnes K, Burn DJ. Effect of levodopa on cognitive function in Parkinson's disease with and without dementia and dementia with Lewy bodies. J Neurol Neurosurg Psychiatry. 2006;77:1323–8.
108. Molloy S, Minett T, O'Brien JT, McKeith IG, Burn DJ. Levodopa use and sleep in patients with dementia with Lewy bodies. Mov Disord. 2009;24:609–12.
109. Goldman JG, Goetz CG, Brandabur M, Sanfilippo M, Stebbins GT. Effects of dopaminergic medications on psychosis and motor function in dementia with Lewy bodies. Mov Disord. 2008;23:2248–50.
110. Takahashi S, Mizukami K, Yasuno F, Asada T. Depression associated with dementia with Lewy bodies (DLB) and the effect of somatotherapy. Psychogeriatrics. 2009;9:56–61.
111. Aurora RN, Zak RS, Maganti RK, Auerbach SH, Casey KR, Chowdhuri S, Karippot A, Ramar K, Kristo DA, Morgenthaler TI. Best practice guide for the treatment of REM sleep behavior disorder (RBDd). J Clin Sleep Med. 2010;6:85–95.
112. Magierski R, Kloszewska I, Sobow TM. The influence of vascular risk factors on the survival rate of patients with dementia with Lewy bodies and Alzheimer disease. Neurol Neurochir Pol. 2010;44:139–47.
113. Hanyu H, Sato T, Hirao K, Kanetaka H, Sakurai H, Iwamoto T. Differences in clinical course between dementia with Lewy bodies and Alzheimer's disease. Eur J Neurol. 2009;16:212–7.
114. Stubendorff K, Hansson O, Minthon L, Londos E. Differences in survival between patients with dementia with Lewy bodies and patients with Alzheimer's disease – measured from a fixed cognitive level. Dement Geriatr Cogn Disord. 2011;32:408–16.
115. Walker Z, Allen RL, Shergill S, Mullan E, Katona CL. Three years survival in patients with a clinical diagnosis of dementia with Lewy bodies. Int J Geriatr Psychiatr. 2000;15:267–73.
116. Lonnroos E, Kyyronen P, Bell JS, van der Cammen TJ, Hartikainen S. Risk of death among persons with Alzheimer's disease: a national register-based nested case-control study. J Alzheimers Dis. 2013;33:157–64.
117. Jellinger KA, Wenning GK, Seppi K. Predictors of survival in dementia with Lewy bodies and Parkinson dementia. Neurodegener Dis. 2007;4:428–30.
118. Olichney JM, Galasko D, Salmon DP, Hofstetter CR, Hansen LA, Katzman R, Thal LJ. Cognitive decline is faster in Lewy body variant than in Alzheimer's disease. Neurology. 1998;51:351–7.
119. de Lau LM, Schipper CM, Hofman A, Koudstaal PJ, Breteler MM. Prognosis of Parkinson disease: risk of dementia and mortality: the Rotterdam study. Arch Neurol. 2005;62:1265–9.
120. Garcia-Ptacek SF, Kåreholt B, Cuadrado I, Religa ML, Eriksdotter M. Mortality risk after dementia diagnosis by dementia type and underlying factors: a cohort of 15209 patients based on the Swedish dementia registry. J Alzheimers Dis. 2014;41(2):467–77.
121. Stubendorff K, Aarsland D, Minthon L, Londos E. The impact of autonomic dysfunction on survival in patients with dementia with Lewy bodies and Parkinson's disease with dementia. PLoS One. 2012;7:e45451.
122. Helmes E, Bowler JV, Merskey H, Munoz DG, Hachinski VC. Rates of cognitive decline in Alzheimer's disease and dementia with Lewy bodies. Dement Geriatr Cogn Disord. 2003;15:67–71.
123. Gill DP, Hubbard RA, Koepsell TD, Borrie MJ, Petrella RJ, Knopman DS, Kukull WA. Differences in rate of functional decline across three dementia types. Alzheimers Dement. 2013;9:S63–71.
124. Gill DP, Koepsell TD, Hubbard RA, Kukull WA. Risk of decline in functional activities in dementia with Lewy bodies and Alzheimer disease. Alzheimer Dis Assoc Disord. 2011;25:17–23.

Toxic-Induced Parkinsonism

21

Pille Taba

Abbreviations

$CaNa_2EDTA$	Calcium salt of ethylenediamine-tetraacetic acid
MDMA	Methylenedioxymethamphetamine
MPTP	1-methyl-4-phenyl-1,2,5,6-tetrahydropyridine
MRI	Magnetic resonance imaging
PET	Positron emission tomography
SPECT	Single-photon emission computed tomography

21.1 Introduction

A large number of neurotoxins have been linked with secondary parkinsonism including metals, organic solvents and illicit drugs (Table 21.1). Manganese was the first substance linked with parkinsonism [1], but the precise cause of its toxicity remains undetermined. An outbreak of 1-methyl-4-phenyl-1,2,5,6-tetrahydropyridine (MPTP) parkinsonism caused by preparation of a designer drug MPPP in California provided several clues to the possible pathogenesis of Parkinson's disease and the development of a non-human primate animal model for drug testing [2]. Improved public health measures designed to prevent exposure to neurotoxins is the most important need as apart from chelation therapy or the promotion of excretion of the toxin by haemodialysis, no efficacious symptomatic treatments are available.

21.2 Metals

21.2.1 Manganese and Manganism

Manganese (Mn) is an essential trace metal in tissues of the body, but its excessive exposure may lead to a toxic syndrome called manganism, first described by John Couper in 1837 in workers inhaling manganese oxide in an ore-grinding plant. He described a distinctive gait disturbance with facial immobility, profuse hypersalivation and slurred speech.

Further reports have added to the clinical description, and it is now recognised that symmetrical hypokinesia with rigidity, a dystonic 'cock walk', postural instability leading to falls often backwards and a characteristic mixed dysarthria are common features. Mild cognitive and neurobehavioural disorders (locura manganica) may also be present. Elevated blood manganese levels and basal ganglia hyperintensities on magnetic reso-

P. Taba, MD, PhD
Department of Neurology and Neurosurgery,
University of Tartu, Puusepa 8 – H452,
Tartu 51014, Estonia
e-mail: Pille.Taba@kliinikum.ee

C. Falup-Pecurariu et al. (eds.), *Movement Disorders Curricula*,
DOI 10.1007/978-3-7091-1628-9_21

Table 21.1 Toxins causing parkinsonism

Category	Toxin	Exposure	Clinical symptomatology
Metals	Manganese (Mn)	Welding, mining industry, smelting; drug abuse ('ephedrone encephalopathy'); total parenteral nutrition; acquired hepatocerebral degeneration; inherited hypermanganesaemia	Manganism: bradykinesia, rigidity, dystonic cock walk, postural instability, falls, mixed dysarthria, cognitive and behavioural disorders
			Cases of inherited hypermanganesaemia: polycytaemia additionally to manganism and hepatic cirrhosis
	Lead (Pb)	Industrial and domestic settings: paints, ointments, leaded petrol, etc.	Neuropathy, gingival lead line, ataxia, neurobehavioural deficits. A case: parkinsonism and dystonia
Illicit drugs	1-methyl-4-phenyl-1,2,5,6-tetrahydropyridine (MPTP)	Historically: drug abuse	Bradykinesia, rigidity; dyskinesias and on-off fluctuations as adverse effects to levodopa therapy
	'Ecstasy' (MDMA)	Drug abuse	Cases of parkinsonism: rigidity and bradykinesia, periodic asymmetric rest tremor
	Methcathinone (ephedrone)	Injected 'designer' drug containing methcathinone and manganese	Bradykinesia, rigidity, postural instability, backward falls, dysarthria, dystonias
	Cocaine	Drug abuse	Chorea; akathisia; tics; orofacial dyskinesias ('crack dancing'). Cases: neuroleptic malignant syndrome; parkinsonism
	Opioids	Inhaled heroin pyrolysate ('chasing the dragon'); meperidine (pethidine)	Cases of parkinsonism: hypokinesia, rigidity
Natural toxins	Kava-kava	Treatment of anxiety	Cases: parkinsonism, dystonias, choreoathetosis, liver damage
Organic solvents	Hydrocarbons: trichloroethylene, hexane, petroleum	Inhalation and dermal exposure in industrial settings (glues, resins manufacturing etc.)	Parkinsonism, speech disorder, polyneuropathy
	Carbon disulphide (CS_2)	Inhalation in rubber and viscose rayon plant workers	Bradykinesia, rigidity, tremor, gait disorder, ataxia, peripheral neuropathy, psychiatric disorders
	Methanol	Inhalation of methanol vapours, dermal exposure, ingestion	Confusion, nausea, ataxia, vision impairment, delayed parkinsonism and dystonias
Other toxins	Carbon monoxide (CO)	Poisoning from parked and enclosed vehicle, kitchen stove, leaky heater	Parkinsonism, chorea, dystonia, athetosis, tremor, cognitive impairment, behavioural disorder
	Cyanide	Ingestion, injection, inhalation	Parkinsonism, gait disorder, dystonias

nance imaging (MRI) T1 sequences indicate current exposure (Fig. 21.1). Sometimes the neurological handicap increases even after the cessation of exposure. Parkinsonism is not responsive to levodopa treatment, but chelation with the calcium salt of ethylenediaminetetraacetic acid ($CaNa_2EDTA$) has demonstrated a limited clinical benefit [3, 4].

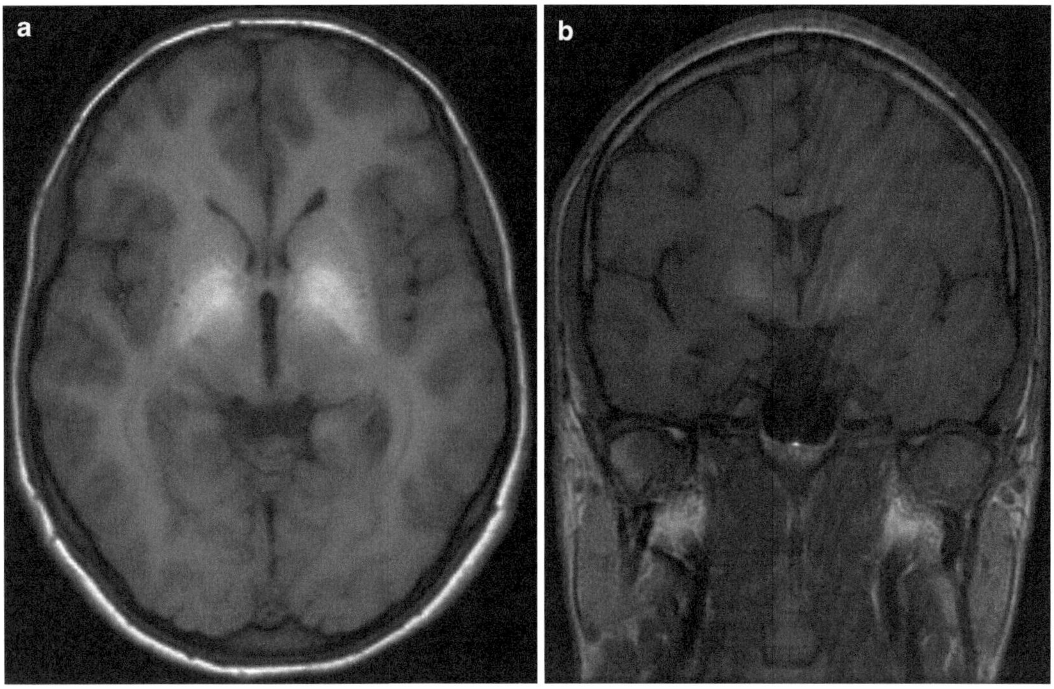

Fig. 21.1 Accumulation of manganese in basal ganglia, causing hyperintensities in T1-weighted sequences in MRI in an ephedrone (methcathinone) abuser

The commonest cause of manganese intoxication is occupational inhalational exposure, especially in the mining industry, ferromanganese smelting and welding [5, 6]. Chronic manganism has also been described in workers in the manufacture of steel and batteries, bactericidal agents and gasoline, in the water purification process and in non-occupational settings including long-term total parenteral nutrition or intoxication by ingestion, chronic renal failure undergoing maintenance haemodialysis and acute or chronic liver failure [7–12]. Despite a number of high profile legal cases in the USA, there is no conclusive evidence that Parkinson's disease occurs more frequently in welders [13, 14]. Chronic acquired hepatocerebral degeneration is a rare disorder characterised by parkinsonism, ataxia, myoclonus, cognitive disorder and accumulation of manganese in basal ganglia in association with hepatic cirrhosis [15, 16]. T1 hyperintensities on MRI suggestive of manganese accumulation have also rarely been reported in patients with chronic iron (Fe) deficiency as it increases gastric absorption of manganese [17].

21.2.2 Inherited Hypermanganesaemia

A rare autosomal recessive disorder affecting mainly children and characterised by hepatic cirrhosis, polycythaemia, a cock-walk gait and early-onset generalised dystonia, with T1 sequence MRI showing hyperintensities caused by manganese deposition, and increased serum manganese concentration and low ferritin, has recently been described. Whole-genome mapping of consanguineous families identified homozygous mutations in the SLC30A10 gene, on chromosome 1q41–q42 that encodes the manganese transporter protein. Early intervention with calcium disodium edetate chelation therapy and oral iron supplementation has been reported to be effective [18–20].

21.2.3 Manganese Overload in Drug Abusers ("Ephedrone Encephalopathy")

Manganese overload can occur following the injection of a 'designer' drug, containing an amphetamine analogue methcathinone (ephedrone) (known as Jeff, Mulka or Cat), synthesised from over-the-counter nasal decongestion remedies containing pseudoephedrine and mixed with potassium permanganate and vinegar. After several weeks of injecting the stimulant, a parkinsonian syndrome associated with postural instability and falls, severe dysarthria and prominent limb dystonia develops within few months of exposure. The biomarkers of manganese exposure, including high serum and hair manganese levels and symmetric hyperintensities of T1-weighted MRI, are present only in active abusers. The syndrome is irreversible, and further clinical deterioration may occur after cessation of exposure. Most of the cases in the literature have been reported from Russia, Estonia, Latvia, Georgia and Ukraine [21–24]. Potassium permanganate, used in the processing of coca-leaf extraction, has also been reported to cause manganese intoxication [25].

21.2.4 Other Metals Affecting Basal Ganglia

Mercury (Hg), bismuth (Bi), lead (Pb), thallium (Tl) and tin (Sn) also rarely damage the basal ganglia and have been associated with tremor, myoclonus, chorea and ataxia, accompanied by psychiatric symptoms – psychotic or behavioural disorders or depression [26–30]. In workers exposed to mercury, a single-photon emission computed tomography (SPECT) Dat Scan study showed a significant decrease of striatal uptake although there were no clear signs of parkinsonism [31]. A single case of parkinsonism, dystonia and frontal dysexecutive syndrome has been linked with bullet fragments in a hip joint that recovered after surgical excision and lead chelating therapy [32].

21.3 Illicit Drugs

21.3.1 1-methyl-4-phenyl-1,2,5,6-tetrahydropyridine (MPTP)

In the early 1980s, a subacute severe parkinsonian syndrome was described in a small number of Californian drug abusers, caused by MPTP, a by-product of the chemical synthesis of a meperidine analogue with potent heroin-like effects. Levodopa and dopamine agonists produced improvement, but typical side effects including dyskinesias and on-off fluctuations occurred very early. MPTP produces selective degeneration of nigral cells and reduction of dopaminergic function in the caudate and putamen as demonstrated by [^{18}F]fluorodopa PET. At autopsy, there was a severe neuronal loss in the substantia nigra, but no Lewy bodies. Research on the mechanism of toxicity of MPTP and the observation that selegiline could prevent MPTP-induced nigral toxicity led to the development of an effective experimental model for the testing of antiparkinsonian drugs [2, 33].

21.3.2 Psychostimulants: Amphetamine and Derivates

Amphetamine and related derivatives (methamphetamine, methylenedioxymethamphetamine MDMA (Ecstasy), methylphenidate, methcathinone, khat) are the most commonly abused drugs in this category. They can induce neurotoxicity in animal models and may lead to lasting chemical changes in the basal ganglia. Chorea, myoclonus and punding have been reported, and there are case reports of parkinsonism after the use of MDMA (Ecstasy) [34–36]. In methamphetamine and methcathinone abusers, a significant reduction of DAT density in caudate nucleus and putamen has been demonstrated with positron emission tomography (PET) [37]. Although it is probable that the neurotoxic effects in ephedrone users are due to manganese overload, it is possible that toxic effects directly related to methcathinone also contribute [22].

21.3.3 Cocaine

Chronic high-dose cocaine exposure can induce slow choreiform limb movements and orofacial dyskinesias, referred as 'crack dancing'. Neuroleptic malignant syndrome has rarely been described in the acute stage and parkinsonism following an abstinence. Cocaine is the most frequent drug of abuse associated with strokes, and extrapyramidal damage may occur in this context [38, 39]. A neuropathological study in chronic cocaine users demonstrated elevated α-synuclein levels in substantia nigra and tegmentum that may show a risk for degenerative changes in cocaine addicts [40].

21.3.4 Opioids

Heroin overdose leading to respiratory depression and brain anoxia-ischaemia may cause globus pallidus and cerebral border-zone infarction with symptoms of tremor and rigidity, myoclonus, dystonias, and ataxia. Inhaled heroin pyrolysate ('chasing the dragon') can cause a spongiform encephalopathy, characterised by ataxia, apathy and confusion. A bradykinetic syndrome may also occur during the recovery phase. Diffuse white matter hyperintensities have been reported on MRI, but also grey matter lesions of the basal ganglia have been demonstrated in cases with akinetic-rigid parkinsonism [39, 41]. Meperidine (pethidine) may cause tremor, myoclonus, delirium and hallucinations. A case of reversible parkinsonism related to meperidine administered during surgery has also been described [42].

21.4 Other Toxic Agents

21.4.1 Natural Toxins

Several plant concoctions used for religious ceremonial purposes and as recreational psychedelic drugs, including the peyote cactus (psilocybin) and angel trumpet flower, can cause chorea and dyskinesias. Cases with parkinsonism and dystonias as side effects of treatment with kava-kava have been described [43, 44].

21.4.2 Organic Solvents

Chronic inhalation and dermal exposure to trichloroethylene and hexane in factory workers, a long-term exposure to carbon disulfide (CS_2) in viscose rayon workers and an accidental ingestion of petroleum have all been linked with cases of parkinsonism [45–49]. Methanol intoxication can also cause parkinsonism, dystonias, confusion and vision impairment. Delayed neurotoxic effects of long-term exposure to methanol vapour in the laboratory have been described [50, 51].

21.4.3 Pesticides

The association between pesticides and parkinsonism is controversial, and despite a great deal of neuroepidemiological endeavour, the link between pesticide exposure and an increased risk of Parkinson's disease remains unproven. Organophosphates and organochlorines have rarely been linked with movement disorders [52–55].

21.4.4 Carbon Monoxide

Carbon monoxide (CO) poisoning may result in delayed onset parkinsonism accompanied by cognitive and behavioural disorder, chorea, dystonia, athetosis and tremor. A parkinsonian syndrome develops typically in one month after the exposure, and response to levodopa is poor, but the majority of patients recover spontaneously over 1 year [56, 57].

21.4.5 Cyanide

Poisoning of cyanide may result due to exposure through ingestion, injection or inhalation; potassium cyanide has been used in suicide attempts. The mortality rate in acute intoxication is 95 %, but in case of survival, parkinsonism with dystonias develops over a period of days, with a poor response to levodopa [58].

Conclusions

Neurotoxin-induced parkinsonism is relatively rare, and many of the cases present as emergencies. Early recognition is important as several complications may be reduced or prevented by early intervention, and improved public health measures may help to reduce the number of cases in the future.

References

1. Couper J. On the effects of black oxide of manganese when inhaled into the lungs. Br Ann Med Pharm. 1837;1:41–2.
2. Langston JW, Ballard P. Chronic parkinsonism in humans due to a product of meperidine-analog synthesis. Science. 1983;219:979–80.
3. Guilarte TR. Manganese neurotoxicity: new perspectives from behavioral, neuroimaging, and neuropathological studies in humans and non-human primates. Front Ageing Neurosci. 2013;5:23.
4. Taba P. Metals and movement disorders. Curr Opin Neurol. 2013;26:435–41.
5. Lucchini RG, Guazzetti S, Zoni S, Donna F, Peter S, Zacco A, Salmistraro M, Bontrmpi E, Zimmermann NJ, Smith DR. Tremor, olfactory and motor changes in Italian adolescents exposed to historical ferro-manganese emission. Neurotoxicology. 2012;33: 687–96.
6. Bowler RM, Gocheva V, Harris M, Ngo L, Abdelouahab N, Wilkinson J, Doty RL, Park R, Roels HA. Prospective study on neurotoxic effects in manganese-exposed bridge construction welders. Neurotoxicology. 2011;32:596–605.
7. Abdalian R, Saqui O, Fernandes G, Allard JP. Effects of manganese from a commercial multi-trace element supplement in a population sample of Canadian patients on long-term parenteral nutrition. JPEN J Parenter Enteral Nutr. 2013;37:410–5.
8. Sanchez B, Casalots-Casado J, Quintana S, Arroyo A, Martin-Fumado C, Galtes I. Fatal mangamese intoxication due to an error in the elaboration of Epsom salts for a liver cleansing diet. Forensic Sci Int. 2012;223:e1–4.
9. Bouchard M, Mergler D, Baldwin ME, Panisset M. Manganese cumulative exposure and symptoms: a follow-up study of alloy workers. Neurotoxicology. 2008;29:577–83.
10. Da Silva CJ, da Rocha AJ, Jeronymo S, Mendes MF, Milani FT, Maia ACM, Braga FT, Sens YAS, Miorin LA. A preliminary study revealing a new association in patients undergoing maintenance hemodialysis: manganism symptoms and T1 hyperintense changes in the basal ganglia. Am J Neuroradiol. 2007;28: 1474–9.
11. Aggarwal A, Vaidya S, Shah S, Singh J, Desai S, Bhatt M. Reversible parkinsonism and T1W pallidal hyperiontensities in acute liver failure. Mov Disord. 2006;21:1986–90.
12. Blumberg K, Walsh MP. Status report concerning the use of MMT in gasoline. International Council on Clean Transportation (ICCT), 2004.
13. Mortimer JA, Borenstein AR, Nelson LM. Associations of welding and manganese exposure with Parkinson's disease. Neurology. 2012;79:1174–80.
14. Racette BA, Criswell S, Lundin JI, Hobson A, Seixas N, Kotzbauer PT, Evanoff BA, Zhang J, Sheppard L, Checkoway H. Increased risk of parkinsonism associated with welding exposure. Neurotoxicology. 2012;33:1356–61.
15. Maffeo E, Montuschi A, Stura G, Giordana MT. Chronic acquired hepatocerebral degeneration, pallidal T1 MRI hyperintensity and manganese in a series of cirrhotic patients. Neurol Sci. 2013;34. doi:10.1007/s10072-013-1458-x.
16. Butterworth RF. Parkinsonism in cirrhosis: pathogenesis and current therapeutic options. Metab Brain Dis. 2013;28:261–7.
17. Herrero Hernandez E, Valentini MC, Discalzi G. T1 weighted hyperintensity in basal ganglia at brain magnetic resonance imaging: are different pathologies sharing a common mechanism? Neurotoxicology. 2002;23:669–74.
18. Tuschl K, Clayton PT, Gospe Jr SM, Gulab S, Ibrahim S, Singhi P, Aulakh R, Ribeiro RT, Barsottini OG, Zaki MS, Del Rosario ML, Dyack S, Price V, Rideout A, Gordon K, Wevers RA, Chong WKK, Milla PB. Syndrome of hepatic cirrhosis, dystonia, polycythemia, and hypermanganesemia caused by mutations in SLC30A10, a manganese transporter in man. Am J Hum Genet. 2012;90:457–66.
19. Quadri M, Federico A, Zhao T, Breedveld GJ, Battisti C, Delnooz C, Severijnen LA, Mammarella LDT, Mignarri A, Monti L, Sanna A, Lu P, Punzo F, Cossu G, Willemsen R, Rasi F, Oostra BA, van de Warrenburg BP, Bonifati V. Mutations in SLC30A10 cause parkinsonism and dystonia with hypermanganesemia, polycythemia, and chronic liver disease. Am J Hum Genet. 2012;90:467–77.
20. Ribeiro RT, Dos Santos-Neto D, Braga-Neto P, Barsottini OG. Inherited manganism. Clin Neurol Neurosurg. 2013;115:1536–8.
21. Levin OS. "Ephedrone" encephalopathy. Zh Nevrol Psikhiatr Im S S Korsakova. 2005;105:12–20.
22. Sikk K, Haldre S, Aquilonius SM, Asser A, Paris M, Roose Ä, Petterson J, Eriksson SL, Bergquist J, Taba P. Manganese-induced parkinsonism in methcathinone abusers: bio-markers of exposure and follow-up. Eur J Neurol. 2013;20:915–20.
23. Stepens A, Groma V, Skuja S, Platkajis A, Aldiņš P, Ekateina I, Martiņsone I, Bricis R, Donaghy M. The outcome of the movement disorder in methcathinone abusers: clinical, MRI and manganesemia changes, and neuropathology. Eur J Neurol. 2013;20. doi:10.1111/ene.12185.
24. Selikhova M, Fedoryshyn L, Matviyenko Y, Komnatska I, Kyrylchuk M, Krolicki L, Friedman A,

Taylor A, Jäger R, Lees A, Sanotsky Y. Parkinsonism and dystonia caused by the illicit use of ephedrone – a longitudinal study. Mov Disord. 2008;23:2224–31.
25. Ensing JG. Bazooka: cocaine-base and manganese carbonate. J Anal Toxicol. 1985;9:45–6.
26. Bernhoft RA. Mercury toxicity and treatment: a review of the literature. J Environ Publ Health. 2012;460508. doi:10.1155/2012/460508.
27. Silbernagel SM, Carpenter DO, Gilbert SG, Gochfeld M, Groth III E, Hightower JM, Schiavone M. Recognizing and preventing overexposure to methylmercury from fish and seafood consumption: information for physicians. J Toxicol. 2011;983072. doi:10.1155/983072.
28. Ovaska H, Wood DM, House I, Dargan PI, Jones AL, Murray S. Severe iatrogenic bismuth poisoning with bismuth iodoform paraffin paste treated with DMPS chelation. Clin Toxicol. 2008;46:855–7.
29. D'souza HS, Dsouza SA, Menezes G, Venkatesh T. Diagnosis, evaluation, and treatment of lead poisoning in general population. Ind J Clin Biochem. 2011;26:197–201.
30. Tsai YT, Huang CC, Kuo HC, Wang HM, Shen WS, Shih TS, Chu NS. Central nervous system effects in acute thallium poisoning. Neurotoxicology. 2006;27:291–5.
31. Lin CY, Liou SH, Hsiech CM, Ku MC, Tsai SY. Dose–response relationship between cumulative mercury exposure index and specific uptake ratio in the striatum on Tc-99m TRODAT SPECT. Clin Nucl Med. 2011;36:689–93.
32. Oomen JW, Smits BW, Swinkels DW, Schreurs BW, Bloem BR, Hedriks MP. A toxic shot from the hip. J Neurol Neurosurg Psychiatry. 2011;82:353–4.
33. Jackson-Lewis V, Ischiropoulos H, Przedborski S. Animal models in Parkinson's disease. Parkinsonism Relat Disord. 2012;18S1:S183–5.
34. Iacovelli L, Fulceri F, De Blasi A, Nicoletti F, Ruggieri S, Fornai F. The neurotoxicity of amphetamines: bridging drugs of abuse and neurodegenerative disorders. Exp Neurol. 2006;201:24–31.
35. Kuniyoshi SM, Jankovic J. MDMA and parkinsonism. N Engl J Med. 2003;349:96–7.
36. O'Suilleabhain P, Giller C. Rapidly progressive parkinsonism in a self- reported user of ecstasy and other drugs. Mov Disord. 2003;18:1378–403.
37. McCann UD, Wong DF, Yokoi F, et al. Reduced striatal dopamine transporte density in abstinent methamphetamine and methcathinone users: evidence from positron emission tomography studies with [^{11}C] WIN-35, 428. J Neurosci. 1998;18:8417–22.
38. Bauer LO. Psychomotor and electroencephalographic sequelae of cocaine dependence. In: D'Haenen H, den Boer JA, Willner P, editors. Biological psychiatry, NIDA Res Monogr, vol. 163. Chichester: Wiley; 1997. p. 66–93.
39. Büttner A. The neuropathology of drug abuse. Neuropathol Appl Neurobiol. 2011;37:118–34.
40. Mash DC, Ouyang Q, Pablo J, et al. Cocaine abusers have an overexpression of α-synuclein in dopamine neurons. J Neurosci. 2003;23:2564–71.
41. Heales S, Crawley F, Rudge P. Reversible parkinsonism following heroin pyrolysate inhalation is associated with tetrahydrobiopterin deficiency. Mov Disord. 2004;19:1248–51.
42. Lieberman AN, Goldstein M. Reversible parkinsonism related to meperidine. N Engl J Med 1985;312:509.
43. Forrester MB. Jimsonweed (Datura stramonium) exposures in Texas 1998–2004. J Toxicol Environ Health. 2006;69:1757–62.
44. Meseguer E, Taboada R, Sánchez V, Mena MA, Campos V, de Yebenes JG. Life-threatening parkinsonism induced by kava-kava. Mov Disord. 2002;17:195–6.
45. Lock EA, Zhang J, Checkoway H. Solvents and Parkinson disease: a systematic review of toxicological and epidemiological evidence. Toxicol Appl Pharmacol. 2013;266:345–55.
46. Gash DM, Rutland K, Hudson NL, et al. Trichloroethylene: Parkinsonism and complex 1 mitochondrial neurotoxicity. Ann Neurol. 2008;63:181–92.
47. Pezzoli G, Strada O, Silani V, Zecchinelli A, Perbellini L, Javoy-Agid F, Ghidoni P, Motti EDF, Masini T, Scarlato G, Agid Y, Hirsch EC. Clinical and pathological features in hydrocarbon-induced parkinsonism. Ann Neurol. 1996;40:922–5.
48. Huang CC, Yen TC, Shih TS, Chang HY, Chu NS. Dopamine transporter binding study in differentiating carbon disulfide induced parkinsonism from idiopathic parkinsonism. Neuro Toxicol. 2004;25:341–7.
49. Tetrud JW, Langston JW, Irwin I, Snow B. Parkinsonism caused by petroleum waste ingestion. Neurology. 1994;44:1051–4.
50. Franquet E, Salvadó-Figueres M, Lorenzo-Bosquet C, Cuberas-Borrós G, Rovira A, Castell-Conesa J, Hernandez-Vara J. Nigrostriatal pathway dysfunction in a methanol-induced delayed dystonia-parkinsonism. Mov Disord. 2012;27:1220–1.
51. Finkelstein Y, Vardi J. Progressive parkinsonism in a young experimental physicist following long-term exposure to methanol. Neurotoxicology. 2002;23:521–5.
52. Casida JE, Durkin KA. Neuroactive insecticides: targets, selectivity, resistance, and secondary effects. Annu Rev Entomol. 2013;58:99–117.
53. Moretto A, Colosio C. The role of pesticide exposure in the genesis of Parkinson's disease: epidemiological studies and experimental data. Toxicology. 2013;307:24–34.
54. Brent J, Schaeffer TH. Systematic review of parkinsonian syndromes in short- and long-term survivors of paraquat poisoning. J Occup Environ Med. 2011;53:1332–8.
55. Freire C, Koifman S. Pesticide exposure and Parkinson's disease: epidemiological evidence of association. Neurotoxicology. 2012;33:947–71.

56. Kao HW, Cho NY, Hsueh CJ, Chou MC, Chung HW, Liou M, Chiang SW, Chen SY, Juan CJ, Huang GS, Chen CY. Delayed parkinsonism after CO intoxication: evaluation of the substantia nigra with inversion-recovery MR imaging. Radiology. 2012;265: 215–21.
57. Chen NC, Lui CC, Huang SH, Huang CW, Lee CC, Chang WN, Chen CH, Lin YT, Chang CC. Pallidoreticular lesion in carbon monoxide intoxication by gradient echo: report of a case with parkinsonism features and review of the literature. Acta Neurol Taiwan. 2012;21:44–8.
58. Di Filippo M, Tambasco N, Muzi G, Balucani C, Saggese E, Parnetti L, Calabresi P, Rossi A. Parkinsonism and cognitive impairment following chronic exposure to potassium cyanide. Mov Disord. 2008;23:468–70.

22 Vascular Parkinsonism

Yacov Balash and Amos D. Korczyn

Abbreviations

BD	Binswanger's disease
BG	Basal ganglia
CSF	Cerebrospinal fluid
LBP	Lower body parkinsonism
MSA	Multiple system atrophy
NPH	Normal pressure hydrocephalus
PD	Parkinson's disease
PSP	Progressive supranuclear palsy
SN	Substantia nigra
SWEDD	Scan without evidence of dopaminergic deficit
TCS	Transcranial ultrasonography
VP	Vascular parkinsonism
WMLs	White matter lesions

22.1 Introduction

Elderly people frequently suffer from gait impairment and falls. There are many causes for these disorders; among which, lower body parkinsonism (LBP) is common. Clinical, pathological, and imaging data support a major contribution of vascular changes and particularly small vessel disease of the brain as the underlying process.

LBP is clinically different from idiopathic Parkinson's disease (PD) by not involving the face and upper limbs (or only minimally), not responding to levodopa, and being predominantly bilateral in onset. Many patients with LBP have, or develop, cognitive impairment and urinary incontinence. On the other hand, there is no involvement of autonomic, olfactory or sleep, as seen in PD.

The main imaging feature of this syndrome is the existence, on MRI, of extensive white matter lesions (WMLs). However, WMLs are not always associated with motor symptoms and may present with cognitive decline. The clinical syndrome of dementia associated with WMLs is attributed to Binswanger's disease (BD). In addition to cognitive impairment, however, patients with BD frequently have gait impairment as well as urinary incontinence. Thus, BD and LBP have strikingly overlapping clinical features, risk factors, and neuroimaging manifestations. Therefore, they could present different manifestations of the same pathology. Long-term follow-up studies of these two groups of patients may reveal the late development of a common phenotype, combining features of both gait disturbances and cognitive decline, but

Y. Balash, MD, PhD
Movement Disorders Unit, Department of Neurology, Tel-Aviv Sourasky Medical Center, Tel-Aviv, Israel

A.D. Korczyn, MD (✉)
Departments of Neurology, Physiology and Pharmacology, Sackler School of Medicine, Tel-Aviv University, Ramat-Aviv 69978, Israel
e-mail: amoskor@post.tau.ac.il

Received: September 18th, 2014.

C. Falup-Pecurariu et al. (eds.), *Movement Disorders Curricula*,
DOI 10.1007/978-3-7091-1628-9_22

so far prospective data are lacking. Although at present no therapy is available for LBP, strict control of vascular risk factors may prevent or slow down the deterioration. Several investigators have demonstrated clinical improvement following cerebrospinal fluid drainage, pointing at a similarity to normal pressure hydrocephalus (NPH), which has similar phenotype as LBP.

22.2 Historical Background

Throughout the twentieth century, the entity of PD underwent many changes. Essential tremor, multiple system atrophy, progressive supranuclear palsy, cortico-basal ganglionic degeneration, dementia-ALS-parkinsonism complex, and others have been defined as separate nosological entities, based on clinical, pathological, and drug response features. The umbrella term of PD today still covers several distinct "subtypes," including tremor predominant, akinetic-rigid, and others. It is not clear to what extent this latter subdivision reflects separate pathogenetic or pathologic processes. The etiology and pathogenesis of PD were actively looked for but still are largely unknown [1].

Progressive gait impairment of the elderly has attracted clinical attention for many years. Its etiology has been unknown, and because of the paucity of other symptoms, many such cases may be labeled as having "gait apraxia," although several other terms have also been used (Table 22.1).

This is the background against which the entity of vascular parkinsonism (VP) must be seen. The idea that parkinsonism can result from environmental causes was suggested forcefully by the appearance of extrapyramidal disorders related to the encephalitis lethargica epidemic in the second and third decades of the last century. At about the same period, the British neurologist MacDonald Critchley suggested that parkinsonian features could result from multiple vascular (arteriosclerotic or syphilitic) changes in the brain. However, he was cautious to indicate that this syndrome was dissimilar in many respects to what he considered idiopathic, or sporadic, PD [2], which was regarded as "abiotrophy." As described by Critchley, VP patients had primarily gait impairment, although more advanced cases had additional features (Table 22.2).

The concept of arteriosclerotic parkinsonism coined by Critchley did not gain popularity up to 1970–1980 as the relations between arteriosclerosis and PD were frequently denied, and superposition of vascular changes in some patients with PD was considered to be coincidental and not relevant to the clinical picture of nigral degeneration. So the number of papers quoting Critchley's work or using the term arteriosclerotic parkinsonism was small, compelling Critchley 52 years later to modify his basic idea of arteriosclerosis as a possible cause of PD, and rename the condition as "arteriosclerotic pseudoparkinsonism," that was considered alien to PD both clinically and pathogenetically [3]. This situation changed rather abruptly after David Marsden, another influential British neurologist, reiterated the idea of arteriosclerotic parkinsonism. Marsden and Thompson suggested that subcortical arteriosclerotic encephalopathy, or BD – then considered primarily a rare dementing disorder – was a prominent cause of gait disorder in the elderly, employing the term LBP [4]. Shortly thereafter, Jankovic et al. [5] used the term VP to describe a clinical phenotype with gait impairment as the leading feature, and stressing a vascular pathogenesis where the subcortical

Table 22.1 Gait disorders in the elderly

Gait apraxia
Senile gait
High-level gait disorder
Psychogenic gait
Fear of falling
Frontal lobe gait
Subcortical disequilibrium

Table 22.2 Vascular parkinsonism subtypes according to Critchley

A. Rigidity, masked face, short-stepped gait
B. Same + pseudobulbar manifestations
C. Same + dementia and incontinence
D. Same + pyramidal signs
E. Same + cerebellar signs

white matter is predominantly affected. Jankovic and colleagues referred to *lower body parkinsonism* and supported the vascular pathogenesis by demonstrating on MRI brain changes in patients with this clinical phenotype [6]. They made the important observation of a poor response to levodopa, although this was originally discussed by Parkes et al. [7].

Parkinsonian features can derive from a number of vascular lesions apart from WMLs, which in some cases may be focal. Hunter et al. [8] provided what may be the first pathological demonstration of stroke-induced parkinsonism, featuring a case of unilateral parkinsonism developed shortly after the occurrence of brain stem ischemia. Surprisingly, the nigral lesion in that case was *ipsilateral* to the hemiparkinsonism. Lazzarino et al. [9] described a case where unilateral parkinsonism followed a lacunar infarct in the contralateral substantia nigra. A recent publication by Harik et al. [10] described a patient with unilateral parkinsonism following a contralateral brain stem hemorrhagic stroke. Tolosa and Santamaria [11] described three cases where a parkinsonian syndrome developed subacutely and improved spontaneously. Brain CT demonstrated the existence of basal ganglia infarcts, and thus they concluded that these cases had "vascular parkinsonism," although none had a history of previous strokes, and long-tract signs were absent [11]. Similar findings were reported by Rieder Groswasser et al. [12] and by Ikeda et al. [13]. However, unlike the cases described by Marsden et al. [5] and by Jankovic et al. [6], these patients presented with unilateral disease while gait impairment was not prominent.

The occurrence of vascular lesions in the brains of PD patients may be coincidental, could be the main cause of the clinical manifestations or contribute to it. Single lacunes in the basal ganglia seem to be irrelevant to the clinical picture [14]. Bilateral basal ganglionic lesions are more likely to be manifested by parkinsonism [15], although it is possible that in these cases there was also coexistent white matter damage.

Nowadays, most cases where parkinsonism is thought to be due to vascular lesions are associated with white matter brain disease and/or lacunes [16].

22.3 Modern Concepts

At present, the term VP is used to describe the entity of elderly patients who have predominantly "lower body parkinsonism" manifested by lower limb bradykinesia, slow, short-stepped gait, which is gradually progressing until patients become wheelchair bound. These patients frequently go on to develop urinary incontinence, and many cases have brisk tendon reflexes in the lower limbs, extensor plantar responses, as well as cognitive decline. Parkinsonian features and pyramidal sings in the upper part of the body are minimal – the speech is relatively unimpaired; bradykinesia and hypokinesia are minimal if at all present in the upper limbs and tremor is typically not present [17].

The vascular risk factors responsible for VP include hypertension, dyslipidemia, diabetes, smoking, etc.; neuroimaging demonstrates damage to the deep white matter, seen either as hypodense lesions on brain CT or hyperintensities on T2 sequences on MRI. Although leucoaraiosis is not always due to vascular changes [18], the association with vascular risk factors supports a vascular etiology. The frequent coexistence of lacunes, mostly in the basal ganglia and thalamus, provides additional support for a vascular pathogenesis.

Thus VP is a variant of small vessel disease of the brain, directly or indirectly affecting the striatonigral system, which manifests neurologically with parkinsonian-like features, and accompanied by additional neurological signs [19].

VP has now entered into the last international classification of illnesses (ICD-10), as a form of secondary parkinsonism (item G21.4) [20].

22.4 Epidemiology

The prevalence of VP is estimated as 2–17.2 % of the total cases of parkinsonism in various population-based studies and clinic cohorts. Published data are heterogenous and may not be accurate because of lack of accepted criteria for clinical diagnosis of VP. Pathological verification was not carried out in most works; however,

Table 22.3 Prevalence of vascular parkinsonism

Author	Year	Prevalence	Criteria of diagnosis
Savica et al.	2013	11/542 (2.02 %)	Not indicated
Horvath et al.	2013	23/261 (8.8 %)	Pathology proved
Glass et al.	2012	28/1375 (2.03 %)	Pathology proved
Seijo-Martinez et al.	2011	7/41 (17.1 %)	Clinical criteria – two of the following: history of repeated strokes with an abrupt onset and stepwise progression of parkinsonism features, hypertension, pseudobulbar palsy, broad-based rigid gait, and widespread pyramidal signs. Information from brain MRI and/or CT studies
Munhoz et al.	2010	60/1528 (3.9 %)	Zijlmans' no agreed clinico-radiological criteria (2004)
Newman et al.	2009	11/64 (17.2 %)	Clinical criteria
The Rotterdam study, De Lau et al.	2004	5 % of 132	Not indicated

when it was performed, the results were significantly different from each other (Table 22.3). The landmark UK Brain Bank [21] data of 100 patients identified 76 cases in whom the diagnosis of PD was supported by the pathological identification of Lewy bodies. However, a quarter of them had in addition vascular changes, which could have contributed to the clinical manifestations. A restrictive definition, where VP would include only "pure" LBP, will give a lower figure than a broader one which will include also patients with dementia and gait impairment associated with subcortical WMLs and lacunes. PD

Table 22.4 Clinical features of vascular parkinsonism

Age of onset above 70 years
Pyramidal signs
Pseudobulbar palsy
Cognitive impairment
Multiple vascular risk factors
Acute onset
Rapid progression
Poor response to dopaminergic therapy
Absence of tremor
History of stroke

has been shown to have an earlier age of onset versus VP. In PD, age of onset can vary from 30 to 80 years, but most commonly the onset is in the sixth or seventh decade. The age of onset is similar to that of PD, or slightly higher [6, 22], and there is male predominance, which probably reflects the fact that vascular disease in general is more common in men (Table 22.4).

22.5 Clinical Features

Clinical features of VP and the disease progression milestones were confirmed by the largest retrospective analysis of 28 parkinsonian cases from the archives of the Queen Square Brain Bank in which cerebrovascular disease was the only pathological finding, i.e., without Lewy bodies [22].

The predominant manifestation of LBP is gait impairment (100 %), which is slow and insecure, similar to that in PD, but the base is not always narrow. The posture is unstable with poor postural responses. The legs are spastic rather than rigid, with brisk tendon reflexes, mainly in the knees, with possible clonus, and the plantar responses are extensor on one or both sides in many cases. While sitting, the feet movements are slow, considerably slower than those of the upper limbs. Patients frequently manifest freezing, but the kinematic characteristics of the gait abnormalities in LBP have not been defined well. Gait ignition failure may be another, rather uncommon, manifestation [23]. Patients may have abnormal glabellar tap responses, and other "release signs" are occasionally present. Bender's face-hand test is frequently seen. Pseudobulbar symptoms are common, particularly in the more advanced cases. Smell loss may occur but rarely [24].

The upper limbs may also be affected, although considerably less so than the legs, with brisk tendon reflexes, but tremor is relatively rare. Speech impairment was seen in 71 % of patients in the London series [22]. Some response to levodopa was seen in a majority of patients, but it was functionally disappointing, and patients rarely reported motor fluctuations or dyskinesias [22]. Urinary symptoms including incontinence were revealed in 68 % of patients, constipation in 56 %, and orthostatic hypotension in 27 % [22].

Mood disorders and dementia were documented in 60 % and 39 % respectively; subjective cognitive complaints were noticed in 64 % of patients. The VP patients performed worse than the PD group on frontal/executive tasks [22]. Visual hallucinations were not reported in any case, suggesting that when present they are likely to point to a diagnosis of PD with associated cerebrovascular pathology or dementia with Lewy bodies.

Most VP patients present with an insidious onset and steadily progressive disease with early milestones and duration shorter than PD. In most cases there is slow deterioration of the gait, with gradual appearance of urinary difficulties and cognitive decline, unless these have been present before. Verghese et al. showed that gait impairment by itself is a significant risk factor for the development of dementia [25].

Disease duration was associated with time to sphincter dysfunction and nursing home admission in nearly two thirds of patients in 5 years [22].

22.6 Differential Diagnosis of Vascular Parkinsonism

22.6.1 Parkinson's Disease (PD)

PD is a main and usual differential diagnostic challenge for VP. Patients with PD are more likely to have a longer duration of illness and slower progression compared to VP. Overall, the majorities of patients with PD present with insidious onset of unilateral symptoms and have a progressive course of their symptoms. The posture in PD is stooped up to camptocormia in some cases, with knees and hips flexion, which is rarely seen in VD because of prominent rigidity in extensor muscles mostly in the lower body. Postural instability and gait disorders (narrow-based, short-step shuffling gait) are usually later symptoms in PD, which become obvious after 7–10 years of the disease. Oppositely, gait disturbances were reported as the initial symptom in 90 % of VP patients and resemble the gait in hydrocephalus.

In PD, tremor, rigidity, and bradykinesia generally present in the upper limbs. The typical 4–5 Hz pill-rolling type resting tremor of the thumb and fingers is significantly more common in PD than in VP, where a non-rolling type of resting tremor may be observed, but it is very rare as the initial symptom. In PD, there are no spasticity, extensor plantar or exaggerated tendon reflexes, hemiparesis, and ataxia.

Usually no cognitive decline can be seen in PD at the beginning or early in the course of the disease. Motor fluctuations, peak of dose dyskinesias as a manifestation of progressive nigrostriatal denervation and adverse effects of levodopa such as confusion and hallucinations, or dopamine dysregulation are relatively specific features of PD. Both snout reflex and palmo-mental reflexes were more frequently positive in the VP patients than in PD patients [26].

22.6.2 Multiple System Atrophy (MSA)

Parkinsonian symptoms can occur frequently in MSA, and 12.6 % of patients with a clinical diagnosis of PD are found to have MSA at autopsy [27]. Clinical differentiation of VP from MSA-predominating Parkinsonism-like symptoms (MSA-P) may be difficult, because both groups have rigidity and bradykinesia more prominent than tremor, rapidly progressive disability, and poor response to levodopa.

Clinical features, pointing to the MSA-P, especially in advanced stages, are younger age

(40–50 years), preserved cognition, severe bulbar disorders – dysphagia, aspirations, dysarthria, inspiratory gasps, or stridor – as well as prominent autonomic disturbances such as urinary retention or incontinence and orthostatic hypotension. There are pronounced balance disorders due to the lack of postural reflexes causing recurrent fallings. Cerebellar syndrome appears eventually in a majority of originally MSA-P patients.

22.6.3 Progressive Supranuclear Palsy (PSP)

PSP is a parkinsonian-like disorder with vertical supranuclear ophthalmoparesis (either moderate to severe upward or any downward gaze abnormalities) and prominent postural instability with falls at the beginning of the disease. PSP patients who have not yet developed vertical gaze palsy, but have falls or postural instability can be difficult to differentiate from VP. Clinical features such as symmetric parkinsonism and pyramidal signs occur in both VP and PSP. The clinical manifestations, which characterize PSP, are early onset of cognitive decline, frequent oculomotor complaints of patients, craniocervical dystonias (retrocollis with extensor axial rigidity, blepharospasm, oromandibular dystonia), and eyelid-opening apraxia.

22.6.4 Normal Pressure Hydrocephalus (NPH)

The classical clinical triad of NPH, gait and posture disturbances, cognitive decline, and urinary incontinence, need not to be present simultaneously. Bradykinesia and gait disorders in NPH may resemble the "frontal lobe gait" with irregular wide base slow and short steps, shuffling, and freezings. However, usually no pyramidal signs are seen in NPH. Brain CT or MRI scan is determinative as well as substantial clinical effect after lumbar cerebrospinal fluid drainage or shunting (but see below).

22.7 Special Cases of Vascular Parkinsonism

22.7.1 VP Associated with Brain Stem Lesions

These anecdotal cases of vascular lesions of the SN or nigrostriatal pathway have features resembling PD, including responsiveness to levodopa. However, the follow-up, long-term prognosis and special features of the dopaminergic treatment are unknown. To illustrate the point, we can discuss a case of a patient in whom right hemiparkinsonism was diagnosed following hemorrhage into the left SN. 99mTc-HMPAO SPECT showed reduced uptake in the left putamen, globus pallidus, and thalamus [28]. The SPECT abnormalities were assumed to be the result of the stroke, rather than a coincidental abnormality [28]. In another report, a patient developed right-sided cogwheel rigidity and resting tremor. In this case the MRI showed a contralateral midbrain hemorrhage affecting the SN, and IMP-SPECT images showed reduced radioisotope uptake in the left striatum, thalamus, and frontal lobe [29]. Sudden onset of stooped posture, small steppage gait, akinesia and freezing of gait, and extrapyramidal rigidity in the arms were seen in a patient with a small high-density lesion in the medial side of right cerebral peduncle and a low-density lesion in the left putamen. On T1- and T2 weighted MRI images, a right peduncular low-signal lesion was seen extending to the SN, which was partially destroyed. Parkinsonism rapidly improved and completely disappeared within 2 weeks. The hemorrhagic high-density lesion of the right peduncle on CT also disappeared [30].

These cases had in common an apoplectic appearance of unilateral parkinsonian signs, which are the logical result of an ischemic or hemorrhagic lesion of the SN or the nigrostriatal tract, and therefore constitute the most straightforward examples of VP. Such cases should have an acute onset, be nonprogressive and even spontaneously improving over time, and be responding to levodopa. At autopsy such cases should not contain synuclein deposits. In patients with clinically suspected VP, the comparison of levodopa response with the pathologically confirmed presence of macroscopic vascular damage in the nigrostriatal pathway and cell loss in the SN showed that the majority of patients with a good or excellent response to levodopa had infarcts or lacunae in the SN in the absence of Lewy bodies [31].

Parkinsonism has been described in patients with central nervous system vasculitis [32], Behçet's disease [33, 34], rheumatoid arthritis [35, 36], lupus erythematosus [37, 38], antiphospholipid syndrome [39–41], disseminated intravascular coagulation [42], Fabry's disease [43], and some infections like syphilis [2, 44, 45] and rarely others [46, 47].

Not unexpectedly, most patients with vascular brain stem lesions had additional manifestations, consistent with the damaged area. Of course, more extensive lesions due to basilar occlusion will also affect the SN, but the extrapyramidal signs will be overshadowed by other manifestations of brain stem dysfunction.

Acute or subacute parkinsonism was also observed as a result of tentorial herniations with brain stem compression in patients with subdural hematomas or as a result of rupture of arterial aneurysms [48–50]. Unilateral rest tremor associated with bilateral extrapyramidal syndrome responsive to levodopa was seen in a 25-year-old man, 7 months after subarachnoid hemorrhage due to rupture of a peduncular subthalamic arteriovenous malformation [51]. In some of these cases, parkinsonism improved following removal of the hematoma [52], but in others it persisted and usually responded to levodopa [53]. Kim [54] reported patients with (hemi) parkinsonism after infarction in the territory of the anterior cerebral artery.

Destruction of the left subthalamic nucleus by hematoma could actually improve preexisting contralateral parkinsonian rigidity after the disappearance of the ballistic movement phase [55].

22.7.2 VP Associated with Basal Ganglia Lesions

Ischemic infarcts in the territory of the lenticulostriate arteries were said to be the most frequent cause of contralateral parkinsonism [56–59]. In these cases, there was an acute onset of the disorder with supportive imaging data to suggest a vascular etiology.

A lateralized subacute parkinsonism with CT evidence of a single lacunar infarct in the contralateral BG was described by Lazzarino et al. [9]. A clinical syndrome indistinguishable from PD, in which postmortem examination revealed extensive lacunar infarctions of the BG without evidence of coexistent PD was reported [60]. Lacunar infarctions in the BG are frequently observed in patients without parkinsonism and even in completely asymptomatic cases. The extrapyramidal signs, if present, can be asymmetrical without consistent relationship to the side of the lacune [14]. Subdivision of parkinsonian patients with lacunar infarcts in the BG into those with lacunes in the caudate nucleus, lentiform nucleus, or both did not correlate with the clinical presentation [11]. However, these CT studies have not evaluated the likely contribution of associated WMLs.

22.7.3 VP Associated with White Matter Lesions

A common picture of VP associated with WMLs is that of short-stepped gait with or without freezing [61]; lead-pipe rigidity; no or mild upper limb involvement; the absence of rest tremor, which develops insidiously; and negative response to levodopa [5, 6, 31, 62]. Pseudobulbar palsy is observed in nearly half of the patients [63]. The patients frequently have cognitive decline and detrusor overactivity [64, 65]. Long-tract signs in the limbs, indicating damage to the corticospinal tracts, are found in more than half of the cases [63]. Many of these patients have vascular risk factors and particularly hypertension. The evolution of this disease is typically slow, occurring over several months or even years [14]. Brain imaging shows diffuse subcortical white matter damage, not unlike that seen in patients with BD, sometimes accompanied by unilateral or bilateral BG infarcts [66]. Loss of postural reflexes and gait abnormalities seen in these cases may indicate "extrapyramidal" features, but are difficult to disassociate from coexisting spasticity, and the slowness may also reflect pyramidal, rather than extrapyramidal, damage.

Comparing the brain pathology in these patients with that in matched patients with BD who had no parkinsonism according to clinical records failed to reveal any significant differences in the extent of BG damage [63], thus pointing to the central role of white matter damage. The number of oligodendrocytes in the frontal white matter of VP patients was significantly less than in age-matched normal control subjects, but the reduction was not as severe as in those with BD. Widespread lesions in the frontal white matter with only meager lesions in the BG were the main pathological features of VP. The extent of frontal white matter pallor tended to be less broad in VP than in BD without parkinsonism [63]. Marked atrophy in the frontal cortex and lacunar lesions around the lateral ventricles in VP were previously shown by Grundl et al. [67]. The exact pathogenesis of these white matter changes is debated and likely heterogeneous but is generally thought to represent areas of chronic or recurrent partial ischemia. While patients with BG lacunar infarct could recover spontaneously, those with frontal lobe infarcts could remain static, and those with periventricular and deep subcortical WMLs usually had progressive deterioration [31].

Diffuse white matter damage typically manifests as a combination of extrapyramidal, pyramidal, and sometimes cognitive decline. These cases would typically not respond to levodopa, because the lesions involve the ascending loop of the BG-thalamic-cortical loop [68], distal to the striatal site of action of dopamine.

White matter disease contributes to the motor features in PD; its severity was shown to be associated with motor impairments. In a recent study of Bohnen et al. [69], parkinsonian patients (Hoehn and Yahr stages 1–3 [70]) underwent brain magnetic resonance and [11C] dihydrotetrabenazine vesicular monoamine transporter PET imaging. White matter signal hyperintensity was robustly associated with axial motor impairment including stooped posture, postural instability, and gait difficulties and less with bradykinesia. However, no significant white matter signal hyperintensity burden effects were found for rigidity or tremor UPDRS sub-scores. Importantly, increased white matter signal hyperintensity burden was associated with worse motor performance *independent* of the degree of nigrostriatal dopaminergic denervation in PD. According to the authors, comorbid leukoaraiosis may be a greater determinant of axial motor impairment than the nigrostriatal dopaminergic denervation itself [69].

22.8 Neuroimaging

Patients with LBP typically demonstrate extensive lesions of the periventricular white matter with lacunes, mainly in the basal ganglia, as well as dilatation of the lateral and third cerebral ventricles. As these changes develop and accumulate over months and years, there is no point in defining quantitatively the extent of these changes. As will be discussed below, similar changes are seen in patients with BD (with or without gait impairment), but little attempt has been made to differentiate those MRI changes which are responsible for cognitive decline from those associated with gait impairment.

By definition, patients with VP must have vascular lesions in their brain, and it would be difficult to make a diagnosis of VP in the face of a normal MRI. However, the mere existence of WML or lacunes in the brain is insufficient to make a diagnosis of VP since these occur commonly in apparently unaffected elderly people and their existence in PD patients does not correlate with gait abnormalities [24, 71].

It is of interest that even when examining cognitively normal elderly, the extent of WML corresponds to gait abnormalities and reduced gait velocity [72]. Baezner et al. [73] found that abnormal gait parameters in otherwise normal elderly had the strongest correlations with disruption of normal-appearing white matter, but there was no brain region which was particularly relevant. Thus it seems that the gait impairment associated with white matter brain lesions starts diffusely throughout the subcortical white matter progresses and as it may develop the cardinal manifestations of the VP syndrome [74]. Elderly subjects with more severe WMLs were particularly likely to demonstrate deterioration of gait [75]. WMLs, similar to those described above, have also been demonstrated in elderly people with cognitive impairment. The cognitive changes are nonspecific and can include memory, executive functions, and general intelligence [76]. The midbrain and the pontine areas in VP patients were significantly smaller than in PD and resembled the brain stem atrophy in PSP [77].

It should be mentioned that the neuroimaging studies reported so far were mainly conventional ones. Advanced imaging, like diffusion tensor imaging, resting-state fMRI, specific examination of normal-appearing white matter, and high-field (e.g., 7 T) examinations, may throw additional light on the pathogenesis and manifestations [78].

Different authors use different nomenclature when describing these lesions. An attempt to reach common standards for research into small vessel disease is therefore urgently needed [79].

22.9 Nuclear Imaging

Small studies failed to find specific changes in VP patients and indeed were not significantly different than in healthy individuals. The characteristic reduction of the uptake 123I-FP-CIT is pronounced in the contralateral putamen of PD patients with unilateral symptoms, but is not seen in VP [80]. Normal striatal 123I-FP-CIT binding with no significant differences in striatal or subregional binding ratios compared with those of controls was seen in patients with VP. PD usually shows abnormal uptake in the striatum, which progresses from the putamen to caudate and contralaterally to the clinically more affected side [81]. However in a case of vascular lesion of the basal ganglia located in lenticular nuclei or putamen, concordant defects on I-123-ioflupane and perfusion brain imaging were also seen [82]. Striatal asymmetry index detected using 123I-FP-CIT SPECT was significantly less in patients with VP compared to PD subjects [83]. As compared to normal controls, patients with VP had significant reduction of the NAA/CRE [(N-acetylaspartate to creatine plus phosphocreatine (CRE)] ratio in the frontal cortex, suggesting a lesion beyond the classical extrapyramidal system [84].

VP may be a probable cause of extrapyramidal disorders in subjects with normal dopamine transporter (DAT) without evidence of dopaminergic deficit (SWEDD) [85], which is considered as a slowly progressive or nonprogressive disorder [86].

22.10 Transcranial Ultrasonography

Typical VP patients do not have hyperechogenic areas at the midbrain, and the basal ganglia are normal (the latter is also found in PD). Normal echogenicity of the SN correlated in 95 % with the clinical impression of VP, reflecting a high positive predictive value of transcranial ultrasonography for VP [87].

22.11 Pathology

Vascular changes in the brain are the hallmarks of VP. These are usually ischemic, rarely hemorrhagic, and affect relevant areas of the brain, i.e., subcortical white matter (mainly periventricular), basal ganglia, thalamus, and upper brain stem. Changes of the blood vessels themselves have not been described in detail but are expected to consist mainly of vessel wall changes, such as lipohyalinosis.

Only a few series of pathological studies focusing on VP patients have been reported.

Among those, the study of Yamanouchi et al. [63] is the most detailed. These investigators performed a detailed examination of VP patients, comparing them to patients with PD and normal controls. Their definition of PD included pallor of the SN, while such changes were not seen in VP. Majorities of VP and BD patients had extensive changes in the white matter, particularly of the frontal lobes, as well as BG lacunes [63]. These could occasionally be seen in PD but were much less severe. The white matter changes were accompanied by severe loss of oligodendrocytes.

While it is customary to assume that pathology should be the gold standard for diagnosis, this is not necessarily the case for VP, for a variety of reasons. Firstly, there are no accepted criteria for the pathologic diagnosis of VP. Secondly, the MRI may be more sensitive to identify WMLs and can be used to quantify the damage (including changes in normal-appearing white matter) than the pathological examination. Of course microscopic examination is important to identify the underlying pathologic process, such as CADASIL, which also can manifest as parkinsonism [88].

22.12 Pathogenesis and Mechanisms

VP is a clinical syndrome that may have similarities to the cardinal motor manifestations of PD. In the pathogenesis of VP without a direct lesion affecting the SN, the dopamine level and its metabolites in the CSF should be normal [89]. Thus, the accepted explanation of the clinical symptoms in VP is related to postsynaptic lesions of the nigrostriatal system mainly as a result of a patchy destruction of neurons or axons at the putamen, globus pallidus, and probably the cerebral white matter.

The vascular lesions affecting the basal ganglia or the subcortical and deep white matter may affect the striato-thalamic-cortical loops, leading to the clinical features of gait impairment and the other features of VP [17, 90].

The white matter changes in VP probably reflect ischemic changes, resulting from repeated hypoxic or ischemic episodes, which lead to inflammatory responses in the affected brain areas, with induction of proteases, free radical generation and consequently opening of the blood-brain barrier, extravasations of noxious elements, and consequently myelin breakdown [91, 92].

The hallmarks of LBP are the gait abnormalities. The most clearly demonstrable anatomical lesions are in the white matter although basal ganglia lacunes are seen very frequently, and it is difficult to define the role of each in the pathogenesis.

BG lacunes and particularly WMLs are very common in elderly individuals, particularly these harboring hypertension and other vascular risk factors, and they commonly co-occur. It is therefore difficult to ascertain which of them are responsible for the motor dysfunction. The basal ganglia are immediate suspects when discussing parkinsonian symptoms. Yet the gait impairment, associated pyramidal signs, and urinary dysfunction make the frontal white matter changes more likely suspects. The bradykinesia and other extrapyramidal features point to a possible involvement of the basal ganglia-thalamocortical circuits [72].

As mentioned above, there is poor correlation between the imaging picture and the corresponding clinical manifestations which may be absent altogether or consist of cognitive impairment, depression, urinary incontinence, or any combination of these. Chronic ischemic changes affecting the subcortical white matter may result in slowly progressing gait impairment, which will fail to respond to dopaminergic medication.

In an attempt to localize the areas of white matter lesions which are responsible for the gait abnormalities, de Laat et al. [74] have examined a large cohort of elderly subjects who had cerebral white matter changes but intact cognition and lacked other parkinsonian signs. They found that voxel-based pathological data also confirmed that in many cases the white matter changes are accompanied by lacunes in the BG and particularly in the thalamus, and they had independent contributions to the parkinsonian signs. Thus, mixed pathology is not unusual [92].

The term "frontal gait disorder" is supported by a recent study showing disruption of the frontal lobe white matter in patients with VP, implying prefrontal cortex outflow damage [93].

22.13 Treatment

Therapy of VP is disappointing. Levodopa, amantadine, dopamine agonists, and other antiparkinsonian drugs are inefficacious or have minor effects especially in cases caused by subcortical white matter damage [7, 19]. Both deep brain stimulation of the globus pallidus or subthalamic nucleus [94] and physical therapy [95] are of limited value. Almost by definition, attention to the vascular risk factors is expected to slow down the rate of decline, yet no studies have been reported which substantiate this.

A long-term history of hypertension, heart disease, diabetes, smoking, cerebrovascular accidents, and other risk factors for stroke support a vascular origin of these symptoms in both groups. It is conceivable that preventive treatment of vascular or inflammatory risk factors in patients with VP, earlier in life well before the first symptoms, could reduce its severity. Similarly, treatment of cerebral inflammatory and ischemic lesions could possibly lessen morbidity associated with parkinsonism [96, 97]. However, the development of such programs depends on the elaboration and implementation of the international diagnostic criteria of VP.

An interesting therapeutic option which has been suggested is of cerebrospinal fluid drainage. The clinical similarity of the gait impairment in VP to NPH has already been mentioned by several authors [4, 5, 88]. Thompson and Marsden [4] also commented that several of their patients with "gait disorder subcortical arteriosclerotic encephalopathy" had dilated ventricles. The white matter changes of BD and NPH are remarkably similar [98]. Attempts to treat patients suffering from VP by CSF shunting have been reported with positive results [98–101]. Recently a small double-blind study has supported these findings, although the follow-up was relatively short, just 3 months [102]. Controlled studies on a large group of patients, with a longer follow-up, are not yet available to support the use of either repeated lumbar punctures or placement of a shunting tube in VP patients except as an experimental procedure. Such studies may also indicate which patients are more or less likely to respond.

Atherosclerotic brain disease is common in the elderly and can affect patients with PD as well. These patients with "mixed disease" are likely to respond to dopaminominetic therapy but less so than patients with "pure" PD. Rarely, acute stroke can result in levodopa-responsive VP [103].

Other treatment modalities, such as repetitive transcranial magnetic stimulation [104], have been suggested.

Conclusions

VP rarely starts abruptly, when a lacune or hemorrhage affects a strategic location [105]. More often, the disorder develops insidiously, frequently starting with gait impairment: slow shuffling gait, with short steps and falls. As the disease develops, additional manifestations are seen, including urinary incontinence and cognitive decline, and later pseudobulbar symptoms.

If the final stages of VP include dementia and urinary incontinence, what about the earliest stages? Important studies, such as the LADIS study, have examined prospectively normal elderly individuals, and they found that age-related white matter changes correlated with gait and balance impairment [23] and also predicted the occurrence of depression [106].

In conclusion, VP, or gait impairment in the elderly, is a common, but not a constant, consequence of subcortical white matter changes and basal ganglia lacunes. The overlap between LBP and BD suggests that these are in fact a single disease entity, but long-term prospective studies of both disorders are necessary to support this conclusion.

References

1. Korczyn AD. Parkinson's disease. In: Heggenhougen K, editor. International encyclopedia of public health. Oxford: Academic; 2008. p. 10–7.
2. Critchley M. Arteriosclerotic parkinsonism. Brain. 1929;52:23–83.
3. Critchley M. Arteriosclerotic pseudoparkinsonism. In: Rose FC, Capildeo R, editors. Research progress in Parkinson's disease. London: Pitman; 1981. p. 745–52.
4. Thompson PD, Marsden CD. Gait disorder of subcortical arteriosclerotic encephalopathy. Binswanger's disease. Mov Disord. 1987;2:1–8.
5. FitzGerald PM, Jankovic J. Lower body parkinsonism, evidence for vascular etiology. Mov Disord. 1989;4:249–60.
6. Winikates J, Jankovic J. Clinical correlates of vascular parkinsonism. Arch Neurol. 1999;56:98–102.
7. Parkes JD, Marsden CD, Rees JE, Curzon G, Kantamaneni BD, Knill-Jones R, et al. Parkinson's disease, cerebral arteriosclerosis, and senile dementia. Clinical features and response to levodopa. Q J Med. 1974;43:49–61.
8. Hunter R, Smith J, Thomson T, Dayan AD. Hemiparkinsonism with infarction of the ipsilateral substantia nigra. Neuropathol Appl Neurobiol. 1978;4:297–301.
9. Lazzarino LG, Nicolai A, Toppani D. Subacute parkinsonism from a single lacunar infarct in the basal ganglia. Acta Neurol (Napoli). 1990;12: 292–5.
10. Harik SI, Al-Hinti JT, Archer RL, Angtuaco EJC. Hemiparkinsonism after unilateral traumatic midbrain hemorrhage in a young woman. Neurol Clin Pract. 2013;3:4–7.
11. Tolosa ES, Santamaría J. Parkinsonism and basal ganglia infarcts. Neurology. 1984;34:1516–8.
12. Rieder-Groswasser I, Bornstein NM, Korczyn AD. Parkinsonism in patients with lacunar infarcts of the basal ganglia. Eur Neurol. 1995;35:46–9.
13. Ikeda K, Kotabe T, Kanbashi S, Kinoshita M. Parkinsonism in lacunar infarcts of the basal ganglia. Eur Neurol. 1996;36:248–9.
14. Inzelberg R, Bornstein NM, Rieder Grosswasser I, Korczyn AD. Basal ganglia lacunes and parkinsonism. Neuroepidemiology. 1994;13:108–12.
15. Bhatia KP, Marsden CD. The behavioural and motor consequences of focal lesions of the basal ganglia in man. Brain. 1994;117:859–76.
16. Balash Y, Korczyn AD. Vascular parkinsonism. Handb Clin Neurol. 2007;84:417–25.
17. Sibon I, Fenelon G, Quinn NP, Tison F. Vascular parkinsonism. J Neurol. 2004;251:513–24.
18. Leys D, Pruvo JP, Parent M, Vermersch P, Soetaert G, Steinling M, et al. Could Wallerian degeneration contribute to "leuko-araiosis" in subjects free of any vascular disorder? J Neurol Neurosurg Psychiatry. 1991;54:46–50.
19. Zijlmans JC, Daniel SE, Hughes AJ, Révész T, Lees AJ. Clinicopathological investigation of vascular parkinsonism, including clinical criteria for diagnosis. Mov Disord. 2004;19:630–40.
20. ICD 10. International Classification of Diseases 10th Revision. PMIC. Los Angeles, CA, 2013.
21. Hughes AJ, Daniel SE, Blankson S, Lees AJ. A clinicopathologic study of 100 cases of Parkinson's disease. Arch Neurol. 1993;50:140–8.
22. Glass PG, Lees AJ, Bacellar A, Zijlmans J, Katzenschlager R, Silveira-Moriyama L. The clinical features of pathologically confirmed vascular parkinsonism. J Neurol Neurosurg Psychiatry. 2012;83:1027–9.
23. Atchison PR, Thompson PD, Frackowiak RS, Marsden CD. The syndrome of gait ignition failure: a report of six cases. Mov Disord. 1993;8:285–92.
24. Herman T, Rosenberg-Katz K, Jacob Y, Auriel E, Gurevich T, Giladi N, et al. White matter hyperintensities in Parkinson's disease, do they explain the disparity between the postural instability gait difficulty and tremor dominant subtypes? PLoS ONE. 2013;8:e55193.
25. Parihar R, Mahoney JR, Verghese J. Relationship of gait and cognition in the elderly. Curr Transl Geriatr Exp Gerontol Rep. 2013;1:2.
26. Okuda B, Kawabata K, Tachibana H, Kamogawa K, Okamoto K. Primitive reflexes distinguish vascular parkinsonism from Parkinson's disease. Clin Neurol Neurosurg. 2008;110:562–5.
27. Joutsa J, Gardberg M, Röyttä M, Kaasinen V. Diagnostic accuracy of parkinsonism syndromes by general neurologists. Parkinsonism Relat Disord. 2014;20:840–4.
28. Abe K, Yanagihara T. Hemiparkinsonism following haemorrhage in the contralateral substantia nigra. Neuroradiology. 1996;38 Suppl 1:S67–9.
29. Inoue H, Udaka F, Takahashi M, Nishinaka K, Kameyama M. Secondary parkinsonism following midbrain hemorrhage. Rinsho Shinkeigaku. 1997;37:266–9.
30. Miyagi K, Imaizumi T, Nagura H, Yamanouchi H. A case of transient parkinsonism due to mesencephalic hemorrhage. Rinsho Shinkeigaku. 1992;32:743–6.
31. Chang CM, Yu YL, Ng HK, Leung SY, Fong KY. Vascular pseudoparkinsonism. Acta Neurol Scand. 1992;86:588–92.
32. Fabiani G, Teive HA, Germiniani FM, Sa DS, Werneck LC. Reversible parkinsonian syndrome in systemic and brain vasculitis. Mov Disord. 2002;17:601–4.
33. Bogdanova D, Milanov I, Georgiev D. Parkinsonian syndrome as a neurological manifestation of Behçet's disease. Can J Neurol Sci. 1998;25:82–5.
34. Joseph FG, Scolding NJ. Neuro-Behçet's disease in Caucasians: a study of 22 patients. Eur J Neurol. 2007;14:174–80.
35. Ertan S, Fresko I, Apaydin H, Ozekmekci S, Yazici H. Extrapyramidal type rigidity in rheumatoid arthritis. Rheumatology (Oxford). 1999;38:627–30.

36. Hrycaj P, Korczowska I, Lacki JK. Severe Parkinson's disease in rheumatoid arthritis patient treated with infliximab. Rheumatology (Oxford). 2003;42:702–3.
37. Tan EK, Chan LL, Auchus AP. Reversible parkinsonism in systemic lupus erythematosus. J Neurol Sci. 2001;193:53–7.
38. Garcia-Moreno JM, Chacon J. Juvenile parkinsonism as a manifestation of systemic lupus erythematosus: case report and review of the literature. Mov Disord. 2002;17:1329–35.
39. Huang YC, Lyu RK, Chen ST, Chu YC, Wu YR. Parkinsonism in a patient with antiphospholipid syndrome – case report and literature review. J Neurol Sci. 2008;267:166–9.
40. Adhiyaman V, Meara RJ, Bhowmick BK. Antiphospholipid syndrome and dystonia-parkinsonism: need for anticoagulation. Parkinsonism Relat Disord. 2002;8:215.
41. Milanov I, Bogdanova D. Antiphospholipid syndrome and dystonia-parkinsonism. A case report. Parkinsonism Relat Disord. 2001;7:139–41.
42. Yoritaka A, Hattori T, Hattori Y, Mori H, Matsuoka S, Shirai T, Kondo T, Mizuno Y. A 85-year-old woman with the onset of progressive gait disturbance at 80 years of the age. No To Shinkei. 1997;49:379–89.
43. Buechner S, De Cristofaro MT, Ramat S, Borsini W. Parkinsonism and Anderson Fabry's disease: a case report. Mov Disord. 2006;21:103–7.
44. Spitz M, Maia FM, Gomes HR, Scaff M, Barbosa ER. Parkinsonism secondary to neurosyphilis. Mov Disord. 2008;23:1948–9.
45. Tong ML, Lin LR, Zhang HL, Huang SJ, Liu GL, Zheng WH, et al. Spectrum and characterization of movement disorders secondary to neurosyphilis. Parkinsonism Relat Disord. 2013;19:441–5.
46. Cassarino DS, Quezado MM, Ghatak NR, Duray PH. Lyme-associated parkinsonism: a neuropathologic case study and review of the literature. Arch Pathol Lab Med. 2003;127:1204–6.
47. Vlajinac H, Dzoljic E, Maksimovic J, Marinkovic J, Sipetic S, Kostic V. Infections as a risk factor for Parkinson's disease: a case-control study. Int J Neurosci. 2013;123:329–32.
48. Cosi V, Tonali P. Acute Parkinson syndrome following subarachnoid hemorrhage in a schizophrenic subject. Riv Patol Nerv Ment. 1964;85:287–301.
49. Pau A, Brambilla M, Cossu M, Schoenhuber R, Siccardi D, Turtas S. Parkinsonism in the presence of intracranial extracerebral haematomas. Acta Neurochir (Wien). 1989;96:159–60.
50. Turjanski N, Pentland B, Lees AJ, Brooks DJ. Parkinsonism associated with acute intracranial hematomas: an [18F] dopa positron-emission tomography study. Mov Disord. 1997;12:1035–8.
51. Defer GL, Remy P, Malapert D, Ricolfi F, Samson Y, Degos JD. Rest tremor and extrapyramidal symptoms after midbrain haemorrhage: clinical and 18F-dopa PET evaluation. J Neurol Neurosurg Psychiatry. 1994;57:987–9.
52. Sunada I, Inoue T, Tamura K, Akano Y, Fu Y. Parkinsonism due to chronic subdural hematoma. Neurol Med Chir (Tokyo). 1996;36:99–101.
53. Trosch RM, Ransom BR. Levodopa-responsive parkinsonism following central herniation due to bilateral subdural hematomas. Neurology. 1990;40:376–7.
54. Kim JS. Involuntary movements after anterior cerebral artery territory infarction. Stroke. 2001;32:258–61.
55. Yamada A, Takeuchi H, Miki H. Unilateral abolition of parkinsonian rigidity after subthalamic nucleus hemorrhage. Rinsho Shinkeigaku. 1992;32:887–9.
56. Friedman A, Kang UJ, Tatemichi TK, Burke RE. A case of parkinsonism following striatal lacunar infarction. J Neurol Neurosurg Psychiatry. 1986;49:1087–8.
57. Kulisevsky J, Berthier ML, Avila A, Roig C. Unilateral parkinsonism and stereotyped movements following a right lenticular infarction. Mov Disord. 1996;11:752–4.
58. Fenelon G, Houeto JL. Unilateral parkinsonism following a large infarct in the territory of the lenticulostriate arteries. Mov Disord. 1997;12:1086–90.
59. Sibon I, Guyot M, Allard M, Tison F. Parkinsonism following anterior choroidal artery stroke. Eur J Neurol. 2004;11:283–4.
60. Murrow RW, Schweiger GD, Kepes JJ, Koller WC. Parkinsonism due to a basal ganglia lacunar state: clinicopathologic correlation. Neurology. 1990;40:897–900.
61. Giladi N, Kao R, Fahn S. Freezing phenomenon in patients with parkinsonian syndromes. Mov Disord. 1997;12:302–5.
62. van Zagten M, Lodder J, Kessels F. Gait disorder and parkinsonian signs in patients with stroke related to small deep infarcts and white matter lesions. Mov Disord. 1998;13:89–95.
63. Yamanouchi H, Nagura H. Neurological signs and frontal white matter lesions in vascular parkinsonism. A clinicopathologic study. Stroke. 1997;28:965–9.
64. Cummings JL. Vascular subcortical dementias: clinical aspects. Dementia. 1994;5:177–80.
65. Holstein J, Chatellier G, Piette F, Moulias R. Prevalence of associated diseases in different types of dementia among elderly institutionalized patients: analysis of 3447 records. J Am Geriatr Soc. 1994;42:972–7.
66. Demirkiran M, Bozdemir H, Sarica Y. Vascular parkinsonism: a distinct, heterogeneous clinical entity. Acta Neurol Scand. 2001;104:63–7.
67. Grundl W, Ziegler R, Westphal KP, Hufnagl M, Szirtes J, Kornhuber HH. Parkinson's syndrome: cranial computed-tomography findings. Their dependence on sex and age. Acta Med Hung. 1991;48:127–36.
68. Bergman H, Deuschl G. Pathophysiology of Parkinson's disease: from clinical neurology to basic neuroscience and back. Mov Disord. 2002;17 Suppl 3:S28–40.

69. Bohnen NI, Müller ML, Zarzhevsky N, Koeppe RA, Bogan CW, Kilbourn MR, et al. Leucoaraiosis, nigrostriatal denervation and motor symptoms in Parkinson's disease. Brain. 2011;134:2358–65.
70. Hoehn MM, Yahr MD. Parkinsonism: onset, progression and mortality. Neurology. 1967;17:427–42.
71. Antonini A, Vitale C, Barone P, Cilia R, Righini A, Bonuccelli U, et al. The relationship between cerebral vascular disease and parkinsonism: the VADO study. Parkinsonism Relat Disord. 2012;18:775–80.
72. Bohnen NI, Albin RL. White matter lesions in Parkinson disease. Nat Rev Neurol. 2011;7:229–36.
73. Baezner H, Blahak C, Poggesi A, Pantoni L, Inzitari D, Chabriat H, et al. Association of gait and balance disorders with age-related white matter changes: the LADIS study. Neurology. 2008;70:935–42.
74. de Laat KF, van Norden AG, Gons RA, van Uden IW, Zwiers MP, Bloem BR, et al. Cerebral white matter lesions and lacunar infarcts contribute to the presence of mild parkinsonian signs. Stroke. 2012;43:2574–9.
75. Kreisel SH, Blahak C, Bäzner H, Inzitari D, Pantoni L, Poggesi A, et al. Deterioration of gait and balance over time: the effects of age-related white matter change – the LADIS study. Cerebrovasc Dis. 2013;35:544–53.
76. Kloppenborg RP, Nederkoorn PJ, Geerlings MI, van den Berg E. Presence and progression of white matter hyperintensities and cognition: a meta-analysis. Neurology. 2014;82:2127–38.
77. Choi SM, Kim BC, Nam TS, Kim JT, Lee SH, Park MS, et al. Midbrain atrophy in vascular Parkinsonism. Eur Neurol. 2011;65:296–301.
78. Van Norden AG, de Laat KF, Gons RA, van Uden IW, van Dijk EJ, van Oudheusden LJ, et al. Causes and consequences of cerebral small vessel disease. The RUN DMC study: a prospective cohort study. Study rationale and protocol. BMC Neurol. 2011;11:29.
79. Wardlaw JM, Smith EE, Biessels GJ, Cordonnier C, Fazekas F, Frayne R, et al. Neuroimaging standards for research into small vessel disease and its contribution to ageing and neurodegeneration. Lancet Neurol. 2013;12:822–38.
80. Tzen KY, Lu CS, Yen TC, Wey SP, Ting G. Differential diagnosis of Parkinson's disease and vascular parkinsonism by (99m) Tc-TRODAT-1. J Nucl Med. 2001;42:408–13.
81. Lorberboym M, Djaldetti R, Melamed E, Sadeh M, Lampl Y. 123I-FP-CIT SPECT imaging of dopamine transporters in patients with cerebrovascular disease and clinical diagnosis of vascular parkinsonism. J Nucl Med. 2004;45:1688–93.
82. Milà M, Cuberas G, Rovira A, Porta F, Negre M, Rossi S, et al. Can I-123-FP-CIT images give us a clue that implies a vascular parkinsonism? Clin Nucl Med. 2007;32:886–8.
83. Contrafatto D, Mostile G, Nicoletti A, Dibilio V, Raciti L, Lanzafame S, et al. [(123) I]FP-CIT-SPECT asymmetry index to differentiate Parkinson's disease from vascular parkinsonism. Acta Neurol Scand. 2012;126:12–6.
84. Abe K, Terakawa H, Takanashi M, Watanabe Y, Tanaka H, Fujita N, et al. Proton magnetic resonance spectroscopy of patients with parkinsonism. Brain Res Bull. 2000;52:589–95.
85. Bajaj N. SWEDD for the general neurologist. ACNR. 2010;10:30–1.
86. Marek K, Seibyl J, Eberly S, Oakes D, Shoulson I, Lang AE, et al. Longitudinal follow-up of SWEDD subjects in the PRECEPT study. Neurology. 2014;82:1791–7.
87. Venegas P, Miranda G, Gomez R, Hudson L, Sinning M. Sensitivity and specificity of transcranial sonography in Parkinson's disease. Rev Chil Neuro-Psiquiat. 2009;47 Suppl 1:S22.
88. Wegner F, Strecker K, Schwarz J, Wagner A, Heinritz W, Sommerer F, et al. Vascular parkinsonism in a CADASIL case with an intact nigrostriatal dopaminergic system. J Neurol. 2007;254:1743–5.
89. Loeffler DA, LeWitt PA, DeMaggio AJ, Juneau PL, Milbury PE, Matson WR. Markers of dopamine depletion and compensatory response in striatum and cerebrospinal fluid. J Neural Transm Park Dis Dement Sect. 1995;9:45–53.
90. Jellinger KA. Prevalence of cerebrovascular lesions in Parkinson's disease. A postmortem study. Acta Neuropathol. 2003;105:415–9.
91. Auriel E, Bornstein NM, Berenyi E, Varkonyi I, Gabor M, Majtenyi K, et al. Clinical, radiological and pathological correlates of leukoaraiosis. Acta Neurol Scand. 2011;123:41–7.
92. Rosenberg GA, Bjerke M, Wallin A. Multimodal markers of inflammation in the subcortical ischemic vascular disease type of vascular cognitive impairment. Stroke. 2014;45:1531–8.
93. Wang HC, Hsu JL, Leemans A. Diffusion tensor imaging of vascular parkinsonism: structural changes in cerebral white matter and the association with clinical severity. Arch Neurol. 2012;69:1340–8.
94. Krack P, Dowsey PL, Benabid AL, Acarin N, Benazzouz A, Künig G, et al. Ineffective subthalamic nucleus stimulation in levodopa-resistant post-ischemic parkinsonism. Neurology. 2000;54:2182–4.
95. Tomlinson CL, Patel S, Meek C, Clarke CE, Stowe R, Shah L, et al. Physiotherapy versus placebo or no intervention in Parkinson's disease. Cochrane Database Syst Rev. 2012;8:CD002817.
96. Gao X, Simon KC, Schwarzschild MA, Ascherio A. Prospective study of statin use and risk of Parkinson disease. Arch Neurol. 2012;69:380–4.
97. Gao X, Chen H, Schwarzschild MA, Ascherio A. Use of ibuprofen and risk of Parkinson disease. Neurology. 2011;76:863–9.
98. Tullberg M, Hultin L, Ekholm S, Månsson JE, Fredman P, Wikkelsö C. White matter changes in normal pressure hydrocephalus and Binswanger disease: specificity, predictive value and correlations to

axonal degeneration and demyelination. Acta Neurol Scand. 2002;105:417–26.
99. Akiguchi I, Ishii M, Watanabe Y, Watanabe T, Kawasaki T, Yagi H, et al. Shunt-responsive parkinsonism and reversible white matter lesions in patients with idiopathic NPH. J Neurol. 2008;255:1392–9.
100. Espay AJ, Narayan RK, Duker AP, Barrett Jr ET, de Courten-Myers G. Lower-body parkinsonism, reconsidering the threshold for external lumbar drainage. Nat Clin Pract Neurol. 2008;4:50–5.
101. Ondo WG, Chan LL, Levy JK. Vascular parkinsonism, clinical correlates predicting motor improvement after lumbar puncture. Mov Disord. 2002;17:91–7.
102. Tisell M, Tullberg M, Hellström P, Edsbagge M, Högfeldt M, Wikkelsö C. Shunt surgery in patients with hydrocephalus and white matter changes. J Neurosurg. 2011;114:1432–8.
103. Ling MJ, Aggarwal A, Morris JG. Dopa-responsive parkinsonism secondary to right temporal lobe haemorrahage. Mov Disord. 2002;17:402–4.
104. Yip CW, Cheong PW, Green A, Prakash PK, Fook-Cheong SK, Tan EK, et al. A prospective pilot study of repetitive transcranial magnetic stimulation for gait dysfunction in vascular parkinsonism. Clin Neurol Neurosurg. 2013;115:887–91.
105. Handley A, Medcalf P, Hellier K, Dutta D. Movement disorders after stroke. Age Ageing. 2009;38:260–6.
106. Teodorczuk A, Firbank MJ, Pantoni L, Poggesi A, Erkinjuntti T, Wallin A, et al. Relationship between baseline white-matter changes and development of late-life depressive symptoms: 3-year results from the LADIS study. Psychol Med. 2010;40:603–10.

23 Stiff Person Syndromes

Sonia Benítez-Rivero and Pablo Mir

23.1 Introduction

The term 'stiff person syndrome' (SPS) was introduced by Moersch and Woltman in 1956 [1] to describe an unusual and previously unrecognised disorder characterised by progressive fluctuating muscular rigidity with superimposed episodes of more intense spasm [2–4]. Co-contractions of agonist and antagonist muscles and continuous involuntary firing of motor units at rest are the clinical and electrophysiological hallmarks of the disease [4, 5]. A significant development in this condition was the discovery of autoantibodies directed against glutamic acid decarboxylase (GAD), a protein that catalyses the decarboxylation of L-glutamate to GABA and is widely expressed in presynaptic GABAergic terminals in the CNS [6]. This has led to a great increase in understanding the probable pathophysiological mechanisms underlying the disorder, prompting the suggestion that SPS is an autoimmune disease [2, 3, 5].

Greater awareness of the condition in recent years has also led to the recognition of different patterns of presentation of stiff person variants, but the classification of stiff persons remains confusing, with the reporting of an increasing number of overlapping syndromes [2]. The most established condition is the classical stiff person syndrome, first described by Moersch and Woltman. Stiff persons with 'plus' signs are reported to have a poorer treatment response and prognosis. Some of them have a paraneoplastic aetiology [6].

Clinically, stiff persons with 'plus' signs may be divided into the following groups according to the aggressiveness of the pathology and its relative distribution:

- Subacute (death within 3 years, long tract signs present): 'progressive encephalomyelitis with rigidity and myoclonus'
- Chronic (survival >3 years, long tract signs absent/few): includes the 'jerking stiff person syndrome' (brainstem form) and 'stiff limb syndrome' (spinal form)

S. Benítez-Rivero
Unidad de Trastornos del Movimiento, Servicio de Neurología y Neurofisiología Clínica, Instituto de Biomedicina de Sevilla, Hospital Universitario Virgen del Rocío/CSIC/Universidad de Sevilla, Avda. Manuel Siurot s/n., Seville 41013, Spain
e-mail: pmir@us.es

P. Mir (✉)
Unidad de Trastornos del Movimiento, Servicio de Neurología y Neurofisiología Clínica, Instituto de Biomedicina de Sevilla, Hospital Universitario Virgen del Rocío/CSIC/Universidad de Sevilla, Avda. Manuel Siurot s/n., Seville 41013, Spain

Centro de Investigación Biomédica en Red sobre Enfermedades Neurodegenerativas (CIBERNED), Seville, Spain

C. Falup-Pecurariu et al. (eds.), *Movement Disorders Curricula*, DOI 10.1007/978-3-7091-1628-9_23

23.2 The Classical Stiff Person Syndrome

The classical SPS begins insidiously in patients in their mid-to-late 30s, usually without antecedent infection or other triggering factors [5]. The disease is characterised by paraspinal and abdominal rigidity with an exaggerated lumbar lordosis and superimposed episodic spasms precipitated by movement, emotional upset, peripheral stimulation or auditory startle. The spasms are frequently painful and may be accompanied by profuse sweating, tachycardia, tachypnoea and hypertension [3] (Table 23.1). The proximal lower limbs are involved in some cases, but this is often apparent only on walking when the patient has a stiff wooden gait. The calf and foot muscles are rarely if ever involved. There is no weakness, sensory loss, sphincter involvement or clinical evidence of brainstem disturbance [6]. Once the disease is established, there follows a slow progression over months or years. Eventually, the condition stabilises and may remain static for several years or even decades [2]. As SPS progresses, the majority of patients have an increasing frequency of falls, require assistance for walking and activities of daily living and frequently lose their ability to work [5].

Previous series of patients with antibodies anti-GAD and SPS have demonstrated an association with autoimmune diseases, including insulin-dependent diabetes mellitus in 30–60 %, autoimmune thyroid disease in 10 % and pernicious anaemia in 5 %. Sjögren syndrome and other autoimmune diseases also may be seen [2].

Table 23.1 The main clinical and electromyographic features of the stiff person syndrome

Clinical features	Electromyographic features
Gradual onset of stiffness in the axial muscles	Continuous motor unit activity
Legs more affected than arms	Normal motor unit morphology
Exaggerated lumbar lordosis	Normal peripheral nerve conduction
Abdominal wall rigidity	EMG activity abolished by sleep, peripheral nerve block, spinal or general anaesthesia
Rigidity abolished by sleep	
Stimulus-sensitive painful muscle spasms	

23.3 Progressive Encephalomyelitis with Rigidity and Myoclonus (PERM)

This is a rare condition characterised by a subacute encephalomyelitis that primarily affects the grey matter, resulting in widespread rigidity and rapid decline of cognitive capacities [5], as well as painful myoclonus, spasms and long tract and brainstem signs [6].

Patients survive less than 3 years, regardless of treatment. Histologically, it may differ from more indolent cases in the presence of demyelination. The relentless progression and the histology suggest a paraneoplastic aetiology, and this has been confirmed in occasional cases [6].

23.4 Jerking Stiff Person Syndrome

This form of stiff person ‘plus’ syndrome is characterised by brainstem myoclonus that involves all four limbs. The jerks may occur in paroxysms which compromise breathing and may be fatal. Patients with this syndrome may survive 10 years or more. The long survival makes a paraneoplastic aetiology seem unlikely [6].

23.5 Stiff Limb Syndrome (SLS)

Patients typically present between the ages of 20 and 50 with a rigid distal limb [7]. The legs are most commonly involved and there is a relative or total sparing of the trunk. The upper limbs may occasionally be involved [6]. About half of the patients follow a relapsing and remitting course, and around a third develop symptoms or signs of brainstem involvement. Similarly, half develop a sphincter disturbance after a mean of 5 years [7, 8].

23.6 Paraneoplastic SPS

In patients with a short history of SPS, investigations for potential neoplasms that include mammography and computerised tomography scans of the chest are mandatory. Neurological symptoms may precede diagnosis of the cancer by several years. Clinical features are almost indistinguishable from typical SPS. However, the arms appear to be involved more frequently than in the classical form [9]. Segmental rigidity and spasm of the trunk and one leg have also been reported as a paraneoplastic phenomenon [4].

Antibodies to amphiphysin, a 128-kd neuronal protein concentrated in nerve terminals, are found in women with breast cancer associated SPS [4, 10, 11]. Autoimmunity to gephyrin, a cytosolic protein at postsynaptic inhibitory synapses, has also been described. SPS has also been reported in association with neoplasia of the colon, Hodgkin's disease, thymoma and lung [4].

Table 23.2 Differential diagnosis of SPS

Neuromyotonia, benign fasciculations and cramps
Generalised myositis fibrosa
Atypical polyradiculitis
Tetanus
Strychnine intoxication
Cramping disease (Satoyoshi's syndrome)
Hyperekplexia
Intramedullary spinal tumour
Atypical multiple sclerosis
Primary lateral sclerosis
Axial dystonia
Orthostatic tremor
Psychogenic movement disorder

23.7 Diagnosis

The diagnosis of SPS is established by clinical findings and exclusion of pyramidal and parkinsonian disorders (Table 23.2), with supportive evidence from serological and cerebrospinal fluid (CSF) testing that shows elevated anti-GAD antibodies and electrophysiological findings on EMG studies [5]. Between 60 % and 80 % of patients with SPS, SLS or PERM have serum and CSF autoantibodies to GAD [4, 7, 9]. In those patients with anti-GAD antibodies, we can find antibodies to pancreatic islet cells (50–60 %), gastric parietal cells (50 %), thyroid microsomes (30–40 %) and thyroglobulin (15 %). Oligoclonal IgG is found in the CSF in 30 % [4]. A crucial finding and an important diagnostic criterion is the presence of continuous motor unit activity that gives rise to the rigidity and persists despite attempted relaxation. It is most prominent in the axial muscles, particularly the thoracolumbar paraspinal and rectus abdominis muscles but can be found in the leg and proximal arm muscles. Peripheral nerve conduction velocities are normal. The rigidity and continuous motor unit activity lessen or even disappear during sleep and after spinal or general anaesthesia, indicating a central source [2].

Conventional magnetic resonance imaging (MRI) studies of the nervous system are usually normal. MR spectroscopy has demonstrated a significant regional decrease in GABA levels in the motor cortex, providing supportive evidence of deficient GABAergic inhibition as a pathophysiological mechanism in SPS [5].

23.8 Therapeutic Considerations

Based on the presumed pathogenesis of SPS, the two main therapeutic approaches are the following: (1) GABA-enhancing drugs and (2) immunomodulating or immunosuppressant agents. At the onset of SPS symptoms and at the time of establishing the appropriate diagnosis, diazepam or other benzodiazepines ($GABA_A$ agonists) are usually the first choice and the mainstay of therapy. Most patients respond favourably to diazepam, baclofen or similar drugs for some period of time, although they eventually require higher doses, which invariably cause drowsiness and other undesirable effects. Several reports have described a substantial beneficial effect of immunotherapies such as prednisone, plasmapheresis and high-dose IVIg in the treatment of SPS [5, 12]. More recently, several case reports have indicated that rituximab, a B-cell depleting monoclonal antibody, is well tolerated and appears to exert long-lasting clinical remissions [5, 13].

References

1. Moersch FP, Woltman HW. Progressive fluctuating muscular rigidity and spasm (stiff-man syndrome): report of a case and some observations in 13 other cases. Mayo Clin Proc. 1956;31:421–7.
2. Meinck HM, Thompson PD. Stiff man syndrome and related conditions. Mov Disord. 2002;17:853–66.
3. Donaldson IV, Marsden CD, Schneider SA, Bhatia KP. Stiff man syndromes. In: Oxford University Press, editors. Marsden's book of movement disorders. New York: Oxford University Press; 2012. p. 1287–307.
4. Thompson PD. The stiff-man syndrome and related disorders. Parkinsonism Relat Disord. 2001;8:147–53.
5. Rakocevic G, Floeter MK. Autoimmune stiff person syndrome and related myelopathies: understanding of electrophysiological and immunological processes. Muscle Nerve. 2012;45:623–34.
6. Brown P, Marsden CD. The stiff man and stiff man plus syndromes. J Neurol. 1999;246:648–52.
7. Barker RA, Revesz T, Thom M, Marsden CD, Brown P. Review of 23 patients affected by the stiff man syndrome: clinical subdivision into stiff trunk (man) syndrome, stiff limb syndrome, and progressive encephalomyelitis with rigidity. J Neurol Neurosurg Psychiatry. 1998;65:633–40.
8. Hajjioui A, Benbouazza K, Faris MA, Missaoui A, Hassouni NH. Stiff limb syndrome: a case report. Cases J. 2010;3:60.
9. Meinck HM. Stiff man syndrome. CNS Drugs. 2001;15:515–26.
10. Murinson B, Guarnaccia JB. Stiff-person syndrome with amphiphysin antibodies. Distinctive features of a rare disease. Neurology. 2008;71:1955–8.
11. Folli F. Stiff man syndrome, 40 years later. J Neurol Neurosurg Psychiatry. 1998;65:618.
12. Dalakas MC, Fujii M, Li M, Lutfi B, Kyhos J, McElroy B. High-dose intravenous immune globulin for stiff-person syndrome. N Engl J Med. 2001;345:1870–6.
13. Baker MR, Das M, Isaacs J, Fawcett PR, Bates D. Treatment of stiff-person syndrome with rituximab. J Neurol Neurosurg Psychiatry. 2005;76:999–1001.

24 Dystonia

Francesca Del Sorbo and Alberto Albanese

24.1 Definition

Dystonia is a movement disorder characterized by sustained or intermittent muscle contractions causing abnormal, often repetitive, movements, postures, or both. Dystonic movements are typically patterned, twisting, and may be tremulous. Dystonia is often initiated or worsened by voluntary action and associated with overflow muscle activation.

This recent definition [1] summarizes the hallmark features of dystonia and its recognizable phenomenology with physical signs characterized by a combination of (tonic) postures and (phasic) movements, including tremor. Dystonia has a special relationship with voluntary movements and involves further clinical features, including overflow, mirror dystonia, and gestes antagonistes (sensory tricks) (Table 24.1). The full house phenomenology typically occurs in the isolated non-acquired dystonia syndromes, particularly in recognized genetic forms (e.g., DYT1 or DYT6). Clinical recognition becomes forthright when the phenomenology is complete. Conversely, incomplete phenomenology may impede the recognition of dystonia and favor misdiagnosis with other hyperkinetic disorders, such as essential tremor, parkinsonian tremor, and myoclonus [2].

This definition takes into account the broad phenomenology of dystonia that may affect any body part. Body regions involved by dystonia are the upper or lower cranial region, the cervical region, the larynx, the trunk, the upper limbs, or the lower limbs. These different territories may be involved individually or in different combinations. The body distribution may change over time, typically with progression to the involvement of previously uninvolved sites. Although in most cases dystonia combines abnormal movements and postures, some forms of dystonia, such as blepharospasm and laryngeal dystonia, are not associated with postures and rather characterized by focal involuntary contractions that interfere with physiological opening or closing of the eyelids or the larynx.

24.2 Classification

The current classification of dystonia is based on two axes. Axis I summarizes the clinical features observed in a given patient (Fig. 24.1), whereas axis II classifies etiologies.

F. Del Sorbo, MD
Istituto Neurologico Carlo Besta,
Via Celoria 11, Milan, Italy
e-mail: francesca.delsorbo@istituto-besta.it

A. Albanese, MD (✉)
Department of Neurology, Istituto Clinico Humanitas,
Via A Manzoni 56, Rozzano, Milan, Italy

Department of Neurology, Università Cattolica del
Sacro Cuore, Milan, Italy
e-mail: alberto.albanese@unicatt.it

C. Falup-Pecurariu et al. (eds.), *Movement Disorders Curricula*,
DOI 10.1007/978-3-7091-1628-9_24

Table 24.1 Clinical hallmarks of dystonia

Clinical sign	Depiction
Dystonic (tonic) postures	A body part is flexed or twisted along its longitudinal axis (not available for blepharospasm or laryngeal dystonia). A sensation of rigidity and traction is present in the affected part
Dystonic (phasic) movements, including dystonic tremor	Movement may be fast or slow and may appear as "tremor," "tic," "chorea," or "myoclonus." The dystonic nature is revealed by recognition of a twisting nature or a pull in a preferred direction, repetitive and patterned attitude (i.e., movements are consistent and predictable); movements are often sustained at their peak to lessen when a given posture (usually opposite to the preferred direction) is identified ("null point")
	Dystonic tremor is defined as a spontaneous oscillatory, rhythmical, although often inconstant, patterned movement produced by contractions of dystonic muscles often exacerbated by an attempt to maintain primary (normal) posture. The dystonic tremor may not be relieved by allowing the abnormal dystonic posture to fully develop without resistance ("null point")
Voluntary action	Purposeful, anticipated, goal-directed movement produced by will. Dystonia is typically influenced by voluntary movement or voluntarily maintained posture, as in antigravity support
Overflow dystonia	Involuntary muscle contraction which accompanies, ipsilaterally or contralaterally, the dystonic movement or dystonic posture but is anatomically distinct from. It commonly occurs at the peak of dystonic movements or postures
Mirror dystonia	Unilateral involuntary posture or movement that is the same or similar in character to a dystonic feature. Mirror dystonia can be elicited in the unaffected or less severely affected body side by dystonia during repetitive tasks of the most affected body side. Typical tasks that can be performed to elicit this sign include finger sequence, writing, or movements resembling piano playing. Mirror dystonia may be present in all limbs, but are most common in the upper limbs, especially the hands
Sensory tricks or gestes antagonistes	Voluntary actions that specifically correct the abnormal posture or alleviate the dystonic movements. Alleviation of dystonia occurs during the geste movement, usually soon after its start and may last for as long as the geste or slowly reverses spontaneously before its end. These are usually simple movements ("gestes") involving, or directed to, the body region affected by dystonia, but not consisting in a forceful opposition to the phenomenology of dystonia. The geste movement does not push or pull the affected body part, but simply touches it ("sensory trick") or accompanies it during alleviation of dystonia

24.2.1 Axis I. Clinical Characteristics

The clinical characteristics describe the phenomenology of dystonia in a given patient. Classification along the first axis is primarily aimed to facilitate clinical recognition, diagnosis, and treatment. Once a patient is classified according to this axis, the identification of the clinical characteristics of dystonia and of the associated features defines the syndromic pattern and helps clinical orientation among the diverse presentation and associations of dystonia. Five descriptors are utilized to specify clinical characteristics: age at onset, body distribution, temporal pattern, coexistence of other movement disorders, and other neurological manifestations.

Classification by age at onset distinguishes five age groups, infancy (birth to 2 years), childhood (3–12 years), adolescence (13–20 years), early adulthood (21–40 years), and late adulthood (>40 years), with the major goal to aid diagnostic testing and determining prognosis. For example, dystonia that begins in childhood is more likely to have a discoverable cause and more likely to progress from focal to generalized. For example, dystonia that emerges during infancy, particularly the first year of life, has a very high probability of being due to an inherited metabolic disorder with specific diagnostic implications and grave prognostic consequences [3]. Dystonia that emerges between 2 and 6 years of age might be more consistent with dystonic

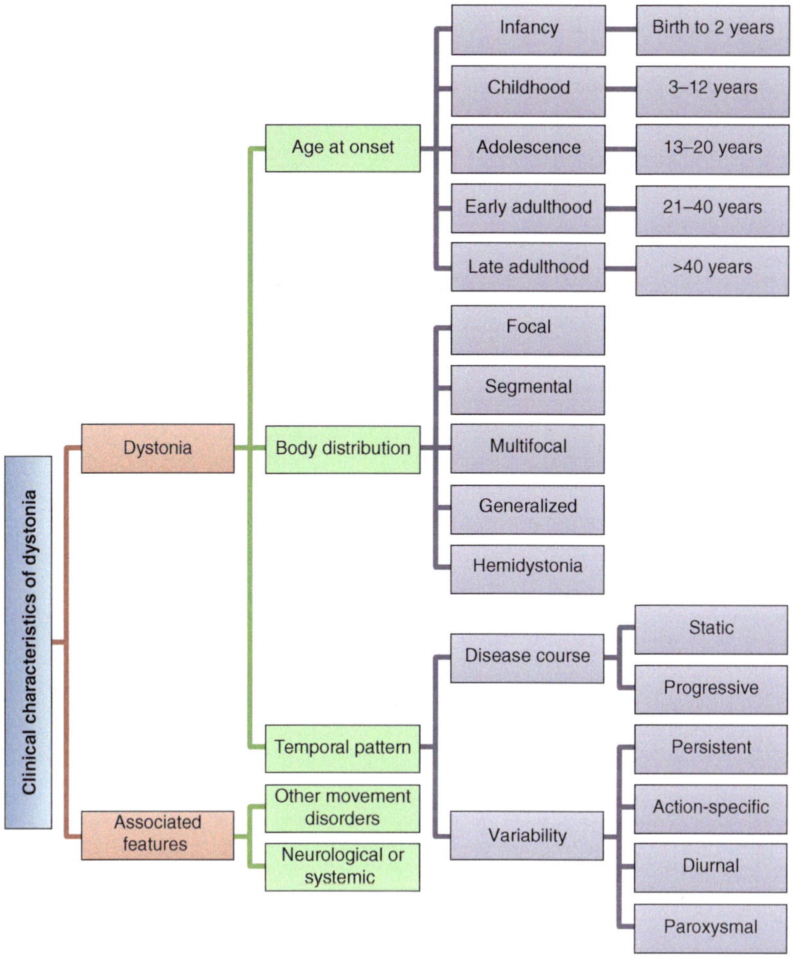

Fig. 24.1 Classification of dystonia along axis I allows to describe the clinical characteristics of dystonia observed in dystonia syndromes. This scheme provides a logical organization of the clinical features that need to be evaluated. If there are no associated movement disorders or systemic manifestations, dystonia is defined "isolated." Otherwise it is "combined" with another movement disorder or "associated" with neurological or systemic manifestations

cerebral palsy, especially if it follows a period of developmental motor delay. Other dystonia syndromes, such as dopa-responsive dystonia, tend to emerge between 6 and 14 years of age. Finally, sporadic focal dystonia usually emerges after 50 years of age.

Considering the body regions affected, dystonia may be focal (e.g., blepharospasm, oromandibular dystonia, cervical dystonia, laryngeal dystonia, and writer's cramp), segmental if two or more contiguous body regions are affected (e.g., blepharospasm with lower facial and jaw or tongue involvement or bi-brachial dystonia), multifocal if two noncontiguous or more (contiguous or not) body regions are involved, or generalized when the trunk and at least two other sites are involved. Hemidystonia is restricted to one body side (typical examples of hemidystonia are due to acquired brain lesions in the contralateral hemisphere). This type of classification has important implications for diagnosis and therapy. For example, the diagnostic considerations in adult-onset focal dystonia are very different from those in young-onset generalized dystonia. The treatment of choice for focal and segmental dystonias involves botulinum neurotoxins, while for generalized dystonias more often involves medications or surgery.

The temporal pattern is an important clinical characteristic that facilitates diagnosis and treatment choices. Important temporal characteristics are related to disease course or variability. The disease course can be either static or progressive. This terminology is particularly used by pediatric neurologists, but it also suits adult cases. In addition, variability provides descriptors on the occurrence of dystonia through the day and can have four different patterns: persistent (dystonia that persists to approximately the same extent throughout the day); action specific (dystonia that occurs only during a particular activity or task); diurnal fluctuations (dystonia fluctuates during the day, with recognizable circadian variations in occurrence, severity, and phenomenology); and paroxysmal (sudden self-limited episodes of dystonia usually induced by a trigger with return to preexisting neurological state). Paroxysmal dystonia should be distinguished from dystonia always triggered by the same activity or action (i.e., task-specific dystonia). In paroxysmal dystonia, the same trigger on different occasions might or might not induce an attack, whereas in action dystonia (including task-specific dystonia), the same motor activity will predictably induce dystonia. Paroxysmal dystonia typically lasts after the trigger has ended, while action (or task-specific) dystonia is no longer evident when the inducing action is completed.

Another important clinical descriptor of dystonia is related to its occurrence in isolation (i.e., dystonia is the only motor feature, with the exception of tremor) or in combination with other movement disorders (such as myoclonus, parkinsonism, etc.). The resulting syndromes may give rise to recognizable associations, such as isolated dystonia or dystonia with myoclonus, parkinsonism, other movement disorders, etc. The term "isolated" or "combined" refers to the phenomenology and does not carry implications about the underlying etiology. In combined forms, dystonia does not necessarily have to be the predominant movement disorder and may not be the prominent motor phenomenology (e.g., foot dystonia in Parkinson disease, mild dystonic features in myoclonus-dystonia).

A relevant step for characterizing dystonia syndromes is outlining the presence or absence of other neurologic or systemic features associated to dystonia. For example, cognitive decline is typically observed in degenerative or progressive dystonia syndromes. Wilson disease is a disorder where dystonia is typically combined with other neurological or psychiatric symptoms and liver disease [4].

24.2.2 Axis II. Etiology

The second axis addresses etiology which is an evolving area as the etiology of many forms of dystonia is still not fully understood. Two complementary characteristics have been recognized as useful for the etiological classification: identifiable anatomical changes and pattern of inheritance. Anatomical causes can be investigated using brain imaging or by pathology. Evidence of degeneration, either at the gross, microscopic, or molecular level, provides a useful means to discriminate subgroups of dystonia into degenerative forms (i.e., progressive structural abnormality, such as neuronal loss), static lesions (i.e., nonprogressive neurodevelopmental anomalies or acquired lesions), and no evidence of degeneration or structural lesion. Pattern of inheritance differentiates inherited (e.g., autosomal dominant, autosomal recessive, X-linked recessive, mitochondrial) from acquired conditions due to a known specific cause (e.g., perinatal brain injury, drugs, vascular, or psychogenic) by means of metabolic, genetic, or other tests. If there is no known cause of dystonia, this is classified as idiopathic, namely, sporadic or familial. Many cases of focal or segmental isolated dystonia with onset in adulthood fall in this category. The most common forms of focal dystonia can have sporadic or familial occurrence.

Inherited dystonias are of proven genetic origin. Dystonia genes are listed with different coding systems, such as the DYTs, the PARKs, the PNKDs, or with non-systematic acronyms. The DYT listing, originally created to encompass the monogenic dystonia syndromes, cannot be considered as comprehensive or exhaustive at present [5, 6] (Table 24.2).

Table 24.2 Synopsis of the most common genetic forms of dystonia

Disease (OMIM)[a]	Gene/locus[b]	Main phenomenology	Transmission[c]
Isolated dystonia			
DYT1 (128100)	TOR1A	Generalized childhood limb-onset dystonia	AD
DYT2 (224500)	None	Childhood/early adulthood-onset generalized dystonia with prominent cranial-cervical involvement	AR
DYT4 (128101)	TUBB4	Adolescence/early adulthood-onset focal, segmental, generalized dystonia with prominent laryngeal involvement (whispering dysphonia)	AD
DYT6 (602629)	THAP1	Adolescence/early adulthood-onset mixed-type dystonia	AD
DYT7 (602124)	18p	Adult-onset focal dystonia	AD
DYT13 (607671)	1p36.13–36.32	Childhood/early adulthood-onset mixed-type dystonia	AD
DYT17 (612406)	20p11.2–q13.12	Adolescent-onset segmental or generalized dystonia with severe dysphonia	AR
DYT21 (614588)	2q14.3–q21.3	Adolescence/adult-onset mixed dystonia	AD
DYT23 (614860)	CIZ1	Adolescence/adult-onset cervical dystonia	AD
DYT24 (615034)	ANO3	Childhood/adult-onset craniocervical, segmental dystonia	AD
DYT25 (615073)	GNAL	Childhood/adult-onset craniocervical, segmental, generalized dystonia	AD
Combined dystonia			
DYT5 (128230)	GCH1	Childhood-onset dopa-responsive dystonia	AD
THD (605407)	TH	Infancy/childhood-onset dopa-responsive dystonia	AR
SPR (612716)	SPR	Dopa-responsive dystonia	AR
DYT11 (159900)	SGCE	Childhood/adolescence-onset myoclonus-dystonia	AD
DYT15 (607488)	18p11	Myoclonus-dystonia	AD
RDP (128235)	ATP1A3	Childhood/adolescence rapid-onset dystonia-parkinsonism	AD
DYT3 (314250)	TAF1	Adult-onset dystonia-parkinsonism	XR
DYT16 (612067)	PRKRA	Childhood/adolescence-onset dystonia-parkinsonism	AR
DTDS (613135)	SLC6A3	Childhood/adult-onset parkinsonism-dystonia	AR
PARK2 (602544)	PRKN	Childhood/early adulthood-onset parkinsonism with limb dystonia	AR
PARK6 (605909)	PINK1	Childhood/late adult-onset parkinsonism with limb dystonia	AR
PARK7 (606324)	DJ1	Childhood/early adulthood-onset parkinsonism with limb dystonia	AR
PNKD1 (118800)	MR1	Infancy/childhood-onset paroxysmal non-kinesigenic dystonia-choreoathetosis	AD
PKD2 (611031)	16q	Childhood/adolescence-onset paroxysmal kinesigenic dystonia-choreoathetosis	AD
Dystonia with other neurological or systemic manifestations			
PNKD2 (611147)	2q31	Childhood/late adult-onset paroxysmal non-kinesigenic dystonia mainly of hands and feet, possible migraines and seizures	AD

(continued)

Table 24.2 (continued)

Disease (OMIM)[a]	Gene/locus[b]	Main phenomenology	Transmission[c]
GLUT1DS2 (612126)	SLC2A1	Childhood-onset paroxysmal exercise-induced dystonia-choreoathetosis with or without epilepsy and/or hemolytic anemia	AD
PKD1 (128200)	PRRT2	Childhood/adolescence-onset paroxysmal kinesigenic dystonia-choreoathetosis and infantile convulsions	AD
AT (208900)	ATM	Childhood-onset cerebellar ataxia, oculocutaneous telangiectases, choreoathetosis, dystonia, myoclonus, oculomotor abnormalities, seizures, short stature, delayed puberty, diabetes mellitus, lymphocytopenia, immune defects, predisposition to neoplasia, and sinopulmonary infections. AT variant with isolated dystonia may be present	AR
CHAC (200150)	VPS13A	Adult-onset parkinsonism, orofacial dyskinesias, dystonia, choreoathetosis, tics, seizures, hyporeflexia, psychosis, possible dementia, acanthocytes, increased creatine kinase	AR
CLF (204200)	CLN3	Childhood-onset cerebral atrophy, macular degeneration, optic atrophy, retinitis pigmentosa, mental retardation, dementia, parkinsonism, myoclonus, cerebellar signs, seizures, concentric hypertrophic cardiomyopathy	AR
DDS (304700)	TIMM8A	Childhood-onset progressive deafness, dystonia, spasticity, mental retardation	XR
DPRLA (125370)	ATN1	Childhood/adult-onset cerebellar ataxia, choreoathetosis, myoclonus, dementia, seizures	AD
FC (230000)	FUCA1	Infancy-onset progressive psychomotor retardation, seizures, neuropathy, spastic quadriplegia, angiokeratoma, coarse facial features, dysostosis multiplex, hearing loss, cardiomegaly, hepatomegaly, splenomegaly, increased urine oligosaccharides, alpha-L-fucosidase deficiency	AR
GA (231670)	GCDH	Infancy-onset encephalopathy, choreoathetosis, dystonia, opisthotonus, spastic diplegia, hepatomegaly, glutaric aciduria, glutaryl-CoA dehydrogenase deficiency, metabolic acidosis, ketonemia, ketonuria, hypoglycemia	AR
HD (143100)	IT-15	Childhood/adult-onset chorea, dystonia, dementia, behavioral disorders, abnormal eye movement; parkinsonism, seizures, ataxic gait (juvenile form)	AD
HDL2 (606438)	JPH3	Adult-onset chorea, dystonia, parkinsonism, dementia	AD

Table 24.2 (continued)

Disease (OMIM)[a]	Gene/locus[b]	Main phenomenology	Transmission[c]
LHON (535000)	Several genes	Childhood/adult-onset optic atrophy, tremor, dystonia, ataxia, neuropathy, cardiac arrhythmia	M
LNS (300322)	HPRT	Mental retardation, motor delay, spasticity, choreoathetosis, dystonia, parkinsonism, self-injurious behavior, hyperuricemia, hyperuricosuria	XR
LS (256000)	Several genes	Infancy/childhood-onset, rapid progression, clinical heterogeneity	M or AR
MLD (250100)	ARSA	Infantile, juvenile, and adult forms with clinical heterogeneity	AR
NFP (606159)	FTL	Neurodegeneration with brain iron accumulation type 3	AD
NPC1 (257220)	NPC1	Infantile, juvenile, or adult forms with clinical heterogeneity. Mental retardation, motor delay, spasticity, ataxia, loss of speech, seizures. myoclonic jerks, dystonia, vertical supranuclear gaze palsy, dementia, and psychiatric manifestations, hepatosplenomegaly, cholestatic jaundice	AR
NPC2 (607625)	HE1	Variable age of onset and phenotype. Developmental delay, loss of speech, mental deterioration, dementia, psychosis, spasticity, dystonia, seizures, cerebellar ataxia, cataplexy, vertical supranuclear gaze palsy, hepatosplenomegaly, pulmonary involvement	AR
PARK14	PLA2G6	Neurodegeneration with brain iron accumulation type 2	AR
PKAN (234200)	PANK2	Neurodegeneration with brain iron accumulation type 1	AR
PMD (312080)	PLP1	Infancy-onset progressive pyramidal and cerebellar signs, optic atrophy, rotary nystagmus, "rolling" head tremor, dystonia, choreoathetosis, parkinsonian, mental retardation, psychomotor delay or deterioration	XR
RTT (312750)	MECP2	Mental retardation, motor delay, autism, seizures, spasticity, ataxia, dystonia, autistic behavior, ECG, respiratory and autonomic abnormalities	XD
SCA17 (607136)	TBP	Adolescence/early adulthood-onset ataxia, parkinsonism, dystonia, chorea, myoclonus, ocular movement abnormalities, seizures, dementia, psychiatric symptoms	AD
SCA3 (109150)	ATXN3	Adult-onset ataxia, spasticity, parkinsonism, dystonia, ocular movement abnormalities, neuropathy, bladder disturbances	AD
SCA6 (183086)	CACNA1A	Adult-onset ataxia, chorea, spasticity, dystonia, ocular movement abnormalities	AD

(continued)

Table 24.2 (continued)

Disease (OMIM)[a]	Gene/locus[b]	Main phenomenology	Transmission[c]
TSD (272800)	HEXA	Infancy-onset paralysis, psychomotor degeneration, dementia, seizures, blindness, Gm2-ganglioside accumulation, hexosaminidase A deficiency	AR
WD (277900)	ATP7B	Tremor, dystonia, parkinsonian features, dementia, visceral and skeletal abnormalities, copper abnormalities, Kayser-Fleischer ring	AR

The gene name is indicated whenever possible; otherwise, the locus is reported

[a]Abbreviations: *AT* ataxia-telangiectasia, *CHAC* choreoacanthocytosis, *CLF* ceroid-lipofuscinosis, *DDS* dystonia-deafness syndrome, *DPRLA* dentatorubral-pallidoluysian atrophy, *DTDS* dopamine transporter deficiency syndrome, *GA* glutaricacidemia, *GLUT1DS2* GLUT1 deficiency syndrome 2, *FC* fucosidosis, *HD* Huntington's disease, *HDL2* Huntington-like disease type 2, *LHON* Leber hereditary optic neuropathy, *LNS* Lesch-Nyhan syndrome, *LS* Leigh syndrome, *MLD* metachromatic leukodystrophy, *NFP* neuroferritinopathy, *NPC1* Niemann-Pick type C1, *NPC2* Niemann-Pick type C2, *PARK2* Parkinson disease 2, *PARK6* Parkinson disease 6, *PKAN* pantothenate kinase-associated neurodegeneration, *PKD1* paroxysmal kinesigenic dyskinesia 1, *PKD2* paroxysmal kinesigenic dyskinesia 2, *PMD* Pelizaeus-Merzbacher disease, *PNKD1* paroxysmal non-kinesigenic dyskinesia 1, *PNKD2* paroxysmal non-kinesigenic dyskinesia 2, *RDP* rapid-onset dystonia-parkinsonism, *RTT* Rett syndrome, *SPR* sepiapterin reductase deficiency, *THD* tyrosine hydroxylase deficiency, *TSD* Tay-Sachs disease, *WD* Wilson disease

[b]Abbreviations: *ARSA* arylsulfatase A, *ATM* ataxia-telangiectasia mutated gene, *ATN1* atrophin 1, *ATP1A3* ATPase, Na+/K+ transporting, *ATP7B* ATPase, Cu^{++}-transporting beta polypeptide, *ATX3* ataxin-3, *CACNA1A* calcium channel, voltage-dependent, *p/q type* alpha-1a subunit, *CLN3* CLN3 gene, *DJ1* oncogene DJ1, *FUCA1* alpha-L-fucosidase 1, *FTL* ferritin light chain, *GCH1* guanosine triphosphate cyclohydrolase 1, *GCDH* glutaryl-CoA dehydrogenase, *HE1* epididymal secretory protein, *HEXA* hexosaminidase A alpha polypeptide, *HPRT* hypoxanthine guanine phosphoribosyltransferase 1, *IT-15* important transcript 15 (huntingtin), *JPH3* junctophilin 3, *MECP2* methyl-CpG-binding protein 2, *MR1* myofibrillogenesis regulator 1 gene, *NPC1* Niemann-Pick type C1 gene, *PANK2* pantothenate kinase 2, *PRKN* parkin, *PRKRA* double-stranded RNA-activated protein kinase, *PRRT2* proline-rich transmembrane protein 2, *PLA2G6* phospholipase A2 group VI, *PLP1* proteolipid protein 1, *SLC2A1* solute carrier family 2 (facilitated glucose transporter), member 1, *SPR* sepiapterin reductase deficiency, *SGCE* ε-sarcoglycan, *TAF1* TATA boxing-binding protein associated factor, *TBP* TATA box-binding protein, *TH* tyrosine hydroxylase, *THAP1* thanatos-associated protein, *TIMM8A* translocase of inner mitochondrial membrane 8, *TOR1A* torsin A gene, *VPS13A* vacuolar protein sorting 13

[c]Transmission: *AD* autosomal dominant, *AR* autosomal recessive, *M* mitochondrial, *XR* X-linked recessive

The most common forms of inherited dystonias are, among the autosomal dominant forms, DYT1, DYT5, DYT6, DYT11, rapid-onset dystonia-parkinsonism (DYT12), neuroferritinopathy (NBIA3), dentatorubral-pallidoluysian atrophy, and Huntington disease. The most common forms of autosomal recessive inherited dystonias encompass Wilson disease, PKAN (NBIA1), PLAN (NBIA2), and type 2 juvenile Parkinson disease (PARK2), and various metabolic disorders. Inherited dystonia with X-linked transmission encompass forms such as Lubag (DYT3), Lesch-Nyhan syndrome, and Mohr-Tranebjaerg syndrome. Finally, mitochondrial forms, such as Leigh syndrome or Leber optic atrophy and dystonia, also give rise to inherited dystonias.

The most common idiopathic forms are the isolated focal dystonias that usually have adult-onset and limited tendency to spread. Cervical dystonia (also called "torticollis") involves the cervical muscles, resulting in abnormal head, neck, and shoulder positions [7]; cranial dystonia may affect the orbicularis oculi ("blepharospasm") and is often accompanied by contractions of the surrounding muscles, such as the procerus and the corrugator [8]; oromandibular dystonia affects the mouth, tongue, or the jaw in isolation or in combination [9, 10]; laryngeal dystonia (also known as "spasmodic dysphonia") affects phonatory muscles [11]; "occupational cramps" (e.g., writer's cramp, musician's cramp) are task-specific forms of dystonia affecting the upper limb [12]. The syndromes of late (adult)-

onset isolated focal dystonia are usually sporadic without an identifiable cause and rarely progress to generalization, although they can spread to involve contiguous body regions (segmental distribution).

The most common forms of acquired dystonias are due to perinatal brain injury (dystonic cerebral palsy, delayed-onset dystonia), infection (viral encephalitis, encephalitis lethargica, subacute sclerosing panencephalitis, human immunodeficiency virus infection, tuberculosis, syphilis, etc.), drug (levodopa and dopamine agonists, neuroleptics (dopamine receptor-blocking drugs), anticonvulsants, and calcium channel blockers), toxic (manganese, cobalt, carbon disulfide, cyanide, methanol, disulfiram, and 3-nitropropionic acid), vascular (ischemia, hemorrhage, and arteriovenous malformation including aneurysm), neoplastic (brain tumor, and paraneoplastic encephalitis), brain injury (head trauma, brain surgery including stereotactic ablations, and electrical injury), and psychogenic (functional).

24.3 Diagnosis

The diagnosis of dystonia is clinical, as there is no specific diagnostic test allowing to confirm the diagnosis. Therefore, expert clinical examination is warranted [13]. The diagnosis is made by searching for the cardinal physical signs that constitute the hallmark of dystonia and are summarized in Table 24.1. These signs have to be looked for in all movement disorders, either fast or slow, also when the immediate clinical impression is that of a "tremor," "tic," "chorea," or "myoclonus." In this diagnostic process, disorders that may mimic dystonia (pseudodystonia), such as those due to spasms, orthopedic, or neuromuscular disorders, should be ruled out [1]. In fact, these conditions result in abnormal movements, postures, or spasm, which are not associated with the specific phenomenology of dystonia.

Although the recognition of dystonia is based on clinical features and neurophysiological tests are not routinely recommended for the diagnosis, electromyography (EMG) mapping from various muscles may contribute to the clinical assessment by showing some characteristic features of dystonia [13]. EMG can complement clinical observation and can be useful to distinguish the three types of abnormal activation (tonic, phasic, and tremulous) that correspond to the homonymous clinical features [14], to detect features of dystonia such as co-activation of agonist muscles with greater detail than allowed by visual inspection, to differentiate different types of tremors from myoclonus and dystonia, and finally to identify the muscles involved and the actual disease topography [15]. Therefore, the observation of EMG abnormalities typical of dystonia is helpful when the clinical features are considered insufficient to the diagnosis [16].

Once a diagnosis of dystonia has been made, the next step is to delineate the clinical dystonia syndrome [17]. A careful delineation of the syndromic pattern, along with neuroimaging characteristics, is important because it aids in narrowing down the long list of potential etiologies for more targeted diagnostic testing.

For patients with isolated dystonia, the investigation process depends on the age at onset, the body distribution, and whether there are affected family members. In adults with focal or segmental dystonia only, no diagnostic tests are required because they usually are unrevealing [18]. In adults with hemidystonia or generalized dystonia, neuroimaging is useful because the likelihood of disclosing a structural cause is higher. The diagnostic approach in younger individuals with isolated dystonia is quite different, because there is a much higher likelihood of disclosing a cause [19]. Neuroimaging is important for all early-onset cases, regardless of body distribution. Genetic testing may be performed after establishing the clinical diagnosis. The EFNS guidelines provide indications for performing genetic testing [13]. TOR1A testing is recommended for patients with early-onset limb isolated dystonia and in those with an affected relative with early-onset dystonia. THAP1 testing is recommended in early-onset or familial cases with craniocervical dystonia or after exclusion of DYT1. Individuals with early-onset myoclonus should be tested for mutations in the SGCE gene. If direct sequencing of the SGCE gene is negative, additional gene dosage is required to improve the proportion of mutations detected. A levodopa trial is warranted in every patient with early-onset isolated dystonia without an alternative diagnosis. In sporadic adult-onset isolated dystonias, the chance of finding a genetic cause is less than 2 %, so genetic testing usually is not cost-effective, unless there are other affected family members [19].

For all patients in whom dystonia is combined with other neurologic or systemic features, some additional investigation work-up is warranted, regardless of the age at onset or body distribution. The laboratory work-up depends on the nature of the associated features and the age at onset. More than 100 different syndromes with combined dystonia have been recognized [17]. Neuroimaging is useful in virtually all combined dystonias, because it can provide important diagnostic clues [20]. Metal deposition can be detected by neuroimaging on computed tomography (e.g., copper) or MRI (e.g., iron) [21]. Presynaptic dopaminergic scan (DAT or ^{18}FDOPA) is useful to differentiate between dopa-responsive dystonia and juvenile Parkinson disease presenting with dystonia [22]. This can also be useful to distinguish dystonic tremor from parkinsonian tremor [13]. In combined dystonia syndromes, laboratory testing is useful and should be targeted on the syndromic pattern. For example, dystonia combined with parkinsonism leads to a list of disorders for more targeted diagnostic testing such as DRD, Wilson disease, genetic forms of parkinsonism which often have young-onset and recessive inheritance (PARK2, 6, and 7), X-linked dystonia-parkinsonism/Lubag (DYT3), rapid-onset dystonia-parkinsonism (DYT12), and neurodegeneration with brain iron accumulation (including PANK2- and PLA2G6-associated neurodegeneration, neuroferritinopathy, and others) [21].

When a specific etiology cannot be determined, it is important to follow patients and revise the diagnosis as additional clinical features are recognized. Many combined dystonic disorders may present first with what appears to be isolated dystonia, and additional clinical features may develop over the following months or years as in the case of parkinsonian syndromes, in which isolated limb dystonia may be the presenting feature [22]. In Parkin disease, particularly, dystonia at onset may occur in over 40 % of cases [23]. It is not until other clinical features emerge that the diagnosis becomes more obvious.

Conclusions

The diagnosis of dystonia remains a difficult exercise. The new classification scheme helps in supporting the identification of dystonia syndromes in the clinical setting. A careful evaluation is needed for all patients with dystonia along axis I guidance, in order to identify uncommon subtypes where specific etiology-based treatments can dramatically alter the course of the disorder. Botulinum toxins are the treatment of choice for most focal and segmental dystonias and may be used also to target specific regions in patients with broader spread. Deep brain stimulation and other surgical procedures are available when oral medications and botulinum toxins provide inadequate relief of symptoms.

References

1. Albanese A, Bhatia K, Bressman SB, Delong MR, Fahn S, Fung VS, et al. Phenomenology and classification of dystonia: a consensus update. Mov Disord. 2013;28(7):863–73.
2. Lalli S, Albanese A. The diagnostic challenge of primary dystonia: evidence from misdiagnosis. Mov Disord. 2010;25(11):1619–26.
3. Sanger TD. Pathophysiology of pediatric movement disorders. J Child Neurol. 2003;18 Suppl 1:S9–24.
4. Weiss EM, Hershey T, Karimi M, Racette B, Tabbal SD, Mink JW, et al. Relative risk of spread of symptoms among the focal onset primary dystonias. Mov Disord. 2006;21(8):1175–81.
5. Elia AE, Lalli S, Albanese A. Differential diagnosis of dystonia. Eur J Neurol. 2010;17 Suppl 1:1–8.
6. Klein C. Genetics in dystonia. Parkinsonism Relat Disord. 2014;20 Suppl 1:S137–42.

7. Stacy M. Epidemiology, clinical presentation, and diagnosis of cervical dystonia. Neurol Clin. 2008;26 Suppl 1:23–42.
8. Peckham EL, Lopez G, Shamim EA, Richardson SP, Sanku S, Malkani R, et al. Clinical features of patients with blepharospasm: a report of 240 patients. Eur J Neurol. 2011;18(3):382–6.
9. Papapetropoulos S, Singer C. Primary focal lingual dystonia. Mov Disord. 2006;21(3):429–30.
10. Singer C, Papapetropoulos S. A comparison of jaw-closing and jaw-opening idiopathic oromandibular dystonia. Parkinsonism Relat Disord. 2006;12(2):115–8.
11. Ludlow CL. Spasmodic dysphonia: a laryngeal control disorder specific to speech. J Neurosci. 2011;31(3):793–7.
12. Torres-Russotto D, Perlmutter JS. Focal dystonias of the hand and upper extremity. J Hand Surg Am. 2008;33(9):1657–8.
13. Albanese A, Asmus F, Bhatia KP, Elia AE, Elibol B, Filippini G, et al. EFNS guidelines on diagnosis and treatment of primary dystonias. Eur J Neurol. 2011; 18(1):5–18.
14. Deuschl G, Heinen F, Kleedorfer B, Wagner M, Lucking CH, Poewe W. Clinical and polymyographic investigation of spasmodic torticollis. J Neurol. 1992;239(1):9–15.
15. Pullman SL, Goodin DS, Marquinez AI, Tabbal S, Rubin M. Clinical utility of surface EMG: report of the therapeutics and technology assessment subcommittee of the American Academy of Neurology. Neurology. 2000;55(2):171–7.
16. Albanese A, Barnes MP, Bhatia KP, Fernandez-Alvarez E, Filippini G, Gasser T, et al. A systematic review on the diagnosis and treatment of primary (idiopathic) dystonia and dystonia plus syndromes: report of an EFNS/MDS-ES task force. Eur J Neurol. 2006;13(5):433–44.
17. Fung VS, Jinnah HA, Bhatia K, Vidailhet M. Assessment of patients with isolated or combined dystonia: an update on dystonia syndromes. Mov Disord. 2013;28(7):889–98.
18. Jinnah HA, Berardelli A, Comella C, Defazio G, Delong MR, Factor S, et al. The focal dystonias: current views and challenges for future research. Mov Disord. 2013;28(7):926–43.
19. Jinnah HA, Factor SA. Diagnosis and treatment of dystonia. Neurol Clin. 2015;33(1):77–100.
20. Stoessl AJ, Lehericy S, Strafella AP. Imaging insights into basal ganglia function, Parkinson's disease, and dystonia. Lancet. 2014;384(9942):532–44.
21. Schneider SA, Bhatia KP. Secondary dystonia-clinical clues and syndromic associations. J Mov Disord. 2009;2(2):58–63.
22. Elia AE, Del SF, Romito LM, Barzaghi C, Garavaglia B, Albanese A. Isolated limb dystonia as presenting feature of Parkin disease. J Neurol Neurosurg Psychiatry. 2014;85(7):827–8.
23. Khan NL, Graham E, Critchley P, Schrag AE, Wood NW, Lees AJ, et al. Parkin disease: a phenotypic study of a large case series. Brain. 2003;126(Pt 6): 1279–92.

Huntington's Disease

25

Michael Orth

25.1 Introduction

George Huntington, in a family from New England, gave a detailed account of the phenotype of an inherited movement disorder with cognitive impairment and behavioural problems that progress relentlessly until death [1]. This disorder now bears his name, Huntington's disease (HD). HD is the most common inherited cause of chorea. The genetic mutation causing HD was first mapped to chromosome 4 in 1983 [2] with the gene and its mutation identified as a CAG repeat expansion in the *HTT* gene in 1993 [3].

25.2 Clinical Manifestations

Most carriers of the *HTT* mutation develop clinical signs of HD between the ages of 30 and 50. However, there are very early, so-called juvenile, forms of HD with onset before the age of 20 [4], as well as late-onset variants with onset later than age 60 [5]. The clinical spectrum of HD comprises progressive motor dysfunction with a mixed movement disorder that consists of chorea, dystonia, bradykinesia and rigidity, clumsiness, a swallowing disorder and gait and balance problems with falls. Patients invariably develop dementia with personality changes and progressive loss of autonomy, while behavioural problems such as depression or irritability are present in many, but not all, patients. In addition, urge incontinence and bowel problems, weight loss, as well as insensitivity to pain may develop; in the absence of an alternative explanation, these clinical features are probably also due to HD. In the following, the clinical features of HD will be divided into clinical domains bearing in mind that in practice this distinction may not always be this clear.

25.2.1 Motor Domain

The motor phenotype consists in most patients of chorea and dystonia. Hence, HD is considered a predominantly hyperkinetic movement disorder. Chorea is generalised and often involves the face, mouth, tongue, trunk and arms more than the legs (Video 25.1). Patients find it difficult to maintain a posture; motor impersistence affects the eyes, the tongue or the limbs. Commonly, chorea is

Disclosure The author reports no conflict of interest.

Electronic supplementary material The online version of this chapter (doi:10.1007/978-3-7091-1628-9_25) contains supplementary material, which is available to authorized users.

M. Orth, MD, PhD
Department of Neurology and European Huntington's Disease Network, Ulm University Hospital, Oberer Eselsberg 45/1, 89081 Ulm, Germany

Department of Neurology, University of Ulm, Ulm, Germany
e-mail: michael.orth@uni-ulm.de

C. Falup-Pecurariu et al. (eds.), *Movement Disorders Curricula*,
DOI 10.1007/978-3-7091-1628-9_25

accompanied by a degree of dystonia in particular cervical dystonia. Parkinsonian features – bradykinesia and rigidity – are also not uncommon and can be the most prominent motor sign in some patients, e.g. those with juvenile onset but also in other patients with a later onset (see Video 25.2) or in late stages of the disease.

A characteristic feature of HD is the oculomotor disorder. In addition to gaze impersistence – the patient finds it difficult to maintain eye contact, and the eyes seem choreatic – patients may have to induce voluntary externally or internally triggered eye movements with a blink or head movements (Video 25.3). These head movements or eye blinking can be suppressed to a certain degree, but eventually patients may be incapable of initiating saccades without turning their head. This can resemble oculomotor apraxia.

25.2.2 Cognitive Domain

Cognition is invariably affected over the course of HD (for a review, see [6]). Some people develop cognitive impairment early on before a diagnosis of motor manifest HD is made [7]. In some this may be the first sign of manifest HD, while others seem less impaired until they are further advanced. Once evident cognitive skills decline until every HD patient has developed dementia. Executive dysfunction is typical in HD. Planning and organising their daily activities and chores becomes increasingly challenging, and patients are easily overwhelmed when mental flexibility is required, e.g. in dealing with multiple tasks that they have to attend to at the same time. This can be a complaint at the workplace where it may be noted that the affected individual has slowed down, achieving less and less even when working more hours. The patient may only be able to deal with one task at a time having difficulty to switch attention efficiently. The patient may note these shortcomings himself; as a consequence, self-esteem may suffer, and frustration may rise with irritability, anger or depression. Mental inflexibility can develop into perseveration and a lack of will, and executive dysfunction can develop into apathy (see below).

As the disease progresses, patients become more self-centred and fail to see other people's point of view. The perception of self and others changes, as does the ability to monitor self-appearance and the consequences of actions, e.g. regarding the social surroundings. Patients may progressively neglect themselves. This includes grooming, personal hygiene and eating but also their relationships with others, in particular their family and carers. This may be related to deficits of emotion recognition abilities [8], in particular concerning negative emotions, as a result of which the relationship with family and carers can suffer a loss of empathy and connectedness when the patient increasingly needs support and, at the same time, changes as a person (for a review, see [9]). Not all cognitive abilities decline at the same speed. Language skills, for instance, may be preserved much longer than executive skills. However, as in other forms of dementia, HD patients gradually lose their autonomy and become dependent on carers and family.

It is important to distinguish attention deficits with subsequent cognitive impairment from primary cognitive deficits [10]. Inattention and loss of energy and drive can be important features of depression and can affect cognitive performance. In any HD patient with cognitive impairment, in particular when this evolved rapidly at early disease stages, a mood disorder has to be considered and treated. Psychosis may be another explanation for a (treatable) loss of cognitive skills and can be difficult to diagnose clinically (see below).

25.2.3 Neuropsychiatric Manifestations

The motor signs of HD may be the most noticeable. However, together with the cognitive features of HD, the main neuropsychiatric aspects of HD – depression, anxiety, irritability and aggression, perseveration, apathy and psychosis – are very often more troublesome. They have a higher negative impact on quality of life for patients, families and caregivers than the motor manifestations [6, 11]. Consistent with clinical impression, systematic data analysis, using, e.g.

principle component analysis, confirms that neuropsychiatric symptoms in HD can be differentiated into those that pertain to affect, irritability/aggression and apathy [12–14]. With the exception of apathy, behavioural abnormalities may be common but are not invariably part of HD. This may relate to the episodic nature of many behavioural problems, e.g. depression or psychosis, which are amenable to treatment.

25.2.4 Affective Disorders

The most common affective disorder in HD is depression. Anxiety may also be very common but is very often part of a depressive disorder from which it is therefore difficult to disentangle. Depression can occur at any point in time during the course of HD, with its severity ranging from sub-threshold depressive symptoms to major depressive disorder (MDD) [15]. The description of George Huntington already emphasised that suicide was a serious risk in HD [1]. Suicidal ideation is probably very common in HD with data suggesting that maybe a third of HD patients entertain suicidal ideas in their lifetime [16–18]. Low mood is a predictor for suicidal ideas; hence, screening for the core symptoms of depression is important. However, many people with HD, in particular in the preclinical phase, consider suicide an option should they lose their autonomy when the disease manifests. Considering the inevitability of a relentlessly progressive loss of abilities once HD manifests suicide as a way out of this conundrum can reassure people with HD that they retain a degree of control over their fate.

25.2.5 Irritability and Aggression

Relatives and carers of HD patients often report that irritability and outbursts of verbal and physical aggression are the most difficult behavioural challenge. People with HD sometimes observe themselves, particularly when insight is preserved, that they have developed mood swings where they feel extreme anger irresistibly welling up within them leading to an explosive outburst with verbal abuse and aggression towards objects or even towards other people. This is then followed by remorse, sadness and, sometimes, even ideas of suicide. This resembles rage attacks in the context of impaired impulse control in other contexts. Often the hostility and aggression is directed towards those closest to the patient. Once insight is lost, it is then mainly the family and carers of patients that report such behaviour. The behaviour can go on for a long time, often hours or even days, and is out of proportion to the preceding, often only very minor, provocation or inconvenience. A simple reminder about a trivial task can suffice to spark an outburst. People around the patient have to change their behaviour, and, when untreated, irritability and aggression can estrange the patient emotionally from those he or she most depends on. As a consequence, family and carers may feel that they cannot cope with the situation so that the patient may no longer be able to live at home.

25.2.6 Apathy

Apathy denotes a lack of interest, feeling, drive, emotion or concern. Some patients experience this as very unpleasant and suffer from apathy, e.g. in the context of depression. Others may have lost insight and are not concerned, quite in contrast to their relatives. If pronounced this cluster of symptoms more resembles abulia in that patients lack the will to do anything. In HD, apathy develops insidiously so that it may take some time for the symptoms to become noticeable. When they do, however, apathy can be a very frustrating problem of HD for family and carers [6]. The patient has lost his interest in his hobbies, spends more time doing very little, and needs a push from those around him. If not reminded by others, the patient may neglect personal hygiene, grooming and even eating. He may spend a lot of time watching TV and may not even be bothered to change the channel. In contrast to family and carers, the patient is not unduly concerned by his lack of will.

25.2.7 Perseveration and Obsessive-Compulsive Disorder

Obsessive-compulsive disorder (OCD) is an anxiety disorder. Patients feel they have to do certain things, dwell on a thought, recall an experience or ruminate on something abstract (ICD-10; http://www.who.int/classifications/icd/en/). Characteristically, at the expense of mounting levels of anxiety, patients need to resist such behaviour or thinking, which is qualified as alien to his or her personality. Some of the obsessive behaviours aim to relieve anxiety, worry, fear, or uneasiness in a ritualistic way, e.g. washing in response to fear of contamination. OCD in patients with HD may not be more common than in the general population. However, repetitive behaviours that do not follow on from anxiety-provoking thoughts and are characteristically not perceived as alien or abnormal are very common in HD [6]. The distinction from OCD is important because the underlying pathophysiological concepts and management differ between OCD and perseveration. Perseverative behaviours are most commonly reported by family and carers. The patient, very often when a degree of dementia has already developed, gets stuck on certain ideas or behaviours and is not easily redirected. He prefers certain routines in his day-to-day life and may react angrily if forced to vary from this routine. Simple things such as an appointment with the doctor can provoke discomfort and sleepless nights, and together with a loss of the sense of time the patient may be restless and urging for the departure for that appointment hours before it would actually be necessary. He may repeatedly ask the same questions or get stuck on a certain topic about which he will go on and on. Without prompting he may return to this topic later in the day, or sometimes even the next day, and will again dwell on this for a long time. While the patient may be unfazed, such perseverative behaviours can cause major distress to family and carers.

25.2.8 Psychosis

Psychosis in HD strikingly resembles schizophrenia with delusions, auditory hallucinations, disordered thinking, social withdrawal and emotional blunting. The prevalence figures for psychosis in HD vary between 3 and 11 % (see [6, 19]). However, the prevalence of psychosis in HD is much lower than for other neuropsychiatric symptoms (see above). Similar to major depressive episodes, the diagnosis of schizophrenia in HD is difficult and, according to the various diagnostic guidelines such as ICD or DSM, not recommended because of the organic basis of HD. Clinically, it can be challenging to distinguish apathy and emotional changes in the context of the degenerative dementia in HD from negative symptoms as a sign of a psychotic episode in particular in the absence of clear evidence of delusions or/and hallucinations. Psychosis can occur at any time in HD including the motor premanifest phase. Hence, prominent negative symptoms and disordered thinking with a rather abrupt onset in an HD patient in whom cognition seemed until then fairly intact raises the possibility of a psychosis in particular if there is no evidence to suggest the presence of a mood disorder. Considering the impact on quality of life, a suspicion of psychosis merits empirical treatment, which can sometimes clarify that distinction.

25.3 Juvenile HD

Juvenile HD (JHD) is often defined as HD with an age at onset before age 20. This age cutoff is arbitrary. More importantly, JHD affects individuals who are still developing intellectually, emotionally and as socially competent independent persons. This may help understand some of the clinical phenomena but also the enormous implications of JHD for the patient and the affected family [4].

Fortunately, JHD is rare. Depending on the epidemiological study, between 1 and 10 % of HD patients have JHD while childhood HD (onset before age 10) may be even rarer [20]. JHD can manifest before unequivocal signs of HD become apparent in a parent; most commonly, JHD is inherited from an affected father.

Clinically, as in adult-onset HD, patients have a mixed movement disorder, cognitive impairment and behavioural abnormalities. However, there are important differences between the phenotype of adult-onset HD and JHD. Instead of chorea, which, if it is present, appears fairly late, a hypokinetic rigid syndrome, dystonia, ataxia and tremor predominate (Videos 25.2 and 25.4). A considerable number of patients with JHD (about 30 %) have epileptic seizures. The cognitive changes and behavioural abnormalities can be particularly troubling. Depending on the age of the child, this becomes apparent as developmental delay or, in older children, as a loss of cognitive abilities and dementia. Children may show a change of character and personality with aggressive, truculent and oppositional or antisocial behaviour; as in adults with HD, depression and apathy are common. It is sometimes difficult to differentiate signs and symptoms that are directly related to the biology of HD from those that may arise as a consequence of the psychologically and emotionally challenging responses from the environment.

The management and treatment of JHD is even more complex than that of adult HD. It always requires close interdisciplinary collaboration of patients and their family and carers, medical doctors, psychologists, teachers and others around the patient and his family. For further reading, the interested reader is referred to an excellent book on JHD [4].

25.4 Differential Diagnosis

The diagnosis in a patient with typical signs of HD and a family history of genetically confirmed HD is straightforward. The clinical diagnosis can then be confirmed by molecular genetic testing for the *HTT* CAG repeat expansion mutation. If the clinical picture is typical for HD but there is no family history, genetic testing for HD is still appropriate. The CAG repeat expansion can be unstable, in particular, when inherited from the father, so that the clinically affected patient may have more repeats than the parent. The parent, therefore, may not have developed manifest HD yet. The parent may also have a CAG repeat length in the reduced penetrance, or intermediate allele, range so may not have had HD. There is also the possibility that the father is not the biological father.

The phenotype may be unusual while the family history suggests an inherited disorder. This could be the case in JHD as discussed above. If genetic testing is negative for the *HTT* mutation, there are several other genetic progressive disorders that can present with a mixed movement disorder and cognitive decline in the first three decades of life (for a review see [21]). These include dentato-rubro-pallido-luysian atrophy (DRPLA), much more common than HD in Japan and rare in people of European descent, neurodegeneration with brain iron accumulation (NBIA; e.g. predominantly childhood-onset PKAN1) or neuroferritinopathy. The presence of myoclonus and epilepsy can point towards DRPLA, while MRI can reveal iron deposits sometimes giving rise to the eye-of-the-tiger sign characteristic for PKAN1. MRI is also very useful in detecting other types of brain metal deposits such as those in Wilson's disease, aceruloplasminaemia, Kufor-Rakeb syndrome or manganism.

A number of HD phenocopies have been identified, some of them within distinct populations. These can be caused by a *PRNP* mutation (HD-like 1) or a mutation in the *JPH3* gene encoding junctaphilin-3 (HD-like 2, in people of African descent) (for a review, see [22]). If the phenotype is suggestive of HD but *HTT* testing is negative, unusual features can point towards an alternative diagnosis. Prominent bucco-oro-lingual chorea and dyskinesias with major eating difficulties because of involuntary tongue protrusion and tongue and lip biting can be indicative of choreoacanthocytosis (Video 25.5). This would be supported by the presence of seizures, neuropathy or myopathy (or just elevated creatine kinase levels) or cardiac involvement and an increase in acanthocytes in the blood. Choreoacanthocytosis can either be caused by mutations in the *VPS13A* gene encoding chorein or the *XK* gene in McLeod's syndrome. Childhood-onset chorea without cognitive decline and little progression can be a manifestation of benign hereditary chorea (BHC) although the phenotype of BHC can be quite variable and may not always be benign. Ataxia can point towards hereditary spinocerebellar ataxias, of which SCA17 can mimic the phenotype of HD. MRI with evidence of cerebellar atrophy can be helpful here.

Finally, from time to time, patients present with adult-onset chorea caused by medical diseases (for a review, see [23]). Sudden onset of hemichorea is suggestive of a vascular cause (often thalamic lesions), including possibly lesions in conjunction with polycythaemia vera or autoimmune-mediated disorders such as systemic lupus erythematosus or antiphospholipid syndrome. In children and adolescents, chorea can be caused by Sydenham's chorea and rheumatic fever following pharyngitis due to group A ß-haemolytic streptococcus. Chorea can occur in pregnancy (chorea gravidarum) and can be associated with taking oral contraceptive pills. Rarely, hyperthyroidism, renal failure and uraemia, hypocalcaemia or non-ketotic hyperglycaemia can cause a hyperkinetic movement disorder including chorea. Medication can cause chorea including L-dopa in Parkinson's disease but also SSRIs or dopamine-receptor antagonists. Taking a careful history often, but not always, gives important clues. These patients usually do not have any oculomotor disorder or dementia.

Subacute onset of chorea can be suggestive of a paraneoplastic disorder, e.g. in the context of small cell lung cancer with anti-CRMP-5 antibodies.

25.5 Treatment and Management of HD

A lot of effort is dedicated to finding causal treatments in HD [24], and the first safety and tolerability trial with an HTT lowering approach is currently under way (http://en.hdbuzz.net/204). While this offers hope that 1 day causal treatment in HD will be possible, the treatment and management options that are currently available in HD target the symptoms of HD. This can improve the quality of life of HD patients and their families even though symptomatic treatment may not influence the biology that underlies HD.

25.5.1 Standards of Care and Multidisciplinary Clinic

HD is not limited to the HD patient but affects the whole family. This includes relatives being at risk of having inherited the HD mutation, those knowing they carry the HD gene, carers and symptomatic family members. This adds to the complexity of HD. Therefore, HD care requires a multidisciplinary approach involving a range of services that can support the symptomatic individual in each stage of HD as well as addressing the needs of those around the symptomatic patient [25]. A multidisciplinary approach to the family with HD comprises a variety of specialised services, such as neurology, psychiatry, neuropsychology, clinical genetics, physiotherapy, speech and language therapy, dietician, social services and dentistry. An HD management clinic can serve as the hub where these specialised services come together to benefit the HD family. The role of the HD clinic is to provide information and to establish a management plan in collaboration with partner agencies outside the clinic. These partner agencies include, for example, acute services and inpatient care, general physicians and primary care services, psychiatric care, psychiatric nursing services, social work and welfare rights, financial advisors, disability employment advisors, peer support groups, housing support services, day care services, personal care, occupational therapy services and drivers' licensing authorities. For examples of multidisciplinary HD clinics and guidelines, the reader is referred to the websites of the Huntington's Disease Society of America (www.hdsa.org) or the European Huntington's Disease Network's Standards of Care working group (EHDN; www.euro-hd.net) or a recent publication [26].

25.5.2 Management of Clinical Manifestations

The majority of patients attending an HD clinic will have manifest HD. However, it is important to recognise that living with the knowledge of carrying a mutated *HTT* gene can be very difficult. Even though there are no clinical signs of manifest HD, people with premanifest HD may be in need of support or pharmacological or non-pharmacological treatment. In the absence of causal, disease-modifying treatment options, the approach to treatment needs to be guided by first establishing a hierarchy of problems. This requires taking a careful history from the patient and, importantly, family and caregivers. It is important to identify who has which problem. In particular, the behavioural problems, such as apathy or irritability, are sometimes much more troublesome for the family and carers than for the patient who may even deny having any problems at all. Listing the problems in their order of relevance determines in which order the problems need to be addressed. It is very important to explain carefully to the patient and caregivers what the pharmacological and non-pharmacological management options are. This should lead to the definition of the treatment goals and how to measure treatment effects. As a general principle for therapy, one should try and address as many problems from the list with a single intervention, often a drug. In the course of the evaluation of treatment effects, one has to be mindful of drug interactions when using more than one drug and of trying to differentiate signs of HD from side effects of medication. It is sometimes useful to consider reducing the amount of pharmacotherapy rather than adding yet another drug or increasing the doses since side effects of medication can be mistaken for signs of HD. Finally, it is always important to consider causes other than HD for a particular problem. There is no evidence to suggest that HD patients are protected from other ailments that may thus affect them just as they affect the rest of the population.

25.5.3 Motor Signs and Symptoms

Once it has been established that motor signs and symptoms impair the patient's day-to-day activities, there are pharmacological and non-pharmacological treatment options (Table 25.1).

Table 25.1 Treatment options in HD

	Treatment options	
Clinical problem	Pharmacological	Non-pharmacological
Chorea	D-RA (tiapride, olanzapine); TBZ	If severe and intractable Huntington chair
	↓SSRI; mirtazapine if restless, clonazepam	
Dystonia	↓D-RA, ↓TBZ; botulinum toxin (focal dystonia)	Physiotherapy
Hypokinesia-rigidity	↓D-RA, ↓TBZ	Physiotherapy
Gait and balance	↓D-RA, ↓TBZ (if dystonic or rigid); D-RA, TBZ if choreic	Physiotherapy
Dysphagia	↓D-RA, ↓TBZ (if dystonic or rigid)	Speech and language therapy, gastric feeding tube, nutritional advice
Weight loss	D-RA (if also choreic or irritable)	Speech and language therapy, hyper-caloric food supplements
Depression/anxiety	SSRI, mirtazapine, agomelatine, D-RA (enhancing SSRI)	Psychotherapy (if cognitively not too impaired)
Irritability	SSRI, mirtazapine, agomelatine, D-RA (e.g. olanzapine)	
Aggression, verbal	SSRI, mirtazapine, agomelatine, D-RA	
Aggression, physical	D-RA (olanzapine, quetiapine)	
Perseveration	Try SSRI; combination of SSRI and D-RA (clomipramine, olanzapine	Behaviour modification
Apathy	SSRI, aripiprazole, bupropion	Establish routines, day care
	↓D-RA, ↓TBZ	
Psychosis	D-RA	
Sleep-wake cycle	Mirtazapine, agomelatine, clonazepam	Sleep hygiene

D-RA dopamine-receptor antagonist, *TBZ* tetrabenazine *SSRI* selective-serotonin reuptake inhibitor, ↓ reduce

When considering the treatment options, it is important to be clear about the type of motor symptom – hyperkinetic, hypokinetic-rigid, gait and balance problems and swallowing – that is to be treated. Symptomatic pharmacological treatment of hyperkinetic motor manifestations most commonly targets the dopaminergic system. Available drugs include dopamine receptor antagonists ('antipsychotics') that target postsynaptic dopamine receptors and tetrabenazine, a reversible inhibitor of the vesicular monoamine transporter 2 (VMAT-2) that concentrates monoamines such as dopamine within presynaptic vesicles. VMAT-2 inhibition leads to the depletion of presynaptic dopamine. The evidence indicating efficacy of these agents is largely empirical even though small clinical trials suggest antipsychotics are effective, and a placebo-controlled trial demonstrated that tetrabenazine was better than placebo in treating chorea [27, 28]. However, a systematic Cochrane review of the available data was unable to recommend any drug solely based on the available evidence [29]. It is further important to note that antipsychotics and tetrabenazine can have substantial side effects; adverse affects on cognition, mood or alertness can outweigh the beneficial effects on chorea. A further option for the treatment of hyperkinesia in conjunction with restlessness and disturbed sleep-wake cycle can be clonazepam.

In the absence of evidence-based guidelines, recent efforts benefited from large clinical networks in North America and Australia (Huntington Study Group, www.hsg.org) and Europe (European Huntington's Network, EHDN; www.euro-hd.net) in capturing expert's experience in the management of HD motor symptoms [30]. This initiative has published an algorithm for the treatment of chorea [30]. This algorithm takes into account that abnormal movements are often accompanied by neuropsychiatric manifestations (see the next section). Hence, the choice of treatment depends also on non-motor problems (Table 25.1). In addition, the movement disorder in HD is mixed. While chorea may respond to some degree to treatment, dystonia and hypokinetic-rigid symptoms are more difficult to treat with medication. While it is always worth a trial, hypokinetic-rigid symptoms often do not respond satisfactorily to dopaminergic therapy, at least in the author's experience. Hypokinetic-rigid symptoms and dystonia can be the side effects of medication, in particular antipsychotics and tetrabenazine. Dystonia and hypokinetic-rigid symptoms can also contribute to gait and balance problems or speech and swallowing difficulties. Sometimes, reducing the dose of these medications can have a beneficial effect on these motor symptoms. Botulinum toxin can be a further option for the treatment of dystonia.

Non-pharmacological approaches such as physiotherapy, occupational therapy and speech and language therapy are very important in the treatment of these motor manifestations. A guideline for physiotherapy published by the EHDN physiotherapy working group can be found on www.euro-hd.net/html/network/groups/physio.

Dysphagia puts patients at risk for aspiration pneumonia. Treatment and prevention of dysphagia remains empirical in the absence of any evidence to support a particular therapeutic strategy [31]. Frequent dysphagia and coughing at meal times suggest the presence of swallowing difficulties. However, it remains unclear if, for example, video-fluoroscopy assessment is more sensitive to predict aspiration than clinical common sense. The option of placing a gastric feeding tube needs to be discussed with the patient and carers/family when, in the judgement of the physician, the risk of aspiration exists. Patients can benefit greatly from counselling by a dietician whenever dysphagia and/or nutrition (including weight loss) become an issue.

25.5.4 Neuropsychiatric and Cognitive Manifestations

For depression, the treatment and management recommendations are essentially the same as for depression in other contexts [32]. Depending on the severity of the depressive disorder, this can include medication and psychotherapy (Table 25.1). If anxiety and loss of energy predominate, the drug of first choice may be a serotonin reuptake inhibitor (SSRI) such as citalopram or a mixed SSRI/noradrenalin uptake inhibitor (NARI) such as venlafaxine. If insomnia, anxiety and restlessness are prominent, a sleep-inducing drug such as mirtazapine or agomelatine (even though the effects of agomelatine may be less convincing than those of mirtazapine) may be a good first choice. Some patients benefit from a combination of an SSRI, or combined SSRI/NARI, and a sleep-inducing antidepressant, or even small doses of clonazepam in particular if there is evidence to suggest disturbed REM sleep. An important distinction is that between insomnia as a biological feature of depression and the fairly common disturbance of the sleep-wake cycle in HD. A sleep-inducing antidepressant can be useful in both situations to improve the quality of sleep. This can have beneficial effects on concentration and thus cognition. It remains to be shown whether improved sleep quality may also contribute to the clearance of unwanted proteins and thus have a biological effect [33].

Apathy can be a particularly troublesome problem in HD since there is no good treatment. Apathy can always, at least in part, occur in the context of depression even if there are no obvious signs of depressed mood. Thus, a trial of an antidepressant, e.g. an SSRI or combined SSRI/NARI like venlafaxine, is warranted (see Table 25.1). If this does not improve the situation, aripiprazole can be tried. In the author's experience, aripiprazole sometimes does improve drive and concentration with beneficial effects also on cognition even though this needs to be investigated more systematically. The same is true for bupropion and other pharmacologic treatments that are used in other neurodegenerative disorders [34]. It is important to bear in mind that sedation and apathy can be side effects of medication in particular with antipsychotics or tetrabenazine. Reducing the dose of these drugs can sometimes have an effect on apathy. Non-pharmacological interventions are very important even though there is no evidence to advocate any particular intervention. These can include scheduled activities, including therapies such as physiotherapy, and chores so that the patient, with help of a carer who can provide a push, adopts a weekly routine.

Irritability and aggression sooner or later cause distress for the patient and his family. Similar to motor treatments and apathy treatments, there is no evidence base that could serve as a treatment guideline. For the same reasons as for chorea, expert opinion has been synthesised into a treatment algorithm for irritability/aggression [35]. Depending on the severity of outbursts, the first choice may be an SSRI if outbursts are verbal but not physical. If depression and insomnia also pose problems, mirtazapine or agomelatine may be good choices. Severe aggression with physical aggression and impulsivity warrant an antipsychotic as first choice (see Table 25.1). The presence of other symptoms also plays a role in the choice of treatment. Concurrent depression, anxiety or OCD may also respond to an antidepressant, whereas concurrent psychosis strongly argues for an antipsychotic as first choice. In some cases, the severity of aggression may require an admission to psychiatry to defuse the situation and avert danger and harm for those around the patient.

Taken together, in each individual patient, treatment should be customised to fit the set of problems the patient presents with. Multiple input including pharmacologic treatments and environmental modifications and also psychosocial support and education for caregivers can help them understand and cope with the situation to the benefit of the HD family. Psychological support for patients and relatives is very important, and psychotherapy, in particular in the preclinical phase of HD and in early manifest HD, can be very helpful.

References

1. Huntington G. On chorea. Med Surg Report. 1872;26:320–1.
2. Gusella JF, Wexler NS, Conneally PM, Naylor SL, Anderson MA, Tanzi RE, et al. A polymorphic DNA marker genetically linked to Huntington's disease. Nature. 1983;306:234–8.
3. The Huntington's Disease Collaborative Research Group. A novel gene containing a trinucleotide repeat that is expanded and unstable on Huntington's disease chromosomes. Cell. 1993;72:971–83.
4. Quarrell OWJ, Brewer HM, Squitieri F, Barker RA, Nance MA, Landwehrmeyer GB, editors. Juvenile

Huntington's disease (and other trinucleotide repeat disorders). Oxford: Oxford University Press; 2009.
5. Kremer B. Clinical neurology of Huntington's disease. In: Bates G, Harper P, Jones L, editors. Clinical neurology of Huntington's disease. 3rd ed. Oxford: Oxford University Press; 2002. p. 28–61.
6. Craufurd D, Snowden J. Neuropsychological and neuropsychiatric aspects of Huntington's disease. In: Bates G, Harper P, Jones L, editors. Neuropsychological and neuropsychiatric aspects of Huntington's disease. Oxford: Oxford University Press; 2002. p. 62–94.
7. Paulsen JS, Smith MM, Long JD. Cognitive decline in prodromal Huntington disease: implications for clinical trials. J Neurol Neurosurg Psychiatry. 2013;84:1233–9.
8. Sprengelmeyer R, Young AW, Calder AJ, Karnat A, Lange H, Homberg V, et al. Loss of disgust. Perception of faces and emotions in Huntington's disease. Brain. 1996;119(Pt 5):1647–65.
9. Henley SM, Novak MJ, Frost C, King J, Tabrizi SJ, Warren JD. Emotion recognition in Huntington's disease: a systematic review. Neurosci Biobehav Rev. 2012;36:237–53.
10. Wolf RC, Gron G, Sambataro F, Vasic N, Wolf ND, Thomann PA, et al. Brain activation and functional connectivity in premanifest Huntington's disease during states of intrinsic and phasic alertness. Hum Brain Mapp. 2012;33:2161–73.
11. Ho AK, Gilbert AS, Mason SL, Goodman AO, Barker RA. Health-related quality of life in Huntington's disease: which factors matter most? Mov Disord. 2009;24:574–8.
12. Kingma EM, van Duijn E, Timman R, van der Mast RC, Roos RA. Behavioural problems in Huntington's disease using the problem behaviours assessment. Gen Hosp Psychiatry. 2008;30:155–61.
13. Rickards H, De Souza J, van Walsem M, van Duijn E, Simpson SA, Squitieri F, et al. Factor analysis of behavioural symptoms in Huntington's disease. J Neurol Neurosurg Psychiatry. 2011;82:411–2.
14. van Duijn E, Craufurd D, Hubers AA, Giltay EJ, Bonelli R, Rickards H, Anderson KE, van Walsem MR, van der Mast RC, Orth M, Landwehrmeyer GB, European Huntington's Disease Network Behavioural Phenotype Working Group. Neuropsychiatric symptoms in a European Huntington's disease cohort (REGISTRY). J Neurol Neurosurg Psychiatry. 2014;85(12):1411–8.
15. Epping EA, Paulsen JS. Depression in the early stages of Huntington disease. Neurodegener Dis Manag. 2011;1:407–14.
16. Paulsen JS, Hoth KF, Nehl C, Stierman L. Critical periods of suicide risk in Huntington's disease. Am J Psychiatry. 2005;162:725–31.
17. Orth M, Handley OJ, Schwenke C, Dunnett SB, Craufurd D, Ho AK, et al. Observing Huntington's disease: the European Huntington's disease network's REGISTRY. PLoS Curr. 2010;2:RRN1184.
18. Hubers AA, van Duijn E, Roos RA, Craufurd D, Rickards H, Bernhard Landwehrmeyer G, et al. Suicidal ideation in a European Huntington's disease population. J Affect Disord. 2013;151:248–58.
19. van Duijn E, Kingma EM, Timman R, Zitman FG, Tibben A, Roos RA, et al. Cross-sectional study on prevalences of psychiatric disorders in mutation carriers of Huntington's disease compared with mutation-negative first-degree relatives. J Clin Psychiatry. 2008;69:1804–10.
20. Quarrell O, O'Donovan KL, Bandmann O, Strong M. The prevalence of juvenile Huntington's disease: a review of the literature and meta-analysis. PLoS Curr. 2012;4:e4f8606b742ef3.
21. Martino D, Stamelou M, Bhatia KP. The differential diagnosis of Huntington's disease-like syndromes: 'red flags' for the clinician. J Neurol Neurosurg Psychiatry. 2013;84:650–6.
22. Wild EJ, Mudanohwo EE, Sweeney MG, Schneider SA, Beck J, Bhatia KP, et al. Huntington's disease phenocopies are clinically and genetically heterogeneous. Mov Disord. 2008;23:716–20.
23. Barton B, Zauber SE, Goetz CG. Movement disorders caused by medical disease. Semin Neurol. 2009;29:97–110.
24. Wild EJ, Tabrizi SJ. Targets for future clinical trials in Huntington's disease: what's in the pipeline? Mov Disord. 2014;29(11):1434–45.
25. Nance MA, Westphal B. Comprehensive care in Huntington's disease. In: Bates G, Harper P, Jones L, editors. Comprehensive care in Huntington's disease. 3rd ed. Oxford: Oxford University Press; 2002. p. 475–500.
26. Neurodegenerative disease management, Feb 2012;2(1):1–87.
27. Venuto CS, McGarry A, Ma Q, Kieburtz K. Pharmacologic approaches to the treatment of Huntington's disease. Mov Disord. 2012;27:31–41.
28. Tetrabenazine as antichorea therapy in Huntington disease: a randomized controlled trial. Neurology 2006;66:366–72.
29. Mestre T, Ferreira J, Coelho MM, Rosa M, Sampaio C. Therapeutic interventions for symptomatic treatment in Huntington's disease. Cochrane Database Syst Rev 2009;(3):CD006456.
30. Burgunder JM, Guttman M, Perlman S, Goodman N, van Kammen DP, Goodman L. An international survey-based algorithm for the pharmacologic treatment of chorea in Huntington's disease. PLoS Curr. 2011;3:RRN1260.
31. Heemskerk AW, Roos RA. Dysphagia in Huntington's disease: a review. Dysphagia. 2011;26:62–6.
32. Geddes JR, Miklowitz DJ. Treatment of bipolar disorder. Lancet. 2013;381:1672–82.
33. Xie L, Kang H, Xu Q, Chen MJ, Liao Y, Thiyagarajan M, et al. Sleep drives metabolite clearance from the adult brain. Science. 2013;342:373–7.
34. Krishnamoorthy A, Craufurd D. Treatment of apathy in Huntington's disease and other movement disorders. Curr Treat Options Neurol. 2011;13:508–19.
35. Groves M, van Duijn E, Anderson K, Craufurd D, Edmondson MC, Goodman N, et al. An international survey-based algorithm for the pharmacologic treatment of irritability in Huntington's disease. PLoS Curr. 2011;3:RRN1259.

Chorea, Ballism, and Athetosis

26

Francisco Cardoso

26.1 Definition

Chorea is defined as a syndrome characterized by the continuous flow of random muscle contractions. This pattern of movement conveys a feeling of restlessness to the observer. When choreic movements are more severe, assuming a flinging, sometimes violent, character, they are called ballism. Neurophysiologic studies show that chorea and ballism share the same neuronal pattern, i.e., hypoactivity of the subthalamic nucleus and increased firing rate of the *globus pallidus pars interna* [26]. Athetosis describes sinuous, slow movements affecting distal limbs, particularly in the arms. There is a clear decline of the use of this term in the contemporary literature. The reason behind this tendency is the realization that athetosis is better defined as dystonia occasionally associated with some degree of chorea.

This chapter provides an overview of the most common causes of chorea in clinical practice with emphasis on clinical features, differential diagnosis, and management. The focus will be on nongenetic causes of chorea since there is one chapter on Huntington's disease.

Electronic supplementary material The online version of this chapter (doi:10.1007/978-3-7091-1628-9_26) contains supplementary material, which is available to authorized users.

F. Cardoso, MD, PhD, FAAN
Movement Disorders Unit, Neurology Service, Internal Medicine Department, Faculty of Medicine, Federal University of Minas Gerias, Av Pasteur 89/1107, 30150-290 Belo Horizonte, MG, Brazil
e-mail: cardosofe@terra.com.br

26.2 Phenomenology

The unpredictable nature of chorea is a feature that distinguishes it from tremor and dystonia. The former is characterized by rhythmic contractions of antagonist muscles, whereas the hallmark of dystonia is the patterned contraction resulting in abnormal postures or torsion movements. Stereotypies are also produced by repetitive contractions but, unlike tremor and dystonia, the resulting movements mimic complex motor behaviors part of the normal human repertoire. Tics can be readily differentiated from chorea because they also reproduce normal human movements or vocalizations, are often preceded by a local unpleasant sensation (sensory tic or prodrome), and can be voluntarily suppressed. One isolated choreic movement can be misinterpreted as myoclonus (a brief, lightning-like contraction with duration inferior to 200 ms), but the latter lacks the continuous flow so typical of chorea.

26.3 Nongenetic Causes of Chorea

Table 26.1 contains a classification of nongenetic choreas by categories of etiology. The most common causes of sporadic chorea are drugs,

C. Falup-Pecurariu et al. (eds.), *Movement Disorders Curricula*,
DOI 10.1007/978-3-7091-1628-9_26

Table 26.1 Etiologic classification of nongenetic chorea

Vascular chorea
Autoimmune chorea
Drug-induced chorea
Metabolic chorea
Infectious chorea

pregnancy, vascular disease, thyrotoxicosis, systemic lupus erythematosus (SLE) and the primary antiphospholipid antibody syndrome (PAPS), polycythemia rubra vera, AIDS, and Sydenham's chorea (SC) [53]. Although population-based epidemiologic studies are not available, a report from a tertiary center in Italy provides an estimate of the relative frequency of the most important causes of nongenetic chorea. The authors identified the following etiologies in 42 consecutive patients with chorea: vascular related (21 cases); drug induced (7 cases); AIDS related (5 cases); hyperglycemia, hyponatremia, and hypoxia (2 cases each); and borreliosis, vasculitis, and SC (1 case each) [52]. This is roughly similar to the numbers in my unit. However, there has been a decline of neurological complications of AIDS in general and, in the particular case of the Movement Disorders Clinic of the Federal University of Minas Gerais (MDC-UFMG), Brazil, SC remains overrepresented in comparison to centers in North America and Western Europe [10].

26.3.1 Vascular Chorea

Chorea is an unusual complication of acute vascular lesion, seen in less than 1 % of patients with acute stroke. This hyperkinesia, often characterized as hemiballism, is usually related to ischemic or hemorrhagic lesion of the basal ganglia and adjacent white matter in the territory of the middle or the posterior cerebral artery (Video 26.1). These cases seem to be more common in Asia where there is a strong association with type II diabetes mellitus. In contrast to common sense, the majority of patients with vascular chorea have lesions outside the subthalamus [22]. Although it often comes into remission spontaneously, in the acute phase patients may require treatment with anti-choreic drugs such as neuroleptics or dopamine depletors. A few patients with vascular chorea may remain with persistent movement disorder. In this circumstance, they can be effectively treated with stereotactic surgery such as thalamotomy or posteroventral pallidotomy [8, 12].

An uncommon cause of chorea is Moyamoya disease, an intracranial vasculopathy that presents with ischemic lesion or, less commonly, hemorrhagic stroke of the basal ganglia [24]. Another rare, but still reported, vascular cause of chorea is the so-called "post-pump chorea" – a complication of extracorporeal circulation. The pathogenesis of this movement disorder is believed to be vascular insult of the basal ganglia during the surgical procedure. The natural history of post-pump chorea is benign with spontaneous remission in most cases [67].

26.3.2 Autoimmune Chorea

26.3.2.1 Sydenham's Chorea (SC)

SC, the neurological manifestation of rheumatic fever (RF), is the prototype of chorea resulting from immune mechanisms. Chorea occurs in 26 % of patients with RF although this figure varies according to time and geographic area [10]. Although largely confined to areas outside North America and Western Europe, it has drawn grown interest lately. This results from the possibility that a similar pathogenic mechanism may be responsible for a subset of patients with Tourette's syndrome (TS) and related conditions – the so-called PANDAS (pediatric autoimmune neuropsychiatric disorders associated with streptococcal infection [59]. However, current evidence strongly pints out against the existence of this entity. Despite the fall in the incidence, SC remains as the most common cause of acute chorea in children worldwide. In fact, occasional outbreaks of RF with occurrence of chorea remain occurring in the USA and Australia [2, 55].

The usual age at onset of SC is 8–9 years, although there are reports of adult-onset SC [10].

One important clinical finding is the observation that SC is very rarely seen below age 5 years [60]. Typically, patients develop this disease 4–8 weeks after an episode of group A β-hemolytic streptococcus (GABHS) pharyngitis. Chorea rapidly spreads, becoming generalized, but 20 % of patients remain with hemichorea [10, 50]. Patients display motor impersistence, particularly noticeable during tongue protrusion and ocular fixation. The muscle tone is usually decreased; in severe and rare cases (8 % of all patients seen at the MDC-UFMG), this is so pronounced that the patient may become bedridden (chorea paralytica) (Video 26.2).

Patients with SC often display other motor findings. There are reports of occurrence of tics in SC. Even vocal tics, reported to be common in SC [47], are not of simple diagnosis in patients with hyperkinesias. Involuntary vocalizations, simply resulting from dystonia or chorea of the pharynx and larynx, have been reported in subjects with oromandibular dystonia, Huntington's disease, or others [30]. In a cohort of 120 SC patients followed up at the MDC-UFMG, we have identified complex tics in fewer than 4 % of subjects.

There has also been growing interest in the behavioral abnormalities present in SC. At the MDC-UFMG, Maia et al. [44] found that obsessive-compulsive behavior (OCB), obsessive-compulsive disorder (OCD), and attention deficit and hyperactivity disorder (ADHD) were more frequent in the SC group (19 %, 23.2 %, 30.4 %) than in the control group (11 %, 4 %, 8 %) and in the RF group (14 %, 6 %, 8 %). In a survey of 100 patients with RF, half of whom had chorea, we found that migraine is more frequent in SC (21.8 %) than in normal controls (8.1 %, $p=0.02$) [66]. This is similar to what has been described in TS [38]. In the older literature, there are also references to papilledema, central retinal artery occlusion, and seizures in a few patients with SC. Another investigation demonstrated that the peripheral nervous system is not targeted in SC [7]. Finally, it must be kept in mind that SC is a major manifestation of RF: 60–80 % of patients display cardiac involvement, particularly mitral valve dysfunction, whereas the association with arthritis is less common, seen in 30 % of subjects; however, in approximately 20 % of the patients, chorea is the sole finding [7]. There is a validated scale to rate SC, the UFMG Sydenham Chorea Rating Scale (USCRS). It is designed to provide a detailed quantitative description of the performance of activities of daily living, behavioral abnormalities, and motor function of patients with SC [64].

There is no investigation directly comparing clinical features of SC with TS. However, the studies of the latter suggest that OCD, ADHD, and others are more common and disabling in TS than in SC [39]. Another important clinical difference between these conditions is the observation that the vast majority of SC subjects present with carditis, whereas this complication has never been reported in TS [10, 39]. Moreover, there is no indication of existence of geographic clusters of TS in contrast with SC. It can be concluded that although there are similarities between SC and tic disorders, there remain important distinctions. These findings go against the existence of PANDAS.

The pathogenesis of SC is related to existence of molecular mimicry between streptococcal and central nervous system antigens. It has been proposed that the GABHS infection in genetically predisposed subjects leads to formation of cross-reactive antibodies that disrupt the basal ganglia function. Several studies have demonstrated the presence of such circulating antibodies in 50–90 % of patients with Sydenham's chorea [14, 29]. In a study of patients seen at the MDC-UFMG, we demonstrated that all patients with active SC have antibasal ganglia antibodies demonstrated by ELISA and Western blot. In subjects with persistent SC, the positivity was about 60 % [14]. It must be emphasized that the biological value of antibasal ganglia antibodies remains to be determined. Two recent studies suggest that they may interfere with neuronal function. In one the authors demonstrated that IgM of one patient with SC induced expression of calcium-dependent calmodulin in a culture of neuroblastoma cells [35]. In another investigation we demonstrated that there is a linear correlation between the increase of intracellular calcium levels in PC12 cells and antibasal ganglia antibody titer in the serum from SC patients. This result suggests that the antibodies have a pathogenic value [63]. More recent evidence indicates that *Streptococcus* can induce antibodies targeting dopamine receptors that induce behavioral abnormalities in rodents [41, 4].

There have also been studies that address the role of immune cellular mechanisms in SC. Investigating sera and CSF samples of SC patients of MDC-UFMG, Church and colleagues [15] found elevation of serum interleukins 4 (IL-4) and 10 (IL-10). The authors concluded that SC is characterized by a Th2 response. We also described an increased concentration of chemokines CXCL9 and CXCL10 in the serum of patients with acute SC [62].

The current diagnostic criteria of SC are a modification of the Jones criteria: chorea with acute or subacute onset and lack of clinical and laboratory evidence of alternative cause are mandatory findings. The diagnosis is further supported by the presence of additional major or minor manifestations of rheumatic fever [10, 11, 25]. The aim of the diagnostic workup in patients suspected to have SC is threefold: (1) to identify evidence of recent streptococcal infection or acute phase reaction, (2) to search for cardiac injury associated with rheumatic fever, and (3) to rule out alternative causes. Tests of acute phase reactants such as erythrocyte sedimentation rate, C-reactive protein, and leukocytosis; other blood tests like rheumatoid factor, mucoproteins, and protein electrophoresis; and supporting evidence of preceding streptococcal infection (increased antistreptolysin O, anti-DNAse-B, or other anti-streptococcal antibodies; positive throat culture for group A *Streptococcus*; recent scarlet fever) are much less helpful in SC than in other forms of RF due to the usual long latency between the infection and onset of the movement disorder. Elevated antistreptolysin O titer may be found in populations with a high prevalence of streptococcal infection. Furthermore, the antistreptolysin O titer declines if the interval between infection and rheumatic fever is greater than 2 months. Anti-DNase-B titers, however, may remain elevated up to 1 year after strep pharyngitis. Heart evaluation (i.e., Doppler echocardiography) is mandatory because of common association of SC with carditis. Serologic studies for SLE and PAPS must be ordered to rule out these conditions. Spinal fluid analysis is usually normal, but it may show a slight increased lymphocyte count. In general, neuroimaging will help rule out structural causes of chorea. CT scan of the brain invariably fails to display abnormalities. Similarly, head MRI is often normal, although there are case reports of reversible hyperintensity in the basal ganglia area. In one study, the authors showed increased signal in just 2 of 24 patients, although morphometric techniques revealed mean values for the size of the striatum and pallidum larger than controls [23]. Another study showed that there is a correlation between the presence of persistent lesions of the basal ganglia on MRI and tendency for a more prolonged course of the disease [20]. PET and SPECT imaging may prove to be useful tools in the evaluation, revealing transient increases in striatal metabolism [69]. In one SPECT study of ten patients with SC, the authors showed that six had hyperperfusion of the basal ganglia [3]. This contrasts with other choreic disorders (such as Huntington's disease) that are associated with hypometabolism. Of note, however, another SPECT investigation showed hyperperfusion in two patients with SC, whereas the remaining five had hypometabolism [16]. It is possible that the inconsistencies in these functional imaging studies reflect heterogeneity of the population of patients. The test of antineuronal antibodies, however, is not commercially available, being just performed for research purposes.

There are no controlled studies of symptomatic treatment of SC. For most authorities, however, the first choice is valproic acid although other anticonvulsants, such as carbamazepine, are also found to be effective and well tolerated [21, 28]. Dopamine receptor blocking agents, usually risperidone, are left for patients who fail to respond to valproic acid or those rare cases with chorea paralytica. The need for caution in the use of neuroleptics in rheumatic chorea is demonstrated by a case-control study, comparing the response to these drugs in patients with SC and TS. The authors demonstrated that 5 % of 100 patients with chorea developed parkinsonism, dystonia, or both, whereas these findings were not observed among patients with tics matched for age and dosage of neuroleptics [61].

Steroids are reserved for patients with persistent disabling chorea refractory to anti-choreic agents. We reported that 25 mg/kg/day in children and 1 g/day in adults of methylprednisolone for 5 days followed by 1 mg/kg/day of prednisone is an effective and well-tolerated treatment for patients with SC refractory to conventional treatment with anti-choreic drugs and penicillin [9]. The same protocol has been shown to control chorea in patients with SC who developed side effects to neuroleptics [65]. There are few reports describing the usefulness of plasma exchange or intravenous immunoglobulin in SC [32]. Because of the efficacy of other therapeutic agents described in the previous paragraph, potential complications, and high cost of the latter treatment modalities, these options are usually not recommended. Finally, the most important measure in the treatment of patients with SC is secondary prophylaxis with penicillin or, if there is allergy, sulfa drugs up to age 21 years.

SC is often described as a self-limited condition, which spontaneously comes into remission after a course of 8–9 months. However, prospective studies have shown that up to 50 % of patients may remain with chorea after a follow-up of 2 years. This has been called persistent SC [11]. Moreover, despite regular use of secondary prophylaxis, recurrences of SC are observed in up to 30 % of subjects [11, 36]. Interestingly, in many of the recurrences, there is lack of association either with streptococcus infection or even antibasal ganglia antibodies [27, 36].

26.3.2.2 Other Autoimmune Choreas

Other immunologic causes of chorea are SLE, PAPS, vasculitis, and paraneoplastic syndromes. SLE and PAPS are classically described as the prototypes of autoimmune choreas [53]. However, several reports show that chorea is seen in no more than 1–2 % of large series of patients with these conditions [1, 56, 68]. Sanna et al. [56] confirmed the notion that chorea and other neuropsychiatric syndromes, present in 185 of their 323 consecutive patients with SLE, are associated with antiphospholipid antibodies. Autoimmune chorea has also been reported in the context of paraneoplastic syndromes associated with anti-Hu, anti-CRMP5, anti-LGI1, and CASPR2 antibodies. This is more commonly seen, but exclusively, in patients with small-cell lung carcinoma [18, 34, 51].

26.3.3 Drug-Induced Chorea

Table 26.2 contains a list of drugs described in association with induction of chorea. Levodopa-induced chorea, the most common form of drug-induced chorea seen by movement disorder specialists, is not tackled in this chapter. There are reports of patients treated with lithium, lamotrigine, or methadone who developed chorea that came into remission after discontinuation of the drugs [17, 42, 58]. Oral contraceptive-induced chorea has traditionally been regarded as a syndrome related to SC. It is hypothesized that hormones could potentially lead a basal ganglia previously injured during the acute phase of rheumatic fever to produce chorea. A report suggests that rather than related to dopamine system dysfunction, oral contraceptive-induced chorea could be mediated by antibasal ganglia antibodies [48].

Table 26.2 Drugs related to induction of chorea

Alcohol
Anticholinergics
Antiepileptic agents (hydantoin, lamotrigine, valproic acid)
Antihypertensive agents (captopril, alpha-methyldopa)
Calcium channel blockers (cinnarizine, flunarizine)
Cocaine
Dopamine agonists
Hormones
Levodopa
Lithium
Methadone
Neuroleptics
Stimulants (amphetamine, methylphenidate, pemoline)
Superselective serotonin reuptake inhibitors (fluoxetine, paroxetine)
Tricyclic antidepressants (imipramine)

Chorea gravidarum, chorea occurring during pregnancy, is also believed to have the same pathogenesis as oral contraceptive-induced chorea [5, 43].

26.3.4 Metabolic Chorea

Chronic-acquired or non-Wilsonian hepatolenticular degeneration was the first well-characterized metabolic cause of chorea thanks to the pioneer work of Adams and Victor. Although first described in the context of complications of alcohol abuse, it can occur in any form of acquired liver disease. The clinical picture is heterogeneous since patients may present with a variable combination of neurological and hepatic manifestations. The neurological findings include apathy, somnolence, parkinsonism, tremor, myoclonus, asterixis, and chorea. In most instances there is a combination of different movement disorders, but a few subjects may present with isolated chorea. MRI of the brain shows not only images compatible with cavitations in the basal ganglia (hyperintense signal on T2 and hypointense on T1) but also hyperintense T1 signal in the pallidum, putamen, and upper brainstem. The latter has been interpreted as caused by deposition of manganese [31].

As already mentioned, there is an association of chorea and nonketotic hyperglycemia in type II diabetes mellitus. This condition seems particularly common among Asians since the reports. Unlike the usual neurological manifestations of nonketotic hyperglycemia, patients do not have change in the level of consciousness and develop unilateral or generalized chorea-ballism. The MRI findings are characteristic with hyperintense signal of the pallidum on T1. Although of controversial interpretation, most studies relate this image to microhemorrhages of the pallidum. Once glycemic control is achieved, there is gradual remission of chorea [13, 40].

A few patients with hyperthyroidism may develop generalized chorea or even ballism related to this endocrine dysfunction. The lack of structural changes in the brain, appearance with onset of thyrotoxicosis, and remission with endocrine control suggest that the basal ganglia dysfunction is induced by hormones [54]. Other possible metabolic causes of chorea are hypoglycemia, renal failure, and ketogenic diet [33].

26.3.5 Infectious Chorea

HIV and its complications has been the most often reported infectious cause of chorea. In one series of 42 consecutive patients with nongenetic chorea, for instance, AIDS was found to be the cause in 12 % of the subjects [52]. In HIV-positive patients, chorea is the result of either the direct action of the virus or other mechanisms such as opportunistic infections (toxoplasmosis, syphilis, and others) or drugs [6]. There is, however, a decline of neurological complications of HIV infection after the introduction of highly active antiretroviral therapy. Other infections related to chorea are new variant Creutzfeldt-Jakob disease and tuberculosis [33, 45, 46].

26.4 Athetosis

As already mentioned in the introduction of the chapter, movement disorder experts use this term less and less. However, there are two situations where it is still used. The first and most common is to describe the combination of dystonia and chorea in the distal portions of limbs in patients with cerebral palsy [49]. Although traditionally described as a complication of kernicterus, athetosis may happen in cerebral palsy of any cause. The phenomenology is characterized by a variable combination of dystonia, chorea, myoclonus, and spasticity. A few patients may improve with levodopa, clonazepam, baclofen, anticholinergics, or tetrabenazine. Most of them, however, are refractory to clinical treatment, and even surgical treatment has not been successful. There is one recent report, for instance, describing failure of deep brain stimulation of the globus pallidus internus in alleviating chorea in four patients with cerebral palsy [37]. Finally, slow, distal, writhing movements of the fingers or toes in patients with proprioception loss are described as pseudoathetosis. This dyskinesia is usually described in association with peripheral neuropathy. However, central lesions resulting in impairment of proprioception (myelopathy, thalamic lesion, or others) may also cause pseudoathetosis [57]. As this movement disorder does not cause significant morbidity, no treatment is required.

References

1. Asherson RA, Cervera R. Unusual manifestations of the antiphospholipid syndrome. Clin Rev Allergy Immunol. 2003;25:61–78.
2. Ayoub EM. Resurgence of rheumatic fever in the United States. The changing picture of a preventable illness. Postgrad Med. 1992;92:133–42.
3. Barsottini OG, Ferraz HB, Seviliano MM, Barbieri A. Brain SPECT imaging in Sydenham's chorea. Braz J Med Biol Res. 2002;35:431–6.
4. Brimberg L, Benhar I, Mascaro-Blanco A, et al. Behavioral, pharmacological, and immunological abnormalities after streptococcal exposure: a novel rat model of Sydenham chorea and related neuropsychiatric disorders. Neuropsychopharmacology. 2012;37:2076–87.
5. Cardoso F. Chorea gravidarum. Arch Neurol. 2002;59:868–70.
6. Cardoso F. HIV-related movement disorders: epidemiology, pathogenesis and management. CNS Drugs. 2002;16:663–8.
7. Cardoso F, Dornas L, Cunningham M, Oliveira JT. Nerve conduction study in Sydenham's chorea. Mov Disord. 2004:360–3. doi:10.1002/mds.20318.
8. Cardoso F, Jankovic J, Grossman RG, Hamilton WJ. Outcome after stereotactic thalamotomy for dystonia and hemiballismus. Neurosurgery. 1995;36:501–7.
9. Cardoso F, Maia D, Cunningham MC, Valença G. Treatment of Sydenham chorea with corticosteroids. Mov Disord. 2003;18:1374–7.
10. Cardoso F, Silva CE, Mota CC. Sydenham's chorea in 50 consecutive patients with rheumatic fever. Mov Disord. 1997;12:701–3.
11. Cardoso F, Vargas AP, Oliveira LD, et al. Persistent Sydenham's chorea. Mov Disord. 1999;14:805–7.
12. Choi SJ, Lee SW, Kim MC, et al. Posteroventral pallidotomy in medically intractable postapoplectic monochorea: case report. Surg Neurol. 2003;59:486–90.
13. Chu K, Kang DW, Kim DE, et al. Diffusion-weighted and gradient echo magnetic resonance findings of hemichorea-hemiballismus associated with diabetic hyperglycemia: a hyperviscosity syndrome? Arch Neurol. 2002;59:448–52.
14. Church AJ, Cardoso F, Dale RC, et al. Anti-basal ganglia antibodies in acute and persistent Sydenham's chorea. Neurology. 2002;59:227–31.
15. Church AJ, Dale RC, Cardoso F, et al. CSF and serum immune parameters in Sydenham's chorea: evidence of an autoimmune syndrome? J Neuroimmunol. 2003;136(1–2):149–53.
16. Citak EC, Gukuyener K, Karabacak NI, et al. Functional brain imaging in Sydenham's chorea and streptococcal tic disorders. J Child Neurol. 2004;19:387–90.
17. Das KB, Harris C, Smyth DP, Cross JH. Unusual side effects of lamotrigine therapy. J Child Neurol. 2003;18:479–80.
18. Dorban S, Gille M, Kessler R, et al. Chorea-athetosis in the anti-Hu syndrome. Rev Neurol (Paris). 2004;160:126–9.
19. Erickson JC, Jabbari B, Difazio MP. Basal ganglia injury as a complication of the ketogenic diet. Mov Disord. 2003;18:448–51.
20. Faustino PC, Terreri MT, da Rocha AJ, et al. Clinical, laboratory, psychiatric and magnetic resonance findings in patients with Sydenham's chorea. Neuroradiology. 2003;45:456–62.
21. Genel F, Arslanoglu S, Uran N, Saylan B. Sydenham's chorea: clinical findings and comparison of the efficacies of sodium valproate and carbamazepine regimens. Brain Dev. 2002;24:73–6.
22. Ghika-Schmid F, Ghika J, Regli F, Bogousslavsky J. Hyperkinetic movement disorders during and after acute stroke: the Lausanne Stroke Registry. J Neurol Sci. 1997;146:109–16.
23. Giedd JN, Rapoport JL, Kruesi MJ, et al. Sydenham's chorea: magnetic resonance imaging of the basal ganglia. Neurology. 1995;45:2199–202.
24. Gonzalez-Alegre P, Ammache Z, Davis PH, Rodnitzky RL. Moyamoya-induced paroxysmal dyskinesia. Mov Disord. 2003;18:1051–6.
25. Guidelines for diagnosis of rheumatic fever, Jones criteria, 1992 update. Special Writing Group of the Committee of Rheumatic Fever, Endocarditis, and Kawasaki Disease of the Council on Cardio-Vascular Disease of the Young of the American Heart Association. Guidelines for the diagnosis of rheumatic fever. JAMA. 1992;268:2069–73.
26. Hamani C, Saint-Cyr JA, Fraser J, et al. The subthalamic nucleus in the context of movement disorders. Brain. 2004;127:4–20.
27. Harrison NA, Church A, Nisbet A, Rudge P, Giovannoni G. Late recurrences of Sydenham's chorea are not associated with anti-basal ganglia antibodies. J Neurol Neurosurg Psychiatry. 2004;75:1478–9.
28. Hernandez-Latorre MA, Roig-Quilis M. The efficiency of carbamazepine in a case of post-streptococcal hemichorea. Rev Neurol (Spain). 2003;37:322–6.
29. Husby G, Van De Rijn U, Zabriskie JB, et al. Antibodies reacting with cytoplasm of subthalamic and caudate nuclei neurons in chorea and acute rheumatic fever. J Exp Med. 1976;144:1094–110.
30. Jankovic J. Differential diagnosis and etiology of tics. Adv Neurol. 2001;85:15–29.
31. Jog MS, Lang AE. Chronic acquired hepatocerebral degeneration: case reports and insights. Mov Disord. 1995;10:714–22.
32. Jordan LC, Singer HS. Sydenham chorea in children. Curr Treat Options Neurol. 2003;5:283–90.
33. Kalita J, Ranjan P, Misra UK, Das BK. Hemichorea: a rare presentation of tuberculoma. J Neurol Sci. 2003;208:109–11.

34. Kinirons P, Fulton A, Keoghan M, et al. Paraneoplastic limbic encephalitis (PLE) and chorea associated with CRMP-5 neuronal antibody. Neurology. 2003;61: 1623–4.
35. Kirvan CA, Swedo SE, Heuser JS, Cunningham MW. Mimicry and autoantibody-mediated neuronal cell signaling in Sydenham chorea. Nat Med. 2003;9(7):914–20.
36. Korn-Lubetzki I, Brand A, Steiner I. Recurrence of Sydenham chorea: implications for pathogenesis. Arch Neurol. 2004;61:1261–4.
37. Krauss JK, Loher TJ, Weigel R, et al. Chronic stimulation of the globus pallidus internus for treatment of non-DYT1 generalized dystonia and choreoathetosis: 2-year follow up. J Neurosurg. 2003;98:785–92.
38. Kwack C, Vuong KD, Jankovic J. Migraine headache in patients with Tourette syndrome. Arch Neurol. 2003;60:1595–8.
39. Leckman JF. Tourette's syndrome. Lancet. 2002;360: 1577–86.
40. Lin JJ, Chang MK. Hemiballism-hemichorea and non-ketotic hyperglycemia. J Neurol Neurosurg Psychiatry. 1994;57:748–50.
41. Lotan D, Benhar I, Alvarez K, et al. Behavioral and neural effects of intra-striatal infusión of anti-streptococcal antibodies in rats. Brain Behav Immun. 2014;38:249–62.
42. Lussier D, Cruciani RA. Choreiform movements after a single dose of methadone. J Pain Symptom Manage. 2003;26:688–91.
43. Maia DP, Fonseca PG, Camargos ST, et al. Pregnancy in patients with Sydenham's chorea. Parkinsonism Relat Disord. 2012;18:458–61.
44. Maia DP, Teixeira Jr AL, Cunningham MCQ, Cardoso F. Obsessive compulsive behavior, hyperactivity and attention deficit disorder in Sydenham's chorea. Neurology. 2005;64:1799–801.
45. Martinelli P, Rizzo G, Scaglione C, Capellari S. Neurosyphilis orofacial dyskinesia: the candy sign. Mov Disord. 2013;28:246–7.
46. McKee D, Talbot P. Chorea as a presenting feature of variant Creutzfeldt-Jakob disease. Mov Disord. 2003;18:837–8.
47. Mercadante MT, Campos MC, Marques-Dias MJ, et al. Vocal tics in Sydenham's chorea. J Am Acad Child Adolesc Psychiatry. 1997;36:305–6.
48. Miranda M, Cardoso F, Giovannoni G, Church A. Oral contraceptive induced chorea: another condition associated with anti-basal ganglia antibodies. J Neurol Neurosurg Psychiatry. 2004;75:327–8.
49. Morris JG, Grattan-Smith P, Jankelowitz SK, et al. Athetosis II: the syndrome of mild athetoid cerebral palsy. Mov Disord. 2002;17:1281–7.
50. Nausieda PA, Grossman BJ, Koller WC, et al. Sydenham's chorea: an update. Neurology. 1980;30: 331–4.
51. O'Toole O, Lennon VA, Ahlskog JE, et al. Autoimmune chorea in adults. Neurology. 2013:80:1133–44.
52. Piccolo I, Defanti CA, Soliveri P, et al. Cause and course in a series of patients with sporadic chorea. J Neurol. 2003;250:429–35.
53. Quinn N, Schrag A. Huntington's disease and other choreas. J Neurol. 1998;245:709–16.
54. Ristic AJ, Svetel M, Dragasevic N, et al. Bilateral chorea-ballism associated with hyperthyroidism. Mov Disord. 2004;19:982–3.
55. Ryan M, Antony JH, Grattan-Smith PJ. Sydenham chorea: a resurgence of the 1990s? J Paediatr Child Health. 2000;36:95–6.
56. Sanna G, Bertolaccini ML, Cuadrado MJ, et al. Neuropsychiatric manifestations in systemic lupus erythematosus: prevalence and association with antiphospholipid antibodies. J Rheumatol. 2003;30: 985–92.
57. Sharp FR, Rando TA, Greenberg SA, et al. Pseudochoreoathetosis. Movements associated with loss of proprioception. Arch Neurol. 1994;51:1103–9.
58. Stemper B, Thurauf N, Neundorfer B, Heckmann JG. Choreoathetosis related to lithium intoxication. Eur J Neurol. 2003;10:743–4.
59. Swedo SE, Leonard HL, Garvey M, et al. Pediatric autoimmune neuropsychiatric disorders associated with streptococcal infections: clinical description of the first 50 cases. Am J Psychiatry. 1998;155:264–71.
60. Tani LY, Veasy LG, Minich LL, Shaddy RE. Rheumatic fever in children younger than 5 years: is the presentation different? Pediatrics. 2003;112:1065–8.
61. Teixeira Jr AL, Cardoso F, Maia DP, Cunningham MC. Sydenham's chorea may be a risk factor for drug induced parkinsonism. J Neurol Neurosurg Psychiatry. 2003;74:1350–1.
62. Teixeira Jr AL, Cardoso F, Souza ALS, Teixeira MM. Increased serum concentrations of monokine induced by interferon-y/CXCL9 and interferon-y-inducible protein 10/CXCL-10 in Sydenham's chorea patients. J Neuroimmunol. 2004;150:157–62.
63. Teixeira-Jr AL, Guimarães MM, Romano-Silva MA, Cardoso F. Serum from Sydenham's chorea patients modifies intracellular calcium levels in PC12 cells by a complement independent mechanism. Mov Disord. 2005;20:843–5.
64. Teixeira Jr AL, Maia DP, Cardoso F. UFMG Sydenham's chorea rating scale (USCRS): reliability and consistency. Mov Disord. 2005:585–91. doi:10.1002/mds.20377.
65. Teixeira Jr AL, Maia DP, Cardoso F. Treatment of acute Sydenham's chorea with methyl-prednisolone pulse-therapy. Parkinsonism Relat Disord. 2005;11: 327–30.
66. Teixeira Jr AL, Meira FCA, Maia DP, Cunningham MC, Cardoso F. Migraine headache in patients with Sydenham's chorea. Cephalalgia. 2005;25: 542–4.
67. Thobois S, Bozio A, Ninet J, Akhavi A, Broussolle E. Chorea after cardiopulmonary bypass. Eur Neurol. 2004;51:46–7.
68. Unterman A, Nolte JE, Boaz M, et al. Neuropsychiatric syndromes in systemic lupus erythematosus: a meta-analysis. Semin Arthritis Rheum. 2011;41:1–11.
69. Weindl A, Kuwert T, Leenders KL, et al. Increased striatal glucose consumption in Sydenham's chorea. Mov Disord. 1993;8:437–44.

27 Tardive Dyskinesia

Sweta Goel and William Ondo

Abbreviation

AIMS	Abnormal Involuntary Movement Scale
ATAs	Atypical antipsychotics
BCAAs	Branched-chain amino acids
BDNF	Brain-derived neurotrophic factor
DBS	Deep brain stimulation
TAs	Typical antipsychotics
TBZ	Tetrabenazine
TD	Tardive dyskinesia

S. Goel, MBBS
Department of Neurology, University of Texas, Houston, 6431 Fannin street, MSB 7.044, Houston, TX 77030, USA
e-mail: sweta.goel@uth.tmc.edu

W. Ondo, MD (✉)
Director of Movement disorders, Methodist Neurological Instituter, Houston, TX, USA
e-mail: wondo@houstonmethodist.org

27.1 Tardive Dyskinesia Phenomenology

The term "tardive dyskinesia" (TD) means any abnormal movement after an event, in this case, the use of a dopaminergic blocking agent. It can occur while on the offending agent or after stopping it for up to a year, the so-called withdrawal dyskinesia. As other medicines are often substituted for the true offending agent, withdrawal dyskinesia can be incorrectly blamed on the new drug. Prognosis is variable. The condition may persist indefinitely or may very gradually improve. Withdrawal dyskinesia tends to be milder and has a better long-term prognosis [1]. A longer duration of continued dopamine antagonist use after the onset of symptoms portends a worse prognosis, so discontinuation of the offending agent is recommended whenever possible.

The most common TD phenotype is stereotype, which is a repetitive, somewhat predictable movement, not oscillatory enough to be considered a tremor. That said many other phenotypes occasionally occur including chorea, dystonia, and tic-like movements. The most common anatomy is the oral-buccal-lingual area; however, the toes are also usually involved, though less noticed. Onset is usually gradual, and frequently the involuntary movements are not as appreciated

C. Falup-Pecurariu et al. (eds.), *Movement Disorders Curricula*,
DOI 10.1007/978-3-7091-1628-9_27

by the patient as one would suspect, based on observing them. Two other distinct phenotypes include tardive dystonia, which usually involves opisthotonic posturing of the whole body and pronation of the arms. This is usually seen in younger males. A tardive pain syndrome may accompany dyskinesia or may be seen in isolation. This is typically a burning or lancinating neuropathic pain and typically experienced in the mouth and/or genitalia.

27.2 Epidemiology and Risk Factors

TD can occur at any point during or after treatment with dopamine antagonists, but the total risk is cumulative. Atypical antipsychotics (ATAs), which have less affinity for dopamine receptors, may be associated with a reduced risk of TD compared to typical antipsychotics (TAs). A prospective, 4-year study of 352 patients by Woods et al. revealed that ATA use reduced the cumulative risk for TD by one-third relative to TA (adjusted RR = 0.68; 95 % CI 0.29–1.64) [2]. Interestingly, despite high penetration of ATA into clinical practice in the 1980s vs 2000s, the incidence of TD appears to be relatively unchanged (5.5 % vs 6.6 % per year) [2]. This has been partly attributed to the increasing off-label uses of these agents.

Relatively lower dopamine receptor affinity most likely decreases the risk of TD with ATA; however, there is marked heterogeneity of actual affinities among marketed ATA. Quetiapine, clozapine, and pimavanserin have by far the lowest and thus may be less culpable compared to others. Nausea medications that block dopamine receptors are common causes of TD. Metoclopramide may be the most culpable agent due to its popularity and extended duration of usage and its easy availability as an over-the-counter medication in certain countries (not including the United States) [3]. The "calcium channel blockers" flunarizine and cinnarizine, which have many receptor interactions, also commonly cause TD [4].

Several studies have looked at predisposing factors for TD. Older age and female sex have been most consistently implicated as risk factors for TD. For example, an 80-year-old woman on dopaminergic blockers has a 20–25 % per year incidence of TD, compared to the average of 5–6 % for younger people. Other factors that have been implicated in increasing the risk of TD are diabetes, alcohol or substance abuse, higher drug dose, long-term treatment, race, preexisting mood, movement or cognitive disorder, and human immunodeficiency virus positivity [1, 5].

Candidate gene studies have recognized several genetic polymorphisms that can increase susceptibility to the development of TD [6]. An overview of the more robust associated gene polymorphisms and the evidence for and against them are provided in Table 27.1. Other genes variably associated with TD include PAWR [7], ADORA2A [8, 9], GRIN2A and GRIN2B [10], COMT, SOD2, PPP1R1B, and RGS2 [6, 11]. Recent genome-wide association studies have to date only corroborated an association with an allele of the heparan sulfate proteoglycan (HSPG) 2 gene [6].

27.3 Pathophysiology

Since Schonecker first described the occurrence of TD with the use of dopamine receptor antagonists [5, 16], several models have been proposed to explain the pathophysiology of TD.

The most commonly accepted explanation for TD involves postsynaptic dopaminergic receptor hypersensitivity [5, 17]. Rodent studies have shown that with the use of neuroleptics, there is upregulation of postsynaptic dopamine receptors in the basal ganglia within a few days, especially D2 receptors [18]. Maximum upregulation requires a constant 80 % receptor occupancy of the drug, and is less robust with intermittent blockade [19–22]. Anatomically, D2 receptors on medium spiny neurons within the striatum inhibit the indirect pathway resulting in disinhibition of the globus pallidus internus and subthalamic nucleus, potentially producing a variety of hyperkinetic movement disorders [23].

Table 27.1 Most studied genetic predispositions in tardive dyskinesia

Gene/receptor	Evidence
Dopamine receptor D2 (DRD2) gene polymorphisms	TaqIA(rs1800497) and −141C Ins/Del have been studied most extensively [6]. A meta-analysis revealed that compared to TD-negative patients, TD-positive patients had a higher A2 allele frequency ($p=0.003$), with an effect size of 1.30 (95 % CI, 1.09–1.55), and higher A2/A2 genotype frequency ($P=0.001$), with an effect size of 1.50 (95 % CI, 1.17–1.92). The −141C Ins/Del alleles and genotypes were not associated with TD [6]
	Another study that investigated 12 polymorphisms spanning the DRD2 gene found that C957T and the adjacent C939T polymorphism were significantly associated with TD ($p=0.013$ and $p=0.022$, respectively) [7]
DRD3 Ser9Gly (rs6280)	A meta-analysis of 13 studies between 1997 and 2008 concluded that there is no or little association between DRD3 Ser9Gly (rs6280) polymorphisms and prevalence of TD [8]
	These findings, however, do not preclude the possible involvement of other DRD3 variants in tardive dyskinesia
APOE 2 allele	Significant difference in APOE 2 allele frequencies noted in Caucasians with TD compared to controls in study of 97 patients [9]. APOE genotype 2/3 with OR 2.29 (1.1–4.9) vs APOE, 2/2 OR 3.55 (0.5–27.1) [9]
	Mechanism by which the APOE 2 allele increases; risk of tardive dyskinesia is unclear [9]
SLC18A2	Encodes for VMAT-2, a vesicular transporter protein that regulates release of dopamine, serotonin, and GABA [10]
	An association study ($N=217$) found significant gene-gene interaction between the high-expression C allele of *SLC18A2* rs363224 and the high-functioning C allele of rs6277 in *DRD2*, supporting the hypothesis of dopamine hyperactivity at the D2 receptor in TD [10]
Heparan sulfate proteoglycan (HSPG) 2 rs2445142	HSPG2 expression may protect against the development of TD via a cholinergic or basic fibroblast growth factor (FGF2)-mediated neuroprotective mechanism. These initial findings with HSPG2 were more recently supported by a reanalysis of genome-wide datasets [11–13]
TNF-α promoter-308A/G	A study of 760 patients showed that total Abnormal Involuntary Movement Scale (AIMS) scores were higher in the group of low-expression GG genotype carriers than in AG genotype carriers for 308A/G (rs1800629) marker in the promoter of the gene coding for TNF-α [14]
5-HT2R gene	The two most commonly studied polymorphisms in the HTR2A receptor gene, namely, 5-HT2A (-1438A > G in the promoter) and HTR2A (102T > C, in exon 1), and one polymorphism in the HTR2C receptor gene (68C > G, Cys23Ser in exon 2) were investigated in a study $N=335$. No significant allelic or genotypic association was observed with TD [15]
Manganese superoxide dismutase (MnSOD) gene	MnSOD gene Ala-9Val polymorphism did not play a major role in the susceptibility to TD in schizophrenic patients

Although this upregulation after DA use is seen in dopamine neuroimaging and postmortem studies in humans, it has not differentiated patients with versus those without TD [23, 24], suggesting receptor upregulation alone does not predict who becomes symptomatic. Therefore, DA receptor upregulation may be necessary but is not solely responsible for TD.

Other neurotransmitter abnormalities including GABA, acetylcholine, and glutamate have also been implicated in humans and animal models of TD. Hypofunction and degeneration of the striatal fast-spiking GABAergic interneurons can lead to imbalance of direct and indirect pathways and have been associated with hyperkinetic movements, including TD [25–27]. A cholinergic deficiency theory originates from the observation that rodents treated with haloperidol have increased vacuous chewing movements (VCM) followed by decreased counts of choline acetyltransferase (ChAT)-positive cells in the ventrolateral striatum and nucleus accumbens [28]. Teo et al. proposed the maladaptive synaptic plasticity theory that hypothesizes that neuroleptics via dopamine receptor sensitization and NMDA receptor alteration can modulate the neurotransmission in the basal ganglia and in turn the sensorimotor cortex [23]. These synaptic modulations can be permanent.

Neurodegeneration has also been postulated to contribute to TD. Neuroleptics can increase free radical damage and cause neuronal degeneration [29]. Excess synaptic dopamine, resulting from receptor blockade, can be oxidized by autoxidation and enzymatic oxidation leading to increased synaptic reactive oxygen species and subsequently neurotoxicity [30, 31]. Zhang et al. have found that patients with TD have decreased serum brain-derived neurotrophic factor (BDNF) compared to non-TD patients and healthy controls, and although the exact role of BDNF in the pathophysiology of TD is not clear, increasing BDNF levels with *Ginkgo biloba* were associated with improved AIMS total scores in one clinical study [32].

27.4 Treatment

Although the seriousness of TD was recognized shortly after the introduction of antipsychotic medications, there is no universally accepted treatment and few positive large-scale trials.

Tetrabenazine (TBZ), a VMAT-2 inhibitor that reduces the release of dopamine and other monoamines, is used to treat a variety of hyperkinetic movement disorders. An analysis of ten retrospective trials, totaling more than a thousand patients, showed that greater than 70 % had marked improvement, excellent improvement, or complete improvement of their TD symptoms using TBZ [33]. That said prospective trials are largely lacking One single blind prospection study did report marked improvement [34]. Adverse events of TBZ generally include sedation, parkinsonism, akathisia, and depression, but not TD, and are usually dose dependent [35]. Prodrug and extended release preparation of TBZ are in various stages of study for TD.

Amantadine, which has multiple mechanisms of action, improved TD by about 40 % in two controlled trials [36, 37]. It is generally well tolerated but may worsen psychosis and often causes livedo reticularis.

Clonazepam, an indirect GABA agonist, was shown to have a 37 % reduction on dyskinesia scores in 1 double-blind, randomized, placebo-controlled study of 19 psychiatric outpatients [38].

Branched-chain amino acids (BCAAs) are postulated to improve TD by competing with dopamine precursors across the blood-brain barrier. One controlled trial showed improved TD and minimal adverse effects with high-dose BCAA therapy (222 mg/kg) [39]. The cohort was exclusively male, and studies including female patients have not reported similar results [24]. Large-scale control trials are needed to further elucidate the therapeutic potential for BCAAs in TD.

One meta-analysis of 17 studies involving 50 patients with TD, mostly tardive dystonia, who underwent deep brain stimulation (DBS) surgery, showed a mean 71.5 % improvement in AIMS [40]. Although the numbers are highly encouraging, caution must be exercised while considering

DBS as a therapeutic option as most of the data collected was from case reports and small trials.

Clozapine and other ATA have shown open-label long-term improvements in TD when substituted for other dopamine blockers. In one 5-year follow-up study, an 87.5 % decrease in Extrapyramidal Symptom Rating Scale scores for TD was observed with mean clozapine dose of 428 mg/day. However, this may be due to natural improvement over time [41].

Vitamin E is the most studied treatment for TD. Unfortunately, most well-designed placebo-controlled trials do not show benefit [42].

Other treatments that have been advocated for TD include *G. biloba* extract (EGb-761) [43], pyridoxine (vitamin B6) [44], botulinum toxin [45, 46], levetiracetam [47], zonisamide [48], melatonin [49, 50], and calcium channel blockers [51].

To conclude, TD is a common, often devastating and permanent condition whose exact pathophysiology is not entirely understood. Treatment strategies are not uniform, and several promising treatments require multicenter, randomized, blinded trials to confirm their efficacy.

References

1. Chaudhuri KR, Ondo WG, Logishetty K, Redyy P, Sherman R. Handbook of movement disorders. London: Current Medicine Group; 2009.
2. Woods SW, Morgenstern H, Saksa JR, Walsh BC, Sullivan MC, Money R, et al. Incidence of tardive dyskinesia with atypical versus conventional antipsychotic medications: a prospective cohort study. J Clin Psychiatry. 2010;71(4):463–74.
3. Pasricha PJ, Pehlivanov N, Sugumar A, Jankovic J. Drug insight: from disturbed motility to disordered movement – a review of the clinical benefits and medicolegal risks of metoclopramide. Nat Clin Pract Gastroenterol Hepatol. 2006;3(3):138–48.
4. Brucke T, Wober C, Podreka I, Wober-Bingol C, Asenbaum S, Aull S, et al. D2 receptor blockade by flunarizine and cinnarizine explains extrapyramidal side effects. A SPECT study. J Cereb Blood Flow Metab Off J Int Soc Cereb Blood Flow Metab. 1995;15(3):513–8.
5. Jankelowitz SK. Treatment of neurolept-induced tardive dyskinesia. Neuropsychiatr Dis Treat. 2013;9:1371–80.
6. Zai CC, De Luca V, Hwang RW, Voineskos A, Muller DJ, Remington G, et al. Meta-analysis of two dopamine D2 receptor gene polymorphisms with tardive dyskinesia in schizophrenia patients. Mol Psychiatry. 2007;12(9):794–5.
7. Zai CC. Association study of tardive dyskinesia and twelve DRD2 polymorphisms in schizo phrenia patients. Int J Neuropsychopharmacol. 2007;10:639–51.
8. Tsai HT, North KE, West SL, Poole C. The DRD3 rs6280 polymorphism and prevalence of tardive dyskinesia: a meta-analysis. Am J Med Genet B Neuropsychiatr Genet Off Publ Int Soc Psychiatr Genet. 2010;153b(1):57–66.
9. Halford J, Mazeika G, Slifer S, Speer M, Saunders AM, Strittmatter WJ, et al. APOE2 allele increased in tardive dyskinesia. Mov Disord. 2006;21(4):540–2.
10. Zai CC, Tiwari AK, Mazzoco M, de Luca V, Muller DJ, Shaikh SA, et al. Association study of the vesicular monoamine transporter gene SLC18A2 with tardive dyskinesia. J Psychiatr Res. 2013;47(11):1760–5.
11. Syu A, Ishiguro H, Inada T, Horiuchi Y, Tanaka S, Ishikawa M, et al. Association of the HSPG2 gene with neuroleptic-induced tardive dyskinesia. Neuropsychopharmacol Off Publ Am Coll Neuropsychopharmacol. 2010;35(5):1155–64.
12. Greenbaum L, Alkelai A, Zozulinsky P, Kohn Y, Lerer B. Support for association of HSPG2 with tardive dyskinesia in Caucasian populations. Pharmacogenomics J. 2012;12(6):513–20.
13. Muller DJ, Chowdhury NI, Zai CC. The pharmacogenetics of antipsychotic-induced adverse events. Curr Opin Psychiatry. 2013;26(2):144–50.
14. Wang F, Fan H, Sun H, Yang F, Luo Y, Liu H, et al. Association between TNF-alpha promoter -308A/G polymorphism and tardive dyskinesian Chinese Han patients with schizophrenia. Prog Neuropsychopharmacol Biol Psychiatry. 2012;37(1):106–10.
15. Deshpande SN, Varma PG, Semwal P, Rao AR, Bhatia T, Nimgaonkar VL, et al. II. Serotonin receptor gene polymorphisms and their association with tardive dyskinesia among schizophrenia patients from North India. Psychiatr Genet. 2005;15(3):157–8.
16. Schonecker M. Paroxysmal dyskinesia as the effect of megaphen. Nervenarzt. 1957;28(12):550–3.
17. Waln O, Jankovic J. An update on tardive dyskinesia: from phenomenology to treatment. Tremor Other Hyperkinetic Mov (NY). 2013;3:p.27 http://tremor-journal.org/article/view/161
18. Schroder J, Bubeck B, Sauer H. D2-dopamine receptor upregulation and treatment response under neuroleptic therapy. Fortschr Neurol Psychiatr. 2000;68 Suppl 1:S42–5.
19. Nyberg S, Nordstrom AL, Halldin C, Farde L. Positron emission tomography studies on D2 dopamine receptor occupancy and plasma antipsychotic drug levels in man. Int Clin Psychopharmacol. 1995;10 Suppl 3:81–5.

20. Farde L, Nordstrom AL, Wiesel FA, Pauli S, Halldin C, Sedvall G. Positron emission tomographic analysis of central D1 and D2 dopamine receptor occupancy in patients treated with classical neuroleptics and clozapine. Relation to extrapyramidal side effects. Arch Gen Psychiatry. 1992;49(7):538–44.
21. Kapur S, Zipursky R, Jones C, Remington G, Houle S. Relationship between dopamine D(2) occupancy, clinical response, and side effects: a double-blind PET study of first-episode schizophrenia. Am J Psychiatry. 2000;157(4):514–20.
22. Ginovart N, Wilson AA, Hussey D, Houle S, Kapur S. D2-receptor upregulation is dependent upon temporal course of D2-occupancy: a longitu dinal [11C]-raclopride PET study in cats. Neuropsychopharmacol Off Publ Am Coll Neuropsychopharmacol. 2009;34(3):662–71.
23. Teo JT, Edwards MJ, Bhatia K. Tardive dyskinesia is caused by maladaptive synaptic plasticity: a hypothesis. Mov Disord Off J Mov Disord Soc. 2012;27(10):1205–15.
24. Rana AQ, Chaudry ZM, Blanchet PJ. New and emerging treatments for symptomatic tardive dyskinesia. Drug Des Devel Ther. 2013;7:1329–40.
25. Gittis AH, Leventhal DK, Fensterheim BA, Pettibone JR, Berke JD, Kreitzer AC. Selective inhibition of striatal fast-spiking interneurons causes dyskinesias. J Neurosci Off J Soc Neurosci. 2011;31(44):15727–31.
26. Gunne LM, Haggstrom JE, Sjoquist B. Association with persistent neuroleptic-induced dyskinesia of regional changes in brain GABA synthesis. Nature. 1984;309(5966):347–9.
27. Margolese HC, Chouinard G, Kolivakis TT, Beauclair L, Miller R. Tardive dyskinesia in the era of typical and atypical antipsychotics. Part 1: pathophysiology and mechanisms of induction. Can J Psychiatry Rev Can Psychiatr. 2005;50(9):541–7.
28. Grimm JW, Chapman MA, Zahm DS, See RE. Decreased choline acetyltransferase immunoreactivity in discrete striatal subregions following chronic haloperidol in rats. Synapse (New York, NY). 2001;39(1):51–7.
29. Elkashef AM, Wyatt RJ. Tardive dyskinesia: possible involvement of free radicals and treatment with vitamin E. Schizophr Bull. 1999;25(4):731–40.
30. Qing H, Xu H, Wei Z, Gibson K, Li XM. The ability of atypical antipsychotic drugs vs. haloperidol to protect PC12 cells against MPP+-induced apoptosis. Eur J Neurosci. 2003;17(8):1563–70.
31. Lohr JB, Kuczenski R, Niculescu AB. Oxidative mechanisms and tardive dyskinesia. CNS Drugs. 2003;17(1):47–62.
32. Zhang XY, Zhang W-F, Zhou D-F, Chen DC, Xiu MH, Wu H-R, et al. Brain-derived neurotrophic factor levels and its Val66Met gene polymorphism predict tardive dyskinesia treatment response to Ginkgo biloba. Biol Psychiatry. 2012;72(8):700–6.
33. Guay DR. Tetrabenazine, a monoamine-depleting drug used in the treatment of hyperkinetic movement disorders. Am J Geriatr Pharmacother. 2010;8(4):331–73.
34. Ondo WG, Tintner R, Thomas M, Jankovic J. Tetrabenazine treatment for Huntington's disease-associated chorea. Clin Neuropharmacol. 2002;25(6):300–2.
35. Jankovic J, Clarence-Smith K. Tetrabenazine for the treatment of chorea and other hyperkinetic movement disorders. Expert Rev Neurother. 2011;11(11):1509–23.
36. Angus S, Sugars J, Boltezar R, Koskewich S, Schneider NM. A controlled trial of amantadine hydrochloride and neuroleptics in the treatment of tardive dyskinesia. J Clin Psychopharmacol. 1997;17(2):88–91.
37. Pappa S, Tsouli S, Apostolou G, Mavreas V, Konitsiotis S. Effects of amantadine on tardive dyskinesia: a randomized, double-blind, placebo-controlled study. Clin Neuropharmacol. 2010;33(6):271–5.
38. Thaker GK, Nguyen JA, Strauss ME, Jacobson R, Kaup BA, Tamminga CA. Clonazepam treatment of tardive dyskinesia: a practical GABAmimetic strategy. Am J Psychiatry. 1990;147(4):445–51.
39. Richardson MA, Bevans ML, Read LL, Chao HM, Clelland JD, Suckow RF, et al. Efficacy of the branched-chain amino acids in the treatment of tardive dyskinesia in men. Am J Psychiatry. 2003;160(6):1117–24.
40. Mentzel CL, Tenback DE, Tijssen MA, Visser-Vandewalle VE, van Harten PN. Efficacy and safety of deep brain stimulation in patients with medication-induced tardive dyskinesia and/or dystonia: a systematic review. J Clin Psychiatry. 2012;73(11):1434–8.
41. Bassitt DP, Louza Neto MR. Clozapine efficacy in tardive dyskinesia in schizophrenic patients.Eur Arch Psychiatry Clin Neurosci. 1998;248(4):209–11.
42. Soares-Weiser K, Maayan N, McGrath J. Vitamin E for neuroleptic-induced tardive dyskinesia. Cochrane Database Syst Rev. 2011;(2):CD000209.
43. Zhang WF, Tan YL, Zhang XY, Chan RC, Wu HR, Zhou DF. Extract of Ginkgo biloba treatment for tardive dyskinesia in schizophrenia: a randomized, double-blind, placebo-controlled trial. J Clin Psychiatry. 2011;72(5):615–21.
44. Lerner V, Miodownik C, Kaptsan A, Bersudsky Y, Libov I, Sela BA, et al. Vitamin B6 treatment for tardive dyskinesia: a randomized, double-blind, placebo-controlled, crossover study. J Clin Psychiatry. 2007;68(11):1648–54.
45. Slotema CW, van Harten PN, Bruggeman R, Hoek HW. Botulinum toxin in the treatment of orofacial tardive dyskinesia: a single blind study. Prog Neuropsychopharmacol Biol Psychiatry. 2008;32(2):507–9.
46. van Harten PN, Hovestadt A. Botulinum toxin as a treatment for tardive dyskinesia. Mov Disord Off J Mov Disord Soc. 2006;21(8):1276–7.

47. Konitsiotis S, Pappa S, Mantas C, Mavreas V. Levetiracetam in tardive dyskinesia: an open label study. Mov Disord Off J Mov Disord Soc. 2006;21(8):1219–21.
48. Iwata Y, Irie S, Uchida H, Suzuki T, Watanabe K, Iwashita S, et al. Effects of zonisamide on tardive dyskinesia: a preliminary open-label trial. J Neurol Sci. 2012;315(1–2):137–40.
49. Castro F, Carrizo E, Prieto de Rincon D, Rincon D, Rincon CA, Asian T, Medina-Leendertz S, et al. Effectiveness of melatonin in tardive dyskinesia. Invest Clin. 2011;52(3):252–60.
50. Nelson LA, McGuire JM, Hausafus SN. Melatonin for the treatment of tardive dyskinesia. Ann Pharmacother. 2003;37(7–8):1128–31.
51. Essali A, Deirawan H, Soares-Weiser K, Adams CE. Calcium channel blockers for neuroleptic-induced tardive dyskinesia. Cochrane Database Syst Rev. 2011(11):CD000206.

Tics and Tourette Syndrome 28

Valerie Cathérine Brandt and Alexander Münchau

Abbreviation

ADHD	Attention-deficit hyperactivity disorder
BG	Basal ganglia
CSTC	Cortico-striato-thalamo-cortical
DA	Dopamine
DBS	Deep brain stimulation
ESSTS	European Society for the Study of Tourette syndrome
GPe	Globus pallidus externus
GPi	Globus pallidus internus
GTS	Gilles de la Tourette syndrome
GWAS	Genome-wide association studies
HRT	Habit reversal therapy
OCD	Obsessive-compulsive disorder
SNPs	Single-nucleotide polymorphisms
THC	Tetra-hydro-cannabinol

28.1 Tics

28.1.1 Definition/Phenomenology

Tics can be divided into motor, phonic (vocal) and cognitive tics [1]. Phonic or vocal tics are sounds that are produced by air movement through the vocal cords, nose or mouth [2]. Cognitive tics, or "impulsions", are repetitive thoughts. In contrast to obsessions, the cardinal feature of obsessive-compulsive disorder (OCD), they are not anxiety driven but are reactions to auditory, visual, tactile or inner stimuli that trigger the urge to tic [3, 4]. Tics are typically associated with a premonitory urge, which grows increasingly unpleasant if the tic is suppressed (see Sect. 28.2.2 for further details).

Tics can range from simple short, repetitive movements (e.g. eye blinking, nasal flare, mouth twitches) or phonic productions (e.g. throat

V.C. Brandt
Department of Paediatric and Adult Movement Disorders and Neuropsychiatry, Institute of Neurogenetics, Center for Brain Behaviour and Metabolism, University of Lübeck, Maria-Curie-Strasse, 23562 Lübeck, Germany
e-mail: valerie.brandt@neuro.uni-luebeck.de

A. Münchau (✉)
Department of Paediatric and Adult Movement Disorders and Neuropsychiatry, Institute of Neurogenetics, Center for Brain Behaviour and Metabolism, University of Lübeck, Maria-Curie-Strasse, 23562 Lübeck, Germany

Neurologische Klinik, Universitätskrankenhaus Hamburg-Eppendorf, Martinistr. 52, Hamburg 20246, Germany
e-mail: alexander.muenchau@neuro.uni-luebeck.de

C. Falup-Pecurariu et al. (eds.), *Movement Disorders Curricula*,
DOI 10.1007/978-3-7091-1628-9_28

clearing, barking, grunting, high-pitched sounds, sniffing) to complex actions, such as gestures, squatting, jumping, repetitive touching or rituals and single words or sentences, which can appear intentional or compulsion-like but are not goal directed [5].

Most tics affect the face, head, shoulders and neck [5]. Single motor tics are difficult to distinguish from single voluntary movements both phenomenologically [6] and electrophysiologically [7] but are misplaced in context and time. Therefore, identifying tics is easier over a longer period of time. For instance, a single eye blink tic is not different from "normal" eye blinking. It is the fact that blinking is excessively repeated and appears exaggerated that sets blink tics apart from physiological blinking [6].

Tics typically exacerbate under strong emotional excitement, irrespective of whether the emotion is negative, such as an emotional trauma or stress, or positive, such as birthdays or a vacation trip [8]. Moreover, focusing attention on tics can increase tic frequency [9, 10], while focusing on a voluntary motor task can decrease it [11].

Tics are partially suppressible for a few minutes up to a few hours [5], and patients frequently suppress their tics in public or "divert" their most obvious tic, such as facial grimacing, to less obvious movements, for instance, leg or foot twitches, to avoid drawing attention. Patients report that tic suppression requires attention, effortful control, and is accompanied by an increasing, uncomfortable urge to execute tics, yet, the majority of patients frequently choose to suppress tics, due to the social friction they may cause.

Sometimes, tics can cause pain or are associated with self-injury, either involuntarily or because, very rarely, the patient uses pain to temporarily relieve the urge to tic [12]. In severe cases, tics can damage joints or result in compressive myelopathy [13].

Tics are usually easy to identify. However, it has been recommended by a European panel of experts to consult an experienced physician for a general physical and neurological examination to avoid misdiagnoses [2].

The most common disorders involving tics are primary tic disorders. A diagnosis in the tic disorder spectrum can fall in one of the following categories: (1) *Tourette syndrome* (*TS*) is characterized as follows: (i) multiple motor tics and one or more phonic tics, (ii) the tics may wax and wane in frequency but have persisted for more than 1 year since first tic onset, (iii) tic onset was before age 18, and (iv) tics are not attributable to drugs or another medical condition [14]. (2) *Persistent (chronic) motor or vocal tic disorder*: the same criteria apply as in TS, but tics are limited to either motor or vocal tics, and the patient has not been diagnosed with TS. (3) *Provisional tic disorder*: the same criteria apply as in chronic tic disorder, but the symptoms have been present for less than 12 months. (4) *Other specified tic disorders*(5) *Unspecified tic disorder*: delineates tics that do not fall into the other categories but cause impairment, e.g. adult onset tics or tics caused by drug intake [14].

28.1.2 Differential Diagnosis

Tics can bear resemblance to other abnormal movements, such as stereotypies, compulsions, myoclonus or chorea. The most conspicuous characteristic distinguishing tics from other abnormal movements is a preceding inner urge or tension, building up, until it is transiently relieved by the tic [15]. This phenomenon is the reason that most patients with tics experience their tics as mostly voluntary actions to relieve an involuntary and uncontrollable urge [16–18]. Hence, tics encompass voluntary as well as involuntary components [16].

Stereotypies are typically more complex than tics and are repeated consecutively. They are not preceded by an inner urge to move. Myoclonus can be distinguished from tics by asking the patient to perform a task that requires fine motor skills. Myoclonus is typically unchanged or becomes more prominent during tasks such as writing or fine finger movements, while tics typically subside during such tasks. Compared to tics, chorea is unpredictable, floating and chaotic but can be difficult to distinguish from rapid tics. In some patients with longer-lasting tonic tics, especially with tics affecting the neck, tics can resemble dystonia [18]. In this case, electromyography can be helpful to detect co-contraction of agonist and antagonist, which is typical for dystonia but not for tics. Again, tics, but not dystonia, are associated with an urge to move. Compulsion-like tics can be differentiated from compulsions because they usually do not serve the purpose of alleviating anxiety. However, some tics are executed to reach a "just-right" feeling, a phenomenon that also occurs in OCD.

Tics can occur in other disorders, such as autism spectrum disorders, and are characteristically present in neuroacanthocytosis and sometimes also in Huntington's disease. Complex tics have also been reported in pantothenate kinase-associated neurodegeneration and a number of X-chromosomal disorders [19]. Acquired causes of tics most typically involve stimulants. Drug intake, especially cocaine, but also amphetamines, anti-depressants, anticonvulsants and antihistamines can induce or exacerbate tics. In rare cases, tics have been reported as a consequence of encephalitis or in association with structural brain lesions, especially to the basal ganglia (BG) [20]. However, the number of reported patients is very small, and their clinical details often lack the information of whether tics were associated with premonitory urges.

28.2 Gilles de la Tourette Syndrome

28.2.1 DSM-V Criteria

Most tic disorders belong to the TS spectrum. TS was named after Georges Edouard Albert Brutus Gilles de la Tourette, who described nine patients suffering from tics in 1885 [21]. The *Diagnostic and Statistical Manual, Fifth Edition* (DSM-5) describes TS as a neurodevelopmental disorder (for diagnostic criteria please see Sect. 28.1.1.) According to DSM-5, it is not necessary for the patient to experience distress or impairment to diagnose TS [22].

Other characteristic phenomena often present in TS encompass echopraxia (automatic imitation of others' actions) [23], echolalia (automatic imitation of others' syllables/words) [24], palilalia (automatic repetition of own syllables/words) and coprolalia/copropraxia (automatic, involuntary swearing/offensive gestures). Coprophenomena are extremely salient but only occur in 10–15 % of TS patients [25].

Up to 90 % of TS patients also suffer from comorbidities. The most common comorbidities are attention-deficit hyperactivity disorder (ADHD) (54 %) and OCD (50 %) [26], while mood and anxiety disorders, disruptive behaviour disorders and sleep disorders are less common [26, 27]. It has been suggested that there may be different subtypes of TS, a "pure TS" subtype and a "TS plus" (comorbidities) subtype, based on the finding that "TS plus" patients showed coprolalia while pure TS patients did not in a sample of 222 patients [28]. However, larger samples, advanced statistical techniques and longitudinal studies will be needed to tease subtypes, associations, causes and consequences apart. For instance, different components of oppositional defiant disorder have been associated with comorbid ADHD and OCD rather than TS per se [29, 30], while psychosocial problems in TS can be predictors for the later occurrence of depressive symptoms [31].

A recent study showed that 68 % of a large sample of 672 participants with a chronic tic disorder had been treated differently because of their symptoms. Over 30 % reported to have been discriminated against rudely, and 17 % had even been asked to leave a public place [32]. Over 40 % reported avoiding social events or group activities because of their tics. It is, thus, not surprising that tic frequency, the severity of premonitory urges and comorbidities have been associated with psychosocial impairment and lower quality of life in TS [33].

In line with these findings, children with TS typically experience more social and educational problems than healthy controls because they often suffer from salient motor and vocal tics or coprolalia. As a result, children with tics are often victims of bullying and stigmatization, which can cause withdrawal, depression and anxiety. Moreover, children with tics report difficulties with school work and unhelpful responses from school staff, especially to phonics tics [34]. Also, children with TS are more susceptible to psychosocial stress than healthy children (see Sect. 28.2.3). Comorbidities can additionally aggravate these problems and commonly cause more objective [35], as well as subjective impairment than the tics [36].

Older TS patients have been reported to experience elevated levels of social impairment compared to younger TS patients, with 25–50 % being single or divorced [37]. Suicide attempts were recorded in 4.8 % of a sample of 524 TS patients in the UK. Symptom severity was higher in this group; comorbidities (especially depression, anxiety and ADHD) were more common, as well as drug or alcohol abuse, unemployment, a forensic history or a family history of suicide attempts [38].

28.2.2 Premonitory Urges

Tic disorders are characterized by involuntary, as well as voluntary, action components [16]. The execution of tics is often perceived as a voluntary response to an uncontrollable urge to move, which has been shown to build up within 10 s before a tic, or a bout of tics, is executed and then transiently subsides [15]. Approximately 80 % of TS patients experience these premonitory urges [25], which have been likened to a strong itch [39] and can present either at the site where the tic is about to occur or can be experienced as a general feeling of rising inner tension. In terms of sensory quality, they have been described as pressure-like, a tickling, cold or warm sensation [40]. Importantly, premonitory urges have a debilitating effect on subjective quality of life [41] and appear to be associated with interoceptive awareness [42] and anxiety-related somatic symptoms [43].

Self-reports suggest that TS patients become aware of their urges on average 3 years after tic onset. However, children aged 5–7 years might have difficulties understanding and describing the concept of urges; hence, this estimate is somewhat questionable [25, 44]. Research has shown that awareness of premonitory sensations increases with age, i.e. cognitive development, not with time since tic onset [40]. Thus, it is still unclear which phenomenon precedes, or causes, which, or whether they are both independent results of a common, underlying cause.

28.2.3 Prevalence and Course

Tics are very common phenomena that can range from single tics (e.g. eye blinking), which, in many cases, may not even be diagnosed as tics, to severe TS, including tics that can cause pain or injury. Epidemiological studies in the UK indicate a prevalence of tic disorders in the range of 3.4–24.4 %, depending on the measure that is used to determine tics and the population that is investigated [45]. The prevalence of TS in children and adolescents aged 5–18 ranges from 0.4 to 3.8 % [45], while the international lifetime prevalence of TS is estimated to be approximately 1 % [25, 45]. TS has been shown to be three to four times more likely to occur in males than in females [45, 46] and appears to occur less frequently in Hispanics, African-Americans and sub-Saharan black Africans [45].

The 2007 US National Survey of Children's Health has estimated a lifetime prevalence of 0.3 % by parent report [46]. This finding underlines the assumption that TS is generally underdiagnosed [47], probably because tics are often not recognized as a neurological symptom. Consequently, the average time until TS is diagnosed is at least 5 years, and patients are often relieved to receive a diagnosis [48].

The average age of motor tic onset is 5–7 years. Phonic tics typically develop several months to years later [25]. Most patients experience their most severe tics around the age of 8–12 [49], followed by a natural decrease until early adulthood. Fifty-nine to 85 % of patients, who were diagnosed with a tic disorders in childhood, are tic-free or only have mild tics as adults [50, 51].

In the remaining 20 %, however, the symptoms continue or can become even more severe, often affecting work and social life [51]. What differentiates the two groups is still largely unknown. The best predictors for tic severity are currently a higher tic severity in childhood, smaller caudate volume, poorer fine motor skills and untreated comorbidities [50] but also psychosocial stress and depression in childhood [31]. Patients with uncomplicated TS tend to have a better prognosis than patients with TS and comorbid ADHD or comorbid ADHD and OCD [52].

28.2.4 Genetic and Environmental Factors

There is a large body of family studies, suggesting that TS is highly heritable [53]. First-degree relatives of TS patients have a 5–17-fold elevated risk of developing TS or a chronic tic disorder, compared to the general population [54–56]. Twin studies showed concordance rates between 53 % and 56 % for monozygotic twins (n=46 pairs) and 8 % for dizygotic twins (n= 13) for TS and 77–94 % and 23 %, respectively, for tics [57, 58]. These results corroborate the assumption that the vulnerability to develop TS has a large genetic component but that the degree, to which symptoms develop, might depend on environmental factors, i.e. the actual cause for developing TS symptoms is probably multifactorial. In line with these results, no single gene or polymorphism has been identified as the main cause of TS [59], suggesting a complex, polygenetic background of the disorder [60].

Genome-wide association studies (GWAS) look for common variants, single-nucleotide polymorphisms (SNPs) that occur in many individuals and only have a small effect concerning the investigated trait. Family studies, on the other hand, search for rare variants, which cause large effects. GWAS have gained popularity, partly because of the common disease – common variant hypothesis – which proposes that common diseases or disorders are the result of a cumulative effect of common alleles that increase susceptibility to the disease. In other words, there are common polymorphisms, which do not normally lead to the development of a disorder, but if several of them accumulate in one person, this person is more likely to develop the disorder [61]. A GWAS in 1285 European TS patients found no significant markers for TS but identified rs7868992 as a strong candidate locus to be implicated in the development of TS. rs7868992 is located in a gene involved in the expression of fibrillar collagen, primarily in the cartilage but also in the cerebellum [55]. Additional analyses implicated rs2060546, a SNP that lies near a gene associated with axon growth and guidance in the developing striatum [62].

A large family study in 2040 individuals identified a region on chromosome 2p to be significantly associated with TS and chronic tic disorder [63]. Rare variants associated with TS have been found in genes associated with dendritic growth [64, 65] and histaminergic and serotonergic pathways [66–68]. Although DA is the neurotransmitter system that has been implicated in TS most consistently, there is no consistent relationship between TS and DA candidate genes [69, 70].

To complicate matters further, there seems to be a genetic association between ODC and TS. TS, chronic tic disorder and OCD are more likely to occur in first-degree family members of TS patients, irrespective of whether patients have symptoms of OCD or not; first-degree family members of OCD patients are more likely to have tics than the general population [54]. The gender distribution of the respective disorders remains stable though. OCD is more likely to occur in female relatives, whereas TS is more likely to occur in male relatives. Although the genetic correlation between TS and OCD was estimated to be 0.41, corroborating the assumption that there is genetic overlap between the two disorders [71], a population-based twin study showed that most of the variance in vulnerability to tics, OCD and ADHD was associated with environmental factors [72].

The first epigenetic study in TS showed that the main alterations in TS were located near genes that are likely relevant for GABA receptors and near genes that have been associated with the development of other neuropsychiatric disorders such as OCD and autism, albeit none of the findings reached the significance threshold [73].

Environmental factors, as well as gene-environment interactions, have been proposed to play a role in the degree, to which TS symptoms develop in a susceptible individual. Several pre- and perinatal factors have been investigated. However, meaningful associations have only been found for low birth weight and maternal smoking [74]. Another study did not find an association between any pre- or perinatal risk factors and tic severity or comorbidities [75]. A study in a large cohort of children showed that maternal prenatal anxiety was related to the likelihood of their children having tics at the age of 13, but it is unclear whether this relationship reflects prenatal influences of maternal mood or a shared genetic vulnerability between mother and child [76].

Although a direct link between stress levels and tic frequency could not be shown in experimental studies [77, 78], children and adolescents with TS experience overall higher levels of psychosocial stress than healthy individuals, which can predict depressive symptoms and OC symptoms in the future [31]. Furthermore, there is evidence that minor negative life events (e.g. relations with family and peers, school achievements, etc.) are related to tic severity, depression and anxiety in children and adolescents with TS [79].

The relationship between the course of tic severity and hormonal development, and the fact that the prevalence in men is higher than in women, led to the assumption that androgenic hormones may play a role during certain stages of development [80].

28.2.5 Pathophysiology

The successful treatment of tics with neuroleptics suggests that the DA transmitter system is primarily affected in TS, although other transmitter systems and their interactions have also yielded promising insights [69]. Structurally, TS has been repeatedly associated with abnormalities in the thalamus, the frontal cortex and the BG, which play an important role in action selection and implementation and performance monitoring in goal-directed behaviour [81, 82]. All of these areas are part of a feedback circle, the "cortico-striato-thalamo-cortical" (CSTC) loop [83]. The CSTC loop can be further subdivided into sensorimotor, associative and limbic loops, because distinct areas of the BG nuclei receive excitatory input from sensorimotor, associative and limbic areas of the cortex [84]. The information is then processed and fed back to the thalamus, either directly, via the globus pallidus internus (GPi), or indirectly, via the globus pallidus externus (GPe), and the subthalamic nucleus, which projects to frontal areas of the neocortex.

There is a wealth of studies, relating abnormalities in CSTC loops to tics. For instance, neuroimaging studies have revealed decreased volumes of the caudate nucleus and the lenticular nucleus (globus pallidus and putamen) in children and adults with TS [85]. Corroborating this finding, postmortem studies found a decrease in the number and an abnormal distribution of cholinergic and GABAergic, inhibitory interneurons in the sensorimotor and associative areas of the striatum in TS patients as compared to healthy controls, suggesting a disrupted inhibitory-excitatory balance within the BG [86, 87]. Transcriptome analysis of the striatum confirmed downregulation of a module, enriched in striatal interneuron transcripts [88].

In line with this finding, bicuculline injections (a GABA-A antagonist) into the anterior or posterior striatum in rats triggered somatotopically related tic-like movements in the fore or hind limbs [89]. A spatiotemporal analysis of tic-related activation in monkeys revealed that activation in cortical motor areas both preceded and followed tic-like movements. Activation of medium spiny neurons in the striatum typically preceded the movement, as well as activation in cortical areas, specifically in the somatotopic area representing the body part, in which the tic was about to occur. Tic-related activation in the GPe followed movement onset and was of larger amplitude, more widespread and more diffuse than activation associated with normal movements, while activation in the GPi was characterized by a significant decrease in firing rate [90].

Direct evidence in humans stems from microelectrode recordings in the GPi of eight TS patients showing that approximately 50 % of the investigated neurons had tic-associated activity [91].

Furthermore, imaging data suggests an association between structural abnormalities in areas connected to the sensorimotor circuit of the CSTC loop and the development of simple tics, while more complex phenotypes of the disorder (e.g. associated OCD) might be related to structural changes in the associative and limbic loops [92, 93]. A study investigating connectivity patterns revealed stronger global functional integration within the CSTC loop in TS patients compared to healthy adults, a pattern similar to that in healthy children. This may point to brain maturation difficulties in TS [93].

A popular model for TS suggests that decreased inhibitory output from the BG may result in excessive cortical activity and, thus, excessive motor output, such as tics [94]. Interestingly, however, it was recently shown that activation in the CSTC loops, preceding tics in adult TS patients, sets off in cortical areas and then spreads to subcortical areas [95]. These data are more congruent with a model, suggesting that certain states can trigger motor plans in the SMA, which trigger the urge to tic [96], at least in adults with TS. Abnormal binding of states to motor plans and motor activation could be due to aberrant motor learning processes on the synaptic level [97].

28.2.6 Therapy

Because TS cannot be cured, the most important part of the treatment is psychoeducation, a point that has been especially emphasized by young TS patients and their parents [98]. Patients and their families should be informed about the neurobiological nature of tics, their fluctuating occurrence, natural course and their relationship with possible environmental triggers, such as stress. Tics can be managed using different methods. However, it is often more important to treat comorbidities because comorbid ADHD, OCD or depression can have a more debilitating effect than tics per se. Tics do not necessarily have to be treated. Especially children do not always suffer from their tics, regardless of their severity, and it is more often their parents, who are concerned. Therefore, subjective impairment should always be assessed before treatment decisions are made. If children experience bullying or problems with teachers, psychoeducation should extend to the school environment. Potent stressors in everyday life can be identified together with the patient, who can then try to avoid them.

There are guidelines for the diagnosis and treatment of TS, developed by experts of the European Society for the Study of Tourette syndrome (ESSTS), including a review of pharmacological treatment studies of the last three decades [2, 99–101]. However, parents of children with TS show high levels of anxiety and depression, both correlated with stress, and may need interventions or preventative measures as well. Social support and coping strategies appear to play a positive role [102].

The most common pharmacological treatment of TS is anti-dopaminergic medication (neuroleptics/antipsychotics). High-quality, placebo-controlled studies suggest that antipsychotics (haloperidol, pimozide, risperidone and ziprasidone) as well as alpha-2 agonists (adrenergic stimulants) are effective in treating tics, as compared to placebo. However, haloperidol appears to cause more side effects than the other drugs, especially long term [103, 104], and is therefore rarely used in TS specialty clinics. TS specialists currently consider tiapride and aripiprazole, followed by sulpiride and risperidone, to be the most useful drugs for treating adults as well as children with TS. Aripiprazole is perceived as most effective with least debilitating side effects by parents of young TS patients, while behavioural therapy is similarly effective, rarely has side effects and is valued by most young patients. However, some children find the techniques difficult to implement [98].

Table 28.1 Medication used as a treatment for tics

Drug	Initial dose (mg)	Average recommended daily dose for adults (mg)	Maximum approved daily dose (mg)	Intake
Typical antipsychotics				
Haloperidol	0.5	1–10	100	2–3×/day
Pimozide	0.5–1	2–8	16	1×/day in the evening
Tiapride	50–100	150–600	1,200	2–3×/day
Sulpiride	50–100	200–600	1,600	2×/day
Atypical antipsychotics				
Risperidone	0.5–1	1–8	16	2×/day
Aripiprazole	2.5	7.5–15	30	1×/day
Noradrenergic agents				
Clonidine	0.025–0.05	0.1–0.15		2–3×/day
Guanfacine	0.5	0.5–1		1×/day at bedtime
Others				
Tetrabenazine	12.5	3 × 25	200	3×/day
Tetrahydrocannabinol	2.5	10–20		2–3×/day

Adapted from Ludolph et al. [117]

Tetrahydrocannabinol (THC) was found to have small but significant effects on symptom severity in TS without affecting cognitive performance (recommendations for drug dosages are given in Table 28.1) [105, 106].

Single, well-localized tics, causing pain or injury, can be treated with botulinum toxin injections, temporarily weakening the muscle [107]. The treatment has been reported to sometimes also reduce premonitory urges. However, some patients report that the respective tics "migrated" to a different body part as a consequence of the treatment; hence, treatment protocols have to be specifically tailored to individual patients and may not always be effective.

In severe cases, TS can be treated using deep brain stimulation [101, 108], particularly of the intralaminar nuclei of the thalamus and the GPi. However, optimal target location, stimulation parameters and inclusion/exclusion criteria for surgery, as well as common side effects, are still unclear.

The most common and well-established behavioural therapy for TS is the "habit reversal therapy" (HRT), alluding to the parallels between tics and habits that have been drawn by some researchers [109]. Like habits, tics are stimulus-driven actions that are not outcome dependent and do not require specific attention. They are both repetitive and subject to change over time. Further, TS patients show increased habit learning compared to healthy controls [110] and tics appear to be strongly over-learned behaviours [111].

HRT trains patients to avoid executing specific tics by producing a motor response that is incompatible with the execution of the tic [112]. A second approach is the "exposure with response prevention" [113], a behavioural approach that stems from behavioural treatments for anxiety disorders and relies on the finding that anxiety is subject to habituation over time [114]. Patients are asked to suppress their tics and expose themselves to the premonitory urge until it subsides. Both approaches have been shown to successfully reduce tic frequency [115]; long-term effects though are unclear.

Only one study has evaluated a relatively new tic intervention by adding an acceptance and commitment therapy component to HRT, which aims to teach patients to accept and handle distressing thoughts and urges instead of avoiding them. The therapy integrates active coping with premonitory urges, negative emotions associated with tics (e.g. embarrassment) as well as cognitive phenomena that are typically related to comorbid OCD and ADHD [116].

Taken together, TS is a common childhood onset neuropsychiatric disorder with a fluctuating course, variable symptoms and signs and a number of typical comorbidities including ADHD and OCD. Severity ranges from very mild to very severe. TS can be challenging because tics often cause stigmatization and distress. TS is usually manageable in a satisfactory way, but it can greatly impair quality of life if not treated adequately.

Acknowledgement A. Münchau was supported by the Possehl-Stiftung, Lübeck. Research support by the Deutsche Forschungsgemeinschaft (SFB 936; MU 1692/4-1), and the University of Lübeck is also gratefully acknowledged.

References

1. DSM-IV. The Tourette syndrome classification study group. Definitions and classification of tic disorders. Arch Neurol. 1993;50:1013–16.
2. Cath DC, Hedderly T, Ludolph AG, et al. European clinical guidelines for Tourette syndrome and other tic disorders. Part I: assessment. Eur Child Adolesc Psychiatry. 2011;20:155–71.
3. Shapiro AK, Shapiro ES, Young JG, Feinberg TE. Gilles de la Tourette syndrome. New York: Raven; 1988.
4. Cath DC, Hoogduin CAL, van de Wetering BJM, van Woerkom TCAM, Roos RAC, Rooymans HGM. Tourette Syndrome and obsessive-compulsive disorder: an analysis of associated phenomena. In: Chase TN FA, Cohen DJ, editors. Adv Neurol. New York: Raven; 1992. p. 33–41.
5. Jankovic J. Tourette syndrome. Phenomenology and classification of tics. Neurol Clin. 1997;15:267–75.
6. Paszek J, Pollok B, Biermann-Ruben K, et al. Is it a tic? Twenty seconds to make a diagnosis. Mov Disord. 2010;25:1106–8.
7. Flanagan JR, Jakobson LS, Munhall KG. Anticipatory grip adjustments are observed in both goal-directed movements and movement tics in an individual with Tourette's syndrome. Exp Brain Res. 1999;128:69–75.
8. Silva RR, Munoz DM, Barickman J, Friedhoff AJ. Environmental factors and related fluctuation of symptoms in children and adolescents with Tourette's disorder. J Child Psychol Psychiatry. 1995;36:305–12.
9. Misirlisoy E, Brandt V, Ganos C, Tubing J, Munchau A, Haggard P. The relation between attention and tic generation in Tourette Syndrome. Neuropsychology. 2015;29(4):658–65.
10. Brandt VC, Lynn MT, Obst M, Brass M, Munchau A. Visual feedback of own tics increases tic frequency in patients with Tourette's syndrome. Cogn Neurosci. 2015;6:1–7.
11. Nixon E, Glazebrook C, Hollis C, Jackson GM. Reduced Tic symptomatology in tourette syndrome after an acute bout of exercise: an observational study. Behav Modif. 2014;38:235–63.
12. Riley DE, Lang AE. Pain in Gilles de la Tourette syndrome and related tic disorders. Can J Neurol Sci. 1989;16:439–41.
13. Krauss JK, Jankovic J. Severe motor tics causing cervical myelopathy in Tourette's syndrome. Mov Disord. 1996;11:563–6.
14. DSM-5. Diagnostic and statistical manual of mental disorders. 5th ed. Arlington: American Psychiatric Publishing; 2013.
15. Brandt VC, Beck C, Sajin V, et al. Temporal relationship between premonitory urges and tics in Gilles de la Tourette syndrome. Cortex. 2016;77:24–37.
16. Cavanna AE, Nani A. Tourette syndrome and consciousness of action. Tremor Other Hyperkinetic Mov. 2013;3:pii: tre-03-181-4368-4361.
17. Kwak C, Dat Vuong K, Jankovic J. Premonitory sensory phenomenon in Tourette's syndrome. Mov Disord. 2003;18:1530–3.
18. Kompoliti K, Goetz CG. Hyperkinetic movement disorders misdiagnosed as tics in Gilles de la Tourette syndrome. Mov Disord. 1998;13:477–80.
19. Kumar R, Lang AE. Tourette syndrome. Secondary tic disorders. Neurol Clin. 1997;15:309–31.
20. Mejia NI, Jankovic J. Secondary tics and tourettism. Rev Bras Psiquiatr. 2005;27:11–7.
21. Gilles de la Tourette G. Etude sur une affection nerveuse caracterisee par le l'incoordination motrice accompagnee d'echolalie et de coprolalie. Arch Neurol. 1885;9:158–200.
22. First MB, Pincus HA. The DSM-IV Text revision: rationale and potential impact on clinical practice. Psychiatr Serv. 2002;53:288–92.
23. Finis J, Moczydlowski A, Pollok B, et al. Echoes from childhood-imitation in Gilles de la Tourette syndrome. Mov Disord. 2012;27:562–5.
24. Ganos C, Ogrzal T, Schnitzler A, Munchau A. The pathophysiology of echopraxia/echolalia: relevance to Gilles de la Tourette syndrome. Mov Disord. 2012;27:1222–9.

25. Robertson MM. Gilles de la Tourette syndrome: the complexities of phenotype and treatment. Br J Hosp Med (Lond). 2011;72:100–7.
26. Hirschtritt ME, Lee PC, Pauls DL, et al. Lifetime prevalence, age of risk, and genetic relationships of comorbid psychiatric disorders in Tourette syndrome. JAMA Psychiatry. 2015;72:325–33.
27. Ghosh D, Rajan PV, Das D, Datta P, Rothner AD, Erenberg G. Sleep disorders in children with Tourette syndrome. Pediatr Neurol. 2014;51:31–5.
28. Eapen V, Robertson MM. Are there distinct subtypes in Tourette syndrome? Pure-Tourette syndrome versus Tourette syndrome-plus, and simple versus complex tics. Neuropsychiatr Dis Treat. 2015;11:1431–6.
29. Thériault M-CG, Lespérance P, Achim A, et al. ODD irritability is associated with obsessive-compulsive behavior and not ADHD in chronic tic disorders. Psychiatry Res. 2014; pii: S0165-1781(0114)00618-00610.
30. Roessner V, Becker A, Banaschewski T, Freeman RD, Rothenberger A, Tourette Syndrome International Database C. Developmental psychopathology of children and adolescents with Tourette syndrome – impact of ADHD. Eur Child Adolesc Psychiatry. 2007;16 Suppl 1:24–35.
31. Lin H, Katsovich L, Ghebremichael M, et al. Psychosocial stress predicts future symptom severities in children and adolescents with Tourette syndrome and/or obsessive-compulsive disorder. J Child Psychol Psychiatry. 2007;48:157–66.
32. Conelea CA, Woods DW, Zinner SH, et al. The impact of Tourette syndrome in adults: results from the Tourette syndrome impact survey. Community Ment Health J. 2013;49:110–20.
33. Eddy CM, Cavanna AE. Premonitory urges in adults with complicated and uncomplicated Tourette syndrome. Behav Modif. 2013;38:264–75.
34. Wadman R, Glazebrook C, Beer C, Jackson GM. Difficulties experienced by young people with Tourette syndrome in secondary school: a mixed methods description of self, parent and staff perspectives. BMC Psychiatry. 2016;16:14.
35. Debes N, Hjalgrim H, Skov L. The presence of attention-deficit hyperactivity disorder (ADHD) and obsessive-compulsive disorder worsen psychosocial and educational problems in Tourette syndrome. J Child Neurol. 2010;25:171–81.
36. Bernard BA, Stebbins GT, Siegel S, et al. Determinants of quality of life in children with Gilles de la Tourette syndrome. Mov Disord. 2009;24:1070–3.
37. Man C, Stern J, Gharatya A, Williams D, Simmons H, Robertson M. Psychosocial characteristics of tourette syndrome in older adults attending a specialist clinic. J Neurol Neurosurg Psychiatry. 2014;85:e3.
38. Gharatya A, Stern J, Man C, Williams D, Simmons H, Robertson M. Suicidality in patients with tourette's syndrome. J Neurol Neurosurg Psychiatry. 2014;85:e3.
39. Lang A. Patient perception of tics and other movement disorders. Neurology. 1991;41:223–8.
40. Banaschewski T, Woerner W, Rothenberger A. Premonitory sensory phenomena and suppressibility of tics in Tourette syndrome: developmental aspects in children and adolescents. Dev Med Child Neurol. 2003;45:700–3.
41. Crossley E, Cavanna AE. Sensory phenomena: clinical correlates and impact on quality of life in adult patients with Tourette syndrome. Psychiatry Res. 2013;209:705–10.
42. Ganos C, Garrido A, Navalpotro-Gomez I, et al. Premonitory urge to tic in tourette's is associated with interoceptive awareness. Mov Disord. 2015;30:1198–202.
43. Rozenman M, Johnson OE, Chang SW, et al. Relationships between premonitory urge and anxiety in youth with chronic tic disorders. Child Health Care. 2015;44:235–48.
44. Leckman JF, Walker DE, Cohen DJ. Premonitory urges in Tourette's syndrome. Am J Psychiatry. 1993;150:98–102.
45. Robertson MM. The prevalence and epidemiology of Gilles de la Tourette syndrome. Part 1: the epidemiological and prevalence studies. J Psychosom Res. 2008;65:461–72.
46. Center for Disease Control & Prevention. Prevalence of diagnosed Tourette syndrome in persons aged 6–17 years – United States, 2007. Morb Mortal Wkly Rep. 2009;58:581–5.
47. Schlander M, Schwarz O, Rothenberger A, Roessner V. Tic disorders: administrative prevalence and co-occurrence with attention-deficit/hyperactivity disorder in a German community sample. Eur Psychiatry. 2011;26:370–4.
48. Mol Debes NM, Hjalgrim H, Skov L. Limited knowledge of Tourette syndrome causes delay in diagnosis. Neuropediatrics. 2008;39:101–5.
49. Leckman JF, Zhang H, Vitale A, et al. Course of tic severity in Tourette syndrome: the first two decades. Pediatrics. 1998;102:14–9.
50. Hassan N, Cavanna AE. The prognosis of Tourette syndrome: implications for clinical practice. Funct Neurol. 2012;27:23–7.
51. Pappert EJ, Goetz CG, Louis ED, Blasucci L, Leurgans S. Objective assessments of longitudinal outcome in Gilles de la Tourette's syndrome. Neurology. 2003;61:936–40.
52. Rizzo R, Gulisano M, Cali PV, Curatolo P. Long term clinical course of Tourette syndrome. Brain Dev. 2012;34:667–73.
53. O'Rourke JA, Scharf JM, Yu D, Pauls DL. The genetics of Tourette syndrome: a review. J Psychosom Res. 2009;67:533–45.
54. Pauls DL, Raymond CL, Stevenson JM, Leckman JF. A family study of Gilles de la Tourette syndrome. Am J Hum Genet. 1991;48:154–63.
55. Scharf JM, Yu D, Mathews CA, et al. Genome-wide association study of Tourette's syndrome. Mol Psychiatry. 2013;18:721–8.

56. Mataix-Cols D, Isomura K, Perez-Vigil A, et al. Familial risks of tourette syndrome and chronic tic disorders. A population-based Cohort study. JAMA Psychiatry. 2015;72:787–93.
57. Price RA, Kidd KK, Cohen DJ, Pauls DL, Leckman JF. A twin study of Tourette syndrome. Arch Gen Psychiatry. 1985;42:815–20.
58. Hyde TM, Aaronson BA, Randolph C, Rickler KC, Weinberger DR. Relationship of birth weight to the phenotypic expression of Gilles de la Tourette's syndrome in monozygotic twins. Neurology. 1992;42:652–8.
59. Dietrich A, Fernandez TV, King RA, et al. The Tourette International Collaborative Genetics (TIC Genetics) study, finding the genes causing Tourette syndrome: objectives and methods. Eur Child Adolesc Psychiatry. 2015;24(2):141–51.
60. Paschou P. The genetic basis of Gilles de la Tour ette syndrome. Neurosci Biobehav Rev. 2013;37:1026–39.
61. Reich DE, Lander ES. On the allelic spectrum of human disease. Trends Genet. 2001;17:502–10.
62. Paschou P, Yu D, Gerber G, et al. Genetic association signal near NTN4 in Tourette syndrome. Ann Neurol. 2014;76:310–5.
63. Tourette Syndrome Association International Consortium for G. Genome scan for Tourette disorder in affected-sibling-pair and multigenerational families. Am J Hum Genet. 2007;80:265–72.
64. Abelson JF, Kwan KY, O'Roak BJ, et al. Sequence variants in SLITRK1 are associated with Tourette's syndrome. Science. 2005;310:317–20.
65. Kajiwara Y, Buxbaum JD, Grice DE. SLITRK1 binds 14-3-3 and regulates neurite outgrowth in a phosphorylation-dependent manner. Biol Psychiatry. 2009;66:918–25.
66. Ercan-Sencicek AG, Stillman AA, Ghosh AK, et al. L-histidine decarboxylase and Tourette's syndrome. N Engl J Med. 2010;362:1901–8.
67. Fernandez TV, Sanders SJ, Yurkiewicz IR, et al. Rare copy number variants in tourette syndrome disrupt genes in histaminergic pathways and overlap with autism. Biol Psychiatry. 2012;71:392–402.
68. Moya PR, Dodman NH, Timpano KR, et al. Rare missense neuronal cadherin gene (CDH2) variants in specific obsessive-compulsive disorder and Tourette disorder phenotypes. Eur J Hum Genet. 2013;21:850–4.
69. Buse J, Schoenefeld K, Munchau A, Roessner V. Neuromodulation in Tourette syndrome: dopamine and beyond. Neurosci Biobehav Rev. 2013;37:1069–84.
70. Paschou P, Fernandez TV, Sharp F, Heiman GA, Hoekstra PJ. Genetic susceptibility and neurotransmitters in Tourette syndrome. Int Rev Neurobiol. 2013;112:155–77.
71. Davis LK, Yu D, Keenan CL, et al. Partitioning the heritability of Tourette syndrome and obsessive compulsive disorder reveals differences in genetic architecture. PLoS Genet. 2013;9:e1003864.
72. Pinto R, Monzani B, Leckman JF, et al. Understanding the covariation of tics, attention-deficit/hyperactivity, and obsessive-compulsive symptoms: a population-based adult twin study. Am J Med Genet B Neuropsychiatr Genet. 2016;171(7):938–47.
73. Zilhao NR, Padmanabhuni SS, Pagliaroli L, et al. Epigenome-wide association study of tic disorders. Twin Res Hum Genet. 2015;18:699–709.
74. Chao TK, Hu J, Pringsheim T. Prenatal risk factors for Tourette syndrome: a systematic review. BMC Pregnancy Childbirth. 2014;14:53.
75. Taylor K, Stern J, Williams D, Simmons H, Robertson M. Do prenatal and perinatal complications influence tic severity in patients with gilles de la tourette syndrome? J Neurol Neurosurg Psychiatry. 2014;85:e3.
76. Ben-Shlomo Y, Scharf JM, Miller LL, Mathews CA. Parental mood during pregnancy and post-natally is associated with offspring risk of Tourette syndrome or chronic tics: prospective data from the Avon Longitudinal Study of Parents and Children (ALSPAC). Eur Child Adolesc Psychiatry. 2016;25:373–81.
77. Conelea CA, Woods DW, Brandt BC. The impact of a stress induction task on tic frequencies in youth with Tourette syndrome. Behav Res Ther. 2011;49:492–7.
78. Conelea CA, Ramanujam K, Walther MR, Freeman JB, Garcia AM. Is there a relationship between tic frequency and physiological arousal? Examination in a sample of children with co-occurring tic and anxiety disorders. Behav Modif. 2014;38:217–34.
79. Steinberg T, Shmuel-Baruch S, Horesh N, Apter A. Life events and Tourette syndrome. Compr Psychiatry. 2013;54:467–73.
80. Leckman JF. Tourette's syndrome. Lancet. 2002;360:1577–86.
81. Leckman JF, Bloch MH, Smith ME, Larabi D, Hampson M. Neurobiological substrates of Tourette's disorder. J Child Adolesc Psychopharmacol. 2010;20:237–47.
82. Ganos C, Roessner V, Munchau A. The functional anatomy of Gilles de la Tourette syndrome. Neurosci Biobehav Rev. 2013;37:1050–62.
83. Alexander GE, DeLong MR. Microstimulation of the primate neostriatum. II. Somatotopic organization of striatal microexcitable zones and their relation to neuronal response properties. J Neurophysiol. 1985;53:1417–30.
84. Alexander GE, DeLong MR, Strick PL. Parallel organization of functionally segregated circuits linking basal ganglia and cortex. Annu Rev Neurosci. 1986;9:357–81.
85. Peterson BS, Thomas P, Kane MJ, et al. Basal Ganglia volumes in patients with Gilles de la Tourette syndrome. Arch Gen Psychiatry. 2003;60:415–24.
86. Kalanithi PS, Zheng W, Kataoka Y, et al. Altered parvalbumin-positive neuron distribution in basal ganglia of individuals with Tourette syndrome. Proc Natl Acad Sci U S A. 2005;102:13307–12.

87. Kataoka Y, Kalanithi PS, Grantz H, et al. Decreased number of parvalbumin and cholinergic interneurons in the striatum of individuals with Tourette syndrome. J Comp Neurol. 2010;518:277–91.
88. Lennington JB, Coppola G, Kataoka-Sasaki Y, et al. Transcriptome analysis of the human striatum in Tourette syndrome. Biol Psychiatry. 2016;79:372–82.
89. Bronfeld M, Yael D, Belelovsky K, Bar-Gad I. Motor tics evoked by striatal disinhibition in the rat. Front Syst Neurosci. 2013;7:50.
90. Bronfeld M, Belelovsky K, Bar-Gad I. Spatial and temporal properties of tic-related neuronal activity in the cortico-basal ganglia loop. J Neurosci. 2011;31:8713–21.
91. Zhuang P, Hallett M, Zhang X, Li J, Zhang Y, Li Y. Neuronal activity in the globus pallidus internus in patients with tics. J Neurol Neurosurg Psychiatry. 2009;80:1075–81.
92. Worbe Y, Gerardin E, Hartmann A, et al. Distinct structural changes underpin clinical phenotypes in patients with Gilles de la Tourette syndrome. Brain. 2010;133:3649–60.
93. Worbe Y, Malherbe C, Hartmann A, et al. Functional immaturity of cortico-basal ganglia networks in Gilles de la Tourette syndrome. Brain. 2012;135:1937–46.
94. Albin RL, Mink JW. Recent advances in Tourette syndrome research. Trends Neurosci. 2006;29:175–82.
95. Neuner I, Werner CJ, Arrubla J, et al. Imaging the where and when of tic generation and resting state networks in adult Tourette patients. Front Hum Neurosci. 2014;8:362.
96. Maia TV, Frank MJ. From reinforcement learning models to psychiatric and neurological disorders. Nat Neurosci. 2011;14:154–62.
97. Brandt VC, Niessen E, Ganos C, Kahl U, Baumer T, Munchau A. Altered synaptic plasticity in Tourette's syndrome and its relationship to motor skill learning. PLoS One. 2014;9:e98417.
98. Hollis C, Pennant M, Cuenca J, et al. Clinical effectiveness and patient perspectives of different treatment strategies for tics in children and adolescents with Tourette syndrome: a systematic review and qualitative analysis. Health Technol Assess. 2016;20:1–450.
99. Roessner V, Plessen KJ, Rothenberger A, et al. European clinical guidelines for Tourette syndrome and other tic disorders. Part II: pharmacological treatment. Eur Child Adolesc Psychiatry. 2011;20:173–96.
100. Verdellen C, van de Griendt J, Hartmann A, Murphy T, Group EG. European clinical guidelines for Tourette syndrome and other tic disorders. Part III: behavioural and psychosocial interventions. Eur Child Adolesc Psychiatry. 2011;20:197–207.
101. Muller-Vahl KR, Cath DC, Cavanna AE, et al. European clinical guidelines for Tourette syndrome and other tic disorders. Part IV: deep brain stimulation. Eur Child Adolesc Psychiatry. 2011;20:209–17.
102. Gousse V, Czernecki V, Denis P, Stilgenbauer JL, Deniau E, Hartmann A. Impact of perceived stress, anxiety-depression and social support on coping strategies of parents having a child with Gilles de la Tourette syndrome. Arch Psychiatr Nurs. 2016;30:109–13.
103. Pringsheim T, Marras C. Pimozide for tics in Tourette's syndrome. Cochrane Database Syst Rev. 2009;(2):CD006996.
104. Weisman H, Qureshi IA, Leckman JF, Scahill L, Bloch MH. Systematic review: pharmacological treatment of tic disorders – efficacy of antipsychotic and alpha-2 adrenergic agonist agents. Neurosci Biobehav Rev. 2013;37:1162–71.
105. Muller-Vahl K, Grotenhermen F. Cannabis therapy. Dtsch Arztebl Int. 2013;110:144.
106. Curtis A, Clarke CE, Rickards HE. Cannabinoids for Tourette's syndrome. Cochrane Database Syst Rev. 2009;(4):CD006565.
107. Marras C, Andrews D, Sime E, Lang AE. Botulinum toxin for simple motor tics: a randomized, double-blind, controlled clinical trial. Neurology. 2001;56:605–10.
108. Zhang XH, Li JY, Zhang YQ, Li YJ. Deep brain stimulation of the globus pallidus internus in patients with intractable Tourette syndrome: a 1-year follow-up study. Chin Med J (Engl). 2016;129:1022–7.
109. Leckman JF, Riddle MA. Tourette's syndrome: when habit-forming systems form habits of their own? Neuron. 2000;28:349–54.
110. Delorme C, Salvador A, Valabregue R, et al. Enhanced habit formation in Gilles de la Tourette syndrome. Brain. 2016;139(Pt 2):605–15.
111. Brandt VC, Patalay P, Baumer T, Brass M, Munchau A. Tics as a model of over-learned behavior-imitation and inhibition of facial tics. Mov Disord. 2016;31(8):1155–62.
112. Azrin NH, Nunn RG. Habit-reversal: a method of eliminating nervous habits and tics. Behav Res Ther. 1973;11:619–28.
113. Hoogduin K, Verdellen C, Cath D. Exposure and response prevention in the treatment of Gilles de la Tourette's syndrome: four case studies. Clin Psychol Psychother. 1997;4:125–37.
114. Foa EB, Chambless DL. Habituation of subjective anxiety during flooding in imagery. Behav Res Ther. 1978;16:391–9.
115. Dutta N, Cavanna AE. The effectiveness of habit reversal therapy in the treatment of Tourette syndrome and other chronic tic disorders: a systematic review. Funct Neurol. 2013;28:7–12.
116. Franklin ME, Best SH, Wilson MA, Loew B, Compton SN. Habit reversal training and acceptance and commitment therapy for Tourette syndrome: a pilot project. J Dev Phys Disabil. 2011;23:49–60.
117. Ludolph AG, Roessner V, Munchau A, Muller-Vahl K. Tourette syndrome and other tic disorders in childhood, adolescence and adulthood. Dtsch Arztebl Int. 2012;109:821–288.

Tremor: Phenomenology, Etiology, Diagnosis, and Treatment

29

Arif Dalvi, Rajesh Pahwa, and Kelly E. Lyons

Tremor is an involuntary rhythmic, oscillatory movement produced by synchronous or alternating contractions of antagonist muscles. Tremor is one of the most common movement disorders and also one of the most common neurological symptoms. A wide variety of etiologies can cause tremor, with essential tremor being the most common. Parkinson's disease, multiple sclerosis, and drug-induced tremors are other etiologies commonly seen in clinical practice. Diagnosis of the specific etiology of tremor is based on the clinical characteristics of the tremor as well as associated symptoms. The phenomenology of tremor including whether the tremor is present at rest, with posture or with action, allows classification of tremor. Imaging studies, while not in themselves diagnostic, can help rule out structural etiologies. Dopamine transporter imaging is a recent modality that can help distinguish essential tremor from parkinsonism. The treatment of tremor is based on etiology and, where possible, treatment of the underlying disease state. Deep brain stimulation of the thalamus can be an effective treatment modality in cases of medication-resistant tremor.

Electronic supplementary material The online version of this chapter (doi:10.1007/978-3-7091-1628 9_29) contains supplementary material, which is available to authorized users.

A. Dalvi, MD, MBA
Movement Disorders Program, Palm Beach Neuroscience Institute, 901 Village Blvd., Suite 702, West Palm Beach, FL 33409, USA
e-mail: dalvi.md@gmail.com

R. Pahwa, MD • K.E. Lyons, PhD (✉)
Department of Neurology, Parkinson's Disease and Movement Disorder Center, University of Kansas Medical Center, 3599 Rainbow Blvd, MS 2012, Kansas City, KS 66160, USA
e-mail: rpahwa@kumc.edu; Kelly.lyons@att.net

29.1 Phenomenology of Tremor

Tremor is one of the most common movement disorders and essential tremor is the most prevalent pathological tremor in adults [1, 2]. Tremor is defined as an involuntary rhythmic, oscillatory movement produced by synchronous or alternating contractions of reciprocally innervated antagonist muscles [3, 4]. The hands are most commonly involved although the legs, voice and head may also be affected. Tremors can be classified by their distribution and frequency, as well as by the "state of activity." The state of activity refers to whether the tremor occurs at rest or with action [3, 5, 6]. The following definitions are often applied:

1. *Rest tremor* is observed when the affected body part is supported against gravity and is not voluntarily activated.

C. Falup-Pecurariu et al. (eds.), *Movement Disorders Curricula*, DOI 10.1007/978-3-7091-1628-9_29

2. *Action tremor* is observed during voluntary contraction of muscles and has the following subtypes:
   (a) *Postural tremor* occurs during voluntary maintenance of a position against gravity (e.g., holding hands outstretched in front of the body).
   (b) *Kinetic tremor* occurs during any aspect of voluntary movement. It can be present when the movement begins, during the course of movement, and as the target is reached (intention tremor).
   (c) *Task-specific tremor* is a type of kinetic tremor that occurs primarily during the execution of a specific task, such as writing or singing.
   (d) *Isometric tremor* is present during muscle contraction that is not accompanied by a change in position of body part (such as maintenance of tightly squeezed fist).

Tremor subtypes and common etiologies are listed in Table 29.1.

29.2 Etiology of Tremor

Essential tremor (ET), Parkinson's disease (PD), multiple sclerosis (MS), and medications are common causes of tremor in clinical practice. However, just as the phenomenology of tremor is varied, the possible etiologies for tremor are numerous, and careful attention to the history and details of the examination are required to ascertain the specific cause.

29.3 Physiological Tremor

A fine action tremor is seen in the majority of people under certain circumstances and is called a physiological tremor [7]. It is a low-amplitude, high-frequency tremor that is often not symptomatic. Enhanced physiological tremor (EPT) refers to a state where the baseline tremor is exacerbated by anxiety, exercise, metabolic disorders such as hyperthyroidism, and drugs including amphetamines, anticonvulsants, antidepressants, beta-receptor agonists, and caffeine [3]. The frequency of EPT ranges from 8 to 12 Hz and is affected by the mechanical properties of the oscillating limb. Unlike ET, the frequency of EPT can be reduced by mass loading, for example, with a lead-weighted wristband.

29.4 Essential Tremor

ET is by far the most common pathological tremor. The term (*tremor semplice essenziale*) was coined by Burressi to describe an isolated action tremor in the absence of other neurological signs [8]. Critchley wrote the first detailed review of ET and considered it to be heredofamilial [9]. Recent observations have raised the issue that it may be a neurodegenerative process with additional symptoms developing over time and with specific genetic etiologies in some cases [2, 10]. Therefore, ET may present in a variety of clinical forms with differing pathological substrates [11, 12]. Video 29.1 demonstrates the postural and intention tremor seen in ET.

ET can be either hereditary or sporadic. The prevalence of ET (0.9 %) is comparable to that of epilepsy (0.7 %). The prevalence increases with age, and ET affects about 4–6 % of people aged 65 years or older [13, 14]. ET presents as a postural and kinetic action tremor, typically bilateral, involving the arms and, in some cases, the head. The voice may also be affected. The tremor may spread to involve the legs, chin, and trunk [15, 16]. Tremor frequency is between 4 and 12 Hz and is inversely related to age with older patients having a lower frequency [15, 17]. Isolated head tremor may also occur, and in such cases cervical dystonia (CD) is a diagnostic consideration, particularly if there is a directional component [6]. Asymmetric hypertrophy of the cervical muscles, especially the sternocleidomastoid, may be observed in CD but is very unusual in ET [18]. CD can coexist with ET and was present in nearly one-third of the ET families in a genetics study, including 10.7 % of ET probands. The dystonic component is often undiagnosed in these individuals [19]. Video 29.2 demonstrates the combination of ET with cervical dystonia. Rest tremor may be seen in the elderly with long-standing

Table 29.1 Tremor diagnosis based on state of activity

	Rest tremor	Postural tremor	Kinetic tremor	Associated symptoms	Common etiologies
Essential tremor	+/–	+++	++	Usually none, occasional difficulty with tandem gait, cognitive changes	ET, FXTAS
Parkinsonian tremor	++	+/–	+/–	Bradykinesia, rigidity, gait, and posture changes	PD, MSA, PSP, DLBD
Cerebellar tremor	+/–	++	++	Based on etiology, for example, optic neuritis in MS, Kaiser-Fleisher rings in Wilson's disease	MS, trauma, Wilson's disease, phenytoin toxicity, alcohol intoxication
Midbrain tremor	+	++	+++	Holmes (rubral) tremor with rest < postural < kinetic tremor	Stroke, midbrain tumor, intracranial hemorrhage

DLBD diffuse Lewy body disease, *ET* essential tremor, *FXTAS* fragile X-associated tremor/ataxia syndrome, *MSA* multiple system atrophy, *PD* Parkinson's disease, *PSP* progressive supranuclear palsy
+++ required feature for diagnosis
++ usually present
+ may be present
+/– may or may not be present, not diagnostic

ET. However, the superimposition of PD or other forms of parkinsonism can also be a possibility [20, 21].

The understanding of the pathological processes underlying ET is limited with inconsistent findings. In one autopsy study, two broad categories of pathology were observed [22]. Prominent cerebellar changes were seen in about 75 %, which included a significant decline in the number of Purkinje cells and a marked increase in the number of swollen Purkinje cell axons called torpedoes. The remaining 25 % of brains showed Lewy bodies confined, for the most part, to the locus coeruleus. Other brain stem structures that show Lewy bodies in PD including the substantia nigra and dorsal vagal nucleus were minimally affected. The authors suggested that the two pathological subtypes were mutually exclusive with the former called cerebellar ET and the latter the Lewy body variant of ET [2]. In contrast, other studies failed to show an increase in Lewy bodies in ET autopsied cases compared to controls [23]. In addition, it is reported that 30 % of persons over the age of 65 years have Lewy bodies at autopsy, raising the question whether some Lewy bodies seen in ET are simply related to aging [24]. At this stage, there are insufficient data to confirm the presence of two pathological subtypes of ET.

In terms of pathophysiology, ET is considered a cerebellar disorder. Pathological changes in ET are seen in the cerebellum itself or in neurons that synapse with Purkinje cells. Functional imaging studies corroborate cerebellar dysfunction in ET [25, 26]. The location of the central oscillator in ET is a matter of debate. The cerebellum and the olivopontocerebellar pathways are favored. However, the ventral intermediate nucleus (VIM) of the thalamus may be an alternative location. Of note the VIM thalamus is the preferred surgical target for deep brain stimulation (DBS) in ET [27]. Noninvasive diffusion tractography from tremor-suppressive VIM DBS electrode contacts demonstrated a highly reproducible network that included motor cortical, subcortical, and cerebellar sites and the brain stem and was felt to be the anatomic basis for the effects of VIM stimulation [28].

29.5 Parkinson's Disease

A "pill-rolling" rest tremor is the typical tremor of PD. In practice, various combinations of rest and postural tremors are seen [5, 29]. Reemergent tremor occasionally seen in PD can resemble the postural tremor of ET. In most cases, the rest tremor of PD subsides when the hands are held outstretched, but in some cases a postural tremor may reemerge after a short duration. The latency from the time the hands are held outstretched to onset of tremor is longer in PD compared to ET [30]. Video 29.3 demonstrates the typical rest tremor seen in PD. PD tremor is usually unilateral in onset and may remain so for several years in contrast to ET. Further clues to a diagnosis of PD tremor include the presence of bradykinesia and rigidity. Often "cogwheel rigidity" is described in PD patients, which refers to the combination of a palpable tremor superimposed on underlying lead pipe rigidity [6]. Tremor is the presenting complaint in 60–70 % of cases of PD and may remain the main manifestation of the condition for several years without development of significant bradykinesia or gait disorder, a condition referred to as benign tremulous PD [31]. Of note, in approximately 10–30 % of PD cases, tremor may be completely absent [32]. The diagnosis of PD is based on clinical symptoms, and the use of formal criteria such as the United Kingdom Parkinson's Disease Society Brain Bank criteria can increase the probability of an accurate diagnosis [33].

The location of the tremor generator in PD is poorly understood, and tremor severity correlates poorly with the nigrostriatal dopaminergic deficit [34]. The loss of particular subgroups of mesencephalic neurons may determine severity of PD tremor [35]. The neurodegeneration of the retrorubral area (A8) is more prominent in tremor-predominant PD, while the lateral substantia nigra (A9) shows more significant degeneration in the akinetic-rigid form. Serotonin systems may also play a role in tremor generation. Reduced 5HT1-A binding has been correlated with tremor but not rigidity or bradykinesia [36]. Possible locations of the central oscillator responsible for PD tremor include the cerebellum, the thalamus, the globus pallidus, and the subthalamic nucleus [37, 38]. During microelectrode recording for DBS, "tremor cells" can be demonstrated in the VIM nucleus of the thalamus, the globus pallidus, and the subthalamic nucleus [39]. It is postulated that these cells form an unstable oscillating network responsible for the tremor. Lesioning in these nuclei or DBS may disrupt this network, resuming normal unsynchronized activity, leading to improved tremor control [37].

29.6 Cerebellar Tremor

Cerebellar tremor is a proximal action tremor of large amplitude with low frequency (3–5 Hz). Lesions of the deep cerebellar nuclei or outflow pathways in the superior cerebellar peduncle cause this tremor [40]. The intention component of kinetic tremor is characteristic of cerebellar tremor. The tremor tends to increase as the target is approached, which is referred to as a terminal tremor [4]. However, various types of postural tremor are also seen. Titubation is a postural tremor of the head and trunk, most pronounced when the patient is standing. It is uncommon for cerebellar tremor to occur in isolation. Associated findings including ataxia and gait disorder are common [5].

The most common causes of cerebellar tremor include MS, mass lesions, and vascular and degenerative diseases. Cerebellar degeneration may result from alcohol abuse or toxicity from drugs such as anticonvulsants, neuroleptics, or lithium. The tremor in these cases tends to be bilateral. In contrast, tremor from a structural lesion such as a mass, infarct, or plaque tends to be unilateral [5]. Cerebellar tremor may occasionally be a delayed sequela to a head injury, either as a result of direct injury to the dentate nucleus or due to shear injury to cerebellar axons in the outflow pathways [41]. Inherited spinocerebellar ataxias [42] and paraneoplastic syndromes [43] are other important causes. Lesions in the deep lateral cerebellar nuclei and their outflow pathways up to the red nucleus can cause cerebellar tremor. Lesions of the red nucleus and beyond cause Holmes tremor. Lesions proximal to the decussation of the outflow pathways result in ipsilateral tremor, and distal lesions result in contralateral tremor. Injury to the cerebellar cortex itself does not cause tremor [44].

29.7 Holmes Tremor

Holmes tremor (rubral tremor or midbrain tremor) refers to a combination of rest, postural, and action tremors due to midbrain lesions. Common causes include strokes, tumors, MS, or vascular malformations. As the lesion is typically in the vicinity of the red nucleus (which is part of the cerebellar outflow tract), the tremor phenotype is similar to that of a cerebellar tremor in that the tremor is irregular with a low frequency [45].

The tremor has a static and dynamic component. The former consists of a coarse tremor with a frequency of 3–5 Hz that increases with attempts at inhibition. The dynamic component consists of an irregular intention tremor similar to that seen in MS. Associated findings may include diplopia, ptosis, oculomotor palsies, hemiparesis, hemianopia, and parkinsonian features [45]. Holmes in 1904 suggested that involvement of the red nucleus was a key anatomic component, leading to the term "rubral tremor" [45]. However, the advent of improved imaging techniques demonstrated that lesions in other midbrain structures as well as the thalamus could also cause this tremor. Hence, the term "rubral tremor" has been abandoned in favor of the term Holmes tremor [4].

29.8 Dystonic Tremor

A dystonic tremor occurs in a body part that is simultaneously affected by dystonia. The tremor is irregular and jerky in nature and interrupted with sustained dystonic spasms. Dystonic tremor is typically position sensitive. For example, when the patient is allowed to move the affected body part to the position of maximal pull, a null point is reached and tremor often ceases [46]. The tremor may be relieved with complete rest or touching the affected body part (*geste antagoniste*) [47].

The pathophysiology of dystonic tremor is poorly understood [48]. Two types of tremor may occur separately or together, an ET-like tremor and a dystonic tremor. The ET-like tremor has a higher frequency with a peak at 9–11 Hz, whereas the dystonic tremor has a peak at about 5 Hz [47].

29.9 Task-Specific Tremor

Task-specific tremor (occupational tremor) is a kinetic tremor that appears during the performance of highly skilled, learned motor tasks such as writing or playing a musical instrument. The most frequent task-specific tremor is primary writing tremor. This tremor often has a dystonic component and may also be classified as a focal dystonia [6, 49]. The tremor may resemble an essential tremor or a dystonic tremor or have features common to both on clinical examination as well as on EMG analysis [47, 50].

29.10 Orthostatic Tremor

Orthostatic tremor (OT) typically involves the legs and trunk and is present when standing still. It generally improves with walking [51]. A latency period of 3–5 min may be present before the tremor is seen. OT is more common in women and usually presents in the sixth or seventh decade. OT has a more rapid frequency than other tremors, in the 13–18 Hz range [52, 53]. While present primarily during standing, OT may also be precipitated by isometric contraction of the upper limbs. Thus, it is more likely related to isometric force control rather than regulation of stance [54]. Orthostatic myoclonus is similar but appears to be a distinct disorder. Patients complain of leg jerking during upright posture. There is a gradual decline of gait, often described as "apraxia" or "gait initiation difficulty" in these patients [55].

29.11 Posttraumatic Tremor

Posttraumatic tremor is a challenging diagnosis with poorly defined criteria. The concept of tremor following a central injury is more accepted than a peripherally induced tremor [56, 57]. Retrospective studies suggest that following closed head injury posttraumatic tremor is the second most common movement disorder after dystonia. Posttraumatic tremor most often follows as a delayed sequela to severe head trauma, and there may be a significant delay between the injury and development of symptoms. In a survey of 289 children with severe head injury, tremor prevalence was about 45 %. The tremor occurred within the first 18 months after injury and subsided spontaneously in over half the cases [58].

29.12 Other Etiologies of Tremor

Expansions of the CGG repeats in the fragile X mental retardation 1 gene (FMR1) lead to clinical manifestations based on the number of repeats. Greater than 200 repeats are associated with developmental delay and autism. However, repeats in the premutation range (55–200) are associated with a tremor resembling ET. Additional symptoms include cerebellar gait ataxia, frontal executive dysfunction, and global brain atrophy and are grouped together as the fragile X-associated tremor/ataxia syndrome (FXTAS). Other associated findings may include mild parkinsonism, peripheral neuropathy, depression, and autonomic dysfunction [59].

Peripheral nerve disorders such as Charcot-Marie-Tooth disease (CMTD) may be associated with tremor. Associated findings include foot deformities, weakness, and atrophy affecting the anterior compartment muscles in the lower leg leading to the "inverted Coke bottle" appearance of the legs. A postural tremor resembling ET is present in about a third of patients with CMTD and can occur in both the demyelinating and axonal forms [60].

Wilson's disease (WD) is an important diagnostic consideration, especially in an adolescent or young adult [6]. Tremor is common in WD and can present as a rest tremor and/or postural tremor. A "wing beating" tremor may be seen when the arms are held in front of the body and flexed at the elbows [61]. Kayser-Fleischer rings may be seen in the cornea on direct exam or by slit-lamp examination and are present in most patients with this neurological disease [62]. Other etiologies of tremor include infectious diseases, trauma, and drugs. These and other rare etiologies of tremor have been reviewed elsewhere by Dalvi and Premkumar [6].

29.13 Psychogenic Tremor

Psychogenic tremor is the most common psychogenic movement disorder. Differentiating between psychogenic tremor and organic tremors can be challenging. The diagnosis is made based on the history as well as careful observation of the tremor [4]. Psychogenic tremors usually have an abrupt onset with maximal disability also often seen at the onset. The clinical course is variable and may include spontaneous remissions and recurrences. Tremors may affect the wrists, elbows, and shoulders but rarely the fingers [63]. The amplitude and frequency of psychogenic tremor is variable in response to attention or distraction. By contrast, with organic tremor although the amplitude may change with stress or emotions, the frequency tends to stay constant. Psychogenic tremor also commonly exhibits an entrainment phenomenon [64]. The frequency of the tremor in a limb may change to match the frequency of voluntary tapping in another limb. Psychiatric evaluation may not always be contributory, but depression and other psychosomatic conditions are common. Psychogenic tremors typically do not respond to conventional anti-tremor medications but may respond to antidepressants or psychotherapy [65].

29.14 Diagnostic Workup

The extent of laboratory investigations depends on the diagnostic certainty after clinical evaluation. Thyroid function tests and routine metabolic tests are usually ordered as screening tests. Screening tests for WD include serum ceruloplasmin, which is usually low, and measurement of 24-h urine copper, which is increased. Further workup for WD includes a slit-lamp examination to look for Kayser-Fleischer rings. Genetic testing/liver biopsy for WD may also be warranted [62]. Electromyography (EMG) and nerve conduction tests are helpful in tremor associated with peripheral neuropathy such as CMTD. Supplementary investigations to consider when tremor and neuropathy coexist include serum protein electrophoresis, urinary Bence-Jones protein, and porphyrin screen. Tremor analysis with accelerometers and surface EMG can help characterize a tremor but has a limited practical role in diagnosis [6].

Brain MRI helps rule out structural etiologies of tremor such as MS or focal midbrain lesions that can lead to Holmes tremor [66]. The role of brain MRI in the diagnosis of parkinsonism is also mainly exclusionary. If present, characteristic radiological abnormalities can assist in the differential diagnosis of parkinsonism [67]. These may include midbrain atrophy in progressive supranuclear palsy, atrophy of the pons and cerebellum as well as the middle cerebellar peduncles (MCPs) in olivopontocerebellar atrophy, and focal cortical atrophy in corticobasal degeneration [68]. Signal hyperintensities within the pons and MCPs in multiple system atrophy (MSA) may occasionally result in the "hot-cross bun" sign [69]. Brain MRI changes in FXTAS include atrophy of the cerebrum, cerebellar cortex, corpus callosum, and pons. A distinctive abnormality of the middle cerebellar peduncles with increased T2 signal is a hallmark of FXTAS [70].

Single-photon computerized emission tomography (SPECT) techniques represent an advance in the ability to distinguish ET from parkinsonism. In cases of diagnostic uncertainty between degenerative parkinsonism and non-degenerative tremor disorders, baseline SPECT imaging with the dopamine transporter ligand (123)I ioflupane (DaTscan™) has shown 78 % sensitivity and 97 % specificity with reference to clinical diagnosis at 3 years, versus 93 % and 46 %, respectively, for baseline clinical diagnosis [71]. However, DaTscan imaging cannot readily differentiate between PD and atypical parkinsonism. Figure 29.1 compares the typical comma-shaped appearance of the DaTscan in ET (1a) with the period-shaped appearance in PD (1b) due to reduced dopamine transporter levels in PD.

29.15 Pharmacological Treatment of Essential Tremor

While no curative treatment for ET is available, medications may improve quality of life. Pharmacological treatment is based on reducing the sympathetic drive that exacerbates tremor, increasing GABAergic inhibition of the central oscillators that drive the tremor, and membrane stabilizing effects. Propranolol, primidone, and alcohol are the prototypical drugs that respectively represent these three mechanisms. Other comorbidities such as diabetes, cardiac failure, glaucoma, and renal failure should be kept in mind when tailoring the choice of drug to a particular patient. The American Academy of Neurology (AAN) has published a practice parameter for the therapy of ET as a guide to treatment [72]. Key pharmacotherapeutic agents are reviewed below.

29.16 Beta-Adrenergic Blockers

Propranolol was one of the earliest agents shown to be effective in ET [73]. It is still a mainstay of treatment and the only medication approved by the FDA for ET. About 50–70 % of patients had substantial relief in randomized controlled trials (RCTs) [73, 74]. The long-acting form of propranolol (propranolol-LA) may help with compliance when high doses are required [75]. Other beta-blockers used include atenolol, metoprolol, nadolol, sotalol, timolol, and arotinol. However, strong clinical evidence for their use is lacking [76]. Contraindications to beta-blockers include asthma, heart blocks, and concurrent calcium-channel blockers. They should be used with caution in diabetics as they can mask the sympathetic response to hypoglycemia [76].

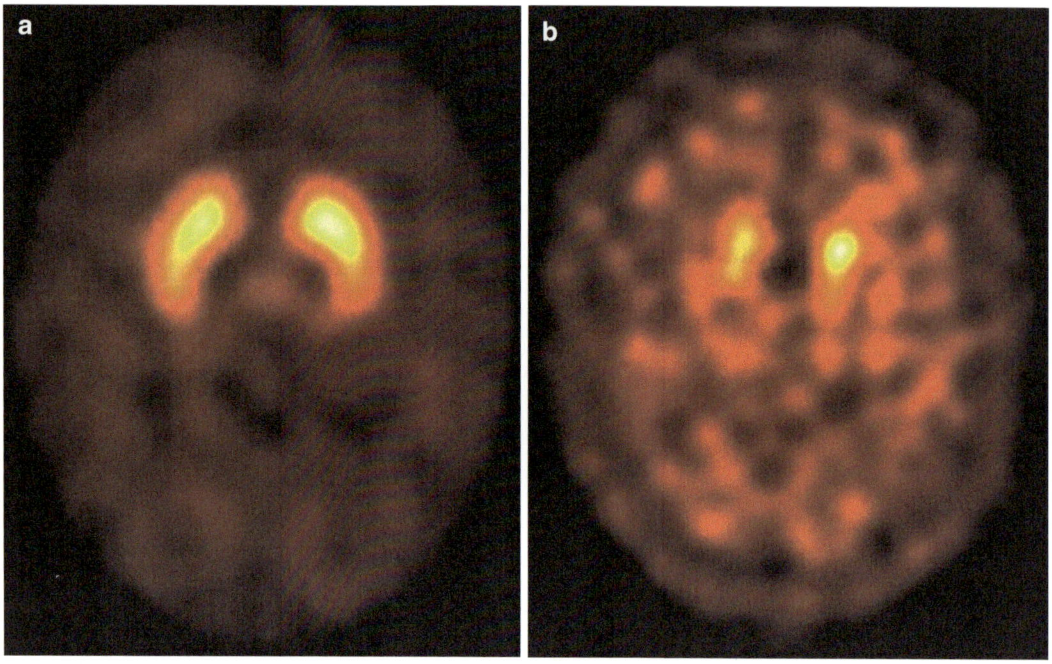

Fig. 29.1 (**a**) DaTscan of an ET patient showing comma-shaped appearance, indicating normal uptake of dopamine. (**b**) DaTscan of a PD patient showing period-shaped appearance, indicating reduced uptake of dopamine

29.17 Primidone

Primidone is as efficacious in ET as propranolol [77]. Doses for ET are lower than typical antiepileptic doses. Primidone is metabolized to phenobarbital and phenylethylmalonamide (PEMA). Primidone was found to be superior to phenobarbital suggesting that it has a direct effect rather than an effect through its metabolites [78]. Combination therapy with propranolol and primidone is useful in refractory tremor [79]. Daytime somnolence can limit the use of primidone, especially in the elderly.

29.18 Gabapentin

Though gabapentin is a structural analog of GABA, it has no affinity for the GABA receptor, and the mechanism of action in ET is unclear. Results from RCTs are mixed with gabapentin shown as equivalent to propranolol [80] or ineffective [81].

29.19 Topiramate

Topiramate has multiple mechanisms of action including glutamate antagonist and GABA-agonist activities. In a RCT, topiramate was found to be superior to placebo for ET [82]. A multicenter study confirmed this finding, when topiramate was used as monotherapy and as an adjunct to one other anti-tremor medication [83]. Topiramate should be avoided in patients with glaucoma or those at risk for nephrolithiasis and should be used with caution in the elderly as it carries a risk of cognitive side effects.

29.20 Benzodiazepines

Alprazolam, clonazepam, and lorazepam may suppress tremor through their GABA-agonist activity. They are especially useful in anxious patients. Alprazolam was shown to be effective in ET in a RCT [84], but clonazepam and lorazepam have not been tested in RCTs. Benzodiazepines are best used as second-line agents due to the potential for tolerance and addiction. Rapid withdrawal should be avoided when these drugs need to be discontinued.

29.21 Botulinum Toxin

A number of patients with head tremor may have CD. The efficacy of botulinum toxins has been unequivocal in this condition. In patients with head tremor without CD, there is limited information from small trials [85]. The use of botulinum toxin in hand tremor is limited by lack of efficacy as demonstrated by functional rating scales, as well as a tendency to affect motor dexterity [86].

29.22 Pharmacological Treatment of Other Tremor Disorders

29.22.1 Parkinson's Disease

The treatment of tremor associated with PD involves addressing the underlying dopaminergic deficit. The mainstay of treatment is levodopa in one of its forms, with dopamine agonists, monoamine oxidase type B inhibitors, catechol-O-methyltransferase inhibitors, and amantadine as adjuncts or alternates in early disease [87]. Anticholinergic drugs can be used but cognitive side effects are a limitation.

29.23 Multiple Sclerosis and Cerebellar Tremor

About 25–60 % of patients with MS have tremor. In addition to the postural tremor, there is an ataxic component, which is harder to treat. Isoniazid in high doses, carbamazepine, propranolol, and glutethimide have been reported to provide some relief [88].

29.24 Dystonic Tremor

Distinguishing ET from dystonic tremor is important in choosing the appropriate therapy. Benzodiazepines including clonazepam, lorazepam, and diazepam are often used. However, the therapeutic dose is often also one at which significant drowsiness or fatigue is observed [47]. As a result, chemodenervation with botulinum toxin has become the first-line treatment for some forms of dystonic tremor such as CD [89]. The dystonic component of primary writing tremor may also respond to clonazepam and EMG-guided botulinum toxin injections [89].

29.25 Holmes Tremor

Holmes tremor has components of rest tremor and postural tremor. As secondary etiologies are frequent, the first step is to treat the underlying etiology if possible. The postural component may respond to ET medications such as propranolol and primidone. The rest tremor component is harder to treat but may respond to levodopa [45].

29.26 Orthostatic Tremor

OT was initially classified as an ET variant. However, first-line drugs for ET are rarely of benefit. Clonazepam may be effective in some cases [90]. The most practical treatment is the use of a walker with a seat that allows the patient to sit when the OT becomes severe.

29.27 Surgical Treatment of Tremor

Surgical treatment is an option for intractable tremor [27]. Video 29.4 demonstrates the impact of DBS on ET. Regardless of etiology, the motor thalamus is the preferred surgical target, which may be explained by its central position between subcortical and cortical tremor networks [91]. Surgical methods for tremor include thalamotomy and DBS. Due to the irreversible nature of thalamotomy and the high risk of hypophonia, dysarthria, and cognitive deficits following bilateral ablation, DBS has become the preferred surgical modality [92]. The surgical treatment of choice for ET is DBS of the VIM nucleus of the thalamus. Lyons and Pahwa reviewed eight outcome studies of DBS for ET, covering 158 patients implanted unilaterally and 68 with bilateral DBS [93]. Across studies, over 33 months of mean follow-up, activities of daily living improved on average by 46 %. There was a reduction in overall tremor of 48 %, including 73 % for hand tremor. Head tremor improved only 35 % in unilaterally implanted patients but 81 % in bilateral patients, and the same was generally true for voice tremor. Complications were rare and generally led to no permanent deficits [93]. A meta-analysis of the complications of DBS for 1,154 patients showed the following common adverse events: mental status or behavioral changes (16.6 %), infection (2.2 %), speech disturbance (2.0 %), symptomatic intracerebral hemorrhage (2.0 %), seizures (1.0 %), misplaced electrodes (1.6 %), and asymptomatic intracerebral hemorrhage (1.2 %). Hardware-related adverse events occurred in 8.7 % of patients [94]. Other tremor etiologies have been shown to be responsive to DBS as well. The mixed rest and tremor components of Holmes tremor have been reported to be amenable to multitarget dual electrode DBS techniques [95, 96]. Dystonic tremor as well as other symptoms of CD were shown to be responsive to pallidal DBS in a sham-controlled trial [97]. Although tremor from PD can be well controlled by VIM DBS, the usual surgical targets in PD are the subthalamic nucleus or the globus pallidus as DBS as these sites can improve other PD symptoms in addition to tremor [98].

References

1. Elble RJ. Tremor: clinical features, pathophysiology, and treatment. Neurol Clin. 2009;27:679–95, v–vi.
2. Louis ED. Essential tremor: evolving clinicopathological concepts in an era of intensive post-mortem enquiry. Lancet Neurol. 2010;9:613–22.
3. Anouti A, Koller WC. Tremor disorders. Diagnosis and management. West J Med. 1995;162:510–3.
4. Deuschl G, Bain P, Brin M. Consensus statement of the movement disorder society on tremor. Ad Hoc Scientific Committee. Mov Disord. 1998;13 Suppl 3:2–23.
5. Bain PG. Parkinsonism & related disorders. Tremor. Parkinsonism Relat Disord. 2007;13 Suppl 3:S369–74.
6. Dalvi A, Premkumar A. Tremor: etiology, phenomenology, and clinical features. Dis Mon. 2011;57:109–26.
7. Elble RJ. Physiologic and essential tremor. Neurology. 1986;36:225–31.
8. Louis ED, Broussolle E, Goetz CG, et al. Historical underpinnings of the term essential tremor in the late 19th century. Neurology. 2008;71:856–9.
9. Critchley M. Observations on essential (heredofamilial) tremor. Brain. 1949;72:113–39.
10. Schmouth JF, Dion PA, Rouleau GA. Genetics of essential tremor: from phenotype to genes, insights from both human and mouse studies. Prog Neurobiol. 2014;119-120C:1–19.
11. Louis ED. Essential tremors: a family of neurodegenerative disorders? Arch Neurol. 2009;66:1202–8.
12. Deuschl G, Elble R. Essential tremor – neurodegenerative or nondegenerative disease towards a working definition of ET. Mov Disord. 2009;24:2033–41.
13. Louis ED, Marder K, Cote L, et al. Prevalence of a history of shaking in persons 65 years of age and older: diagnostic and functional correlates. Mov Disord. 1996;11:63–9.
14. Deuschl G, Raethjen J, Hellriegel H, Elble R. Treatment of patients with essential tremor. Lancet Neurol. 2011;10:148–61.
15. Lou JS, Jankovic J. Essential tremor: clinical correlates in 350 patients. Neurology. 1991;41:234–8.
16. Bain PG, Findley LJ, Thompson PD, et al. A study of hereditary essential tremor. Brain. 1994;117(Pt 4):805–24.
17. Louis ED. Essential tremor. Lancet Neurol. 2005;4:100–10.
18. Pal PK, Samii A, Schulzer M, et al. Head tremor in cervical dystonia. Can J Neurol Sci. 2000;27:137–42.
19. Louis ED, Galecki M, Rao AK. Four essential tremor cases with moderately impaired gait: how impaired can gait be in this disease? From pubmed: Tremor Other Hyperkinet Mov (NY). 2013 Nov 4;3.
20. Shahed J, Jankovic J. Exploring the relationship between essential tremor and Parkinson's disease. Parkinsonism Relat Disord. 2007;13:67–76.
21. Minen MT, Louis ED. Emergence of Parkinson's disease in essential tremor: a study of the clinical correlates in 53 patients. Mov Disord. 2008;23:1602–5.
22. Louis ED, Faust PL, Vonsattel JP, et al. Neuropathological changes in essential tremor: 33 cases compared with 21 controls. Brain. 2007;130:3297–307.
23. Adler CH, Shill HA, Beach TG. Essential tremor and Parkinson's disease: lack of a link. Mov Disord. 2011;26:372–7.
24. Rajput AH, Adler CH, Shill HA, Rajput A. Essential tremor is not a neurodegenerative disease. Neurodegener Dis Manag. 2012;2:259–68.

25. Bucher SF, Seelos KC, Dodel RC, et al. Activation mapping in essential tremor with functional magnetic resonance imaging. Ann Neurol. 1997;41:32–40.
26. Louis ED, Shungu DC, Chan S, et al. Metabolic abnormality in the cerebellum in patients with essential tremor: a proton magnetic resonance spectroscopic imaging study. Neurosci Lett. 2002;333:17–20.
27. Benabid AL, Pollak P, Gervason C, et al. Long-term suppression of tremor by chronic stimulation of the ventral intermediate thalamic nucleus. Lancet. 1991;337:403–6.
28. Klein JC, Barbe MT, Seifried C, et al. The tremor network targeted by successful VIM deep brain stimulation in humans. Neurology. 2012;78:787–95.
29. Deuschl G, Papengut F, Hellriegel H. The phenomenology of parkinsonian tremor. Parkinsonism Relat Disord. 2012;18 Suppl 1:S87–9.
30. Jankovic J, Schwartz KS, Ondo W. Re-emergent tremor of Parkinson's disease. J Neurol Neurosurg Psychiatry. 1999;67:646–50.
31. Josephs KA, Matsumoto JY, Ahlskog JE. Benign tremulous parkinsonism. Arch Neurol. 2006;63:354–7.
32. Hughes AJ, Daniel SE, Blankson S, Lees AJ. A clinicopathologic study of 100 cases of Parkinson's disease. Arch Neurol. 1993;50:140–8.
33. Pahwa R, Lyons KE. Early diagnosis of Parkinson's disease: recommendations from diagnostic clinical guidelines. Am J Manag Care. 2010;16(Suppl Implications):S94–9.
34. Vingerhoets FJ, Schulzer M, Calne DB, Snow BJ. Which clinical sign of Parkinson's disease best reflects the nigrostriatal lesion? Ann Neurol. 1997;41:58–64.
35. Paulus W, Jellinger K. The neuropathologic basis of different clinical subgroups of Parkinson's disease. J Neuropathol Exp Neurol. 1991;50:743–55.
36. Jellinger KA. Post mortem studies in Parkinson's disease – is it possible to detect brain areas for specific symptoms? J Neural Transm Suppl. 1999;56:1–29.
37. Bergman H, Deuschl G. Pathophysiology of Parkinson's disease: from clinical neurology to basic neuroscience and back. Mov Disord. 2002;17 Suppl 3:S28–40.
38. Hallett M. Tremor: pathophysiology. Parkinsonism Relat Disord. 2014;20 Suppl 1:S118–22.
39. Brodkey JA, Tasker RR, Hamani C, et al. Tremor cells in the human thalamus: differences among neurological disorders. J Neurosurg. 2004;101:43–7.
40. Elble RJ. What is essential tremor? Curr Neurol Neurosci Rep. 2013;13:353.
41. Krauss JK, Wakhloo AK, Nobbe F, et al. Lesion of dentatothalamic pathways in severe post-traumatic tremor. Neurol Res. 1995;17:409–16.
42. Manto MU. The wide spectrum of spinocerebellar ataxias (SCAs). Cerebellum. 2005;4:2–6.
43. Mehta SH, Morgan JC, Sethi KD. Paraneoplastic movement disorders. Curr Neurol Neurosci Rep. 2009;9:285–91.
44. Elble RJ. Central mechanisms of tremor. J Clin Neurophysiol. 1996;13:133–44.
45. Dalvi A. Holmes tremor. In: Lyons KE, Pahwa R, editors. Handbook of essential tremor and other tremor disorders. Boca Raton: Taylor and Francis; 2005. p. 243–50.
46. Jain S, Lo SE, Louis ED. Common misdiagnosis of a common neurological disorder: how are we misdiagnosing essential tremor? Arch Neurol. 2006;63:1100–4.
47. Deuschl G. Dystonic tremor. Rev Neurol (Paris). 2003;159:900–5.
48. Deuschl G, Bergman H. Pathophysiology of nonparkinsonian tremors. Mov Disord. 2002;17 Suppl 3:S41–8.
49. Bain PG, Findley LJ, Britton TC, et al. Primary writing tremor. Brain. 1995;118(Pt 6):1461–72.
50. Lee A, Chadde M, Altenmüller E, Schoonderwaldt E. Characteristics of task-specific tremor in string instrument players. Tremor Other Hyperkinetic Mov (NY). 2014;4:198.
51. Yaltho TC, Ondo WG. Orthostatic tremor: a review of 45 cases. Parkinsonism Relat Disord. 2014;20:723–5.
52. Heilman KM. Orthostatic tremor. Arch Neurol. 1984;41:880–1.
53. Littmann L. Fact or artifact? The electrocardiographic diagnosis of orthostatic tremor. J Electrocardiol. 2010;43:270–3.
54. Boroojerdi B, Ferbert A, Foltys H, et al. Evidence for a non-orthostatic origin of orthostatic tremor. J Neurol Neurosurg Psychiatry. 1999;66:284–8.
55. Glass GA, Ahlskog JE, Matsumoto JY. Orthostatic myoclonus: a contributor to gait decline in selected elderly. Neurology. 2007;68:1826–30.
56. Krauss JK, Jankovic J. Head injury and posttraumatic movement disorders. Neurosurgery. 2002;50:927–39; discussion 939–40.
57. Jankovic J. Peripherally induced movement disorders. Neurol Clin. 2009;27:821–32, vii.
58. Johnson SL, Hall DM. Post-traumatic tremor in head injured children. Arch Dis Child. 1992;67:227–8.
59. Leehey MA. Fragile X-associated tremor/ataxia syndrome: clinical phenotype, diagnosis, and treatment. J Investig Med. 2009;57:830–6.
60. Cardoso FE, Jankovic J. Hereditary motor-sensory neuropathy and movement disorders. Muscle Nerve. 1993;16:904–10.
61. Aggarwal A, Bhatt M. Update on Wilson disease. Int Rev Neurobiol. 2013;110:313–48.
62. Huster D. Wilson disease. Best Pract Res Clin Gastroenterol. 2010;24:531–9.
63. Kim YJ, Pakiam AS, Lang AE. Historical and clinical features of psychogenic tremor: a review of 70 cases. Can J Neurol Sci. 1999;26:190–5.
64. Hallett M, Weiner WJ, Kompoliti K. Psychogenic movement disorders. Parkinsonism Relat Disord. 2012;18 Suppl 1:S155–7.
65. Ricciardi L, Edwards MJ. Treatment of functional (psychogenic) movement disorders. Neurotherapeutics. 2014;11:201–7.
66. Paviour DC, Jäger HR, Wilkinson L, et al. Holmes tremor: application of modern neuroimaging techniques. Mov Disord. 2006;21:2260–2.

67. Holtbernd F, Eidelberg D. The utility of neuroimaging in the differential diagnosis of parkinsonian syndromes. Semin Neurol. 2014;34:202–9.
68. Savoiardo M. Differential diagnosis of Parkinson's disease and atypical parkinsonian disorders by magnetic resonance imaging. Neurol Sci. 2003;24 Suppl 1:S35–7.
69. Massano J, Costa F, Nadais G. Teaching neuroImage: MRI in multiple system atrophy: "hot cross bun" sign and hyperintense rim bordering the putamina. Neurology. 2008;71:e38.
70. Berry-Kravis E, Abrams L, Coffey SM, et al. Fragile X-associated tremor/ataxia syndrome: clinical features, genetics, and testing guidelines. Mov Disord. 2007;22:2018–30, quiz 2140.
71. Cummings JL, Henchcliffe C, Schaier S, et al. The role of dopaminergic imaging in patients with symptoms of dopaminergic system neurodegeneration. Brain. 2011;134:3146–66.
72. Zesiewicz TA, Elble RJ, Louis ED, et al. Evidence-based guideline update: treatment of essential tremor: report of the quality standards subcommittee of the American academy of neurology. Neurology. 2011;77:1752–5.
73. Winkler GF, Young RR. Efficacy of chronic propranolol therapy in action tremors of the familial, senile or essential varieties. N Engl J Med. 1974;290:984–8.
74. Calzetti S, Findley LJ, Perucca E, Richens A. The response of essential tremor to propranolol: evaluation of clinical variables governing its efficacy on prolonged administration. J Neurol Neurosurg Psychiatry. 1983;46:393–8.
75. Koller WC. Long-acting propranolol in essential tremor. Neurology. 1985;35:108–10.
76. Ferreira JJ, Sampaio C. Essential tremor. BMJ Clin Evid. 2007 May 1;2007.
77. Koller WC, Royse VL. Efficacy of primidone in essential tremor. Neurology. 1986;36:121–4.
78. Sasso E, Perucca E, Calzetti S. Double-blind comparison of primidone and phenobarbital in essential tremor. Neurology. 1988;38:808–10.
79. Lyons KE, Pahwa R, Comella CL, et al. Benefits and risks of pharmacological treatments for essential tremor. Drug Saf. 2003;26:461–81.
80. Gironell A, Kulisevsky J, Barbanoj M, et al. A randomized placebo-controlled comparative trial of gabapentin and propranolol in essential tremor. Arch Neurol. 1999;56:475–80.
81. Pahwa R, Lyons K, Hubble JP, et al. Double-blind controlled trial of gabapentin in essential tremor. Mov Disord. 1998;13:465–7.
82. Connor GS, Edwards K, Tarsy D. Topiramate in essential tremor: findings from double-blind, placebo-controlled, crossover trials. Clin Neuropharmacol. 2008;31:97–103.
83. Ondo WG, Jankovic J, Connor GS, et al. Topiramate in essential tremor: a double-blind, placebo-controlled trial. Neurology. 2006;66:672–7.
84. Huber SJ, Paulson GW. Efficacy of alprazolam for essential tremor. Neurology. 1988;38:241–3.
85. Pahwa R, Busenbark K, Swanson-Hyland EF, et al. Botulinum toxin treatment of essential head tremor. Neurology. 1995;45:822–4.
86. Jankovic J, Schwartz K, Clemence W, et al. A randomized, double-blind, placebo-controlled study to evaluate botulinum toxin type A in essential hand tremor. Mov Disord. 1996;11:250–6.
87. Diaz NL, Waters CH. Current strategies in the treatment of Parkinson's disease and a personalized approach to management. Expert Rev Neurother. 2009;9:1781–9.
88. Koch M, Mostert J, Heersema D, De Keyser J. Tremor in multiple sclerosis. J Neurol. 2007;254:133–45.
89. Papapetropoulos S, Singer C. Botulinum toxin in movement disorders. Semin Neurol. 2007;27:183–94.
90. Ramtahal J, Larner AJ. Shaky legs? Think POT! Age Ageing. 2009;38:352–3.
91. Schuurman PR, Bosch DA, Merkus MP, Speelman JD. Long-term follow-up of thalamic stimulation versus thalamotomy for tremor suppression. Mov Disord. 2008;23:1146–53.
92. Novak KE, Dalvi A, Nenonene EK, Bernstein LP. Surgical treatment of tremor. Dis Mon. 2011;57:142–59.
93. Lyons KE, Pahwa R. Deep brain stimulation and tremor. Neurotherapeutics. 2008;5:331–8.
94. Videnovic A, Metman LV. Deep brain stimulation for Parkinson's disease: prevalence of adverse events and need for standardized reporting. Mov Disord. 2008;23:343–9.
95. Lim DA, Khandhar SM, Heath S, et al. Multiple target deep brain stimulation for multiple sclerosis related and poststroke Holmes' tremor. Stereotact Funct Neurosurg. 2007;85:144–9.
96. Kobayashi K, Katayama Y, Oshima H, et al. Multitarget, dual-electrode deep brain stimulation of the thalamus and subthalamic area for treatment of Holmes' tremor. J Neurosurg. 2014;120:1025–32.
97. Volkmann J, Mueller J, Deuschl G, et al. Pallidal neurostimulation in patients with medication-refractory cervical dystonia: a randomised, sham-controlled trial. Lancet Neurol. 2014;13:875–84.
98. Larson PS. Deep brain stimulation for movement disorders. Neurotherapeutics. 2014;11:465–74.

Myoclonus and Startle Syndromes

30

Roongroj Bhidayasiri and Onanong Jitkritsadakul

Myoclonus presents as the most rapid and brief movements of all hyperkinetic disorders, characterized by sudden, brief, shock-like involuntary movements [1]. The duration of the movement, or jerk, is usually between 10 and 50 milliseconds (ms) and rarely lasts longer than 100 ms. Positive myoclonus is a term used for these shock-like movements that are caused by active muscle contractions. Negative myoclonus, conversely, occurs when the movements are produced by a sudden brief interruption of muscle activity [2]. "Asterixis" is a type of negative myoclonus that generally occurs in toxic-metabolic encephalopathies, often associated with reduced alertness. Considered as a separate form of negative myoclonus, "postural lapses" are characterized by interruptions of tonic activity of postural muscles, including the neck, trunk, and proximal muscles, lasting between 200 and 500 ms [2]. Both positive and negative myoclonus may be identified in the same patient, such as in posthypoxic myoclonus, and can affect the same muscle group, appearing superficially identical. However, negative myoclonus usually involves muscles, which are tonically recruited, and the interruptions of muscle activity generally result in a loss of antigravitational activity and downward joint displacement. In contrast, positive myoclonus usually involves both flexor and extensor muscles, and the abnormal activation of muscles results in both upward and downward joint displacement [3].

In this chapter, we focus on the differentiation of myoclonus from other movement disorders, clinical approaches, and treatment strategies in patients who present primarily with myoclonus. Selected reviews are provided at the end of this chapter for readers who wish to expand their knowledge on specific aspects of myoclonus.

Electronic supplementary material The online version of this chapter (doi:10.1007/978-3-7091-1628-9_30) contains supplementary material, which is available to authorized users.

R. Bhidayasiri, MD, FRCP, FRCPI (✉)
Professor of Neurology and Director,
Chulalongkorn Centre of Excellence for Parkinson's Disease and Related Disorders, Chulalongkorn University and King Chulalongkorn Memorial Hospital, Thai Red Cross Society, 1873 Rama 4 Road, Bangkok 10330, Thailand

Department of Rehabilitation Medicine, Faculty of Medicine, Juntendo University, Tokyo, Japan
e-mail: rbh@chulapd.org; parkinsondoctor@gmail.com

O. Jitkritsadakul, MD
Department of Medicine, Faculty of Medicine, Chulalongkorn Center of Excellence for Parkinson's Disease & Related Disorders, Chulalongkorn University and King Chulalongkorn Memorial Hospital, Thai Red Cross Society,
1873 Rama 4 Road, Bangkok 10330, Thailand

C. Falup-Pecurariu et al. (eds.), *Movement Disorders Curricula*,
DOI 10.1007/978-3-7091-1628-9_30

30.1 Distinguishing Myoclonus from Other Movement Disorders

Myoclonus is usually distinguishable from other hyperkinesias by its distinct clinical characteristics of rapid onset, short duration, and single-event muscular activation. However, in many cases, it can be quite challenging to establish the distinctive characteristics of muscle activation solely on clinical observations. As myoclonus is one type of jerky movements, other possibilities include tics, dystonic jerks, chorea, ballism, and spasm. Visual examination of the jerks has certain limitations since saccadic latency of human eyes may already be too long to catch the first part of the jerks. Therefore, only the later jerky components may be available for visual inspection. Moreover, visual examination alone may not be sensitive enough to differentiate various types of jerks when the duration is less than 1,000 ms [4]. In these particular situations, electrophysiological studies are often needed to evaluate the physiological profiles of these jerks, thus assisting clinicians in the differentiation.

Careful characterization of the phenomenology helps differentiate myoclonus from its mimics (Table 30.1). Focal tics can look very much like segmental myoclonus. However, stereotypic movements, frequently accompanied by an urge to move, their relative suppressibility, and the relief of the inner urge after the movements help distinguish tics from myoclonus. Differentiation between myoclonic jerks and simple partial seizures can be difficult, often requiring neurophysiologic confirmation. However, consistent focality, unilaterality, or jacksonian spread, which can take many seconds to minutes, strongly support simple partial seizures. The typical movements in epilepsia partialis continua, a form of focal status epilepticus, are usually a combination of repetitive myoclonic jerks with hemiparesis or, less frequently, with other cortically generated deficits. In addition, the long continuing movements of the EPC are frequently rhythmic with a predilection for facial and finger flexors involvement [5, 6]. These findings are in contrast to myoclonus in which the muscle topography tends to be stable in each patient without spreading. Myoclonus can be rhythmic and, if repetitive, can be mistaken for tremor. A form of cortical tremor is considered as a variant of cortical reflex myoclonus [7]. Dystonia can be differentiated from myoclonus due to its characters of intermittent or sustained muscle contractions resulting in abnormal posture or

Table 30.1 Comparison of the main characteristics of myoclonus and other jerky hyperkinetic movements

	Myoclonus	Tics	Dystonic jerk	Chorea and ballism	EPC
Duration	Very brief	Brief	Could be brief	Could be brief	Brief
Pattern	Nonrhythmic jerk	Stereotyped jerk	Paroxysmal jerk accompany the abnormal posture	Randomly flowing jerk	Repetitively, continuous, focal jerky movement
Urge to move	No	Yes	No	No	No
Suppressible	No	Partially	Partially	Partially	No
Vocalization	No	Present	No	No	No
Involvement	Any body part	Predominant craniofacial or upper extremity	Any body part with abnormal posture	Distal – chorea Proximal – ballism	Usually localized to a distal limb
Epileptic seizure or discharge	No	No	No	No	Present

EPC epilepsia partialis continua

twisting. However, dystonic jerks, which are the brief reinforcements of dystonic posturing, can look like myoclonus, particularly if dystonic posturing is subtle. Moreover, dystonia can occur with myoclonus in the same patient as in myoclonus-dystonia (M-D), which is a genetically heterogeneous movement disorder due to the epsilon-sarcoglycan gene mutation [8].

30.2 Classifications of Myoclonus

There are several methods of classifying myoclonus based on clinical appearance, the anatomical origin of the jerks, and etiology (Table 30.2) [1, 9, 10]. Clinically, myoclonus can be described by its distribution as focal, multifocal, segmental, or generalized, whereas myoclonic jerks may also occur spontaneously, in response to various stimuli, or with action. In addition, temporal patterns of myoclonic jerks should also be analyzed to determine if they are irregular (arrhythmic), rhythmic (as in some forms of segmental myoclonus), or oscillatory when the jerks occur as a burst of oscillations. Despite its simplicity, this clinical classification remains useful to practicing neurologists in properly identifying the clinical characteristics of myoclonus with a good assessment of the site of origin in the nervous system (Table 30.3). For example, cortical myoclonus tends to be more prominent in the hands, fingers, and face and is more commonly provoked by tactile stimuli. Brainstem reflex myoclonus, also known as reticular myoclonus, is more likely to affect the arms bilaterally and is manifested as proximal, synchronous, flexor-greater-than-extensor jerky movements, which are frequently induced with variable latency of auditory stimuli, or tapping on the face [11]. Lastly, segmental, unilateral arrhythmic jerking in the arm and/or the trunk is typical of spinal myoclonus, while repetitive flexor arrhythmic jerking of the trunk, hip, knee, and abdomen bilaterally may be due to propriospinal myoclonus [12].

Although the etiology of myoclonus is complex, symptomatic (secondary) causes of myoclonus (72 %) are the most common, followed by epileptic myoclonus (17 %) and essential myoclonus (11 %), respectively [13]. Among those with symptomatic myoclonus,

Table 30.2 Different classifications of myoclonus

Clinical	Anatomical/physiological	Etiological
Related to action At rest With action Reflex induced	Cortical Focal Multifocal Generalized Epilepsia partialis continua	Physiologic myoclonus Sleep jerks Hiccup
Body part Focal Multifocal Segmental Generalized	Cortical-subcortical Epileptic myoclonus	Essential myoclonus Myoclonus-dystonia
Temporal pattern Irregular Regular Oscillatory	Subcortical-supraspinal (brainstem) Startle/hyperekplexia Reticular reflex myoclonus Opsoclonus-myoclonus Palatal tremor	Epileptic myoclonus Childhood myoclonic epilepsy Juvenile myoclonic epilepsy Progressive myoclonic epilepsy Fragments of epilepsy
	Spinal Spinal segmental myoclonus Propriospinal myoclonus	Symptomatic myoclonus CNS infection Neurodegenerative Toxic/metabolic Posthypoxia Storage disease
	Peripheral myoclonus	Psychogenic myoclonus

Table 30.3 Clinical features and electrophysiological findings in different forms of myoclonus [1, 9, 10, 22, 41]

Classification	Clinical features	Electrophysiological findings	Etiology
Cortical	Focal or multifocal myoclonus Stimulus sensitive (tactile, vision) Rhythmic in case of EPC	Brief EMG bursts (<75 ms) Enlarged cortical SEP (common) Timed-locked cortical event (focal sharp wave 10–40 ms) preceding the jerks May be presented C reflex at rest	Posthypoxic action myoclonus (Lance-Adams syndrome) Toxic-metabolic-induced myoclonus PME/PMA Myoclonus in neurodegenerative disease: AD, CBD, DLB, and CJD
Cortical-subcortical	Multifocal or bilaterally synchronized or generalized	Brief EMG bursts (<100 ms) Enlarged cortical SEP (possible) Time-locked association May be presented C reflex at rest	Absence seizures Primary generalized myoclonic epilepsy
Subcortical-supraspinal (brainstem)	Generalized jerks with axial or proximal muscles involvement Stimulus sensitive (auditory)	Brief EMG bursts (10–30 ms) Normal SEPs No EEG correlates Reflex response to sound (sometime)	Essential myoclonus Startle/hyperekplexia Reticular reflex myoclonus Opsoclonus-myoclonus syndrome Palatal myoclonus (tremor): essential and symptomatic
Spinal	A specific dermatomal or segmental axial location (spinal segmental myoclonus) Usually rhythmic and symmetrical May be elicited by taps to the trunk and limbs	EMG bursts >100 ms, spreading rostrally or caudally from generator Normal SEPs Normal EEG	Segmental spinal myoclonus Propriospinal myoclonus
Peripheral	Jerks in the distribution of peripheral nerve/lesion	EMG with marked duration variability Normal SEPs Normal EEG	Hemifacial spasm
Psychogenic	Jerks frequently occurs at the resting state	EMG with marked duration	Conversion disorders
	Variability interference of myoclonus with action	Presence of premovement EEG potential (Bereitschaftspotentials)	Malingering

SEP somatosensory evoked potential, *EEG* electroencephalogram, *EMG* electromyography, *PME* progressive myoclonic epilepsy, *PMA* progressive myoclonic ataxia, *AD* Alzheimer's disease, *CBD* corticobasal degeneration, *DLB* dementia with Lewy bodies, *CJD* Creutzfeldt-Jakob disease

common causes are metabolic encephalopathies, drug intoxication, and hypoxemia. Epileptic myoclonus is the presence of myoclonus in the setting of epilepsy in which myoclonus occurs as only one component of a seizure (myoclonic seizure) or as one of multiple seizure types within an epileptic syndrome [14]. "Essential myoclonus," often familial, is the entity of multifocal myoclonus that occurs without any other neurologic deficits except tremor or mild dystonia [15]. The terms "myoclonic-dystonia" and "myoclonus-dystonia" (M-D) may represent disorders that are part of the essential myoclonus spectrum [8].

30.3 Clinical Diagnostic Approach to Myoclonus

Since myoclonus is a clinical sign, an organized framework is necessary for the diagnosis of the underlying disorder. Therefore, myoclonus should be viewed within the context of the total clinical picture. After obtaining the relevant clinical history, clinical goals should be shaped by information about drug exposure and seizures, identification of myoclonic jerks with clinical distinctions, location of distribution, and temporal patterns (Table 30.2). This information is essential for providing anatomical correlates, which further lead to the recognition of major clinical syndromes (Table 30.3). In the clinical settings, the evaluation of a patient with myoclonus is a stepwise process, beginning with the physiological classification of myoclonus to determine the anatomical localization from which it originates, then formulation of the myoclonic syndrome, which, in turn, leads to a targeted etiological differential diagnosis. Additional prominent neurological or systemic symptoms, signs, and associations help narrow the differential diagnosis further. The properties of myoclonus and other aspects of clinical presentations determine what types of evaluation and testing should be performed. Diagnostic studies can then be guided according to the clinical features of that syndrome. For example, a focal myoclonus of a distal limb induced by stimuli usually represents a form of cortical reflex myoclonus, which may occur as part of an epileptic syndrome or cortical lesions. In contrast, generalized myoclonus or its spread along the body away from the source in time-related, sequential fashion suggests brainstem (reticular) myoclonus.

It is important to characterize the phenomenology carefully to determine whether myoclonus is the only movement disorder (isolated myoclonus) or is combined with another movement disorder (combined myoclonus). As variety of movement disorders can manifest itself as jerky movements (see above), misdiagnosis of myoclonus as another movement disorder is possible, leading to incorrect syndromic diagnosis and inappropriate etiological diagnoses. With the appropriate information, the identification of a correct syndrome limits the list of etiological differential diagnoses and avoids unnecessary investigations. If myoclonus is combined with other features, then we need to determine the dominant phenomenology. For example, myoclonus may also occur in patients with M-D. However, myoclonic jerks of the limb can pose diagnostic challenges if the appearance of dystonia is very subtle or overshadowed by rapid jerky movements.

30.4 Investigations in Myoclonus

A number of medications can induce myoclonus, and the potential agents should be explored in patients with a history of polypharmacy and develop a subacute onset of myoclonus (Table 30.4). In cases where the etiology of myoclonus is unclear, basic ancillary investigations should be considered to cover at least a list of common electrolyte disturbances and metabolic disorders (Table 30.5). Electroencephalography (EEG) is needed in cases of suspected epileptic myoclonus. Certain EEG features are diagnostic of the underlying disorder, such as generalized spikes and 3–6 Hz spike and wave in primary generalized myoclonic epilepsy and 3 Hz spike and wave in absence epileptic syndromes. The loss of normal background rhythm and abnormal slow waves are very suggestive of diffuse encephalopathy. A MRI of the brain is often indicated in patients with focal myoclonus, while imaging of the spinal cord is frequently performed in patients with spinal segmental myoclonus. Table 30.5 provides a list of investigations to be considered in patients who primarily present with myoclonus. (The full details of this type of assessment are not within the scope of this chapter.) Advanced testing should be sought once basic testing is inconclusive and a specific diagnosis is considered in a consultation with movement disorders specialists. The functions of neurophysiologic tests in myoclonus include defining the physiological classification of myoclonus, offering additional information in

Table 30.4 Medication-induced myoclonus (only common ones and selected groups of medications are listed) [1, 10, 42, 43]

Psychiatric medications	Cyclic antidepressants
	Selective serotonin uptake inhibitors
	Monoamine oxidase inhibitors
	Lithium
Antimicrobial medications	Quinolones
	Penicillin
	Cephalosporins
	Imipenem
	Isoniazid
	Acyclovir
Antiepileptic medications	Carbamazepine
	Phenytoin
	Gabapentin
	Lamotrigine
Opiate medications	Morphine and its derivatives
	Fentanyl
	Tramadol
Antiparkinsonian medications	Levodopa
	Dopamine agonists
	Amantadine
	Entacapone
Dopamine-blocking agents	Typical and atypical antipsychotics
	Metoclopramide
Medications for dementia	Cholinesterase inhibitors
Anesthetic agents	Propofol
Others	Antihistamines
	Physostigmine
	Tryptophan
	Amiodarone
	Contrast media

anatomical localization, and ascertaining the physiologic characteristics for certain disorders in order to direct physicians toward the most effective treatments. Several neurophysiologic methods are currently used in the study of myoclonus, including multichannel surface electromyography (EMG) with long latency responses to mixed nerve averaging and evoked potentials (e.g., median nerve stimulation, somatosensory evoked potentials, SEPs). Positive and negative findings from these methods can provide further evidence for determining the physiologic type of myoclonus (Table 30.3).

30.5 Selected Forms of Myoclonus

30.5.1 Postanoxic Myoclonus

Myoclonus can occur in two main settings after an anoxic event [16]. First, during the first 24 h, generalized myoclonic jerking may be evident in a comatose patient, known as myoclonic status, which usually indicates a poor prognosis. Second, a subcortical myoclonus may emerge within days to weeks after recovery of consciousness in survivors of cardiorespiratory arrest, most frequently when severe respiratory dysfunction antedates the cardiac arrest [17]. The definitive description of this entity is that of Lance and Adams, who described four patients who recovered from hypoxic coma, but were left with a permanent disabling neurological syndrome dominated by action or intention myoclonus [18]. Their observation was that generalized spontaneous myoclonus is a feature of an early stage of recovery from an episode of cerebral hypoxia, but that later on myoclonus is precipitated particularly by voluntary movements. They further observed that if myoclonus develops when coordination is required, it supports the presence of cerebellar dysfunction. Myoclonus was particularly aggravated more as the task required increasing precision and as the target of aim was approached. Moreover, negative myoclonus, characterized by abrupt lapses in muscle tone that often result in falls, frequently occurs when patients attempt to ambulate. Among all clinical spectrums of this syndrome, ataxia and negative myoclonus create considerable risk of falling and make transfers exceptionally challenging for these patients.

30.5.2 Myoclonus-Dystonia (M-D)

The term "myoclonic-dystonia" was originally proposed to describe a syndrome of idiopathic dystonia with prominent myoclonic jerks [19].

Table 30.5 Basic ancillary testing and advanced testing of myoclonus

Tests	Suspected disorders
Basic ancillary testing	
Glucose, renal function tests, hepatic function tests, electrolytes	Metabolic-induced myoclonus
Thyroid function and antibodies (antithyroglobulin and antimicrosomal antibodies)	Hyperthyroidism, Hashimoto's encephalopathy
Paraneoplastic antibodies (Anti-Ri, ANNA-2)	Opsoclonus-myoclonus ataxia syndrome
Drug and toxin screening (such as bismuth)	Drug- or toxin-induced myoclonus
Electroencephalography	Epileptic myoclonus
Brain imaging/ spine imaging	Symptomatic myoclonus (related with a focal lesion)
Advanced testing	
14-3-3 protein in cerebrospinal fluid	Creutzfeldt-Jakob disease
Serum ceruloplasmin and copper studies	Wilson's disease
Anti-tissue transglutaminase antibodies (tTGA), endomysial antibodies (EMA), deamidated gliadin peptide antibodies (DGP), small intestinal biopsy	Celiac disease
Anti-T. whipplei antibodies, small intestinal biopsy with periodic acid-Schiff (PAS) staining and polymerase chain reaction (PCR) assay for detecting T. whipplei	Whipple's disease
Skin biopsy for intracytoplasmic periodic acid-Schiff-positive inclusions (Lafora bodies)	Lafora's disease
Enzyme assays for deficiency	Neuraminidase deficiency (sialidosis), biotinidase deficiency
Leukocyte peroxidase assay, skin punch biopsy	Neuronal ceroid lipofuscinosis
Serum alpha fetoprotein (AFP), radiosensitivity testing	Ataxia-telangiectasia
Mitochondrial studied (lactate level, muscle biopsy)	Mitochondrial disease
Genetic testing	Inherited disorders
Body imaging (positron emission tomography; PET scan)	Occult malignancy in patients with suspected paraneoplastic neurological syndromes

However, the term "myoclonus-dystonia" (M-D) was proposed to emphasize the coexistence of myoclonus and dystonia, rather than dominance, of one movement disorder over the other [20]. Many kindred with autosomal dominantly inherited M-D have mutations in the gene for epsilon sarcoglycan [21]. Mutation-positive patients usually present in the first one or two decades of life with predominant myoclonus, which is of subcortical origin [8]. Dystonia usually occurs later and remains mild.

30.5.3 Myoclonus in Parkinsonian Disorders

Myoclonus may occur in a variety of parkinsonian disorders. In Parkinson's disease (PD), myoclonus usually develops as an adverse effect of treatment with levodopa or amantadine or as a feature of dementia in the advanced stage of the disease [22]. Levodopa-induced myoclonus tends to be multifocal and may occur at rest or is induced by action. It is usually observed at the onset of dyskinesia and disappears once optimal clinical efficacy is achieved [23]. In multiple system atrophy (MSA), myoclonus is of low amplitude, irregular, and arrhythmic involving several fingers or the hands when the arms are held outstretched or during movements [22]. This type of myoclonus in MSA is called minipolymyoclonus or jerky, myoclonic postural/action tremor in the second consensus statement on the diagnosis of MSA [24, 25]. Myoclonus, which is stimulus sensitive involving a dystonic limb, has been reported in 25 % of patients with autopsy-proven corticobasal degeneration (CBD) [26, 27].

30.5.4 Brainstem Myoclonus

There are two types of myoclonus that arise from the brainstem reticular formation, which take the form of generalized predominantly axial body jerks. Characteristically, these jerks are very sensitive to auditory stimuli.

30.5.4.1 Brainstem Reticular Myoclonus

In brainstem myoclonus, muscle jerks arise from activity in neuronal centers within the lower brainstem. The neural activity spreads down from the brainstem via a relatively slow spinal efferent motor pathway, while the cranial nerve nuclei are activated by rapid spread up the brainstem. This produces the distinctive caudo-rostral pattern of recruitment of cranial nerve innervated muscles.

30.5.4.2 Exaggerated Startle Response

The exaggerated startle syndrome is characterized by an excessive motor response or "jump" to unexpected auditory and, sometimes, somesthetic and visual stimuli. The "jump" characteristically consists of a blink, contortion of the face, flexion of the neck and trunk, and abduction and flexion of the arms [28]. A good example of a startle syndrome is hyperekplexia, which is a form of hereditary startle disorder, characterized by exaggerated startle responses and neonatal hypertonia. Anatomically, the nucleus reticularis caudalis pontis has been implicated as the primary center activating the acoustic startle reflex, since it receives dense somatosensory inputs from the skin of the face and is also the origin of the reticulospinal tracts, which end monosynaptically at the brainstem and spinal α–motoneurons [29].

30.5.5 Propriospinal Myoclonus

Propriospinal myoclonus is a rare disorder with repetitive, usually flexor arrhythmic brief jerks of the trunk, hips, and knees in a fixed pattern that are often stimulus sensitive and typically increase when supine [30]. It has a presumed generation in the spinal cord in which the neural activity spreads simultaneously rostrally and caudally via propriospinal pathways. However, structural lesions reported to underlie propriospinal myoclonus are scarce, and recent studies have suggested that the majority of cases with propriospinal myoclonus are psychogenic origin with clinical overlaps with adult-onset tics [12, 31, 32].

30.5.6 Psychogenic Myoclonus

Jerks are one of the common movement disorders observed in patients with psychogenic (functional) disorders [33]. With the clinical observation alone, jerks that occur in patients with a conversion disorder or malingering may appear quick enough to be confused with myoclonus. However, certain clinical clues have been proposed as suggestive features of psychogenic jerks, including (1) inconsistent character of the movements (amplitude, frequency, and distribution) and features that are incongruous with typical organic myoclonus, (2) associated psychogenic symptomatology, (3) pronounced reduction of myoclonus with distraction, (4) exacerbation and relief with placebo and suggestion, (5) spontaneous periods of remission, (6) acute onset and sudden resolution, and (7) evidence of underlying psychopathology [34]. Psychogenic myoclonus is associated with a normal Bereitschaftspotential, a slowly rising negativity occurring 1–2 s before the EMG motor onset, indicating involvement of the premotor cortex and supplementary motor area in preparation for movement [35].

30.6 Treatment of Myoclonus

The best strategy for the treatment of myoclonus is to treat the underlying disorder. A thorough evaluation of the etiology of myoclonus is essential for developing a treatment strategy. This frequently will involve correction of metabolic abnormalities or removal of an offending drug (Table 30.4). However, in many cases, treatment of an underlying disorder is not possible, and a recommended

Table 30.6 Pharmacologic treatment of myoclonus based on myoclonic classification [1, 36–38]

Myoclonic classification	Treatment	Recommended daily dosages
1. Cortical myoclonus	Sodium valproate Clonazepam Piracetam Levetiracetam Zonisamide	1,200–2,000 mg Up to 15 mg (slow titration) 2.4–21.6 g 1,000–3,000 mg 200–600 mg
2. Cortical-subcortical myoclonus (especially for juvenile myoclonic epilepsy)	Sodium valproate Levetiracetam Lamotrigine Topiramate Zonisamide Clonazepam	1,000–2,000 mg 1,000–3,000 mg 100–200 mg 100–300 mg 300–500 mg 4–8 mg
3. Brainstem myoclonus and startle	Clonazepam	Up to 15 mg (slow titration)
4. Spinal myoclonus	Clonazepam	Up to 6 mg
5. Peripheral myoclonus	Botulinum toxin (in case of hemifacial spasm)	10–50 μ of Botox® 30–220 μ of Dysport®
6. Psychogenic myoclonus	Combination of psychotherapy treatment	Cognitive behavioral therapy (CBT) Stress management Relaxation techniques Pharmacological treatment

approach to symptomatic treatment comes from its physiological classification based on the involved neurotransmitter systems (Table 30.6) [36–38]. Because of limited clinical evidence, multiple drug trials are frequently necessary, and combinations of therapeutic regimens are often indicated to obtain beneficial responses. For cortical myoclonus, levetiracetam is suggested as first-line treatment although valproic acid and clonazepam are commonly used in clinical practice. Cortical-subcortical myoclonus is the physiology, frequently dominated by myoclonic seizures, such as primary epileptic myoclonus. Valproic acid demonstrated efficacy in such epileptic syndromes with other medications providing an adjunctive role. Clonazepam is used for brainstem and startle myoclonus. Propriospinal myoclonus is difficult to treat, and psychogenic component should be carefully explored. Clonazepam and botulinum toxin are currently considered as the primary treatment for patients with hemifacial spasm [39, 40]. The use of these medications should be weighed against clinical responsiveness and side effects.

Conclusion

Myoclonus is viewed as an instantaneous and involuntary jerk representing one of the common hyperkinetic disorders. Certain characteristics of myoclonus, including sudden, very brief, intermittent, jerky, and non-suppressible movements, help distinguish myoclonus from its common mimics. While a number of classifications have been proposed for different purposes, useful clinically adopted classifications are based on the physiologic localization and the etiology. An organized framework is essential for the diagnostic approach for myoclonus and should be viewed within the context of the full clinical picture. A careful characterization of myoclonus to determine whether myoclonus is the only movement disorder (isolated myoclonus) or is combined with another movement disorder (combined myoclonus) is helpful in leading physicians to establish a possible clinical syndrome and finally the etiology. Investigations in patients with myoclonus can be myriad. Therefore, a stepwise approach is recommended starting from basic ancillary investigations. Despite few controlled trials for the treatment of myoclonus, therapeutic selection is not solely evidence based but also considers the pathophysiology and the mechanism of action of frequently used anticonvulsants.

References

1. Caviness JN, Brown P. Myoclonus: current concepts and recent advances. Lancet Neurol. 2004;3(10): 598–607.
2. Shibasaki H. Physiology of negative myoclonus. Adv Neurol. 2002;89:103–13.
3. Obeso JA, Artieda J, Burleigh A. Clinical aspects of negative myoclonus. Adv Neurol. 1995;67:1–7.
4. Vercueil L. Myoclonus and movement disorders. Neurophysiol Clin. 2006;36(5–6):327–31.
5. Cockerell OC, Rothwell J, Thompson PD, Marsden CD, Shorvon SD. Clinical and physiological features of epilepsia partialis continua. Cases ascertained in the UK. Brain. 1996;119(Pt 2):393–407.
6. Bien CG, Elger CE. Epilepsia partialis continua: semiology and differential diagnoses. Epileptic Disord. 2008;10(1):3–7.
7. Toro C, Pascual-Leone A, Deuschl G, Tate E, Pranzatelli MR, Hallett M. Cortical tremor. A common manifestation of cortical myoclonus. Neurology. 1993;43(11):2346–53.
8. Ritz K, Gerrits MC, Foncke EM, van Ruissen F, van der Linden C, Vergouwen MD, et al. Myoclonus-dystonia: clinical and genetic evaluation of a large cohort. J Neurol Neurosurg Psychiatry. 2009;80(6): 653–8.
9. Shibasaki H. Neurophysiological classification of myoclonus. Neurophysiol Clin. 2006;36(5–6):267–9.
10. Caviness JN. Myoclonus. Parkinsonism Relat Disord. 2007;13 Suppl 3:S375–84.
11. Shibasaki H, Kakigi R, Oda K, Masukawa S. Somatosensory and acoustic brain stem reflex myoclonus. J Neurol Neurosurg Psychiatry. 1988;51(4):572–5. Pubmed Central PMCID: 1032977, Epub 1988/04/01. eng.
12. van der Salm SM, Erro R, Cordivari C, Edwards MJ, Koelman JH, Ende TV, et al. Propriospinal myoclonus: clinical reappraisal and review of literature. Neurology. 2014;83(20):1862–70.
13. Caviness JN, Alving LI, Maraganore DM, Black RA, McDonnell SK, Rocca WA. The incidence and prevalence of myoclonus in Olmsted County. Minn Mayo Clin Proc. 1999;74(6):565–9.
14. Guerrini R, Takahashi T. Myoclonus and epilepsy. Handb Clin Neurol. 2013;111:667–79.
15. Quinn NP. Essential myoclonus and myoclonic dystonia. Mov Disord. 1996;11(2):119–24.
16. English WA, Giffin NJ, Nolan JP. Myoclonus after cardiac arrest: pitfalls in diagnosis and prognosis. Anaesthesia. 2009;64(8):908–11.
17. Frucht S, Fahn S. The clinical spectrum of posthypoxic myoclonus. Mov Disord. 2000;15 Suppl 1:2–7.
18. Lance JW, Adams RD. The syndrome of intention or action myoclonus as a sequel to hypoxic encephalopathy. Brain. 1963;86:111–36.
19. Obeso JA, Rothwell JC, Lang AE, Marsden CD. Myoclonic dystonia. Neurology. 1983;33(7): 825–30.
20. Gasser T. Inherited myoclonus-dystonia syndrome. Adv Neurol. 1998;78:325–34.
21. Zimprich A, Grabowski M, Asmus F, Naumann M, Berg D, Bertram M, et al. Mutations in the gene encoding epsilon-sarcoglycan cause myoclonus-dystonia syndrome. Nat Genet. 2001;29(1):66–9.
22. Truong DD, Bhidayasiri R. Myoclonus and parkinsonism. Handb Clin Neurol. 2007;84:549–60.
23. Defebvre L. Myoclonus and extrapyramidal diseases. Neurophysiol Clin. 2006;36(5–6):319–25.
24. Salazar G, Valls-Sole J, Marti MJ, Chang H, Tolosa ES. Postural and action myoclonus in patients with parkinsonian type multiple system atrophy. Mov Disord. 2000;15(1):77–83.
25. Gilman S, Wenning GK, Low PA, Brooks DJ, Mathias CJ, Trojanowski JQ, et al. Second consensus statement on the diagnosis of multiple system atrophy. Neurology. 2008;71(9):670–6. Pubmed Central PMCID: 2676993, Epub 2008/08/30. eng.
26. Hu WT, Rippon GW, Boeve BF, Knopman DS, Petersen RC, Parisi JE, et al. Alzheimer's disease and corticobasal degeneration presenting as corticobasal syndrome. Mov Disord. 2009;24(9):1375–9.
27. Brunt ER, van Weerden TW, Pruim J, Lakke JW. Unique myoclonic pattern in corticobasal degeneration. Mov Disord. 1995;10(2):132–42.
28. Bhidayasiri R, Truong DD. Startle syndromes. Handb Clin Neurol. 2011;100:421–30.
29. Koch M. The neurobiology of startle. Prog Neurobiol. 1999;59(2):107–28. Epub 1999/08/27. eng.
30. Brown P, Thompson PD, Rothwell JC, Day BL, Marsden CD. Axial myoclonus of propriospinal origin. Brain. 1991;114(Pt 1A):197–214.
31. van der Salm SM, Koelman JH, Henneke S, van Rootselaar AF, Tijssen MA. Axial jerks: a clinical spectrum ranging from propriospinal to psychogenic myoclonus. J Neurol. 2010;257(8):1349–55. Pubmed Central PMCID: 2910307.
32. Kang SY, Sohn YH. Electromyography patterns of propriospinal myoclonus can be mimicked voluntarily. Mov Disord. 2006;21(8):1241–4.
33. Lang AE, Voon V. Psychogenic movement disorders: past developments, current status, and future directions. Mov Disord. 2011;26(6):1175–86.
34. Monday K, Jankovic J. Psychogenic myoclonus. Neurology. 1993;43(2):349–52.
35. Terada K, Ikeda A, Van Ness PC, Nagamine T, Kaji R, Kimura J, et al. Presence of Bereitschaftspotential preceding psychogenic myoclonus: clinical application of jerk-locked back averaging. J Neurol Neurosurg Psychiatry. 1995;58(6):745–7. Pubmed Central PMCID: 1073560.
36. Caviness JN. Treatment of myoclonus. Neurotherapeutics. 2014;11(1):188–200. Pubmed Central PMCID: 3899494.
37. Dijk JM, Tijssen MA. Management of patients with myoclonus: available therapies and the need for an evidence-based approach. Lancet Neurol. 2010;9(10): 1028–36.

38. Kojovic M, Cordivari C, Bhatia K. Myoclonic disorders: a practical approach for diagnosis and treatment. Ther Adv Neurol Disord. 2011;4(1):47–62. Pubmed Central PMCID: 3036960.
39. Simpson DM, Blitzer A, Brashear A, Comella C, Dubinsky R, Hallett M, et al. Assessment: botulinum neurotoxin for the treatment of movement disorders (an evidence-based review): report of the therapeutics and technology assessment subcommittee of the American academy of neurology. Neurology. 2008;70(19):1699–706.
40. Hallett M, Albanese A, Dressler D, Segal KR, Simpson DM, Truong D, et al. Evidence-based review and assessment of botulinum neurotoxin for the treatment of movement disorders. Toxicon. 2013;67:94–114.
41. Pranzatelli MR. Myoclonus in childhood. Semin Pediatr Neurol. 2003;10(1):41–51.
42. Brefel-Courbon C, Gardette V, Ory F, Montastruc JL. Drug-induced myoclonus: a French pharmacovigilance database study. Neurophysiol Clin. 2006;36(5–6):333–6.
43. Jimenez-Jimenez FJ, Puertas I, de Toledo-Heras M. Drug-induced myoclonus: frequency, mechanisms and management. CNS Drugs. 2004;18(2):93–104.

Recommended Reading List

Bhidayasiri R, Truong DD. Startle syndromes. Handb Clin Neurol. 2011;100:421–30.

Caviness JN. Treatment of myoclonus. Neurotherapeutics. 2014;11(1):188–200. Pubmed Central PMCID: 3899494.

Caviness JN, Brown P. Myoclonus: current concepts and recent advances. Lancet Neurol. 2004;3(10): 598–607.

Cockerell OC, Rothwell J, Thompson PD, Marsden CD, Shorvon SD. Clinical and physiological features of epilepsia partialis continua. Cases ascertained in the UK. Brain. 1996;119(Pt 2):393–407.

Shibasaki H. Neurophysiological classification of myoclonus. Neurophysiol Clin. 2006;36(5–6): 267–9.

van der Salm SM, Erro R, Cordivari C, Edwards MJ, Koelman JH, Ende TV, et al. Propriospinal myoclonus: clinical reappraisal and review of literature. Neurology. 2014;83(20):1862–70.

31 Ataxias: A Clinical Synopsis

Ella M.R. Fonteyn and Bart P.C. van de Warrenburg

31.1 Introduction

Ataxia is characterized by irregular, uncoordinated movements of the extremities and by imbalance during stance and walking. Cerebellar ataxia needs to be distinguished from sensory ataxia. The latter is due to loss of proprioception, generally caused by large-fiber peripheral neuropathies and conditions causing dysfunction of the dorsal columns of the spinal cord. Typically, sensory ataxia worsens upon eye closure. Cerebellar ataxia is the result of dysfunction of the cerebellum and its connections. In contrast to sensory ataxia, cerebellar ataxia is often accompanied by other cerebellar signs, such as eye movement abnormalities (jerky pursuit, gaze-evoked nystagmus, dysmetric saccades) and dysarthria. Sensory and cerebellar ataxia can sometimes coexist, for example, in some genetic ataxias.

The causes of cerebellar ataxia are numerous, and even some of the relatively more frequent causes are quite rare, which makes the diagnostic work-up of patients with ataxia in daily practice challenging and rather complicated [1, 2]. For a focused differential diagnosis and targeted work-up, carefully taking a history and looking for relevant clues during the physical examination are crucial. The objective of this chapter is to present a line of thinking for daily practice, rather than enumerating all causes of ataxia. The emphasis will be on adult-onset ataxias, that is, not on congenital- or childhood-onset ataxias (although some diseases that typically start in adulthood can start earlier). For a comprehensive evaluation of cerebellar ataxia in children, we refer to a recent review [3].

31.2 Relevant Information from the History

31.2.1 Continuous or Episodic

When ataxia appears to be episodic, the differential diagnosis is very limited and mainly includes migraine and the genetic episodic ataxias. Basilar-type migraine can cause episodic ataxia, which is most often accompanied by vertigo, dysarthria, and visual disturbances, typically followed by a pounding occipital headache and nausea, which completely resolve after some hours. About half of the families with familial

E.M.R. Fonteyn, MD (✉) • B.P.C. van de Warrenburg, MD, PhD
Department of Neurology (935) and Donders Institute for Brain, Cognition and Behaviour, Radboud University Medical Center,
PO Box 9101, Nijmegen 6500 HB, The Netherlands
e-mail: e.fonteyn@gmail.com; bart.vandewarrenburg@radboudumc.nl

C. Falup-Pecurariu et al. (eds.), *Movement Disorders Curricula*,
DOI 10.1007/978-3-7091-1628-9_31

hemiplegic migraine (FHM1) have cerebellar involvement, including gaze-evoked nystagmus, ataxia, and atrophy of the vermis. Some families have severe attacks with coma or prolonged hemiplegia, with full recovery.

There are seven genotypes of dominantly inherited episodic ataxias (EAs), of which EA1 and EA2 are most common. Onset is usually in late childhood or adolescence. Mutations can be de novo, leading to a negative family history. Depending on the mutation, patients experience episodes of ataxia lasting minutes to hours, occasionally days. There may be other accompanying features, such as vertigo or tinnitus, which sometimes predominate. Interictal findings are indicative, as myokymia points to EA1 and nystagmus to EA2. In EA2, there may be a slowly progressive cerebellar syndrome that evolves over the years.

31.2.2 Speed of Onset and Progression Rate

A really acute onset obviously suggests a stroke of the cerebellum or brainstem. Ataxia developing over hours may be due to Wernicke's encephalopathy (B1 deficiency) or alcohol intoxication. Symptoms that develop over days may be the result of Miller Fisher syndrome or postinfectious cerebellitis (which is rare in adults). Progression in weeks to months is seen in structural lesions of the cerebellum or brainstem, ataxia due to drugs, paraneoplastic cerebellar degeneration, steroid-responsive encephalopathy with antithyroid antibodies (SREAT, formerly known as Hashimoto's encephalopathy), Creutzfeldt-Jakob disease, and antiglutamic acid decarboxylase (anti-GAD)-associated cerebellar ataxia. A gradual onset and progression over years often points to a degenerative cause. There are obvious exceptions to these lists, but the message is that onset speed and progression rate clearly make some diseases far more likely than others.

31.2.3 Onset at Age

Particularly for the genetic ataxias, age at onset seems to become less of a useful indicator. For example, some of the recessive ataxias – of which we previously assumed to always manifest in early life – can start really late. Still, an onset below age 40 years has an increased likelihood of a genetic origin, in comparison with an onset after that age. Multiple system atrophy (MSA) does not need to be considered before age 30 years, and the fragile X tremor/ataxia syndrome (FXTAS) generally starts after age 50 years.

31.2.4 Family History

A genetic cause is of course evident if there is a family history of cerebellar ataxia. The mode of inheritance, suggested by the pedigree, determines which genetic mutations should be looked for. A negative history does not exclude a genetic cause. It is important not only to ask for ataxia in other family members, but also for other movement disorders (e.g., parkinsonism is relatively common in SCA2, and chorea can be part of the SCA17 phenotype) [4], for mental retardation and premature ovarian failure (for FXTAS), and for deafness and diabetes mellitus (for mitochondrial disorders).

31.2.5 General Medical Status

Changes in bodyweight and diarrhea can point toward a thyroid problem or celiac disease. Patients with a history of malignancy may suffer from paraneoplastic cerebellar degeneration. HIV patients may develop a cerebellar ataxia due to various reasons (opportunistic infections, primary CNS lymphoma, etc.). Autonomic problems, such as urinary incontinence or postural faintness, suggest MSA. If the patient has a history of alcohol abuse, the likely diagnosis is alcoholic cerebellar degeneration.

31.2.6 Exogenous Substances

Longstanding alcohol abuse is the most common exogenous substance that causes chronic ataxia. A concomitant vitamin B1 deficiency can cause Wernicke's encephalopathy, with encephalopathy, oculomotor dysfunction, and gait ataxia as the classic triad, requiring immediate vitamin B1 replacement. Although alcohol is the most frequent cause of sporadic ataxias in middle-aged men, a search for other causes still needs to be considered if the alcohol abuse has not been too excessive, or if there is progression after stopping alcohol. Other exogenous substances that can cause ataxia are cannabis, NMDA receptor antagonists, and heavy metals such as mercury, organolead components, and methylmercury.

Various prescription drugs, such as antiepileptic drugs, amiodarone, benzodiazepines, and lithium, can cause ataxia, which is reversible in the majority. Chemotherapy, especially 5-fluorouracil, cytarabine, and methotrexate, is associated with both reversible and permanent cerebellar ataxia.

31.3 Relevant Clues from the Physical Examination

The neurological examination should firstly confirm that there is indeed a cerebellar ataxia. Relevant other elements of the neurological examination include assessing whether there is a peripheral neuropathy, spasticity (the spastic ataxias have a limited number of underlying causes), or any other movement disorder [4–6]. It is worthwhile to invest in the examination of eye movements. There could be some more "standard" cerebellar eye movement abnormalities as mentioned in the introduction. However, some other eye signs are very indicative. For example, a severe difficulty to generate saccades (sometimes referred to as oculomotor apraxia) has a limited differential (of ataxia telangiectasia and ataxia with oculomotor apraxia type 2). A gaze limitation in the vertical plane might suggest Niemann-Pick type C. Some dominant ataxias (e.g., SCA1) and mitochondrial disorders are accompanied by a more extensive ophthalmoplegia.

The non-neurological signs to check are skeletal abnormalities like scoliosis (e.g., Friedreich ataxia), telangiectasias (ataxia telangiectasia), and orthostatic hypotension (MSA).

31.4 Investigations

Tables 31.1 and 31.2 show possible causes of non-genetic and genetic ataxias, respectively, including associated symptoms, abnormalities on MRI imaging, and suggestions for further investigation. Not included in the table are ataxias due to traumatic brain injury, hypoxic encephalopathy, radiation, high-altitude cerebral edema, and heat stroke, which are evident from the history.

In our view, the investigation of patients with cerebellar ataxia should always begin with an MRI brain scan, or a CT brain scan in acute-onset ataxias. The only exception might be the patient in whom there is a known genetic ataxia with a compatible clinical presentation. If the MRI shows no structural lesion, there may be hallmarks of specific ataxia causes.

For further phenotyping, electrophysiological investigations need to be considered, and particularly the presence or absence of a peripheral neuropathy is useful. Also, an ophthalmology referral is sometimes required to exclude or confirm abnormalities of the optic nerves (atrophy, edema), retinal pigmentary changes, macular dystrophy, and Kayser-Fleischer rings.

With regard to the genetic ataxias, the diagnostic approach is changing rapidly. Given the genetic heterogeneity, combined with the clinical overlap, very selective gene testing is being replaced by techniques that analyze multiple genes at once, for example, with a targeted array or with exome sequencing.

Table 31.1 Acquired and (non-genetic) degenerative causes of cerebellar ataxia

Cause	Clues	Suggestions for investigation
Structural lesions		
Stroke, MS, space-occupying lesions, Chiari type I malformation	Focal neurological signs, headache	Investigations depend on findings on CT or MRI brain scan
Toxic		
Alcohol	Medical history, concomitant neuropathy	Liver enzymes, MCV, vitamin B1 MRI: anterior vermis atrophy
Drugs, heavy metals	Medical history	Blood level drug, stop use or exposure
Inflammatory		
Paraneoplastic cerebellar degeneration	Rapid progression, history of malignancy	Anti-neuronal antibodies, tumor screen MRI: cerebellar atrophy (later stages)
Anti-GAD ataxia	Subacute, type 1 diabetes mellitus	Anti-GAD antibodies MRI: cerebellar atrophy (later stages)
Steroid-responsive encephalopathy with antithyroid antibodies	Subacute, seizures, myoclonus, rapid response to steroids	Anti-thyroperoxidase antibodies
Gluten ataxia	Gastrointestinal symptoms	Anti-tissue transglutaminase and anti-endomysium antibodies, bowel biopsy
(Para)infectious		
Epstein-Barr virus	Subacute, preceding infection	Serologic testing, CSF
Miller Fisher syndrome	Subacute, ophthalmoplegia, areflexia	Anti-GQ1b antibodies, EMG
HIV-related ataxia	History of HIV infection Opportunistic infections such as toxoplasmosis, PML	MRI, CSF, search for opportunistic infections
Whipple's disease	Fever, weight loss, diarrhea, abdominal pain, arthritis	PCR finding of *Tropheryma whipplei* in duodenal biopsy
Tabetic neurosyphilis	History of syphilis, sensory ataxia	TPHA, CSF
Metabolic		
Vitamin B1 deficiency (Wernicke's encephalopathy)	Confusion, nystagmus, ophthalmoplegia	Vitamin B1 level MRI: bilateral increased T2 signal in the thalamus, hypothalamus, mammillary bodies, periaqueductal region, fourth ventricle floor, and midline cerebellum
Vitamin B12 deficiency	Sensory ataxia, pyramidal signs	Vitamin B12 level MRI: increased signal in cervical posterior columns on spinal T2-weighted MRI
Vitamin E deficiency	Diarrhea	Vitamin E level, celiac screen, serum amylase
Hypothyroidism	Fatigue, weight gain, constipation	Thyroid-stimulating hormone, free T4
Hypoparathyroidism	Cataract, extrapyramidal symptoms	Parathyroid hormone, calcium, phosphate CT: cerebellar and basal ganglia calcifications

Table 31.1 (continued)

Cause	Clues	Suggestions for investigation
Other		
Superficial siderosis	Sensorineural deafness, pyramidal signs	Audiogram, xanthochromic CSF MRI: linear hypointensity in the posterior fossa on T2-weighted gradient-recalled echo
Degenerative		
Multiple system atrophy	Autonomic failure, parkinsonism	Autonomic testing, nuclear imaging MRI: hot cross bun sign (pontocerebellar fiber degeneration) and putaminal rim (high signal line extending laterally from slightly darkened putamen)
Idiopathic late-onset cerebellar ataxia/ sporadic adult-onset ataxia	Relatively pure ataxia, slow progression	MRI: cerebellar atrophy
Sporadic Creutzfeldt-Jakob disease	Rapid progression, cognitive disturbances, myoclonus, pyramidal tract signs	14-3-3 and tau protein CSF, EEG MRI: Increased signal in basal ganglia and cortex on FLAIR and diffusion-weighted MRI

31.5 Treatment

For only a small number of cerebellar disorders, there is a specific treatment (see below). Most often, however, this is not the case. The aim is then to provide symptomatic relief and supportive care and to prevent further complications. Other specialist doctors that are often needed include rehabilitation specialists, clinical geneticists, and urologists. Recently, a randomized controlled trial with riluzole in SCA and Friedreich patients indicated a symptomatic benefit [7]. With regard to other symptomatic, anti-ataxia drugs, the number of well-conducted studies is disappointingly low, and therefore evidence to support their standard use is lacking [2]. Drugs for the potential other disease manifestations are available, for example, spasticity, nystagmus, parkinsonism, orthostatic hypotension, and urinary urgency.

31.5.1 Specific Interventions

Some specific interventions include stopping the offending substance in toxic ataxia; starting vitamin supplements in vitamin deficiencies; specific dietary recommendations in celiac disease and Refsum's disease; starting corticosteroids in patients with SREAT or ataxia associated with anti-GAD antibodies; treating the underlying tumor and starting immunomodulatory treatment in paraneoplastic cerebellar degeneration; and giving bile acid replacement in cerebrotendinous xanthomatosis.

31.5.2 Allied Health Care

Physical therapy and occupational therapy are recommended in cerebellar disease. Studies suggest that training should be intensive to start with and that patients should be encouraged to practice at home for maximum results. Treatment in patients with degenerative ataxia can already start in earlier stages of disease, since those patients seem to be more likely to benefit. In more complicated cases, especially those with extended comorbidity, referral to a rehabilitation specialist and a more multidisciplinary approach seem warranted.

Table 31.2 Some important genetic causes of cerebellar ataxia

Cause	Clues	Suggestions for investigation
Dominant		
Spinocerebellar ataxias	Family history, slow progression, non-ataxia symptoms, some genotype-specific features	Mutation analysis of SCA genes, repeat expansion SCAs first MRI: cerebellar atrophy
Dentatorubropallidoluysian atrophy	Family history, chorea, dementia, myoclonus, Japanese descent	Mutation analysis of ATN1 gene
Alexander disease	(Pseudo)bulbar signs, spasticity	Mutation analysis of GFAP gene MRI: tadpole sign (atrophy of the medulla and cervical cord with a preserved pontine volume)
Gerstmann-Straussler syndrome	Family history, pyramidal signs, adult-onset dementia	Mutation analysis of PRNP gene
Recessive		
Autosomal recessive cerebellar ataxias (in general)	Family history, often neuropathy, systemic features	Mutation analysis of recessive genes, lysosomal enzymes, metabolic investigation, α-fetoprotein
Wilson's disease	Kayser-Fleischer rings, dystonia, parkinsonism, renal tubular acidosis, cardiomyopathy	Ceruloplasmin, serum and urine copper, liver enzymes, renal function Mutation analyses of ATP7B gene MRI: hyperintense T2 signal changes in basal ganglia
Friedreich ataxia	Age at onset 5–25 years, late onset possible. Mixed cerebellar/sensory ataxia, areflexia, pyramidal weakness, scoliosis	Mutation analysis of FRDA gene
Ataxia telangiectasia	Age of onset 2–3 years. Oculomotor apraxia, conjunctival telangiectasias, extrapyramidal signs, predisposition to cancer. Milder variants exist	α-Fetoprotein Mutation analysis of ATM gene
Ataxia with oculomotor apraxia type 1	Like ataxia telangiectasia, sensorimotor neuropathy, chorea, mental retardation	Albumin, cholesterol Mutation analysis of APTX
Ataxia with oculomotor apraxia type 2	Ataxia with oculomotor apraxia type 1, some features in lesser degree, oculomotor apraxia	Serum α-fetoprotein Mutation analysis of SETX
Autosomal recessive cerebellar ataxia (ARCA) with psychomotor retardation	Psychomotor retardation in early life, late-onset ataxia	Mutation analysis of SYT14
ARCA1	Relatively pure cerebellar syndrome	Mutation analysis of SYNE1
ARCA3	Downbeat nystagmus, lower motor neuron involvement	Mutation analysis of ANO10
Autosomal recessive spastic ataxia of Charlevoix-Saguenay	Spasticity, severe neuropathy, onset below age 10 years	Mutation analysis of SACS

Table 31.2 (continued)

Cause	Clues	Suggestions for investigation
SANDO/MIRAS	Ophthalmoplegia, myoclonus, dystonia, neuropathy	Mutation analysis of POLG1 MRI: cerebellar white matter high-signal changes
Late-onset Tay-Sachs disease	Proximal muscle weakness and atrophy, behavioral problems, areflexia	Enzyme assay hexosaminidase A Mutation analysis of HEXA
Cerebrotendinous xanthomatosis	Tendon xanthomas, diarrhea, pyramidal or extrapyramidal signs, seizures, dementia, cataract	Cholestanol Bile alcohols in urine Mutation analysis of CYP27 MRI: cerebellar white matter high-signal changes
Refsum's disease	Demyelinating polyneuropathy, sensorineural deafness, retinitis pigmentosa, anosmia	Phytanic acid Mutation analysis of PHYH and PEX7
Other		
Fragile X-associated tremor/ataxia syndrome	Family history (learning disability premature ovarian failure), mostly men, action tremor, behavioral changes, autonomic dysfunction	Mutation analysis of FMR1 gene MRI: hyperintense signal changes lateral to dentate nucleus extending into middle cerebral peduncles, often generalized atrophy
Mitochondrial disorders	Family history, diabetes, deafness, multisystem involvement	Mutation analysis of mitochondrial DNA and POLG1, muscle biopsy

References

1. van Gaalen J, van de Warrenburg BP. A practical approach to late-onset cerebellar ataxias. Pract Neurol. 2012;12(1):14–24.
2. van de Warrenburg BP, van Gaalen J, Boesch S, Burgunder J-M, Dürr A, Giunti P, et al. EFNS/ENS consensus for the diagnosis and management of chronic ataxias in adulthood. Eur J Neurol. 2014;21:552–62.
3. Fogel B. Childhood cerebellar ataxia. J Child Neurol. 2012;27(9):1138–45.
4. van Gaalen J, Giunti P, van de Warrenburg BP. Movement disorders in spinocerebellar ataxias. Mov Disord. 2011;26(5):792–800.
5. de Bot ST, Willemsen MA, Vermeer S, Kremer HP, van de Warrenburg BP. Reviewing the genetic causes of spastic-ataxias. Neurology. 2012;79(14):1507–14.
6. Vermeer S, van de Warrenburg BP, Willemsen MA, Cluitmans M, Scheffer H, Kremer BP, et al. Autosomal recessive cerebellar ataxias: the current state of affairs. J Med Genet. 2011;48(10):651–9.
7. Romano S, Coarelli G, Marcotulli C, Leonardi L, Piccolo F, Frontali M, et al. Riluzole in patients with hereditary cerebellar ataxia: a randomized, double-blind, placebo controlled trial. Lancet Neurol. 2015;14:985–91.

Paroxysmal Dyskinesias

32

Panagiotis Zis, Davide Martino,
and Tiziano Tamburini

32.1 Introduction

Paroxysmal dyskinesias are a rare heterogeneous group of conditions manifesting as abnormal involuntary movements that recur episodically and last for only a brief duration [1, 2]. Paroxysmal dyskinesias can broadly be classified to primary or idiopathic and secondary. An overview of the secondary forms is presented in Table 32.1 [3, 4]. However, in this chapter we will only review the main forms of genetically determined paroxysmal dyskinesias.

32.2 Paroxysmal Dyskinesias with Established Genetic Aetiology

This type of paroxysmal dyskinesias can be further classified to three main groups: paroxysmal nonkinesigenic dyskinesias (PNKDs), paroxysmal kinesigenic dyskinesias (PKDs) and paroxysmal exercise-induced dyskinesias (PEDs). Table 32.2 summarizes the clinical characteristics and suggested treatment of all three groups, and Table 32.3 summarizes the known genes that are involved.

P. Zis, MD, PhD (✉)
Department of Neurology, Evangelismos General Hospital, 45-47 Ipsilantou Str, Athens 10676, Greece

International Parkinson's Centre of Excellence, King's College Hospital NHS Foundation Trust, Denmark Hill Campus, London, UK
e-mail: takiszis@gmail.com

D. Martino, PhD (✉)
Queen Elizabeth Hospital, Woolwich, Lewisham & Greenwich NHS Trust, London, UK

International Parkinson's Centre of Excellence, King's College Hospital NHS Foundation Trust, Denmark Hill Campus, London, UK
e-mail: davide_martino@hotmail.it

T. Tamburini, MD, PhD
International Parkinson's Centre of Excellence, King's College Hospital NHS Foundation Trust, Denmark Hill Campus, London, UK

Department of Neuroscience, Rehabilitation, Ophthalmology, Genetics, Maternal and Child Health (DiNOGMI), University of Genoa, Genoa, Italy
e-mail: tizianotamburini@hotmail.it

Received: September 18th, 2014.

C. Falup-Pecurariu et al. (eds.), *Movement Disorders Curricula*,
DOI 10.1007/978-3-7091-1628-9_32

Table 32.1 Overview of the secondary paroxysmal dyskinesias

Causes	Stroke
	Multiple sclerosis
	Peripheral trauma (peripheral nerve damage)
	Central trauma
	Anoxic brain injury
	Kernicterus
	Cytomegalovirus
	Anti-VGKC encephalitis
	Meningovascular syphilis
	Migraine
	Hypnogenic
Phenomenology	Unilateral dystonia
	Rarely chorea, ballism, athetosis, and various hyperkinesias can occur, usually concurrently with dystonia
	Presence of both kinesigenic and nonkinesigenic symptoms in some patients
	Sensory precipitants
	Anti-VGKC encephalitis can lead to faciobrachial dystonic seizures
Latency from insult to symptom	Varies significantly from days (such as cases of trauma) to many years (such as cases of kernicterus)
Treatment	Anticonvulsants
	Clonazepam
	Tetrabenazine and trihexyphenidyl (evidence from case series)
	Botulinum toxin

32.2.1 Paroxysmal Nonkinesigenic Dyskinesias

The first case of paroxysmal dyskinesia was described as early as 1940, when Mount and Reback described a 23-year-old man who had episodes of "choreo-dystonia" that could last several hours [16], which became known as paroxysmal dystonic choreoathetosis [2]. However, years later, Demirkiran and Jankovic pointed out that the attacks in these disorders were not necessarily choreic or dystonic, applying to them the more encompassing term of dyskinesia [17].

PNKD consist of attacks of spontaneous, severe dystonia that may be precipitated by alcohol, caffeine and stress [17, 18]. Movements usually begin unilaterally and tend to spread or even generalize [2]. PNKD usually occurs few times per year with a variable duration of each attack from as short as few minutes to many hours, although usually not longer than 1 h.

The onset of primary PNKD is in early childhood [16]. Male predominance of 2:1 has been observed in sporadic cases, when there is no gender predominance in gene-proven cases [2]. Female patients may experience attacks more frequently during menstruation or ovulation periods [2].

Most cases of PNKD are familial with autosomal dominant inheritance linked to the myofibrillogenesis regulator gene (MR1) or PNKD gene, located on chromosome 2q35. It encodes a protein of 385 amino acids associated to the cell membrane [19, 20]. Another mutation responsible for PNKD was detected in one large family with 16 individuals, variably presenting PNKD or generalized epilepsy or both (generalized epilepsy and paroxysmal dyskinesia, GEPD). This gene, named KCNMA1, is located on chromosome 10q22 and encodes for the α-subunit of the calcium-sensitive potassium channel BK [21, 22]. A third different mutation, named PNKD2, has been identified on chromosome 2q31 in a Canadian family, where ten individuals presented symmetrical paroxysmal nonkinesigenic dyskinesia in the hands and feet with an autosomal dominant inheritance pattern [23].

In terms of management, avoiding triggering factors is crucial along with symptomatic treatment, with clonazepam being the drug of choice [2, 24]. Clonazepam may be effective in up to 30% of patients, and other anticonvulsants, like carbamazepine, should be considered as a further possible treatment option [17]. Some case reports have revealed deep brain stimulation as a potential therapeutic option in medically refractory PKND [5, 10]. Also, symptomatic cases may also benefit from benzodiazepines as described by Mirsattari, who reported effectiveness in three of four patients with PKND symptomatic to HIV infection [6]. Finally, levetiracetam was effective

Table 32.2 Clinical characteristics and suggested treatment of primary paroxysmal dyskinesias

Type	Phenomenology	Triggering factors	Duration	Frequency	Onset	Predominance	Management
Paroxysmal nonkinesigenic dyskinesias	Attacks of spontaneous, severe dystonia, usually unilateral	Alcohol, caffeine, stress	Usually < 1 h	Few times a year	Childhood	Male (2:1)	Avoiding triggering factors
							Clonazepam
Paroxysmal kinesigenic dyskinesias	Attacks of dystonic, choreic or ballistic movements, or a combination of these, usually unilateral	Sudden changes in movement	Seconds	Daily	Childhood – adolescence	Male (4:1)	Carbamazepine
							Phenytoin
Paroxysmal exercise-induced dyskinesias	Attacks of dystonic, movements, usually unilateral	Several minutes of exercise	Usually <5 min	Depends on the level of exercise	Childhood	Female (3:2)	Gabapentin
							Ketogenic diet (in GLUT1-related cases)

Table 32.3 Genes involved in primary paroxysmal dyskinesias

Type	Inheritance	Gene	Location	Role
Paroxysmal nonkinesigenic dyskinesias				
Paroxysmal nonkinesigenic dyskinesia (PKND) [5, 6]	AD	MR1	2q35	Controls glutathione levels Encodes a protein of 385 amino acids associated to the cell membrane
Paroxysmal nonkinesigenic dyskinesia 2 (PKND 2) [7]	ÅD	PNKD2	2q31 (1 family reported)	
Generalized epilepsy and paroxysmal dyskinesia (GEPD) [8, 9]	AD	KCNMA1	10q22.3 (1 family reported)	Encodes the α-subunit of the calcium-sensitive potassium channel BK
Paroxysmal kinesigenic dyskinesias				
Episodic kinesigenic dyskinesia 1 (EKD 1) [10]	AD	PRRT2	16p11.2	Possible involvement in the presynaptic release of neurotransmitter via interaction with synaptosome-associated protein 25 (SNAP-25)
Episodic kinesigenic dyskinesia 2 (EKD 2) [11]	AD	-	16q13-q22.1 (1 family reported)	Unknown
Paroxysmal exercise-induced dyskinesias				
Paroxysmal exercise-induced dyskinesia (isolated) [12]	AD	SLC2A1	1p34.2	Encodes the major glucose transporter type 1 (GLUT1) in brain, placenta and erythrocytes
Paroxysmal exercise-induced dyskinesia with or without epilepsy and/or haemolytic anaemia (GLUT1DS2) [13]	AD	SLC2A1	1p34.2	Same as above
Glucose transport protein type 1 deficiency syndrome (GLUT1DS1) [13]	AD	SLC2A1	1p34.2	Same as above
Paroxysmal choreoathetosis and progressive spastic paraplegia [12, 14]	AD	SLC2A1	1p34.2	Same as above
Rolandic epilepsy with paroxysmal exercise-induced dyskinesia and writer's cramp (RE-PED-WC) [15]	AR	–	16p12-11.2 (1 family reported)	–

AD autosomal dominant, *AR* autosomal recessive

in symptomatic PKND secondarily to hypoparathyroidism, where initial treatment with valproic acid failed [13].

32.2.2 Paroxysmal Kinesigenic Dyskinesias

In 1967, Kertesz was the first to describe PKD, highlighting that attacks in those affected were induced by sudden movement (kinesigenic) [7].

PKD consists of very brief attacks, which are precipitated by sudden changes in movement such as getting up from a chair, getting out of a car, setting off for a sprint race, etc. [8, 9] The clinical manifestation includes dystonic, choreic and ballistic movements, or a combination of these. Movements are usually unilateral but may also be bilateral [2]. Unlike PNKD, PKD occurs daily and some patients can have more than 20 attacks per day [8].

Onset age in PKD varies, but it usually is between 7 and 15 years. There appears to be a higher prevalence in males (estimated ration of 4:1) in the sporadic form but not in familial cases [2].

Interestingly, many individuals may have a brief, non-specific warning or aura prior to an attack. This usually consists of paraesthesia in the affected limb or epigastric discomfort [8]. Some patients learn to positively use the aura as warning sign and prevent attacks by slowing down or "holding tight" to the affected limb.

The major cause of PKD is mutations involving the PRRT2 gene, which is located on chromosome 16 and consists of 4 exons. The gene encodes the 340 amino acids proline-rich transmembrane protein 2, whose function is not completely understood, but some authors reported a possible involvement in the presynaptic release of neurotransmitter via interaction with synaptosome-associated protein 25 (SNAP-25). Heterozygous PRRT2 mutations generally result in truncation and haploinsufficiency and can be associated with both familial and sporadic cases, though familial PKD, BFIS and ICCA show a higher prevalence of genetic changes [11]. Another syndrome characterized by paroxysmal kinesigenic dyskinesia (EKD2) was mapped in 1 Indian family again on chromosome 16 [12].

In terms of treatment, and in contrast to PKND, PKD responds excellent to anticonvulsant treatment [24]. Carbamazepine is the drug of choice [2], when phenytoin is also highly effective [8]. Other evidence of treatment of PKDs is scarce and mainly coming from single case reports or small open series [24]. Thus, oxcarbazepine [14], lamotrigine [15] and topiramate [25] were effective. Other drugs used as an alternative treatment for PKD are risperidone [26], acetazolamide, levodopa, flunarizine and tetrabenazine [27].

32.2.3 Paroxysmal Exercise-Induced Dyskinesias

A third type of paroxysmal dyskinesia, the PED, was introduced by Lance in 1977. He reported a family that had attacks lasting between 5 and 30 min provoked by prolonged exercise [28].

Paroxysmal exercise-induced dyskinesias consist of brief episodes, usually dystonic, that occur after several minutes of physical exercise, rather than at the beginning of movement as in PKD [17, 18], and involve the body parts mostly involved in the physical exertion.

The duration of each attack is on average less than 5 min, and the abnormal movement resolves gradually with cessation of the exercise [18]. The frequency of the episodes depends on the level of the exercise. PED is a rare form of paroxysmal movement disorder, with a male-female ratio of 2:3 [29]. The usual onset age is in childhood (mean age 5 years) [2].

Paroxysms of involuntary movements induced by prolonged exercise may be present in various clinical conditions and show marked etiologic heterogeneity. Familial and sporadic cases of PED were reported with mutations in the SLC2A1 gene, encoding for glucose transport protein type 1 (GLUT1) [30]. The same gene is involved in a number of other autosomal dominant syndromes within the spectrum of GLUT1 deficiency syndromes (GLUT1-DS), where PED can be associated to epilepsy, different levels of cognitive impairment and spastic paraplegia [31, 32]. PED was also reported in 1 family with a different genetic locus mutation and autosomal recessive inheritance pattern, associated to rolandic epilepsy and writer's cramp (RE-PED-WC) [33].

In terms of management, avoiding precipitating events, like prolonged physical exercise, may prevent attacks [24]. Gabapentin may reduce the frequency and severity of attacks. Clonazepam and carbamazepine were found to be of limited benefit [17, 29]. Isolated cases found the use of levodopa, acetazolamide, and trihexiphenidyl successful [29]. Finally, based on the molecular findings in GLUT1-related (see below) cases, a ketogenic diet might be beneficial [34].

References

1. Fahn S. The paroxysmal dyskinesias. In: Marsden CD, Fahn S, editors. Movement disorders. Oxford: Butterworth Heinemann Ltd; 1994. p. 310–45.
2. Bhatia KP. Paroxysmal dyskinesias. Mov Disord. 2011;26(6):1157–65.
3. Blakeley J, Jankovic J. Secondary causes of paroxysmal dyskinesia. Adv Neurol. 2002;89:401–20.
4. Blakeley J, Jankovic J. Secondary paroxysmal dyskinesias. Mov Disord. 2002;17(4):726–34.
5. Loher TJ, Krauss JK, Burgunder JM, Taub E, Siegfried J. Chronic thalamic stimulation for treatment of dystonic paroxysmal nonkinesigenic dyskinesia. Neurology. 2001;56(2):268–70.
6. Mirsattari SM, Berry ME, Holden JK, Ni W, Nath A, Power C. Paroxysmal dyskinesias in patients with HIV infection. Neurology. 1999;52(1):109–14.
7. Kertesz A. Paroxysmal kinesigenic choreoathetosis. An entity within the paroxysmal choreoathetosis syndrome. Description of 10 cases, including 1 autopsied. Neurology. 1967;17:680–90.
8. Bruno MK, Hallett M, Gwinn-Hardy K, Sorensen B, Considine E, Tucker S, Lynch DR, Mathews KD, Swoboda KJ, Harris J, Soong BW, Ashizawa T, Jankovic J, Renner D, Fu YH, Ptacek LJ. Clinical evaluation of idiopathic paroxysmal kinesigenic dyskinesia: new diagnostic criteria. Neurology. 2004;63(12):2280–7.
9. Lotze T, Jankovic J. Paroxysmal kinesigenic dyskinesias. Semin Pediatr Neurol. 2003;10(1):68–79.
10. Yamada K, Goto S, Soyama N, Shimoda O, Kudo M, Kuratsu J, Murase N, Kaji R. Complete suppression of paroxysmal nonkinesigenic dyskinesia by globus pallidus internus pallidal stimulation. Mov Disord. 2006;21(4):576–9.
11. Groffen AJ, Klapwijk T, van Rootselaar AF, Groen JL, Tijssen MA. Genetic and phenotypic heterogeneity in sporadic and familial forms of paroxysmal dyskinesia. J Neurol. 2013;260(1):93–9.
12. Valente EM, Spacey SD, Wali GM, Bhatia KP, Dixon PH, Wood NW, Davis MB. A second paroxysmal kinesigenic choreoathetosis locus (EKD2) mapping on 16q13-q22.1 indicates a family of genes which give rise to paroxysmal disorders on human chromosome 16. Brain. 2000;123(Pt 10):2040–5.
13. Alemdar M, Iseri P, Selekler M, Komsuoğlu SS. Levetiracetam-responding paroxysmal nonkinesigenic dyskinesia. Clin Neuropharmacol. 2007;30(4):241–4.
14. Tsao CY. Effective treatment with oxcarbazepine in paroxysmal kinesigenic choreoathetosis. J Child Neurol. 2004;19(4):300–1.
15. Uberall MA, Wenzel D. Effectiveness of lamotrigine in children with paroxysmal kinesigenic choreoathetosis. Dev Med Child Neurol. 2000;42(10):699–700.
16. Mount LA, Reback S. Familial paroxysmal choreoathetosis. Arch Neurol Psychol. 1940;44:841–7.
17. Demirkiran M, Jankovic J. Paroxysmal dyskinesias: clinical features and classification. Ann Neurol. 1995;38:571–9.
18. Bhatia KP. The paroxysmal dyskinesias. J Neurol. 1999;246(3):149–55.
19. Bruno MK, Lee HY, Auburger GW, Friedman A, Nielsen JE, Lang AE, Bertini E, Van Bogaert P, Averyanov Y, Hallett M, Gwinn-Hardy K, Sorenson B, Pandolfo M, Kwiecinski H, Servidei S, Fu YH, Ptácek L. Genotype-phenotype correlation of paroxysmal nonkinesigenic dyskinesia. Neurology. 2007;68(21):1782–9.
20. Ghezzi D, Viscomi C, Ferlini A, Gualandi F, Mereghetti P, DeGrandis D, Zeviani M. Paroxysmal non-kinesigenic dyskinesia is caused by mutations of the MR-1 mitochondrial targeting sequence. Hum Mol Genet. 2009;18(6):1058–64.
21. Du W, Bautista JF, Yang H, Diez-Sampedro A, You SA, Wang L, Kotagal P, Lüders HO, Shi J, Cui J, Richerson GB, Wang QK. Calcium-sensitive potassium channelopathy in human epilepsy and paroxysmal movement disorder. Nat Genet. 2005;37(7):733–8.
22. Browne DL, Gancher ST, Nutt JG, Brunt ER, Smith EA, Kramer P, Litt M. Episodic ataxia/myokymia syndrome is associated with point mutations in the human potassium channel gene, KCNA1. Nat Genet. 1994;8(2):136–40.
23. Spacey SD, Adams PJ, Lam PC, Materek LA, Stoessl AJ, Snutch TP, Hsiung GY. Genetic heterogeneity in paroxysmal nonkinesigenic dyskinesia. Neurology. 2006;66(10):1588–90.
24. Unterberger I, Trinka E. Diagnosis and treatment of paroxysmal dyskinesias revisited. Ther Adv Neurol Dis. 2008;1(2):4–11.
25. Huang YG, Chen YC, Du F, Li R, Xu GL, Jiang W, Huang J. Topiramate therapy for paroxysmal kinesigenic choreoathetosis. Mov Disord. 2005;20(1):75–7.
26. Karakurum B, Karatas M, Yildirim T. Risperidone as an alternative treatment for paroxysmal kinesigenic dyskinesia. Neurol Sci. 2003;24(2):92–3.

27. Jankovic J, Demirkiran M. Classification of paroxysmal dyskinesias and ataxias. Adv Neurol. 2002;89:387–400.
28. Lance JW. Familial paroxysmal dystonic choreoathetosis and its differentiation from related syndromes. Ann Neurol. 1977;2:285–93.
29. Bhatia KP, Soland VL, Bhatt MH, Quinn NP, Marsden CD. Paroxysmal exercise-induced dystonia: eight new sporadic cases and a review of the literature. Mov Disord. 1997;12:1007–12.
30. Pearson TS, Akman C, Hinton VJ, Engelstad K, De Vivo DC. Phenotypic spectrum of glucose transporter type 1 deficiency syndrome (Glut1 DS). Curr Neurol Neurosci Rep. 2013;13(4):342.
31. Brockmann K. Episodic movement disorders: from phenotype to genotype and back. Curr Neurol Neurosci Rep. 2013;13(10):379.
32. Brockmann K. The expanding phenotype of GLUT1-deficiency syndrome. Brain Dev. 2009;31(7):545–52.
33. Guerrini R, Bonanni P, Nardocci N, Parmeggiani L, Piccirilli M, De Fusco M, Aridon P, Ballabio A, Carrozzo R, Casari G. Autosomal recessive rolandic epilepsy with paroxysmal exercise-induced dystonia and writer's cramp: delineation of the syndrome and gene mapping to chromosome 16p12-11.2. Ann Neurol. 1999;45(3):344–52.
34. Weber YG, Storch A, Wuttke TV, Brockmann K, Kempfle J, Maljevic S, Margari L, Kamm C, Schneider SA, Huber SM, Pekrun A, Roebling R, Seebohm G, Koka S, Lang C, Kraft E, Blazevic D, Salvo-Vargas A, Fauler M, Mottaghy FM, Münchau A, Edwards MJ, Presicci A, Margari F, Gasser T, Lang F, Bhatia KP, Lehmann-Horn F, Lerche H. GLUT1 mutations are a cause of paroxysmal exertion-induced dyskinesias and induce hemolytic anemia by a cation leak. J Clin Invest. 2008;118(6):2157–68.

Wilson's Disease: Neurological Aspects, Clinical Manifestations, and Treatment Considerations

33

Sevasti Bostantjopoulou, Pantelis Stathis, and Spiros Konitsiotis

33.1 Introduction

Wilson's disease (WD), also known as hepatolenticular degeneration, is an autosomal recessive genetic disorder of copper metabolism caused by mutations in the ATP7B gene which leads to accumulation of copper in the body [1, 2]. In 1912, Kinnier Wilson in his landmark paper first described the disorder as a familial nervous system disease characterized by progressive lenticular degeneration associated with cirrhosis of the liver [3]. In 1948, Cummings reported the excess of copper in the brain and liver in patients with WD [4]. Later on (1993), three groups of scientists identified the gene for the disease located on chromosome 13q14 [4]. The ATP7B gene encodes a transmembrane protein ATPase (copper-transporting P-type ATPase 7B) which regulates the bioavailability of intracellular copper [1, 2]. The first efforts for the treatment of the disease started with Cummings (1951) using dimercaprol and continued with the use of penicillamine by Walshe (1956) [4].

33.2 Epidemiology

WD is a relatively rare disorder, and there is a continuous debate about the real frequency of the disease. The worldwide prevalence of WD is estimated to be between 1:30,000 and 1:100,000 population [1, 2] with a gene frequency of about 1 in 90–150 [2]. However, in a recent study, the calculated frequency of individuals predicted to carry two pathogenic mutations was 1:7,026 [5]. High prevalence of WD was found in Sardinia, in Gran Canaria, in a mountain area in Crete and in East Asian population [6, 7]. Although the disease affects equally men and women, the hepatic form occurs more frequently in women, while the neuropsychiatric manifestations are more frequent in men [8]. WD may present at any age from early childhood to late adulthood with a peak incidence of around 17 years [6, 9]. However, the range of age at disease onset is considerably larger than previously reported, with case reports in the literature including patients from 3 years old (even 9 months) to 72 years old [2, 6, 9–11].

S. Bostantjopoulou (✉)
3rd University Department of Neurology, G. Papanikolaou Hospital, Exohi, Thessaloniki 57010, Greece
e-mail: bostkamb@otenet.gr

P. Stathis, MD, PhD
Neurology, Mediterraneo, Spirou Merkouri 25, Athens, Attiki 11634, Greece
e-mail: stathis.pantelis@gmail.com

S. Konitsiotis, MD, PhD
Professor of Neurology, Department of Neurology, University Hospital of Ioannina, 30, 28th October str, Ioannina 45444, Greece

C. Falup-Pecurariu et al. (eds.), *Movement Disorders Curricula*,
DOI 10.1007/978-3-7091-1628-9_33

33.3 Clinical Manifestations

There is a great variability of phenotypic manifestations in WD ranging from asymptomatic individuals to severe acute or chronic liver and neurological disease. The most common clinical manifestations are hepatic, neurologic, and psychiatric. The neurological and hepatic symptoms generally present in equal proportions; however, neurological symptoms present later than the hepatic disease usually in the second to third decade of life. Mean age at onset for hepatic symptomatology is 11–15 years and for neurological manifestations 15–21 years [1, 9, 12, 13].

33.3.1 Presymptomatic WD

Patients may remain asymptomatic for decades, and they are usually discovered incidentally in screening examination because they have an affected sib or during routine liver test function. Initial symptoms can be unspecific and subtle thus delaying the diagnosis. Deterioration in grades at school, behavioral change, hand clumsiness, handwriting difficulty (Fig. 33.1a, b), unexplained pathological liver tests or anemia, bone pains, and arthralgia are some of the nonspecific initial symptoms of the disease [14].

33.3.2 Neurological Manifestations

Neurological signs have been reported at initial examination in 18–68 % of patients [12]. Walshe and Yealland [15] classified the patients with neurological manifestations in four types: (1) parkinsonian, (2) pseudosclerotic, (3) dystonic, and (4) choreic. Recently, three overlapping neurological syndromes have been recognized: (1) akinetic–rigid syndrome resembling parkinsonism, (2) generalized dystonic syndrome, and (3) postural and intention tremor with ataxia, titubation, and dysarthria (pseudosclerosis) [16].

Dysarthria is the most common symptom in WD reported in 85–97 % of the patients [12, 17]. It is usually of mixed type with dystonic, ataxic, and hypokinetic components [9, 12, 14, 17]. In advanced disease, patients become virtually mute [14].

33.4 Movement Disorders

Parkinsonism is found in 19–62 % of the patients [12]. It is of the akinetic–rigid type with rigidity and bradykinesia, usually asymmetric, gait disturbance and postural instability [10, 12, 16]. If rest tremor is present, it usually has a postural and kinetic component [9, 12]. *Dystonic syndrome* is found in 11–65 % of the patients [2, 9, 12, 17, 18]. Dystonia can be focal (blepharospasm, torticollis, writer cramp, dysphonia, oromandibular), segmental, multifocal, or generalized leading to severe contractions. Lesions in the putamen were frequently found in WD patients with dystonia suggesting relationship between dystonia in WD and abnormalities in this brain region [18]. A characteristic focal dystonia of WD is the dystonic facial

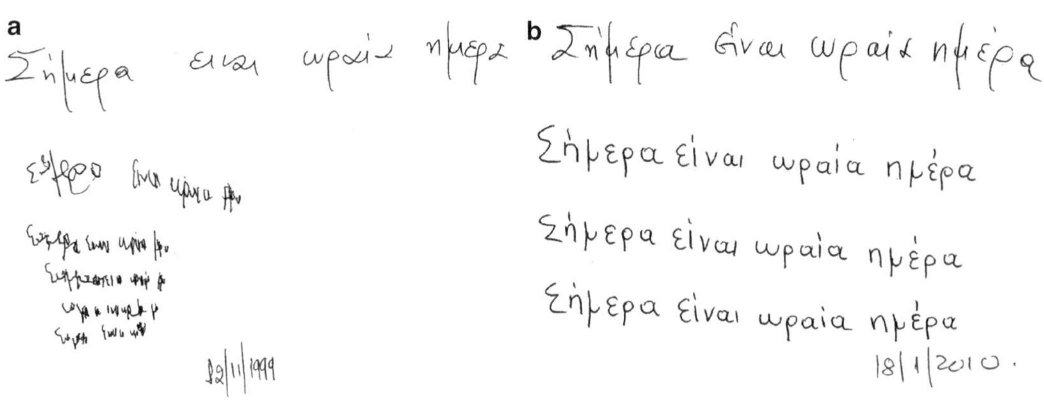

Fig. 33.1 (**a**) Impaired handwriting in the beginning of the disease. (**b**) Same patient, after 11 years on penicillamine

expression – fixed pseudo-smile or risus sardonicus [12, 14, 17]. Risus sardonicus is the result of retraction of the upper lip and mouth opening due to dystonia of the facial and oral muscles [16]. Patients have a typical facial appearance – Wilson's face – with open mouth, facetious smile, reduced eye blinking, drooling saliva, and dull look [14].

Tremor has been reported in 22–60 % of the patients [9, 17]. The tremor can be postural, intentional, or at rest. The tremor usually starts in one limb and later on may spread to the whole body [17]. Most commonly, one or both hands are affected but also the legs, the trunk, the head, and the tongue [9, 14, 17, 19, 20]. During the early phase, there is fine upper limb tremor that may become dramatically worsen for several minutes [20]. Sometimes, early in the disease the tremor has the characteristics of essential tremor [9]. The wing-beating tremor, that is, a proximal upper extremity coarse tremor of lower frequency and higher amplitude elicited by sustained abduction of the arms at 90° with flexed elbows and palms facing downward, is less frequently observed [2, 9, 16, 19–21].

Ataxia has been reported in 30 % of the patients [9, 12]. Cerebellar involvement is associated with scanning speech, ocular motor abnormalities, limb dysmetria, intention tremor, and wide-based gait [9, 22].

Other movement disorders including chorea and athetosis (6–16 %), respiratory dyskinesias with cough, myoclonus (focal or generalized with encephalopathy), tics, painless legs moving toes syndrome, paroxysmal kinesigenic dyskinesia, eyelid apraxia, oculogyric crisis, isolated tongue protrusion syndrome, and stereotyped movements have also been reported [6, 12, 17, 19, 22, 23].

33.5 Cognitive Function

Cognitive impairment in WD has been described even in the first paper from Wilson. Neuropsychological testing reveals cognitive deficits in many domains including attention, visuospatial processing, executive function, and some aspects of memory in neurologically symptomatic patients with WD [24–26]. Patients show lower performance on global cognitive tests compared with controls, but still they remain in the normal limits [25, 27]. Verbal and abstract reasoning and construction, tested by Raven's Progressive Matrices, arithmetics, comprehension, similarities, picture arrangement, object assembly, and block design, show great impairment [26]. Other tests for executive function had controversial results: performances on Wisconsin Card Sorting Test and semantic verbal fluency were normal, while phonemic fluency was abnormal [26]. However, a recent study stresses the executive dysfunction in patients with WD suggesting the involvement of the frontostriatal circuit [27]. Furthermore, patients exhibit impaired conceptual flexibility in the Trail Making Test. Concerning memory, patients have impaired coding difficulties and not increased forgetting [24]. Visual perception and reasoning are also impaired. Attention deficit is one of the most frequent symptoms of cognitive impairment [26]. This has been reported in various studies using different tests. In a recent study, alterations were found on the alerting domain of the attention network and not on the orienting and executive domain [26]. No correlation was found between cognitive deficits and motor symptoms as well as cognitive deficits and copper or ceruloplasmin levels [25]. Dementia of subcortical type is reported in a small percentage of patients (4.2–5 %) [17, 27].

Other neurological manifestations include ocular motor abnormalities (conjugate ocular palsy, upward gaze restriction, saccadic alterations), pyramidal syndrome, seizures (6 %) mainly partial, benign epilepsy of childhood with centrotemporal spikes and even status epilepticus, pseudobulbar palsy with dysphagia, dysautonomia (orthostatic hypotension, abnormal response to Valsalva maneuver, abnormal sympathetic skin responses, sphincter, and sexual dysfunction), migraine, headaches, peripheral sensorimotor polyneuropathy, stroke-like episodes, olfactory impairment, muscle cramps, insomnia, hypersomnia, and altered REM sleep function [12, 14, 17, 19, 22, 28, 29].

33.5.1 Psychiatric Manifestations

Psychiatric symptoms are common in WD and can precede neurologic or hepatic signs. Thirty to 65 % of WD patients have psychiatric manifestations at the time of diagnosis, and 20–50 % of them had visited a psychiatrist prior to the WD diagnosis [30]. Depression and personality change are the most frequent behavioral symptoms in WD. Psychiatric disorders include major depression (4–47 %), bipolar disorder (18–39 %), and psychosis (delusions, hallucinations, thought disorder, and even catatonia in 1.4–11.3 %) [30]. A variety of other psychiatric symptoms have been reported in WD including changes in school performance, obsessive–compulsive disorder, impulsiveness, aggressiveness, emotional liability, disinhibition, irritability, reckless and child-like behavior, anxiety, anorexia nervosa, substance abuse, and antisocial and criminal behavior [1, 12, 17, 22, 30].

33.5.2 Hepatic Manifestations

The spectrum of liver disease in WD ranges from asymptomatic hepatomegaly , isolated splenomegaly, only biochemical abnormalities (elevated serum aminotransferase activity) to acute liver failure [2, 14, 31]. Clinical symptoms in patients with liver disease include jaundice, anorexia, vomiting, ascites, variceal hemorrhage, hemolysis, and acute liver failure [2]. Acute transient hepatitis mimicking viral hepatitis is reported in 25 % of the patients with hepatic symptomatology, while other patients present with symptoms resembling autoimmune hepatitis [2, 19, 31]. The most common hepatic presentation is chronic silent progressive cirrhosis (compensated or decompensated) with isolated splenomegaly and portal hypertension [2, 14, 31, 32]. It is very important to have in mind that there is high prevalence of cirrhosis in patients with neurological symptoms but without clinical signs of liver disease [32]. Acute liver failure is a severe condition with high mortality rate (95 % mortality if left untreated) associated with Coombs' negative hemolytic anemia, coagulopathy, and acute renal failure [2, 14, 19, 31]. It occurs usually in females and in young patients. The liver fails acutely releasing large amount of copper in the blood that results in hemolytic anemia. Other clinical features include chronic hepatitis, rarely hepatocellular carcinoma, pancreatitis, cholelithiasis and cholestasis with pigmented gallstone production, cholangitis, transient episodes of jaundice to hemolysis [1, 2, 31, 33].

33.5.3 Ophthalmological Manifestations

Kayser–Fleischer ring, caused by deposition of copper in Descemet's membrane of the cornea, is found in 44–62 % of patients with liver disease but in almost 95 % of patients with neurological manifestations [2, 14, 31]. However, some studies reported that only 77.8–85.2 % of neurological patients had Kayser–Fleischer ring [34]. Youn et al. [34] found that patients with neurological involvement and without Kayser–Fleischer ring had higher ceruloplasmin and serum copper levels and less common liver cirrhosis and brain lesion in MRI. The Kayser–Fleischer ring is almost always bilateral, but there are some reports with unilateral Kayser–Fleischer ring [19]. The color of the ring ranges from gold to brown and green. It is best visualized with the use of slit lamp as a green discoloration at the outer corneal circumference [12, 14, 19]. The ring first appears in the upper part of the cornea, then in the lower part, and finally all around the cornea. Copper-containing corneal ring can be found in conditions other than WD (false positive) such as hepatic diseases (cirrhosis, hepatitis, chronic cholestatic jaundice, primary biliary cirrhosis and partial biliary atresia), multiple myeloma, pulmonary carcinoma, and copper foreign body in the eye [35]. Another ocular finding in WD is the sunflower cataract caused by deposits of copper in the lens. It is a relatively rare finding (17 %) [12, 19]. It has a green, brown gray, or gold color and a sunflower-like appearance with a central powder-like disk and radiating petal-like spokes [19]. Both the Kayser–Fleischer ring and the sunflower cataract disappear with the treatment.

Other clinical findings include [1, 6, 13, 19, 22, 36–38]:

(a) *Renal disorders* – hypercalciuria and nephrolithiasis, aminociduria, proteinuria, hyperphosphaturia, glomerulonephritis, hematuria, renal tubulopathy, renal acidosis, and Fanconi syndrome.
(b) *Bone and joint disorders* are common and usually large joints (especially the knee) and vertebral column are involved. Skeletal abnormalities include osteoporosis (radiographic evidence in 85% of the patients), osteomalacia, osteochondritis, osteoarthritis, spondylopathy, chondrocalcinosis, subchondral cyst formation, spontaneous fractures, and joint dislocation. Quemeneur et al. suggested that risk factors for fractures in WD are patients with severe neurological involvement, low BMI, and amenorrhea [36].
(c) *Hematological disorders* – hemolytic anemia, thrombocytopenia, leucopenia, and antiphospholipid syndrome.
(d) *Cardiac abnormalities* – arrhythmias, left ventricular and biventricular hypertrophy, early repolarization, cardiomyopathy, and Takotsubo cardiomyopathy.
(e) *Skin hyperpigmentation* of the anterior surface of the limbs and azure lunulae of the fingernails.
(f) *Endocrine disorders* – hypoparathyroidism, hypoglycemia, amenorrhea, infertility, and miscarriages.

33.5.4 Global Clinical Evaluation

Two scales have been developed for assessing semiquantitatively the whole spectrum of neurological, psychiatric, and hepatic symptoms of WD, thus evaluating disease severity, quantifying disability, and monitoring disease progression and drug efficacy: the Unified Wilson's Disease Rating Scale (UWDRS) [39] and the Global Scale for Wilson's Disease (GAS for WD) [40]. The Unified Wilson's Disease Rating Scale consists of three subscales: neurologic, hepatic, and psychiatric. It contains 55 items (27 neurological, 9 hepatic, and 19 psychiatric) with a maximal score of 320 points. Some items are reported by the patients or the family and some come up from the physical examination. The Unified Wilson's Disease Rating Scale consists of two tiers: Tier 1 (global disability) measures the disease burden and covers four domains, that is, liver, cognition and behavior, motor, and osseomuscular, and Tier 2 (neurological assessment) is a multidimensional neurological evaluation that assesses all aspects of neurological dysfunction in WD and contains 14 items.

33.6 Diagnostic Testing

33.6.1 Biochemical Liver Test and Uric Acid

Serum aminotransferase activities are generally abnormal in WD [1, 31]. The levels of aminotransferase activity do not correlate with disease severity. Serum uric acid may be decreased at the same time with hepatic or neurological symptoms [31].

33.6.2 Ceruloplasmin

Ceruloplasmin is a 132-kDa protein synthesized mainly in the liver and is the major carrier for copper in the blood. Ceruloplasmin levels can be estimated by enzymatic or antibody-dependent assay methods. Although the results are roughly equivalent, radioimmunoassays may overestimate ceruloplasmin concentrations [2, 31]. The normal limits of ceruloplasmin vary among laboratories. Although an extremely low serum ceruloplasmin level (<50 mg/L or 5 mg/dL) is a strong evidence for the diagnosis of WD, modestly abnormal levels can lead to diagnostic confusion [41]. In general, serum ceruloplasmin level <200 mg/L (<20 mg/dL) has been considered consistent with WD and diagnostic if associated with Kayser–Fleischer rings and increased 24-h Cu excretion [42]. Serum ceruloplasmin within the normal range does not exclude the diagnosis [31]. In addition, screening for diagnosis of WD in the setting of acute liver failure using ceruloplasmin measurements and serum copper levels is unreliable [43]. False positive results can be found in severe protein loss, in severe liver disease, and in Menkes disease, while false negative results can be found in pregnancy and in estrogen treatment [35, 40].

33.6.3 Serum Copper

Most individuals with Wilson's disease have a subnormal total serum copper concentration that is proportional to the serum ceruloplasmin concentration [2, 31]. The serum non-ceruloplasmin-bound copper concentration, calculated by subtracting the amount of copper associated with ceruloplasmin, determined by the enzymatic assay (ceruloplasmin in mg/L × 3.15) from the total serum copper concentration has been proposed as a diagnostic test for WD. It is elevated above 25 μg/dL (250 μg/L) in most untreated patients (normal<15 μg/dL or <150 μg/L) [2, 31, 42]. Elevated serum copper concentrations are seen in portal cirrhosis, biliary tract disease such as primary sclerosing cholangitis, and hepatitis, probably because excess copper that would normally be excreted in the bile is retained in circulation [44]. In primary biliary cirrhosis, ceruloplasmin is high, resulting in high serum copper. Lesser elevations of hepatic copper are found in chronic copper poisoning, obstructive jaundice, and certain cases of hepatic cirrhosis [31, 43, 44].

33.6.4 Urinary Copper Excretion

The most useful screening test is the 24-h urine measurement. The 24-h urinary excretion of copper reflects the amount of non-ceruloplasmin-bound copper in the circulation and is useful both as a diagnostic and also as a treatment monitoring tool. Although many laboratories take 40 μg/24 h (0.6 μmol/24 h) as the upper limit of normal, the conventional level taken as diagnostic of WD is >100 μg/24 h (>1.6 μmol/24 h) in symptomatic patients [2, 31, 42]. Raised 24-h urinary copper excretion can be found increased in obstructive liver disease, primary biliary cirrhosis, cholestasis, autoimmune hepatitis, and acute hepatic failure of any etiology [2, 13, 31, 35]. Penicillamine challenge studies of urinary copper excretion may be useful in obtaining further evidence of WD, especially in symptomatic children [45].

33.6.5 Hepatic Parenchymal Copper Concentration and Histological Abnormalities in the Liver

Hepatic parenchymal copper content >250 μg/g dry weight provides critical diagnostic information and should be obtained in unclear cases. In untreated patients, normal hepatic copper content (<40–50 μg/g dry weight) almost always excludes a diagnosis of WD [46]. Liver copper concentration can found falsely low in extensive fibrosis and few parenchymal cells and on the other hand can be found falsely high in biliary cirrhosis, autoimmune hepatitis, and cholestasis [1, 19]. The early histological abnormalities in the liver include mild steatosis, glycogenated nuclei in hepatocytes, and focal hepatocellular necrosis [2, 31]. Occasionally, the liver may show histological features of autoimmune hepatitis. With disease progression fibrosis and cirrhosis develop [2, 31]. Rhodanine stain is used to demonstrate excess copper in hepatocytes. However, the positive rhodanine granules are found in less than 10% of patients with WD, and this method cannot substitute quantitative liver copper content [47].

33.6.6 Brain Imaging

Computerized tomography or magnetic resonance imaging (MRI) of the brain may reveal structural abnormalities; however, MRI is a more sensitive method for revealing these abnormalities. Almost all patients with WD and neurological dysfunction have MRI abnormalities. Brain MRI demonstrates widespread lesions (hyperintensities on T2-weighted images and hypointensities on T1-weighted images) in the caudate,

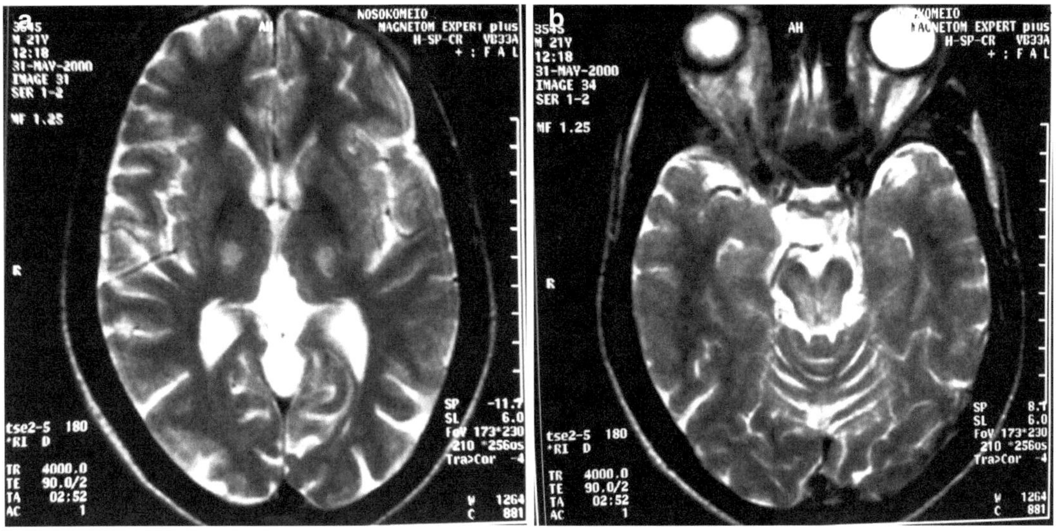

Fig. 33.2 (**a**) T2-weighted MRI shows hyperintense signal in the thalamus bilaterally. (**b**) T2-weighted MRI shows hyperintense signal in the midbrain

putamen, globus pallidum, midbrain, pons, cerebellum, thalamus, and cerebral white matter (Fig. 33.2a, b) [22, 48–50]. Particularly in the putamen, lesions have a pattern of bilateral, symmetrical, concentric-laminar hyperintensities on T2-weighted images [49]. Occasionally, hypointensities on T2-weighted images have been reported in the basal ganglia due to deposition of iron. Some characteristic images, although infrequently found, have been described on MRI such as the "face of the giant panda" in the midbrain (high signal intensity in the tegmentum, preservation of signal intensity of the lateral portion of the pars reticulata of the substantia nigra, and red nucleus and hypointensity of the superior colliculus), the "face of the miniature panda" or "panda cup sign" in the pontine tegmentum (hypointensity of the medial longitudinal fasciculi and central tegmental tracts and hyperintensities of the aqueduct opening in the fourth ventricle), and the "bright claustrum" sign (focal hyperintense signal of the claustrum in long-TR sequences) [22, 48–50]. According to Prashanth et al. [51], the "face of the giant panda" sign together with hyperintensities in the tectal plate and central pons and signal changes in the basal ganglia, thalamus, and brainstem are pathognomonic for WD. Furthermore, cerebral and cerebellar atrophy and central pontine myelinolysis-like changes have been described [48–51]. MRI findings can be similar to those seen in other neurological disorders. It is crucial, therefore, to correlate the imaging data with clinical features and biochemical markers of WD. Diffusion abnormalities (DWI studies) have also been reported in patients with WD, especially in the putamen, pallidum, and subcortical white matter [52]. Some researchers focused their attention to white matter lesions in WD. So Jada et al. [52] reported widespread lobar white matter abnormalities (increased mean diffusivity and decreased fractional anisotropy) using the technique of diffusion tensor imaging. Proton magnetic resonance spectroscopy (MRS) was used for getting information about the biochemistry of the brain in WD. ^{1}H MRS revealed reduction of the N-acetylaspartate (NAA)/choline and NAA/creatine ratio in the basal ganglia and increased ratio of phosphomonoesters/ phosphodiesters in ^{31}P MRS [53]. Transcranial brain parenchyma sonography showed lenticular hyperechogenicity in patients with neurological dysfunction. SPECT studies evaluating dopamine transporter function and integrity of D2 receptors proved symmetrically disturbed presynaptic and postsynaptic function in neurological WD patients [54]. PET studies evaluating glucose metabolic rate showed cortical and subcortical disturbances mainly in the caudate in patients with neurological dysfunction [54].

33.6.7 Neurophysiological Studies

Electroencephalographic abnormalities, usually slight and nonspecific, have been found in patients with WD. Most severe alterations have been reported in patients with severe disease and white matter lesions [55]. Somatosensory evoked potentials, brainstem auditory evoked potentials, and visual evoked potentials were abnormal particularly in patients with neurological dysfunction [55, 56]. Furthermore, studies with transcranial magnetic stimulation revealed reduced cortical excitability and prolonged central motor conduction time [57].

33.6.8 Genetic Studies

WD is an autosomal recessive disorder caused by homozygous or compound heterozygous mutations of the ATP7B gene that encodes a transmembrane adenosine triphosphatase (ATPase) which functions as a copper-dependent P-type ATPase. The gene is located on chromosome 13q14 and consists of 21 exons. More than 600 mutations of the ATP7B gene have been identified so far which are distributed across the ATP7B gene [1, 11, 40]. The most common mutations of the ATP7B gene are missense mutations; however, deletions, insertions, nonsense and intronic splice site have also been reported [40]. The most common mutation in Europe and North America is the H1068Q, while the R778L mutation is more common in China, Japan, and Korea [1, 11, 40]. The wide spectrum of phenotypic and genotypic heterogeneities in WD prevents a direct correlation between genotype and phenotype. In some studies, homozygous H1069Q has been associated with neurological manifestations and late disease onset [11]. However, other factors (environmental, epigenetic, and genetic modulators) seem to play a role in the phenotype of the disease. Mutation analysis by whole-gene sequencing should be performed on individuals in whom the diagnosis is difficult to establish by clinical and biochemical testing [31]. Haplotype analysis or specific testing for known mutations (identification of the disease-causing mutations in the family) can be used for screening of first-degree relatives of patients with WD [31].

33.7 Establishing Diagnosis

Establishing the diagnosis of WD is challenging due to varied and nonspecific clinical manifestations. The disease frequently is underdiagnosed or the diagnosis is delayed (mean delay of 12.8 months) [15]. Since the disease is treatable, accurate and early diagnosis is critical for better prognosis. Diagnosis of WD is based on the combination of clinical features, the presence of Kayser–Fleischer ring, the biochemical and MRI findings, and the results of mutation analysis. Symptomatic patients according to the organ involved in their presenting symptoms are classified into two broad categories: (1) hepatic presentation (acute hepatic WD or chronic hepatic WD) and (2) neurological presentation (associated with or without liver disease) [47]. Ferenci and coworkers [47] proposed a scoring system based on the clinical features and the laboratory findings (Kayser–Fleischer ring, neuropsychiatric symptoms, Coombs' negative hemolytic anemia, urinary copper, serum ceruloplasmin, liver copper, rhodanine staining of hepatocytes, and mutation analysis). If the total score of this scale is four or above, the diagnosis of WD is very likely. Roberts and Schilsky [31] provided guidelines for the diagnosis and treatment of WD approved by the American Association for the Study of Liver Diseases.

33.8 Treatment

Once the diagnosis of WD has been established, proper chelation therapy should be initiated. Treatment should be dedicated, persistent, and lifelong. Currently, there are four drugs available for the treatment of WD, namely D-penicillamine, trientine, zinc, and tetrathiomolybdate. Unfortunately, there is a lack of high-quality, multicenter, prospective, double-blind, randomized trials of the available drugs, and consequently the treatment effects reported and the level of recommendations should be viewed under this prism. The European Association for the Study of the Liver and the American Association for the Study of Liver Diseases developed guidelines for the treatment of patients with WD [2, 31].

33.8.1 D-Penicillamine

Historically, D-penicillamine was the first treatment introduced for WD, and its main mechanism of action is to promote the urinary excretion of copper [58]. However, penicillamine has many other effects including induction of metallothionein, interference with collagen cross-linking, immunosuppressant effects, and inhibition of pyridoxine action [59]. The maintenance dose is 750–1,500 mg/day, administered in two or three divided doses. Preferably, it is administered 1 h prior to meals, because food inhibits its absorption by about 50 %. After absorption, D-penicillamine circulates bound to plasma proteins and 80 % is excreted through the kidneys, with an elimination half-life ranging considerably between 2 and 7 h [60]. D-penicillamine may interfere with pyridoxine, and therefore supplemental pyridoxine should also be provided at a dose of 25–50 mg/day.

The effectiveness of D-penicillamine as treatment for WD is well established. In patients with liver disease, recovery of liver functions and symptomatic improvement occurs within the first 6 months. For neurological WD though, improvement of symptoms is slower that in patients with liver disease, it could take several months, and in some cases it has been observed only after 3 years of continuous penicillamine treatment [61]. A specific matter of concern is worsening of neurological symptoms occurring during the initial phase of treatment which has been described with all three treatments used for WD (D-penicillamine, trientine, zinc) but mainly with D-penicillamine, where up to 50 % of the treated patients is adversely affected. For many of the patients who will deteriorate in the beginning, the neurological worsening is nonreversible, leaving permanent disability. High doses (≥1,500 mg/day) and a rapid increase bear higher risk for this phenomenon, while starting with lower doses and following a slow titration could offer better tolerability. For example, two to four divided doses starting at 125–250 mg/day and increasing by 250 mg every week to a maximum of 1,000–1,500 mg/day could be safer.

In addition, D-penicillamine is associated with numerous side effects, some of them being quite severe, requiring the drug to be discontinued in approximately 30 % of patients. Commonly observed side effects during the first 3 weeks of treatment include sensitivity reactions with fever and rash, lymphadenopathy, proteinuria, and bone marrow toxicity with neutropenia, thrombocytopenia, or total aplasia [62]. In that case, D-penicillamine should be discontinued immediately. Late reactions have also been described including nephrotoxicity, in the context of a lupus-like syndrome with antinuclear antibodies, and hematuria. Proteinuria and cellular elements in the urine usually precede severe nephrotoxicity and should lead to immediate discontinuation of the drug. In addition, some very late side effects have been reported but it seems they are rare and include myasthenia gravis, polymyositis, and serous retinitis.

33.8.2 Trientine

Trientine (triethylenetetramine dihydrochloride or 2,2,2-tetramine) was introduced in 1969 as an alternative for patients who could not tolerate D-penicillamine. It is a chelator with a chemical structure distinct from D-penicillamine that promotes urinary copper excretion. Although introduced as alternative, second-choice drug, it proved to be an effective initial therapy as well, even with patients with decompensated liver disease at presentation [63]. In patients who have developed adverse effects with penicillamine, substitution with trientine will usually resolve them and prevent from recurrence even after prolonged treatment with trientine.

Trientine is absorbed incompletely from the gastrointestinal tract and then metabolized and inactivated, with a minimal amount of 1 % finally appearing in the urine [64].

Dosages of trientine range from 900 to 2,700 mg/day in two or three divided doses, with 900–1,500 mg/day used for maintenance therapy, and should be administered in an empty stomach. Neurological deterioration soon after treatment initiation has also been reported with trientine but appears less common than with D-penicillamine.

33.8.3 Ammonium Tetrathiomolybdate (TM)

Ammonium tetrathiomolybdate is a newer decoppering agent that acts by forming complexes with copper in the intestinal tract, thus preventing its absorption, while in the circulation makes copper unavailable for cellular uptake [65]. TM is still not available commercially for routine use and therefore considered an experimental therapy. From published data, it seems that TM is less likely to cause neurological deterioration in the beginning [66]. Adverse effects reported include bone marrow depression and hepatotoxicity.

33.8.4 Zinc

Zinc was first used in the treatment of Wilson's disease by Schouwink in Holland in the early 1960s. Zinc acts by inducing intestinal metallothionein that is an endogenous chelator of metals. Metallothionein binds copper stored in the enterocytes, preventing its entry into the portal circulation. Once bound, the copper is not absorbed and is excreted with the fecal contents [67].

The recommended dose is 150 mg of zinc/day administered in three divided doses, 30 min before meals. Zinc has very few side effects. Gastric upset is a common complain which could subside by changing the zinc salt employed. Some studies indicate that zinc may reduce leukocyte chemotaxis implying that it may possess immunosuppressant properties. Elevations in serum lipase and/or amylase have also been reported but without clinical or radiologic evidence of pancreatitis. Neurological deterioration is uncommon with zinc [68].

The clinical efficacy of zinc has been tested in limited uncontrolled studies. From the data available, it seems that zinc is less effective than traditional chelating agents (D-penicillamine and trientine) for the treatment of established neurological WD [69]. The current tendency is zinc to be reserved for maintenance treatment, following successful copper removal with a chelator (penicillamine or trientine). In addition, it seems to be effective and safe when used as preventive therapy in yet asymptomatic siblings. Although zinc monotherapy could have a role as first-line therapy in neurologic WD, exclusive monotherapy with zinc in symptomatic liver Wilson's disease is still controversial. Hepatic deterioration has been occasionally reported when zinc was started on those patients and was fatal in one case [70].

33.8.5 Liver Transplantation

Transplantation is frequently necessary for patients presenting with acute liver failure or decompensated cirrhosis due to WD. The procedure selected is orthotopic liver transplantation. The survival in transplanted patients is satisfactory and improving with the longest survival reported being 20 years. The outcome appears to be better for patients with chronic advanced liver disease than for those with acute liver failure [71]. It seems that the neurologic symptoms of patients who need a liver transplant may also improve as a result of the transplantation, but severe neurological deterioration was also observed after successful liver transplantation

33.8.6 Monitoring of Treatment

Adequacy of treatment can be monitored by measuring 24-h urinary copper excretion. After starting chelation treatment, copper excretion in urine increases significantly and may exceed 1,000 μg per 24 h at that time. In maintenance treatment, urinary copper excretion should be around 200–500 μg per 24 h. To document therapeutic efficiency and compliance to treatment, urinary copper excretion after 2 days of chelator cessation should be 100 μg/24 h [72].

References

1. Ala A, et al. Wilson's disease. Lancet. 2007;369:397–408.
2. European Association for the Study of Liver. EALS clinical practice guidelines: Wilson's disease. J Hepatol. 2012;56:671–85.
3. Wilson SAK. Progressive lenticular degeneration: a familial nervous disease associated with cirrhosis of the liver. Brain. 1912;34:295–507.
4. Walshe J. History of Wilson's disease: 1912 to 2000. Mov Disord. 2006;21:142–7.
5. Coffey A, et al. A genetic study of Wilson's disease in the United Kingdom. Brain. 2013;136:1476–87.
6. Mak C, Lam C-W. Diagnosis of Wilson's disease: a comprehensive review. Crit Rev Clin Lab. 2008;45:263–90.
7. Dedousis G, et al. Wilson disease: high prevalence in a mountainous area of Crete. Ann Hum Genet. 2005;69:268–74.
8. Litwin T, et al. Gender differences in Wilson's disease. J Neurol Sci. 2012;312:31–5.
9. Lorincz M. Recognition and treatment of neurologic Wilson's disease. Semin Neurol. 2012;32:538–43.
10. Ferenci P, et al. Late-onset Wilson's disease. Gastroenterology. 2007;132:1294–198.
11. Ferenci P. Phenotype genotype correlations in patients with Wilson's disease. Ann N Y Acad Sci. 2014;1315:1–5.
12. Lorincz M. Neurologic Wilson's disease. Ann N Y Acad Sci. 2010;1184:173–87.
13. Brewer G, Yuzbasiyan-Gurkan V. Wilson disease. Medicine. 1992;71:139–64.
14. Aggarwal A, Bhatt M. Update on Wilson disease. Inter Rev Neurobiol. 2013;10:313–48.
15. Walshe J, Yealland M. Wilson's disease: the problem of delayed diagnosis. J Neurol Neurosurg Psychiatry. 1992;55:692–6.
16. Fahn S, Jankovic J, Hallett M, editors. Principles and practice of movement disorders. 2nd ed. Edinburgh: Elsevier/Saunders; 2011. p. 507–12.
17. Machado A, et al. Neurological manifestations in Wilson's disease: report of 119 cases. Mov Disord. 2006;21:2192–6.
18. Svetel M, et al. Dystonia in Wilson's disease. Mov Disord. 2001;16:719–23.
19. Pfeiffer R. Wilson's disease. Semin Neurol. 2007;27:123–32.
20. Rajput A. Clinical features of tremor in extrapyramidal syndromes. In: Findley L, Koller W, editors. Handbook of tremor disorders. New York: Marcel Dekker; 1995. p. 275–91.
21. Mahajan R, Zachariah U. Images in clinical medicine: wing-beating tremor. N Engl J Med. 2014;37:e1.
22. Das SK, Ray K. Wilson's disease: an update. Nat Clin Pract Neurol. 2006;2:482–93.
23. Michel F, et al. Oxcarbazepine – responsive paroxysmal kinesigenic dyskinesia. Clin Neuropharmacol. 2011;34:262–4.
24. Seniów J, et al. Cognitive functioning in neurologically symptomatic and asymptomatic forms of Wilson's disease. Mov Disord. 2002;17:1077–83.
25. Frota N, et al. Cognitive impairment in Wilson's disease. Dement Neuropsychologia. 2009;3:16–21.
26. Han Y, et al. Selective impairment of attentional networks of alerting in Wilson's disease. PLoS One. 2014;9:e100454.
27. Wenisch E, et al. Cognitive profile in Wilson's disease: a case series of 31 patients. Rev Neurol. 2013;169:944–9.
28. Prashanth LK, et al. Spectrum of epilepsy in Wilson's disease with electroence-phalographic, MR imaging and pathological correlates. J Neurol Sci. 2010;29:44–51.
29. Pestan Knight EM, et al. Status epilepticus in Wilson's disease. Epileptic Disord. 2009;11:138–43.
30. Zimbrean PC, Schilsky ML. Psychiatric aspects of Wilson disease: a review. Gen Hosp Psychiatry. 2014;36:53–62.
31. Roberts E, Schilsky M, American Association for Study of Liver Disease (AASLD). Diagnosis and treatment of Wilson disease: an update. Hepatology. 2008;47:2089–111.
32. Przybylkowski A, et al. Liver cirrhosis in patients newly diagnosed with neurological phenotype of Wilson's disease. Funct Neurol. 2014;29:23–9.
33. Nussinson E, et al. Diagnostic challenges of Wilson's disease presenting as acute pancreatitis, cholangitis and jaundice. World J Hepatol. 2013;5:649–53.
34. Youn J, et al. Characteristics of neurological Wilson's disease without Kayser-Fleischer ring. J Neuropsychol Sci. 2012;323:183–6.
35. Pfeiffer RF. Wilson's disease. In: Watts RL, Koller WC, editors. Movement disorders. Neurologic principles and practice. New York: McGraw-Hill Medical Publishers; 2004. p. 779–97.
36. Quemeneur A-S, et al. Bone status and fractures in 85 adults with Wilson's disease. Osteoporos Int. 2014;25:2573. Epub ahead of print.
37. Adar T, et al. A heartbreaking case of Wilson's disease: Takotsubo cardiomyopathy complicating fulminant hepatic failure. Transpl Int. 2014;27:e109. Epub ahead of print.
38. Krysiak R, et al. Endocrine symptoms as initial manifestations of Wilson's disease. Yale J Biol Med. 2012;85:249–54.
39. Leinweber B, et al. Evaluation of the Unified Wilson's Disease Rating Scale (UWDRS) in German patients with treated Wilson's disease. Mov Disord. 2008;23:54–62.

40. Aggarwal A, et al. A novel global assessment scale for Wilson's disease (GAS for WD). Mov Disord. 2009;24:509–18.
41. Walshe JM. Diagnostic significance of reduced serum ceruloplasmin concentration in neurological disease. Mov Disord. 2005;20:1658–61.
42. Gow PJ, et al. Diagnosis of Wilson's disease: an experience over three decades. Gut. 2000;46:415–9.
43. Korman J, et al. Screening for Wilson disease in acute liver failure: a comparison of currently available diagnostic tests. Hepatology. 2008;48:1167–74.
44. Gross Jr JB, et al. Abnormalities in tests of copper metabolism in primary sclerosis cholangitis. Gastroenterology. 1985;89:272–8.
45. Martins da Costa C, et al. Value of urinary copper excretion after penicillamine challenge in the diagnosis of Wilson's disease. Hepatology. 1992;15: 609–15.
46. Ferenci P, et al. Diagnostic value of quantitative hepatic copper determination in patients with Wilson's disease. Clin Gastroenterol Hepatol. 2005;3:811–8.
47. Ferenci P, et al. Diagnosis and phenotypic classification of Wilson disease. Liver Int. 2003;23:139–42.
48. Aisen AM, et al. Wilson disease of the brain: MR imaging. Radiology. 1985;157:137–41.
49. Sinha S, et al. Wilson's disease: cranial MRI observations and clinical correlation. Neuroradiology. 2006;48:613–21.
50. Parekh J, Aggrawal P. Wilson's disease 'face of giant panda' and 'trident' signs together. Oxf Med Case Rep. 2014;1:16–7.
51. Prashanth LK, et al. Do MRI features distinguish Wilson's disease from other early onset extrapyramidal disorders? An analysis of 100 cases. Mov Disord. 2010;25:672–8.
52. Jadav R, et al. Diffusion Tensor Imaging (DTI) and its clinical correlates in drug naïve Wilson's disease. Metab Brain Dis. 2013;28:455–62.
53. Sinha S, et al. ^{31}P and ^{1}H MR spectroscopy and clinical correlation. Neuroradiology. 2010;52:477–85.
54. Hermann W. Morphological and functional imaging in neurological and non-neurological Wilson's patients. Ann N Y Acad Sci. 2014;1315:24–9.
55. Giagheddu M, et al. Comparison of MRI, EEG, EPs and ECD-SPECT in Wilson's disease. Acta Neurol Scand. 2001;103:71–81.
56. Das M, et al. A study of clinical, MRI and multimodality evoked potentials in neurological Wilson's disease. Eur J Neurol. 2007;14:498–504.
57. Jhunjhunwala K, et al. Alterations of cortical excitability and central motor conduction time in Wilson's disease. Neurosci Lett. 2013;553:90–4.
58. Scheinberg IH, et al. Penicillamine may detoxify copper in Wilson's disease. Lancet. 1987;2:95.
59. Czlonkowska A. The influence of prolonged treatment with D-penicillamine on the immune response in Wilson's disease. Eur J Clin Pharmacol. 1977;12:265–71.
60. Kukovetz WR, et al. Bioavailability and pharmacokinetics of D-penicillamine. J Rheumatol. 1983;10:90–4.
61. Brewer GJ, et al. Worsening of neurologic syndrome in patients with Wilson's disease with initial penicillamine therapy. Arch Neurol. 1987;44:490–3.
62. Medici V, et al. Diagnosis and management of Wilson's disease: results of a single center experience. J Clin Gastroenterol. 2006;40:936–41.
63. Scheinberg IH, et al. The use of trientine in preventing the effects of interrupting penicillamine therapy in Wilson's disease. N Engl J Med. 1987;317:209–13.
64. Kodama H, et al. Metabolism of administered triethylene tetramine dihydrochloride in humans. Life Sci. 1997;61:899–907.
65. Brewer GJ, et al. Treatment of Wilson's disease with ammonium tetrathio-molybdate: I. Initial therapy in 17 neurologically affected patients. Arch Neurol. 1994;51:545–54.
66. Brewer GJ, et al. Treatment of Wilson disease with ammonium tetrathiomolybdate. IV: comparison of tetrathiomolybdate and trientine in a double-blind study of treatment of the neurologic presentation of Wilson disease. Arch Neurol. 2006;63:521–7.
67. Hoogenraad TU. Zinc treatment of Wilson's disease. J Lab Clin Med. 1998;132:240–1.
68. Czlonkowska A, et al. Effects of long-term treatment in Wilson's disease with D-penicillamine and zinc sulphate. J Neurol. 1996;243:269–73.
69. Weiss KH, et al. Zinc monotherapy is not as effective as chelating agents in treatment of Wilson disease. Gastroenterology. 2011;140:1189–98.
70. Walshe JM, Munro NA. Zinc-induced deterioration in Wilson's disease aborted by treatment with penicillamine, dimercaprol, and a novel zero copper diet. Arch Neurol. 1995;52:10–1.
71. Schilsky ML, et al. Liver transplantation for Wilson's disease: indications and outcome. Hepatology. 1994; 19:583–7.
72. Brewer GJ, et al. Treatment of Wilson's disease with zinc. VI: initial treatment studies. J Lab Clin Med. 1989;114:633–8.

Functional (Psychogenic) Movement Disorders: Phenomenology, Diagnosis and Treatment

34

A. Macerollo and M.J. Edwards

34.1 Introduction

Functional (psychogenic) movement disorders (FMD) are part of the spectrum of functional neurological disorders [1], one of the commonest reasons for a neurological outpatient consultation [2, 3].

There is limited consensus on what to call functional/psychogenic disorders. 'Psychogenic' is the most commonly used phrase. However, this presupposes a psychological formulation can always be made which is not supported by current evidence [4]. It also suggests that biological factors are not relevant, in contrast to the biopsychosocial model of all other illnesses. The term psychogenic has poor acceptance amongst patients [5]. We prefer the term 'functional', for reasons that are outlined in detail here [6], although there are opposing views, summarised here [7].

Electronic supplementary material The online version of this chapter (doi:10.1007/978-3-7091-1628-9_34) contains supplementary material, which is available to authorized users.

A. Macerollo, MD (✉)
Sobell Department of Motor Neuroscience and Movement Disorders, National Hospital of Neurology and Neurosurgery, Institute of Neurology, University College London, London WC1N 3BG, UK
e-mail: a.macerollo@ucl.ac.uk

M.J. Edwards, MBBS, BSc (Hons), PhD
Institute of Molecular and Clinical Sciences, St George's University of London, London, UK
e-mail: m.j.edwards@ucl.ac.uk

FMD occupy a grey area between neurology and psychiatry characterized by complex pathophysiology, difficulties in making and communicating the diagnosis to the patients and management for which there is a limited evidence base and which often needs the cooperation of different specialists. This difficult situation has been termed a 'crisis for neurology' [8].

The commonest FMD are tremor and dystonia that together account for about 70% of patients, followed by myoclonus and gait disturbance. Functional parkinsonism, tics and chorea are rare [9].

Women are more often affected than men, and the mean age at onset ranges from 37 to 50 years [9, 10]. FMD are characterized by level of disability and impairment in quality of life equivalent to that reported by patients affected by Parkinson's disease [11]. Consequentially, considerable health and social care costs are associated with this group of patients [12].

In this chapter, we provide an update on the current knowledge on clinical phenomenology, diagnosis and management of FMD.

34.2 Phenomenology

In broad terms, FMD are disorders of movement which, commonly, implies additional movements but in some cases also a reduction of movement associated with abnormal postures.

C. Falup-Pecurariu et al. (eds.), *Movement Disorders Curricula*,
DOI 10.1007/978-3-7091-1628-9_34

Gait disturbance is a common accompaniment to FMD. A variety of gait patterns are described; the most common is the *astasia/abasia* known as 'tightrope walker gait' or 'walking on ice gait'. The patient shifts their centre of gravity quickly from side to side when walking without falling, thus showing excellent balance despite their subjective complaint. Furthermore, in contrast to other patients with poor balance, patients with functional gait disorder tend to walk with a *narrow base* and may show a *dramatic response to Romberg's test*. Other features of functional gait disturbance are *hesitation*, where small forward and backward movements of the leg may be observed while the feet seem to stick on the ground, *fluctuations* in gait impairment and *excessive slowness of movements*, resembling walking in slow motion. A monoplegic dragging gait is commonly seen in patients with functional leg weakness [13–15].

Functional tremor (FT) most frequently involves *hands and arms*, but functional tremor of the head, legs and palate can also occur. Patients typically direct visual attention towards their affected limb, and tremor often worsens significantly *during examination* [16]. FT is typically present *at rest, on posture and on action*. It is characterized by *variability in amplitude and frequency*, clear *distractibility and entrainment* with clinical manoeuvres [17] and *pauses with ballistic movement* [18, 19]. Furthermore it may paradoxically *worsen with loading and restraint* [20].

Functional dystonia (FD) is the second most common presentation in patients with FMD [9]. The typical presentation is with *fixed abnormal postures*, rather than the typical mobile postures of organic dystonia. These commonly have an *unusual distribution* given the age at onset (e.g. leg dystonia in an adult) [21, 22]. *Severe pain*, similar to that present in chronic regional pain syndrome type 1 (CRPS1), is commonly associated [23]. The usual *precipitating factor is a minor peripheral trauma*, and the term 'causalgia-dystonia' was previously coined [24]. The spread of abnormal postures to other body parts without further injury is seen. Important features of FD are the *absence of task or position specificity*, the *absence of a sensory geste* and *poor response to botulinum toxin* [21]. *Limbs* are usually involved, but FD affecting the neck and face is also commonly reported and has specific patterns of muscle involvement [22, 25].

Functional myoclonus (FM) is characterized by *marked daily variability in distribution* and frequency of jerks. It is typically exacerbated by movement [26]. Jerks may be *dramatically stimulus sensitive*, exaggerated compared to the stimulus sensitivity seen in organic myoclonus and associated with a *lack of habituation* [27]. If the limb involved is restrained by the examiner, the myoclonus may worsen and spread to other parts of the body [26].

A small group of patients present with *functional parkinsonism* (FP). The average age at onset is 47 years, *younger* than typical Parkinson's disease (PD). *Symptoms are typically symmetrical*, and tremor, showing features typical of FT, is prominent; rigidity is similar to *voluntary stiffness*, and the resistance may paradoxically decrease with performance of synkinetic movements of an opposite limb. The progressive fatiguing and slowing of repetitive movements seen in true bradykinesia is absent. Postural stability assessment using the *pull test typically leads to dramatic loss of balance and falls* [28, 29].

34.3 Diagnosis

The diagnosis of FMD should not be regarded as a diagnosis of exclusion, nor a diagnosis made on the basis of co-existence of a movement disorder with psychological disorder. Ideally, the diagnosis should be a positive diagnosis, based on positive features from history, examination and appropriate investigations.

Formal *diagnostic criteria* have been developed by Fahn and Williams (the most widely used) [30], recently revised by Gupta and Lang (Table 34.1) [31]. These criteria combined, when appropriate, with additional electrophysiological and imaging testing provide different levels of certainty of diagnosis.

Table 34.1 Fahn-Williams and Gupta-Lang criteria for diagnosis of functional movement disorders [30, 31]

Category	Criteria
Fahn-Williams criteria	
Documented	Persistent relief by psychotherapy, suggestion of placebo response, which may be helped by physiotherapy, or absence of abnormal postures when patient is unobserved
Clinically established	The posture is inconsistent over time, or it is incongruent with classical dystonia (e.g. impossibility to move limbs on request and great resistance during passive movements), plus one of the following manifestations: other psychogenic signs, multiple somatizations, or an obvious psychiatric disorder
Probable	The dystonia is incongruent or inconsistent with typical organic dystonia or there are psychogenic signs or multiple somatizations
Possible	Evidence of an emotional disturbance
Gupta-Lang criteria	
Clinically definite	Documented category
	Clinically established category
	Incongruent and/or inconsistent movement disorders (even without the additional presence of psychogenic signs, multiple somatisations or psychiatric disturbance)
Laboratory-supported definite	Electrophysiological tests proving a FMD (primarily evidence of premovement potentials before jerks or data from tremor studies)

The key clues in the *medical history* that suggest the diagnosis of FMD are an *abrupt onset* with rapid progression to *maximum severity*, previous episodes of movement disorders in the same or different body part with complete or partial *remissions* associated with *paroxysmal exacerbations*. The phenotype is often *inconsistent over time*, with complete change in the pattern of abnormal movements. Previous *somatisations* are common. Physical precipitating events (illness, injury) are common before the onset of functional symptoms [32].

Positive findings on physical examination commonly relate to the normalisation of symptoms with the distraction of attention, for example, the change in tremor with entrainment manoeuvres (see above). Other signs also represent normalisation of movement by distraction of attention, for example, *Hoover's sign* [33–35]. *Fluctuation* in the severity of symptoms during examination is typical.

Positive diagnosis in FMD may be helped by appropriate investigations. *Electromyography* with *accelerometry* can be used to assess tremor frequency and to evaluate the effect on tremor frequency of tapping at a different frequency or during ballistic movements with another limb [36, 37]. It is useful also in the presence of jerks to exclude an organic myoclonus, which is characterized by brief bursts (<50 ms) of muscle activity [38]. *EEG/EMG back averaging* is useful to detect a Bereitschaftspotential (BP), which is a slow-rising wave in the EEG before voluntary movements [39]. This is often present before functional myoclonic jerks. *Nuclear imaging*, DAT-scan (dopamine transporter imaging) [29] and 123I-Ioflupane SPECT [40] are helpful in patients with suspected FT or FP. Such tests need to be considered in association with clinical examination since such scans are normal in many organic tremor (e.g. essential and dystonic tremor) and parkinsonian (e.g. dopa-responsive dystonia, drug-induced parkinsonism) conditions.

34.4 Treatment

The best start to the treatment of FMD is the clear and effective communication of the diagnosis. Failure to do so often results in multiple referrals, repeated unnecessary diagnostic tests and harmful treatment including surgical interventions [21, 41].

There is no good evidence to support the use of drugs in FMD. Intrathecal baclofen has been proposed as helpful for patients with fixed dystonia, but this evidence is uncertain, and treatment-related complications are common [42, 43]. Antidepressants may be helpful and should be used when functional symptoms are associated with anxiety or depression [44].

Psychological therapy, in the form of psychodynamic psychotherapy [45] or cognitive behavioural therapy [46], has some limited evidence for benefit. Physical rehabilitation has face validity as a treatment for motor symptoms, and there is some evidence to support this approach from two previous case-control studies [47, 48] and one randomised trial [49]. Transcranial magnetic stimulation has been reported to have positive impact in patients with FMD, but it sees most likely given the protocols used that this operates via a placebo effect [44, 47]. For severely affected patients, a multidisciplinary inpatient treatment approach may be of benefit, but evidence on which patients are most likely to benefit is limited [50].

References

1. Stone J. Functional neurological symptoms. Clin Med. 2013;13:80–3.
2. Stone J, Carson A, Duncan R, et al. Symptoms 'unexplained by organic disease' in 1144 new neurology out-patients: how often does the diagnosis change at follow-up? Brain. 2009;132:2878–88.
3. Stone J, Carson A, Duncan R, et al. Who is referred to neurology clinics? The diagnoses made in 3781 new patients. Clin Neurol Neurosurg. 2010;112:747–51.
4. Espay AJ, Goldenhar LM, Voon V, et al. Opinions and clinical practices related to diagnosing and managing patients with psychogenic movement disorders: an international survey of movement disorder society members. Mov Disord. 2009;24:1366–74.
5. Stone J, Wojcik W, Durrance D, et al. What should we say to patients with symptoms unexplained by disease? The "number needed to offend". BMJ. 2002;325:1449–50.
6. Edwards MJ, Stone J, Lang AE. From psychogenic movement disorder to functional movement disorder: it's time to change the name. Mov Disord. 2014;29:849–52.
7. Fahn S, Olanow CW. "Psychogenic movement disorders": they are what they are. Mov Disord. 2014;29:853–6.
8. Hallett M. Psychogenic movement disorders: a crisis for neurology. Curr Neurol Neurosci Rep. 2006;6:269–71.
9. Factor SA, Podskalny GD, Molho ES. Psychogenic movement disorders: frequency, clinical profile, and characteristics. J Neurol Neurosurg Psychiatry. 1995;59:406–12.
10. Williams DT, Ford B, Fahn S. Phenomenology and psychopathology related to psychogenic movement disorders. Adv Neurol. 1995;65:231–57.
11. Anderson KE, Gruber-Baldini AL, Vaughan CG, et al. Impact of psychogenic movement disorders versus Parkinson's on disability, quality of life, and psychopathology. Mov Disord. 2007;22:2204–9.
12. Carson A, Stone J, Hibberd C, et al. Disability, distress and unemployment in neurology outpatients with symptoms 'unexplained by organic disease'. J Neurol Neurosurg Psychiatry. 2011;82:810–3.
13. Lempert T, Brandt T, Dieterich M, et al. How to identify psychogenic disorders of stance and gait. A video study in 37 patients. J Neurol. 1991;238:140–6.
14. Baik JS, Lang AE. Gait abnormalities in psychogenic movement disorders. Mov Disord. 2007;22:395–9.
15. Stone J, Warlow C, Sharpe M. The symptom of functional weakness: a controlled study of 107 patients. Brain. 2010;133:1537–51.
16. van Poppelen D, Saifee TA, Schwingenschuh P, et al. Attention to self in psychogenic tremor. Mov Disord. 2011;26:2575–6.
17. Kenney C, Diamond A, Mejia N, et al. Distinguishing psychogenic and essential tremor. J Neurol Sci. 2007;263:94–9.
18. Kumru H, Valls-Sole J, Valldeoriola F, et al. Transient arrest of psychogenic tremor induced by contralateral ballistic movements. Neurosci Lett. 2004;370:135–9.
19. Roper LS, Saifee TA, Parees I, et al. How to use the entrainment test in the diagnosis of functional tremor. Pract Neurol. 2013;13(6):396–8.
20. Deuschl G, Koster B, Lucking CH, et al. Diagnostic and pathophysiological aspects of psychogenic tremors. Mov Disord. 1998;13:294–302.
21. Schrag A, Trimble M, Quinn N, et al. The syndrome of fixed dystonia: an evaluation of 103 patients. Brain. 2004;127:2360–72.
22. Lang AE. Psychogenic dystonia: a review of 18 cases. Can J Neurol Sci. 1995;22:136–43.
23. van Hilten JJ, van de Beek WJ, Roep BO. Multifocal or generalized tonic dystonia of complex regional pain syndrome: a distinct clinical entity associated with HLA-DR13. Ann Neurol. 2000;48:113–6.
24. Bhatia KP, Bhatt MH, Marsden CD. The causalgia-dystonia syndrome. Brain. 1993;116:843–51.
25. Sa DS, Mailis-Gagnon A, Nicholson K, et al. Posttraumatic painful torticollis. Mov Disord. 2003;18:1482–91.
26. Monday K, Jankovic J. Psychogenic myoclonus. Neurology. 1993;43:349–52.
27. Thompson PD, Colebatch JG, Brown P, et al. Voluntary stimulus sensitive jerks and jumps mimicking myoclonus or pathological startle syndromes. Mov Disord. 1992;7:257–62.
28. Lang AE, Koller WC, Fahn S. Psychogenic parkinsonism. Arch Neurol. 1995;52:802–10.
29. Benaderette S, Zanotti FP, Apartis E, et al. Psychogenic parkinsonism: a combination of clinical, electrophysiological, and [(123)I]-FP-CIT SPECT scan explorations improves diagnostic accuracy. Mov Disord. 2006;21:310–7.

30. Fahn S, Williams DT. Psychogenic dystonia. Adv Neurol. 1988;50:431–55.
31. Gupta A, Lang AE. Psychogenic movement disorders. Curr Opin Neurol. 2009;22:430–6.
32. Pareés I, Kojovic M, Pires C, Rubio-Agusti I, Saifee TA, Sadnicka A, Kassavetis P, Macerollo A, Bhatia KP, Carson A, Stone J, Edwards MJ. Physical precipitating factors in functional movement disorders. J Neurol Sci. 2014;338:174–7.
33. McWhirter L, Stone J, Sandercock P, et al. Hoover's sign for the diagnosis of functional weakness: a prospective unblinded cohort study in patients with suspected stroke. J Psychosom Res. 2011;71:384–6.
34. Ziv I, Djaldetti R, Zoldan Y, et al. Diagnosis of "non-organic" limb paresis by a novel objective motor assessment: the quantitative Hoover's test. J Neurol. 1998;245:797–802.
35. Stone J, Zeman A, Sharpe M. Functional weakness and sensory disturbance. J Neurol Neurosurg Psychiatry. 2002;73:241.
36. Zeuner KE, Shoge RO, Goldstein SR, et al. Accelerometry to distinguish psychogenic from essential or parkinsonian tremor. Neurology. 2003;61:548–50.
37. Schwingenschuh P, Katschnig P, Seiler S, et al. Moving toward "laboratory-supported" criteria for psychogenic tremor. Mov Disord. 2011;26:2509–15.
38. Brown P, Thompson PD. Electrophysiological aids to the diagnosis of psychogenic jerks, spasms, and tremor. Mov Disord. 2001;16:595–9.
39. Esposito M, Edwards MJ, Bhatia KP, et al. Idiopathic spinal myoclonus: a clinical and neurophysiological assessment of a movement disorder of uncertain origin. Mov Disord. 2009;24:2344–9.
40. Gaig C, Martí MJ, Tolosa E, Valldeoriola F, Paredes P, Lomeña FJ, Nakamae F. 123I-Ioflupane SPECT in the diagnosis of suspected psychogenic Parkinsonism. Mov Disord. 2006;21:1994–8.
41. Edwards MJ, Alonso-Canovas A, Schrag A, Bloem BR, Thompson PD, Bhatia K. Limb amputations in fixed dystonia: a form of body integrity identity disorder? Mov Disord. 2011;26:1410–4.
42. van Hilten BJ, van de Beek WJ, Hoff JI, et al. Intrathecal baclofen for the treatment of dystonia in patients with reflex sympathetic dystrophy. N Engl J Med. 2000;343:625–30.
43. van Rijn MA, Munts AG, Marinus J, et al. Intrathecal baclofen for dystonia of complex regional pain syndrome. Pain. 2009;143:41–7.
44. Voon V, Lang AE. Antidepressant treatment outcomes of psychogenic movement disorder. J Clin Psychiatry. 2005;66:1529–34.
45. Hinson VK, Weinstein S, Bernard B, et al. Single-blind clinical trial of psychotherapy for treatment of psychogenic movement disorders. Parkinsonism Relat Disord. 2006;12:177–80.
46. Sharpe M, Walker J, Williams C, et al. Guided self-help for functional (psychogenic) symptoms: a randomized controlled efficacy trial. Neurology. 2011;77:564–72.
47. Czarnecki K, Thompson JM, Seime R, et al. Functional movement disorders: successful treatment with a physical therapy rehabilitation protocol. Parkinsonism Relat Disord. 2012;18:247–51.
48. Dallocchio C, Arbasino C, Klersy C, et al. The effects of physical activity on psychogenic movement disorders. Mov Disord. 2010;25:421–5.
49. Jordbru AA, Smedstad LM, Klungsøyr O, Martinsen EW. Psychogenic gait disorder: a randomized controlled trial of physical rehabilitation with one-year follow-up. J Rehabil Med. 2014;46:181–7.
50. Saifee TA, Kassavetis P, Pareés I, Kojovic M, Fisher L, Morton L, Foong J, Price G, Joyce EM, Edwards MJ. Inpatient treatment of functional motor symptoms: a long-term follow-up study. J Neurol. 2012;259:1958–63.

REM Sleep Behavior Disorder

35

Alex Iranzo de Riquer

REM sleep behavior disorder (RBD) is a parasomnia characterized by dream-enacting behaviors and nightmares linked to REM sleep without muscle atonia. The diagnosis of RBD requires confirmation with video-polysomnography because other sleep disorders (e.g., severe obstructive sleep apnea, periodic leg movement disorder, nocturnal frontal lobe epilepsy and sleepwalking) may also present with nightmares and abnormal sleep behaviors. RBD can be classified into an idiopathic form (IRBD) and a secondary form. Available data indicate that most patients with IRBD will eventually be diagnosed with a neurodegenerative disorder including Parkinson disease (PD), dementia with Lewy bodies (DLB), and multiple system atrophy (MSA). Patients with IRBD represent the prodromal stage of these synucleinopathies. The secondary form of RBD is related to neurodegenerative diseases, autoimmune diseases, focal structural lesions in the brain, and the use of some medications. Psychiatric disorders are not linked to RBD [1–3]. In this chapter, we will review IRBD and RBD secondary to neurodegenerative diseases linked to movement disorders, namely PD and MSA.

35.1 Idiopathic REM Sleep Behavior Disorder (IRBD)

The diagnosis of IRBD requires a history of dream-enacting behaviors, video-polysomnography detection of REM sleep with increased muscular activity associated with abnormal behaviors, absence of known neurodegenerative diseases, lack of motor and cognitive complaints, normal neurological examination, normal brain magnetic resonance imaging, and RBD not explained by a brain lesion (e.g., stroke, demyelinating plaque, encephalitis) or by the introduction or withdrawal of any medication or substance (e.g., antidepressants, beta-blockers) [1–3]. In many IRBD patients, subclinical abnormalities can be detected such as olfactory deficits, cognitive deficits on neuropsychological tests, and decreased dopamine transporters imaging in the striatum on functional neuroimaging (Table 35.1). These findings suggest that when IRBD is diagnosed, a neurodegenerative process is already widespread in the nervous system. Of these abnormalities, hyposmia, color vision impairment, substantia nigra hyperechogenicity, and decreased striatal dopamine transporter uptake identify those IRBD patients who are at

A. Iranzo de Riquer, MD, PhD
Multidisciplinary Sleep Unit, Neurology Service, Hospital Clínic de Barcelona and Institut d'Investigació Biomèdiques August Pi i Sunyer (IDIBAPS), C/Villarroel 170, scale 8-4th floor, Barcelona 08036, Spain
e-mail: airanzo@clinic.ub.es

C. Falup-Pecurariu et al. (eds.), *Movement Disorders Curricula*,
DOI 10.1007/978-3-7091-1628-9_35

Table 35.1 Clinical and subclinical abnormalities in idiopathic REM sleep behavior disorder

Reduced arm swinging
Akinesia
Depression
Impaired olfaction
Color vision impairment
Asymptomatic cognitive abnormalities on cognitive tests, especially in the executive, memory, and visuospatial domains
Cortical electroencephalographic slowing
Orthostatic hypotension
Systolic blood pressure drop
Decreased beat-to-beat variability in the cardiac rhythm
Constipation
Reduced postprandial ghrelin response
Urinary incontinence and retention
Erectile impotence
Episodes of acute psychosis after minor or major surgery
Reduced cardiac scintigraphy 123I-MBIG
Decreased dopamine transporter in the striatum, particularly in the left putamen
Substantia nigra hyperechogenicity
Loss of nigral hyperintensity on 3.0 Tesla MRI
Brainstem changes in diffusion tensor imaging
Decreased cortical and increased pontine perfusion

increased short-term risk (2.5–5 years) for being diagnosed with a synucleinopathy according to accepted clinical criteria [4, 5]. Prospective studies have further shown that the echogenic size of the substantia nigra [6], color vision, olfactory dysfunction [5], and dysautonomic changes [7] remain stable over time. In contrast, dopamine transporter imaging shows progressive decline in striatal tracer uptake [8]. Thus, dopamine transporter imaging serves better as a marker of subclinical progression in IRBD. The same happens with cognitive testing that shows worsening in executive, visuospatial, and memory domains with time.

It has been shown that PD, DLB, and MSA frequently develop in IRBD patients who are followed at sleep centers. In the seminal study, Schenck et al. found that parkinsonism developed in 11 of 29 (38 %) IRBD subjects nearly 4 years after the diagnosis of IRBD and almost 13 years after the onset of RBD [9]. After 16 additional years of follow-up, 21 (72.4 %) IRBD patients from the original cohort were diagnosed with PD in 13 cases, DLB in 3, MSA in 2, unspecified dementia in 1, and Alzheimer's disease with autopsy-confirmed combined Alzheimer's disease pathology plus Lewy pathology in 2 cases. Three IRBD subjects were lost during the follow-up period [10]. In a second series, the authors found that 26 of 93 (28 %) IRBD patients developed a neurodegenerative disorder after a mean follow-up of 5 years: PD in 14, DLB in 7, dementia that met clinical criteria for Alzheimer's disease (but also for possible DLB) in 4, and MSA in 1. Survival curves showed that the estimated risk of a neurodegenerative disease after RBD diagnosis was 17.7 % at 5 years, 40.6 % at 10 years, and 52.4 % at 12 years [7]. We reported that 20 of 44 (45 %) IRBD patients developed a neurological disorder after a mean interval of 11.5 years from RBD onset and after a mean follow-up of 5.1 years from the diagnosis of IRBD. Emerging disorders were PD in nine patients (two with associated dementia), DLB in six, MSA with predominant cerebellar syndrome in one, and mild cognitive impairment (MCI) in four in whom visuospatial dysfunction was prominent. The finding that patients who developed a disorder were those with longer follow-up suggested that conversion rate (45 %) could increase with the passage of time [11]. This was confirmed after 7 additional years of follow-up of this original cohort of subjects who were initially diagnosed with IRBD between 1991 and 2003. We found that after a median follow-up of 10.5 years, 82 % were diagnosed with PD ($n = 16$), DLB ($n = 14$) and less frequently MSA ($n = 1$) and mild cognitive impairment ($n = 5$). The estimated risk of defined neurodegenerative syndrome from the diagnosis of IRBD was 34.8 % at 5 years, 73.4 % at 10 years, and 92.5 % at 14 years [12]. These findings, in a group of 44 individuals with long and close follow-up, indicate that most IRBD subjects develop a synucleinopathy with time. Since additional IRBD patients were diagnosed and followed in our sleep center, we aimed to confirm our initial observation in a larger cohort of subjects that comprised all the 174 consecutive IRBD cases diagnosed up to July 2013 in our sleep center. The risk of a defined neurodegenerative syndrome from the time of IRBD diagnosis was 33.1 % at 5 years, 75.7 % at 10 years, and 90.9 % at 14 years. Emerging diagnoses (37.4 %) were DLB in 29 subjects, PD in 22, MSA in 2, and MCI in 12. In six cases who were diagnosed with PD, DLB, and MCI, neuropathological examination disclosed neuronal loss and widespread Lewy-type pathology in the brain in each case [13]. Biopsy of the colon and submandibular gland shows deposits of synuclein in subjects with IRBD [14, 15].

35.2 The Transition Between IRBD and Clinical Diagnosis of PD, DLB, and MSA

PD has a prodromal period of several years where progressive neuronal loss occurs before parkinsonism becomes clinically manifest and the disease can be clinically diagnosed. Olfactory loss, depression, constipation, and RBD may be present during the prodromal period of PD [16]. We have just described the case of a 63-year-old man that presented with IRBD, and a 10-year clinical follow-up showed the development of constipation, hyposmia, depression, and mild cognitive impairment. The patient died without clinical parkinsonism and without dementia and postmortem examination showed neuronal loss and Lewy bodies in the entire brainstem including the substantia nigra, olfactory bulb, and limbic system [17].

In patients with IRBD that developed PD with time, voice and face akinesia appeared earliest (estimated prodromal interval of nearly 10 years) followed by rigidity (4.4 years), gait abnormalities (4.4 years), and limb bradykinesia (4.2 years) [18]. In one prospective study following clinically 44 IRBD patients, 16 (13 men and 3 women) were diagnosed with PD [12]. Mean age at PD diagnosis was 75 years, RBD duration at the time of the diagnosis of PD was 13 years, and the interval between diagnosis of RBD and diagnosis of PD was 5.5 years. Five PD patients developed dementia. In these five patients, the median interval between diagnosis of PD and development of dementia was 6 years. Patients with IRBD seen at sleep centers who later develop PD present a progressive parkinsonian syndrome where rigidity, bradykinesia, and hypomimia are prominent. This rigid-akinetic syndrome responds to levodopa. Resting tremor is not usually the presenting sign but this may appear at later stages of the disease. In these subjects, constipation and self-reported loss of smell is common before the emergence of parkinsonian signs. In some patients, parkinsonism appears in parallel with MCI onset. MCI, in fact, is more common in PD subjects with RBD than without RBD.

In IRBD patients who later develop DLB, the first presentation may be (1) severe acute episodes of agitation, hallucinations, and delirium after elective surgery (knee, hip, abdominal) that resolve spontaneously or with small doses of neuroleptics after 1 or 2 weeks; (2) acute episodes of paranoid delusions; (3) isolated visual hallucinations such as bugs running on the floor or the sensation of having someone or a shadow behind his or her back; and (4) MCI. MCI is an intermediate stage between normal cognitive function and dementia where individuals have cognitive complaints, deficits in neuropsychological tests, and their daily living activities are preserved. In the particular setting of IRBD, MCI can be considered an abnormal condition which frequently evolves into DLB and sometimes into PD. This is based on the following data. First, MCI occurs in nearly 20 % of untreated PD patients at the time of initial diagnosis and predicts conversion to dementia. Second, most IRBD patients seen in sleep centers who develop MCI are eventually diagnosed with DLB. Third, IRBD patients that develop MCI but no dementia show markers of a synucleinopathy such as decreased striatal dopamine transporter, hyperechogenicity of the substantia nigra, and hyposmia. Finally, in patients with MCI with comorbid RBD who later develop dementia, postmortem examination shows Lewy body pathology.

In patients with IRBD who later developed MSA with cerebellar signs, brain MRI may show atrophy of the pons and cerebellum before the emergence of a cerebellar syndrome. In these patients, urinary problems and falls due to cerebellar ataxia may be one of the initial manifestations of the disease. Nocturnal stridor may also appear before the appearance of parkinsonism or ataxia in MSA.

35.3 RBD in Parkinson Disease

RBD is common among the synucleinopathies PD, DLB, and MSA because in these diseases cell loss is common within the neuronal structures that regulate REM sleep atonia, namely the subcoeruleus nucleus and magnocellularis nucleus in the brainstem and the amygdala. RBD occurs in PD patients whether treated or untreated with dopaminergic agents. RBD is more common in MSA (90–100 %) and DLB (70–80 %) than in PD (25–58 %). Type of RBD-related unpleasant dreams, dream-enacting behaviors, and polysomnographic abnormalities are similar among sporadic PD, MSA, and IRBD [19]. RBD has also been described in small series involving other neurodegenerative disorders such as progressive supranuclear palsy and Machado-Joseph disease (Table 35.2).

RBD occurs in 25–58 % of the patients with sporadic PD, antedating the onset of parkinsonism by several years in about 20 % of them RBD [19–23]. RBD may precede parkinsonism or may develop concomitant or after the onset of parkinsonism. In drug-naïve, newly diagnosed PD patients, RBD is seen in 25–30 % of them. RBD occurs in sporadic PD patients whether treated or untreated with dopaminergic agents. RBD confirmed by PSG may also occur in patients with PD linked to Parkin 2 mutations, but in this condition RBD-related clinical manifestations are usually mild. RBD was not detected in one PARK 6 family, an autosomal recessive disorder that manifests as early-onset PD with a particularly mild progression. RBD occurs in PD associated with LRRK2 G2019S mutations. One study showed that in subjects with sporadic PD, the report of sleep-related falling out of bed was clinically suggestive of RBD [24]. In a study involving non-demented PD patients with RBD, VPSG analysis and bed partners' reports demonstrated alleviation of parkinsonism during elaborated and complex RBD episodes. Movements during RBD episodes were faster, stronger, and smoother

Table 35.2 Conditions associated with REM sleep behavior disorder

A. Neurodegenerative diseases
Idiopathic Parkinson disease (25–58 % of the cases)
Parkin 2 mutation (a few descriptions)
LRRK2 mutations (a few descriptions)
Dementia with Lewy bodies (70–80 % of the cases)
Multiple system atrophy (90–100 % of the cases)
Mild cognitive impairment (a few descriptions)
Pure autonomic failure (a few descriptions)
Alzheimer's disease (anecdotal cases)
Progressive supranuclear palsy (a few descriptions)
Guadeloupean parkinsonism (a few descriptions)
Frontotemporal dementia (anecdotal descriptions)
Corticobasal syndrome (anecdotal descriptions)
DJ-1 mutations and parkinsonism-dementia-ALS complex (anecdotal descriptions)
Amyotrophic lateral sclerosis (anecdotal descriptions)
Neurodegeneration with brain accumulation type 1 (anecdotal descriptions)
Huntington disease (a few descriptions)
Spinocerebellar ataxia type 3 (a few descriptions)
Spinocerebellar ataxia type 2 (a few descriptions)
B. Autoimmune disorders
Narcolepsy (30 % of the cases)
Limbic encephalitis associated with antibodies to voltage-gated potassium channels/LIG-1 (a few descriptions)
Anti-NMDAR encephalitis (anecdotal descriptions)
Anti-Ma1 and anti-Ma2 encephalitis (anecdotal descriptions)
Guillain-Barre syndrome (anecdotal descriptions)
C. Other neurological conditions
Myotonic dystrophy type 2 (anecdotal descriptions)
Autism (anecdotal descriptions)
Tourette's syndrome (anecdotal descriptions)
Chiari malformations (anecdotal description)
Smith-Magenis syndrome (anecdotal description)
Moebius syndrome (anecdotal description)
Attention deficit hyperactive disorder (anecdotal description)
Focal brainstem lesions (stroke, cavernoma, tumor, multiple sclerosis plaques) (few descriptions)
D. Medications
Antidepressants
Beta-blockers

than those seen when the PD patient was awake. In the same manner, speech during RBD was more intelligible, better articulated, and louder than during wakefulness [22].

RBD in PD is associated with cognitive impairment, the rigid-akinetic motor subtype, older age, male predominance, autonomic dysfunction, and an increased risk to develop dementia over time. This suggests that the presence of RBD in PD predicts development of widespread neuropathological changes in the brain. Most studies have shown that in non-demented, nonhallucinator sporadic PD patients, the presence of RBD in PD is neither associated with hypersomnia, sleep benefit, sleep architecture disruption, olfactory dysfunction, or lower daily levodopa equivalent dose. When sporadic PD patients exhibit RBD, this parasomnia precedes the onset of parkinsonism in 18–22 % of the cases [19, 21].

35.4 RBD in Multiple System Atrophy

The majority of patients with MSA have RBD [25–27]. The finding that in MSA brainstem cell loss is consistently widespread and severe may explain the high prevalence of RBD in this disease. RBD is currently considered a red flag for the diagnosis of MSA. In one study, 21 consecutive MSA patients without sleep behavioral complaints underwent video-PSG that demonstrated RBD in 19 (90.5 %) [26]. In another study, video-PSG showed RBD in 35 out of 37 (95 %) consecutive patients [25].

Self-awareness of abnormal sleep behaviors and unpleasant dream recall is variable among MSA subjects with RBD. In one study, 27 of 39 (69 %) consecutive MSA patients with RBD or their relatives reported dream-enacting behaviors. Interestingly, most of the 12 that did not report dream-enacting behaviors were sleeping alone at their home [25]. In another study, only 7 of 21 (33 %) MSA patients with RBD recalled vivid dreams [28]. In our first published case series comprising 26 consecutive MSA cases with RBD free of psychoactive drugs, 77 % of the patients were unaware of their abnormal behaviors, which were only noticed by bed partners. Recall of unpleasant dreams was absent in 35 % of the patients [19]. Like in PD, bed partners report that RBD-related movements are faster, stronger, and smother than during wakefulness [26].

RBD may be the first symptom of MSA. In one study of 27 RBD patients aware of their dream-enacting behaviors, RBD preceded the waking motor symptoms in 12 (44 %) [19]. In another study with 19 patients, RBD features were reported by the patients or their relatives as the first manifestation of the disease in 3, concomitant with other symptoms in 9, and developed after the onset of waking symptoms in the remaining 7. In our series, RBD onset antedated parkinsonian, cerebellar, and dysautonomic onset in 35 of 67 (52 %) patients by a mean of 7 years (range, 1–38 years). MSA is eventually diagnosed in only a few subjects with the initial diagnosis of idiopathic RBD (most of them are diagnosed with PD and DLB), probably because in the general population MSA is much more rare than PD and DLB. We reported a patient presenting with dysautonomia, stridor during sleep, and RBD without parkinsonism or cerebellar syndrome in whom brain pathology disclosed MSA after sudden death during wakefulness [29].

References

1. Iranzo A, Santamaria J, Tolosa E. Idiopathic rapid eye movement sleep behaviour disorder: diagnosis, management, and the need for neuroprotective interventions. Lancet Neurol. 2016;15:405–19.
2. Boeve B. REM sleep behaviour disorder. Updated review of the core features, the REM sleep behaviour disorder-neurodegenerative disease association, evolving concepts, controversies, and future directions. Ann NY Acad Sci. 2010;1184:15–54.
3. Arnulf I. REM sleep behaviour disorder: motor manifestations and pathophysiology. Mov Disord. 2012;27:677–89.
4. Iranzo A, Lomeña F, Stockner H, for the Sleep Innsbruck Barcelona (SINBAR) group, et al. Decreased striatal dopamine transporter uptake and substantia nigra hyperechogenicity as risk markers of synucleinopathy in patients with idiopathic rapid-eye-movement sleep behaviour disorder: a prospective study. Lancet Neurol. 2010;9:1070–7.
5. Postuma RB, Gagnon JF, Vendette M, Desjardins C, Montplaisir JY. Olfaction and color vision identify

impending neurodegeneration in rapid eye movement sleep behavior disorder. Ann Neurol. 2011;69:811–8.
6. Iranzo A, Stockner H, Serradell M, et al. Five year follow-up of substantia nigra echogenicity in idiopathic REM sleep behavior disorder. Mov Disord. 2014;29:1774–80.
7. Postuma RB, Gagnon JF, Vendette M, Montplaisir JY. Markers of neurodegeneration in idiopathic rapid eye movement sleep behavior disorder and Parkinson's disease. Brain. 2009;13:3298–307.
8. Iranzo A, Valldeoriola F, Lomeña F, et al. Serial dopamine transporter imaging of nigrostriatal function in patients with idiopathic rapid-eye-movement sleep behaviour disorder: a prospective study. Lancet Neurol. 2011;10:797–805.
9. Schenck CH, Bundlie SR, Mahowald MW. Delayed emergence of a parkinsonian disorder in 38% of 29 older men initially diagnosed with idiopathic rapid eye movement sleep behavior disorder. Neurology. 1996;46:388–92.
10. Schenck CH, Boeve BF, Mahowald MW. Delayed emergence of a parkinsonian disorder or dementia in 81% of older males initially diagnosed with idiopathic REM sleep behavior disorder (IBD): 16 year update on a previously reported series. Sleep Med. 2013;14:744–8.
11. Iranzo A, Molinuevo JL, Santamaria J, et al. Rapid-eye-movement sleep behaviour disorder as an early marker for a neurodegenerative disease: a descriptive study. Lancet Neurol. 2006;5:572–7.
12. Iranzo A, Tolosa E, Gelpi E, et al. Neurodegenerative status and post-mortem pathology in idiopathic rapid-eye-movement disorder: an observational cohort study. Lancet Neurol. 2013;12:443–53.
13. Iranzo A, Fernández-Arcos A, Tolosa E, et al. Neurodegenerative disorder risk in idiopathic REM sleep behavior disorder: study in 174 patients. PLoS One. 2014;9(2):e89741. doi:10.1371/journal.pone.0089741.29.
14. Vilas D, Iranzo A, Tolosa E, et al. Assessment of α-synuclein in submandibular glands of patients with idiopathic rapid-eye-movement sleep behaviour disorder: a case-control study. Lancet Neurol 2016;15:708–18.
15. Sprenger FS, Stefanova N, Gelpi E, et al. Enteric nervous system α-synuclein immunoreactivity in idiopathic REM sleep behavior disorder. Neurology. 2015;85:1761–8.
16. Tolosa E, Pont-Sunyer C. Progress in defining the premotor phase of Parkinson's disease. J Neurol Sci. 2011;310:4–8.
17. Iranzo A, Gelpi E, Tolosa E, Molinuevo JL, Serradell M, Gaig M, Santamaria J. Neuropathology of prodromal Lewy body disease. Mov Disord. 2014;29:410–5.
18. Postuma RN, Lang AE, Gagnon JF, Pelletier A, Montplaisir JY. How does parkinsonism start? Prodromal parkinsonism motor changes in idiopathic REM sleep behaviour disorder. Brain. 2012;27:617–26.
19. Iranzo A, Rye DB, Santamaria J, et al. Characteristics of idiopathic REM sleep behavior disorder and that associated with MSA and PD. Neurology. 2005;65:247–52.
20. Wetter TC, Trenkwalder C, Gershanik O, Högl B. Polysomnographic measures in Parkinson's disease: a comparison between patients with and without REM sleep disturbances. Wien Klin Wochenschr. 2001;113:249–53.
21. Gagnon JF, Vendette M, Postuma R, et al. Mild cognitive impairment in rapid eye movement sleep behaviour disorder and Parkinson disease. Ann Neurol. 2009;66:39–47.
22. De Cock VC, Vidailhet M, Leu S, et al. Restoration of normal muscle control in Parkinson's disease during REM sleep. Brain. 2007;130:450–6.
23. Sixel-Doring F, Trautmann E, Mollenhauer B, Trenkwalder C. Associated factors for REM sleep behaviour disorder in Parkinson disease. Neurology. 2011;77:1048–54.
24. Wallace DM, Shafazand S, Carvalho DZ, et al. Sleep-related falling out of bed in Parkinson's disease. J Clin Neurol. 2012;8:51–7.
25. Plazzi G, Corsini R, Provini F, et al. REM sleep behavior disorders in multiple system atrophy. Neurology. 1997;48:1094–7.
26. De Cock V, Debs R, Oudiette D, et al. The improvement of movement of speech during rapid eye movement sleep behavior disorder in multiple system atrophy. Brain. 2011;134:856–62.
27. Palma JA, Fernandez-Cordon C, Coon EA, et al. Prevalence of REM sleep behavior disorder in multiple system atrophy: a multicenter study and meta-analysis. Clin Auton Res. 2015;25:69–75.
28. Gaig C, Iranzo A, Tolosa E, Vilaseca I, Rey MJ, Santamaria J. Pathologically description of a non-motor variant of multiple system atrophy. J Neurol Neurosurg Psychiatry. 2008;79:1399–400.
29. Tachibana N, Kimura K, Kitajama K, Shinde A, Kimura J, Shibasaki H. REM sleep motor dysfunction in multiple system atrophy: with special emphasis on sleep talk as its early clinical manifestation. J Neurol Neurosurg Psychiatry. 1997;63:678–81.

Restless Legs Syndrome and Painful Legs/Moving Toes

36

Luigi Ferini-Strambi, Sara Marelli, and Romina Combi

List of Abbreviations

CSF	Cerebrospinal fluid
EMG	Electromyography
ICSD-3	International classification of sleep disorders, 3rd edition
PLMS	Periodic limb movements in sleep
PLMTS	Painful legs and moving toes syndrome
PLMW	Periodic limb movements in wakefulness
RLS	Restless legs syndrome
SIT	Suggested Immobilization Test
WED	Willis–Ekbom disease

L. Ferini-Strambi, MD, PhD (✉)
Department of Clinical Neurosciences, San Raffaele Scientific Institute, Sleep Disorders Center, Milan, Italy

Faculty of Psychology, Vita-Salute San Raffaele University, Milan, Italy

Sleep Disorders Center, Università Vita-Salute San Raffaele, Milan, Italy
e-mail: ferinistrambi.luigi@hsr.it

S. Marelli, PhD
Department of Clinical Neurosciences, San Raffaele Scientific Institute, Sleep Disorders Center, Milan, Italy
e-mail: marelli.sara@hsr.it

R. Combi, PhD
Department of Surgery and Traslational Medicine, Università of Milano-Bicocca, Milan, Italy
e-mail: romina.combi@unimib.it

36.1 Restless Legs Syndrome

Restless legs syndrome (RLS), recently renamed Willis–Ekbom disease (WED), is a neurological disorder characterized by paresthesia in the legs, with an urge to move. The most common adult RLS descriptors are "restless," "uncomfortable," "twitchy," "need to stretch," "urge to move," and "legs want to move on their own," and about half of patients express their RLS sensations as painful.

The symptoms begin or worsen during periods of rest or inactivity such as lying down or sitting, while the activity may typically relieve the urge to move and the unpleasant leg sensations. Symptoms may also involve arms and other body parts (20% of patients) [1]. Another important characteristic of RLS is the worsening of symptoms in the evening or during the night. The circadian pattern in the occurrence of RLS symptoms has been investigated by using a method called the "Suggested Immobilization Test" (SIT), administered every 2–4 h during 24–28 h [2]. These studies showed that the severity of leg discomfort followed a circadian rhythm with a maximum occurring after midnight. Moreover, the peak intensity of symptoms occurred on the falling limb of the core body temperature rhythm. Interestingly, it has been reported that changes in melatonin secretion precede the increase in sensory or motor symptoms of RLS [3].

C. Falup-Pecurariu et al. (eds.), *Movement Disorders Curricula*,
DOI 10.1007/978-3-7091-1628-9_36

The majority of RLS patient complain of poor sleep [4]: most patients report difficulty falling asleep, but some patients fall asleep rapidly and wake up shortly after with unpleasant legs sensations that force them to get up and walk around.

The clinical spectrum of RLS is very wide. Some patients may report symptoms during only short periods in their lives, while the severely affected cases have daily symptoms. Interestingly, the age of RLS onset appears to be the only characteristic item qualifying as an endophenotype [5]. Specifically, two different RLS phenotypes of RLS have been reported: (1) Early-onset idiopathic RLS, the most frequent form, with a prevalence onset around 20–40 years, very frequent RLS familial history, slow disease progression, and low cerebrospinal fluid (CSF) ferritin level [5, 6]; (2) Late-onset RLS with the onset after 40 years of age, less frequent RLS familial history, more rapid disease evolution, and more frequent association with other diseases, such as renal failure, diabetes, anemia, neuropathy, and myelopathy [5–7].

RLS prevalence in the general population has been estimated to be approximately 5 % [8]. However, studies conducted in Asian countries thus far indicate a lower prevalence. Prevalence is about twice as high in women as in men. In most studies, prevalence increases with age up to 60–70 years, except in Asian populations where an age-related increase has not been found. In an epidemiological survey conducted in the United States and five European countries [9], RLS symptoms of any frequency were reported by 7.2 % of the general population: symptoms occurred at least two times/week and were reported as moderately or severely distressing by 2.7 %: these subjects were defined RLS sufferers and probably represented the ones that should be adequately treated.

A recent study [10] that evaluated the incidence and correlates of RLS in a US population-based sample (535 participants aged ≥40 years) found an incidence of RLS of 1.7 % per year. Use of estrogen and history of obstructive lung disease were associated with a significantly higher incidence of RLS. RLS, in turn, was associated with insomnia and increased sleepiness.
Incidence of RLS has been recently evaluated also in two population-based cohort prospective studies in Germany: the cumulative incidence was 9.1 and 7.0 %, and the persistence of RLS symptoms from baseline to follow-up was 47.4 % in one study (mean follow-up = 2.2 years) and 41.5 % in the second one (mean follow-up = 5.2 years) [11]. Another prospective study conducted in Japan showed that RLS may not be persistent in more than 50 % of the affected population: the frequency of RLS symptoms, but not the severity, may predict the persistence of the disorder [12].

36.2 Diagnostic Criteria

According to the International classification of sleep disorders, third edition (ICSD-3) [13] five essential criteria are required for the diagnosis of RLS (Table 36.1).

Criteria A1-3 specify the necessary characteristics of the RLS sensations. Interestingly, the results obtained in some circadian rhythm studies showing a worsening of symptoms at night, independently from the activity, have allowed the separation of worsening at rest (criterion A1) from worsening in the evening/night (criterion A3). Criterion B indicates that RLS must be differentiated from other conditions that may mimic RLS. According to the criterion C, clinically significant RLS is defined by RLS symptoms causing substantial distress, sleep disturbance, or impairment of function.

Moreover, other supportive RLS diagnostic criteria may be considered in addition to the essential criteria. They include positive family history, presence of periodic leg movements, and positive response to dopaminergic drugs. Periodic limb movements may occur in sleep (PLMS) or wakefulness (PLMW). PLMW occur during quiet rest and particularly at the transition between waking and sleep, disrupting sleep onset, or the return to sleep. PLMS, mainly associated with arousal from sleep, are repetitive flexions of the legs (hips, knees, and ankles)

Table 36.1 ICSSD-3 diagnostic criteria for RLS

A. An urge to move the legs, usually accompanied by or felt to be caused by uncomfortable and unpleasant sensations in the legs[a, b]. These symptoms must:	
	1. Begin or worsen during periods of rest or inactivity such as lying down or sitting
	2. Be partially or totally relieved by movement, such as walking or stretching, at least as long as the activity continues[c]; and
	3. Occur exclusively or predominantly in the evening or night rather than during the day[d]
B. The above features are not solely accounted for as symptoms of another medical or a behavioral condition (e.g., leg cramps, positional discomfort, myalgia, venous stasis, leg edema, arthritis, habitual foot tapping)	
C. The symptoms of RLS cause concern, distress, sleep disturbance, or impairment in mental, physical, social, occupational, educational, behavioral, or other important areas of functioning[e]	

[a]Sometimes the urge to move the legs is present without the uncomfortable sensations and sometimes the arms or other parts of the body are involved in addition to the legs
[b]For children, the description of these symptoms should be in the child's own words
[c]When symptoms are very severe, relief by activity may not be noticeable but must have been previously present
[d]As a result of severity, treatment intervention, or treatment-induced augmentation, the worsening in the evening or night may not be noticeable but must have been previously present
[e]For certain research applications, such as genetic or epidemiological studies, it may be appropriate to omit criterion C. If so, this should be clearly stated in the research report

during sleep. PLMS are scored only in the case of a series of four or more consecutive movements lasting 0.5–10 s, with an intermovement interval of 5–90 s, recorded on limb electromyography (EMG) [7, 14]. A PLMS index (number of PLMS per hour of sleep) above five per hour is considered abnormal. Interestingly, an abnormal PLMS index may be observed in more than 80 % of RLS patients.

The differentiation of RLS from other conditions that may have similar characteristics is crucial, since about 40 % of individuals without RLS/WED will report some urge or need to move the legs while at rest [13]. The most important "mimics" of RLS are leg cramps, positional discomfort, arthralgias/arthritis, myalgias, leg edema, peripheral neuropathy, radiculopathy, and habitual foot tapping. Fulfilling ICSD-3 diagnostic criteria A2 (better with movement) and A3 (worse in the evening/night) improves specificity for an RLS diagnosis. However, it should also be appreciated that any of RLS mimics can occur in an individual who also has RLS. For example, some patients may have both RLS and leg cramps. When the diagnosis of RLS is not certain, evaluation for the supportive features such as the presence of PLMS or a family history of RLS may be clearly helpful.

36.3 Pathology and Pathophysiology

Brain iron deficiency, central nervous system dopamine regulation, and genetics seem to be primary factors in the pathophysiology of RLS, of which understanding remains incomplete. Decreased iron levels in the substantia nigra and putamen of patients affected by a severe form of RLS have been reported in some brain MRI studies, as well as in ultrasound studies [15, 16]. Moreover, neuropathological studies showed marked decreases in iron, ferritin heavy chain, transferrin receptor, and iron transport proteins contrasting with normal ferritin light chain and tyrosine hydroxylase in the substantia nigra of RLS patients [17].

Concerning the dopamine hypothesis, it is well known that dopaminergic drugs, preferential D3 receptor agonists, are markedly effective in RLS. On the contrary, neuroleptics (dopamine antagonists) may trigger or aggravate RLS. Moreover, a neuropathological study showed some dopaminergic abnormalities in RLS brain tissue, and in particular a significant decrease in D2 receptors in the putamen (correlated with RLS severity), as well as significant increases in tyrosine hydroxylase in the substantia nigra, but not in the putamen [18].

Interestingly, it has been reported that 48 % of patients with Parkinson's disease who were taking domperidone (a dopamine antagonist that does not cross the blood–brain barrier) had RLS compared with 21 % not taking domperidone, suggesting that peripheral dopaminergic influences may be part of RLS pathophysiology [19].

Association of gene variants BTBD9, MEIS1, MAP2K5/LBXCOR, and PTPRD with RLS has been found and replicated, indicating a genetic substrate upon which environmental factors might act. BTBD9 is estimated to confer a population attributable risk (PAR) of 50 % for RLS. Together, BTBD9, MEIS1, and MAP2K5/LBXCOR account for 70 % of the PAR for RLS in individuals with European ancestry. Thus far, two of the variants, BTBD9 and MEIS1, appear to influence expression of PLMS, as well as iron homeostasis. However, the full role of RLS gene variants has not been adequately defined.

36.4 Pharmacological Treatment

In the last years, important changes in the RLS treatment of RLS have been observed. In several studies, different classes of drugs have demonstrated efficacy, including the dopaminergic agents, the alpha-2-delta ligands, and opioids. According to Oertel and colleagues [20] and Garcia-Borreguero and colleagues [21], pharmacological therapy should be limited to those patients who suffer from clinically relevant RLS symptoms including intermittent RLS with impaired sleep quality or quality of life.

Levodopa is the drug most frequently studied in earlier small RLS trials. The immediate response to levodopa without a long titration period is really appreciated by the patient, and a positive response to this drug with the first dosage strongly supports the diagnosis of RLS [22]. However, it is well known that two possible side effects of levodopa are morning rebound and augmentation. Augmentation [23] is characterized by the worsening of RLS symptom severity from pretreatment levels. After an initial therapeutic benefit, the patient refers an earlier onset of symptoms by at least 2–4 h, often associated with a shorter latency to RLS symptoms at rest, extension of symptoms to other body parts, and increased severity of symptoms. Some open-label trials showed prevalence rates of augmentation with levodopa between 18.6 and 72 % [24–26].

More recently, three nonergoline derivatives agonists – pramipexole, ropinirole, and transdermal rotigotine – have been extensively studied for the RLS treatment (Table 36.2). Overall, short- and longer-duration placebo-controlled studies showed that dopamine agonists are effective for treating RLS and PLMS [27].

Another class of drugs that has demonstrated efficacy for RLS and PLMS is the α-2-δ ligands, including gabapentin, gabapentin enacarbil, and pregabalin [28] (Table 36.2). In a recent double-blind study, a greater reduction in the RLS symptoms was seen with 300 mg/day pregabalin than with pramipexole at a dose of either 0.25 or 0.5 mg, over a period of 12 weeks and 52 weeks. Augmentation rates were significantly lower with pregabalin than with 0.5 mg of pramipexole [29].

Some open-label and controlled clinical trials evaluated the effects of opioids in RLS patients [20]. A recent 12-week, placebo-controlled trial studied a fixed dose combination drug, oxycodone–naloxone, administered twice a day in RLS patients who had failed previous treatments owing to lack of benefit or side effects [30]. In this study, 265 patients were randomized to either placebo or oxycodone 5 mg–naloxone 2.5 mg twice a day and titrated up to either benefit or a maximal dose of oxycodone 40 mg–naloxone 20 mg twice a day. After the double-blind phase, all patients entered a 40-week open-label extension. Oxycodone–naloxone was superior to placebo, and in the extension period, provided continued benefit for a median of 281 days at a mean dose of oxycodone 18.1 mg and naloxone 9.1 mg. The active treatment caused some side effects, such as fatigue, constipation, nausea, somnolence, and headache. Interestingly, augmentation was not observed [30].

In conclusion, according to Silber and coworkers [31] chronic/persistent RLS should be treated with either a nonergot dopamine agonist or a α-2-δ calcium channel ligand. Since the α-2-δ ligands can cause depression and weight gain, a dopamine agonist is a more appropriate choice in the presence of these conditions. On the other hand, α-2-δ ligands can alleviate chronic pain and may be helpful in treating anxiety and

Table 36.2 Drugs more frequently used in RLS

Drug	Time to maximum blood level (h)	Elimination half-life	Initial daily dose (mg)	Usual dose range (mg)
Dopaminergic agonists				
Ropinirole	1–1.5	6	0.25 (–0.5)	0.50–4.00 mg daily approximately 1–3 h before bedtime
Pramipexole	2	8–12 (increase with decreasing glomerular filtration rate and age)	0.125	0.125–1.000 mg daily approximately 1–3 h before bedtime
Rotigotine	Stable plasma levels over 24 h	Stable plasma levels over 24 h (elimination half-life biphasic: 3 and 6)	1	1–3 mg daily
Alpha-2-delta ligands				
Gabapentin	2	5–7	300	300–1200 mg daily; may be in split dosing with an afternoon and bedtime dose
Gabapentin enacarbil	7–9	Relatively stable plasma levels over 18–24 h (elimination half-life:6)	600	600–1800 mg daily about 1 h before bedtime
Pregabalin	1.5	6	100	Up to 300 mg

insomnia, so the presence of any of these comorbidities may favor their use. Another important aspect that can influence the choice of the treatment is the duration of RLS symptoms. For RLS present through much of the day and night, the use of long-acting agents, such as the rotigotine patch or gabapentin enacarbil, should be considered. In refractory RLS, a combination therapy with drugs of different classes or oral prolonged release of oxycodone–naloxone should be considered.

36.5 Painful Legs/Moving Toes Syndrome

Painful legs and moving toes syndrome (PLMTS) is a rare and underdiagnosed disorder characterized by pain, typically of a neuropathic quality, in the feet or legs, associated with writhing movements of one or more toes. The pain usually precedes the onset of the involuntary movements and may vary in constancy and intensity [32]. The toe and foot movements are complex, repetitive, and nonrhythmic. PLMTS may be unilateral or bilateral. Diagnosis is based on clinical presentation.

The pathophysiology of PLMTS is unknown. However, some authors have suggested an association with a peripheral lesion, mainly at the level of the root or nerve. Possibly, a peripheral lesion causes aberrant input leading to "central reorganization," at the level of the spinal cord. This reorganization may be the responsible for the pain and movement [33].

In PLMTS, the treatment is usually unsatisfactory. The compounds commonly used for neuropathic pain, such as gabapentin, pregabalin, clonazepam, carbamazepine, and baclofen, have been reported anecdotally to improve the symptoms. Other anecdotal therapies include spinal blocks, spinal cord stimulation, and local injection of botulinum toxin. A recent report described a sustained improvement over the years with toxin treatment [34].

Another recent study describes the long-term beneficial effect of pramipexole in the treatment of PLMTS [35]. Interestingly, an analgesic effect of pramipexole has been already reported in patients with fibromyalgia. It is known that dopamine agonists can decrease N-methyl-D-aspartate-mediated pain through activation of a receptor tyrosine kinase.

Rarity, as well as usually unsatisfactory treatment, clearly differentiates PLMTS from RLS. Clinically, unlike RLS pain in PLMTS is not necessarily increased at night or relieved by movement.

References

1. Trenkwalder C, Paulus W. Restless legs syndrome: pathophysiology, clinical presentation and management. Nat Rev Neurol. 2010;6:337–46.
2. Montplaisir J, Allen R, Walters A, Ferini-Strambi L. Restless legs syndrome and periodic limb movements during sleep. In: Kryger H, Roth T, Dement WC, editors. Principles and practice of sleep medicine. 4th ed. Philadelphia: Elsevier; 2005. p. 839–52.
3. Michaud M, Dumont M, Selmaoui B, Paquet J, Fantini ML, Montplaisir J. Circadian rhythm of restless legs syndrome: relationship with biological markers. Ann Neurol. 2004;55:372–80.
4. Hening W, Walters A, Allen RP, Montplaisir J, Myers A, Ferini-Strambi L. Impact, diagnosis and treatment of restless legs syndrome (RLS) in a primary care population: the REST (RLS epidemiology, symptoms and treatment) primary care study. Sleep Med. 2004;5:237–46.
5. Winkelmann J, Wetter TC, Collado-Seidel V, Gasser T, Dichgans M, Yassouridis A, Trenkwalder C. Clinical characteristics and frequency of the hereditary restless legs syndrome in a population of 300 patients. Sleep. 2000;23:597–602.
6. Whittom S, Dauvilliers Y, Pennestri MH, Vercauteren F, Molinari N, Petit D, Montplaisir J. Age-at-onset in restless legs syndrome: a clinical and polysomnographic study. Sleep Med. 2007;9:54–9.
7. Allen RP, Picchietti D, Hening WA, Trenkwalder C, Walters AS, Montplaisir J, Restless Legs Syndrome Diagnosis and Epidemiology workshop at the National Institutes of Health, International Restless Legs Syndrome Study Group. Restless legs syndrome: diagnostic criteria, special considerations, and epidemiology. A report from the restless legs syndrome diagnosis and epidemiology workshop at the National Institute of Health. Sleep Med. 2003;4:101–19.
8. Garcia-Borreguero D, Egatz R, Winkelmann J, Berger K. Epidemiology of restless legs syndrome: the current status. Sleep Med Rev. 2006;10:153–67.
9. Allen RP, Walters A, Montplaisir J, Hening W, Myers A, Bell TJ, Ferini-Strambi L. Restless legs syndrome prevalence and impact: REST general population study. Arch Intern Med. 2005;165:1286–92.
10. Budhiraja P, Budhiraja R, Goodwin JL, Allen RP, Newman AB, Koo BB, Quan SF. Incidence of restless legs syndrome and its correlates. J Clin Sleep Med. 2012;8(2):119–24.
11. Szentkiralyi A, Fendrich K, Hoffmann W, Happe S, Berger K. Incidence of restless legs syndrome in two population-based cohort studies in Germany. Sleep Med. 2011;12(9):815–20.
12. Kagimura T, Nomura T, Kusumi M, Nakashima K, Inoue Y. Prospective survey on the natural course of restless legs syndrome over two years in a closed cohort. Sleep Med. 2011;12(9):821–6.
13. American Academy of Sleep Medicine. International classification of sleep disorders. 3rd ed. Darien: American Academy of Sleep Medicine; 2014.
14. Zucconi M, Ferri R, Allen R, Baier PC, Bruni O, Chokroverty S, Ferini-Strambi L, Fulda S, Garcia-Borreguero D, Hening WA, Hirshkowitz M, Högl B, Hornyak M, King M, Montagna P, Parrino L, Plazzi G, Terzano MG, International Restless Legs Syndrome Study Group (IRLSSG). The official World Association of Sleep Medicine (WASM) standards for recording and scoring periodic leg movements in sleep (PLMS) and wakefulness (PLMW) developed in collaboration with a task force from the International Restless Legs Syndrome Study Group (IRLSSG). Sleep Med. 2006;7:175–83.
15. Allen RP, Barker PB, Wehrl F, Song HK, Earley CJ. MRI measurement of brain iron in patients with restless legs syndrome. Neurology. 2001;56:263–5.
16. Earley CJ, Barker P, Horska A, Allen RP. MRI-determined regional brain iron concentrations in early- and late-onset restless legs syndrome. Sleep Med. 2006;7:458–61.
17. Connor JR, Wang XS, Patton SM, Enzies SL, Troncoso JC, Earley CJ, Allen RP. Decreased transferrin receptor expression by neuromelanin cells in restless legs syndrome. Neurology. 2004;62:1563–7.
18. Connor JR, Wang XS, Allen RP, Beard JL, Wiesinger JA, Felt BT, Earley CJ. Altered dopaminergic profile in the putamen and substantia nigra in restless leg syndrome. Brain. 2009;132:2403–12.
19. Rios Romenets S, Dauvilliers Y, Cochen de Cock V, Carlander B, Bayard S, Galatas C, Wolfson C, Postuma RB. Restless legs syndrome outside the blood–brain barrier-exacerbation by domperidone in Parkinson's disease. Parkinsonism Relat Disord. 2013;19:92–4.
20. Oertel WH, Trenkwalder C, Zucconi M, Benes H, Borreguero DG, Bassetti C, Partinen M, Ferini-Strambi L, Stiasny-Kolster K. State of the art in restless legs syndrome: practice recommendations for treating restless legs syndrome. Mov Disord. 2007;22 Suppl 18:S466–75.
21. Garcia-Borreguero D, Stillman P, Benes H, Buschmann H, Chaudhuri KR, Gonzalez Rodríguez VM, Högl B, Kohnen R, Monti GC, Stiasny-Kolster K, Trenkwalder C, Williams AM, Zucconi M. Algorithms for the diagnosis and treatment of restless legs syndrome in primary care. BMC Neurol. 2011;11:28.
22. Stiasny-Kolster K, Kohnen R, Moller JC, Oertel W. Validation of "L-dopa test" for diagnosis of restless legs syndrome. Mov Disord. 2006;21:1333–9.

23. Garcia-Borreguero D, Allen RP, Kohnen R, Högl B, Trenkwalder C, Oertel W, Hening WA, Paulus W, Rye D, Walters A, Winkelmann J, Earley CJ, International Restless Legs Syndrome Study Group. Diagnostic standards for dopaminergic augmentation of restless legs syndrome: report from World Association of Sleep Medicine-International Restless Legs Syndrome Study Group consensus conference at the Max Planck Institute. Sleep Med. 2007;8:520–30.
24. Vignatelli L, Billiard M, Clarenbach P, Garcia-Borreguero D, Kaynak D, Liesiene V, Trenkwalder C, Montagna P, Task Force EFNS. EFNS guidelines on management of restless legs syndrome and periodic limb movement disorder in sleep. Eur J Neurol. 2006;13:1049–65.
25. Collado-Seidel V, Kazenwadel J, Wetter TC, Kohnen R, Winkelmann J, Selzer R, Oertel WH, Trenkwalder C. A controlled study of additional sr-L-dopa in L-dopa-responsive restless legs syndrome with late-night symptoms. Neurology. 1999;52:285–90.
26. Garcia-Borreguero D, Kohnen R, Hogl B, Ferini-Strambi L, Hadjigeorgiou GM, Hornyak M, de Weerd AW, Happe S, Stiasny-Kolster K, Gschliesser V, Egatz R, Cabrero B, Frauscher B, Trenkwalder C, Hening WA, Allen RP. Validation of the Augmentation Severity Rating Scale (ASRS): a multicentric, prospective study with levo-dopa in RLS. Sleep Med. 2007;8:455–63.
27. Ferini-Strambi L, Marelli S. Pharmacotherapy for restless legs syndrome. Expert Opin Pharmacother. 2014;15(8):1127–38.
28. Garcia-Borreguero D, Larrosa O, de la Llave Y, Verger K, Masramon X, Hernandez G. Treatment of restless legs syndrome with gabapentin. Neurology. 2002;59:1573–9.
29. Allen RP, Chen C, Garcia-Borreguero D, Polo O, DuBrava S, Miceli J, Knapp L, Winkelman JW. Comparison of pregabalin with pramipexole for restless legs syndrome. N Engl J Med. 2014;370(7):621–31.
30. Trenkwalder C, Benes H, Grote L, García-Borreguero D, Högl B, Hopp M, Bosse B, Oksche A, Reimer K, Winkelmann J, Allen RP, Kohnen R, RELOXYN Study Group. Prolonged release oxycodone-naloxone for treatment of severe restless legs syndrome after failure of previous treatment: a double-blind, randomised, placebo-controlled trial with an open-label extension. Lancet Neurol. 2013;12:1141–50.
31. Silber MH, Becker PM, Earley C, Garcia-Borreguero D, Ondo WG, Medical Advisory Board of the Willis-Ekbom Disease Foundation. Willis-Ekbom Disease Foundation revised consensus statement on the management of restless legs syndrome. Mayo Clin Proc. 2013;88(9):977–86.
32. Liu R, Moizuddin M, Hung S. Painful legs and moving toes-case report and review of literature. BJMP. 2011;4(3):431–4.
33. Jabbari B, Molloy FM, Erickson M, Floeter MK. Bilateral painful hand-moving fingers: electrophysiological assessment of the central nervous system oscillator. Mov Disord. 2000;6:1259–63.
34. Rodriguez RL, Fernandez HH. Sustained benefit of painful legs moving toes syndrome with botulinum toxin type A. J Clin Neurosci. 2013;20(7):1031–2.
35. Beckmann Y1, Gürgör N, Bülbül NG, Seçil Y, Türkmen N. Painful legs and moving toes syndrome: responsive to dopaminergic treatment. Acta Neurol Belg. 2015;115(1):87–8.

37 Botulinum Toxin Use in Movement Disorders and Spasticity

Karen Frei and Daniel Truong

Botulinum toxin was first used as a treatment for strabismus by Alan Scott published in 1980 [23]. Soon thereafter, botulinum toxin was developed as a treatment for many different conditions including strabismus, hemifacial spasm, blepharospasm, and cervical dystonia. Over time botulinum toxin injections have been considered to treat any condition with focal muscle overactivity including cosmetic uses to reduce wrinkles.

Botulinum toxin is the protein product of the bacterium *Clostridium botulinum*. There are seven serotypes of botulinum toxin denoted as A through G. However, only serotypes A and B have been developed commercially. Commercially available forms of botulinum toxin in the USA include Botox (onabotulinum toxin), Dysport (abobotulinum toxin), Xeomin (incobotulinum toxin), and Myobloc (rimabotulinum toxin). Botox, Dysport, and Xeomin are all serotype A, and Myobloc is serotype B.

K. Frei, MD
Department of Neurology, Loma Linda University Medical Center, 11370 Anderson St. Suite B-100, Loma Linda, CA, USA
e-mail: kfrei@llu.edu

D. Truong, MD (✉)
Parkinson's and Movement Disorder Institute, 9940 Talbert Avenue, Suite 204, Fountain Valley, CA 92708, USA
e-mail: dtruong@pmdi.org

Botulinum toxin acts to inhibit the release of acetylcholine from the neuromuscular synapses. There are three steps to this process. The toxin first binds to the receptors on the presynaptic chain. The toxin is internalized into the neuron, and then an enzymatic cleavage takes place. The toxin's light chain cleaves proteins involved in the acetylcholine transport protein cascade also known as SNARE proteins. SNARE proteins act to regulate fusion of the vesicle containing acetylcholine to the plasma membrane, Botulinum toxin type A cleaves SNAP 25, and botulinum toxin type B cleaves synaptophysin-2 also known as VAMP (vesicle-associated membrane protein). The vesicles containing acetylcholine are prevented from binding to the membrane, and acetylcholine is not released. The reduced acetylcholine release results in muscle weakness, the expected therapeutic result. After 3 months, the presynaptic neuron forms sprouts restoring the neuromuscular synapse which then can act at the muscle restoring the acetylcholine activity to normal [10, 16].

In the majority of cases, the botulinum toxin is injected into muscles that are overly active, usually the muscles producing the aberrant movement. The toxin's beneficial effect takes up to 2 weeks to begin and lasts up to 3 months. Recurrent injections are required to produce and maintain optimum effect. Time intervals between injections are generally 3 months. It is thought that giving doses at 3-month intervals will prevent

C. Falup-Pecurariu et al. (eds.), *Movement Disorders Curricula*,
DOI 10.1007/978-3-7091-1628-9_37

antibody production against the toxin. Antibodies to the toxin render the toxin inactive, and a patient will appear not to respond to the injections. Antibody tests or a simple forehead test can be performed to assess for antibodies to the toxin. The forehead test consists of a small amount of the botulinum toxin injected into one side of the forehead and the effect of toxin evaluated by the inability to raise the eyebrow on the side of the injection.

Adverse effects from botulinum toxin injections are also transient with many of them resolving within 2 weeks following injection. Side effects include excessive muscle weakness, shortness of breath, head drop, ptosis, diplopia, and dysphagia. At times, these adverse effects can persist for 3 months.

Botulinum toxin has many therapeutic uses from treatment of spasticity to cosmetic uses. It is used for hyperhidrosis and has been injected into the urinary bladder for hyperactivity of the detrusor muscle. Refractory migraine headaches have responded to botulinum toxin. We will discuss botulinum toxin injections as it relates to the treatment of movement disorders and spasticity.

37.1 Dystonia

Botulinum toxin injections have become the mainstay of treatment for dystonia. Dystonia is one of the most common movement disorders treated. Dystonia is a movement disorder characterized by sustained or intermittent muscle contractions causing abnormal, often repetitive, movements, postures, or both. Dystonic movements are typically patterned, twisting, and may be tremulous. Dystonia is often initiated or worsened by voluntary action and associated with overflow muscle activation [2]. Dystonia can be focal affecting one part of the body, segmental in which two or more adjacent body parts are affected or generalized in which the entire body appears to be affected. Dystonic tremor can be present, especially early in the disorder. The tremor is inconstant, patterned movement produced by contractions of dystonic muscles often exacerbated by an attempt to maintain normal posture [2]. The dystonic tremor tends to be more irregular in timing and amplitude compared to other types of tremor due to irregular underlying muscle bursts [17]. However, dystonic tremor can appear to be postural, intentional, or rarely resting tremors. Dystonic tremor can be confused with myoclonus. However, when occurring in the setting of dystonia, myoclonus usually involves the unaffected limb [14].

Dystonic symptoms can be present only when performing a certain activity such as handwriting in writer's cramp. Most overuse forms of dystonia, also denoted as task-specific dystonia, occur in this manner. Sometimes task-specific dystonia can generalize or be present with other activities. For example, writer's cramp which begins only with handwriting may become present when performing any activity requiring fine motor skill.

Oftentimes a light touch on the face can reduce cervical dystonia, or a touch on the forehead can reduce blepharospasm. This is known as a sensory trick. Sensory tricks are seen in up to 70% of patients with cervical dystonia and to a lesser degree in the other dystonias [28]. Sensory tricks, also called geste antagoniste, can sometimes be used to alleviate symptoms of dystonia. An example is when a cervical collar is worn to treat cervical dystonia. The touch of the collar can reduce the symptoms. Sensory tricks do not produce complete alleviation of symptoms, however, and the response can wane. In the majority of cases, botulinum toxin is the best treatment for dystonia. Infrequent transient side effects from botulinum toxin injections including dry mouth, ptosis, head drop, or dysphagia may occur dependent upon location of the injections. Generalized dystonia which usually requires too great of a dose of botulinum toxin is an exception. Alternative therapies such as medication and deep brain stimulation can be helpful in these cases.

37.2 Blepharospasm

Blepharospasm is a form of adult onset focal dystonia affecting the eyes. Involuntary contraction of the periocular muscles produces forced eye closure and impaired ability to open the eyes.

Patients can present with a range of symptoms from excessive blinking to prolonged spasms of eye closure which may result in functional blindness. At times dry eye may precede the onset of blepharospasm. Bright light and walking tend to exacerbate the condition. The photophobia can also be referred to as photo-oculodynia in which there is pain induced by light. Blue light appears to be most uncomfortable. It is thought that the melanopsin pathway may be involved in photo-oculodynia. Wearing dark glasses can be helpful [18]. Sensory tricks in blepharospasm are usually touching the forehead or around the eyes.

Singing and dancing can be helpful in alleviating symptoms for a short period of time. Two examples are a patient who would sing in order to be able to perform housework and a patient who was a professional ballroom dancer who could not walk without his eyes closed tightly but who had no trouble when dancing. Treatment of blepharospasm with botulinum toxin allows the patient to keep the eyes open more easily. The targeted muscles for botulinum toxin injection include the orbicularis oculi, procerus, corrugator, and frontalis muscles. The orbicularis oculi is divided into three parts: orbital, preseptal, and pretarsal. The pretarsal portion of the orbicularis oculi is located in the eyelid. Injections in the middle of the upper lid should always be avoided in order to prevent ptosis [8]. The pretarsal portion of the orbicularis oculi may require injections in severe cases. These injections are more painful but produce fewer side effects [1, 4, 8]. Side effects of the botulinum toxin injections are usually transient and include diplopia, ptosis, tearing, blurred vision, and local hematoma. Side effects often resolve within 2 weeks [16].

37.3 Oromandibular Dystonia

Oromandibular dystonia is a form of focal dystonia which involves the lower facial musculature, jaw, and/or tongue. Patients may have difficulty with speaking or chewing, and oftentimes they will bite their cheek or tongue. Pain can accompany this disorder and is usually temporomandibular joint syndrome or tension headache. Dental wear and rarely TMJ dislocation may occur [5]. These regions can be affected in isolation or in combination. Dystonia involving the lower facial muscles produces a grimacing appearance, pursing of the lips, mouth pulling to one side, and other facial contortions. Jaw-opening and jaw-closing dystonia are also included in this category. Targeted muscles are dependent upon the particular facial appearance with the goal of treatment to restore the symmetry of the face and upon the particular movement that predominates. Jaw-closing dystonia involves the symmetric contraction of jaw closers (the medial pterygoids, masseters, and temporalis muscles). In this case, the jaw is held closed and is not able to be opened. This can lead to a form of bruxism known as dystonic bruxism. Jaw-opening dystonia involves the symmetric contraction of jaw openers (the lateral pterygoids and digastric muscles). In this case, the mouth is held open and not able to be closed or the jaw protrudes. The jaw can deviate to one side as well which occurs when there is asymmetric contraction of the jaw openers and closers [29]. Botulinum toxin injections are reasonable first-line treatment for oromandibular dystonia. Jaw-closing dystonia tends to respond best to this treatment [5]. Side effects from botulinum toxin injections include transient dysphagia and facial weakness.

Sensory tricks in oromandibular dystonia are usually oral and can be as simple as holding a toothpick in the mouth. Chewing gum and touching the lips or chin are other examples. Dental appliances have been made which also help manage the symptoms in this manner.

The combination of blepharospasm, orofacial dystonia, and cervical dystonia comprises Meige's syndrome. Treatment of this syndrome consists of botulinum toxin injections where needed.

37.4 Embouchure Dystonia

Embouchure dystonia is a focal task-specific form of dystonia. It is seen in musicians who play woodwind and brass instruments. Embouchure refers to the pattern of perioral and jaw muscles used to initiate and control the amplitude and force of airflow into the mouthpiece of a woodwind or brass instrument. Patients present with complaints of "difficulty performing." Loss of embouchure control, lip fatigue, lip tremor, and other involuntary facial movements were the most common initial complaints in a study looking at 26 and 89 patients [12, 13]. Symptoms tend to persist and can spread to occur during other tasks involving the perioral musculature such as drinking from a bottle, speaking, or eating. There are some cases of spread of the dystonia to involve the hands and/or neck [13]. Muscles involved in embouchure dystonia include the paired levator and depressor anguli oris, levator labii superioris, depressor labii inferioris, zygomaticus major and minor, buccinators, and the mentalis. Botulinum toxin injections have been performed but have had variable success, and professional musicians rarely see dramatic improvement. Very small doses and precise targeting of the muscles are required in this case in order to prevent dysarthria or trouble with chewing. There have been some reports of improvement of this condition with dental appliances [22]. No real improvement with increased practice or periods of abstention from playing the instrument has been noted [12]. In most instances, this form of dystonia results in significant professional disability.

37.5 Cervical Dystonia

Cervical dystonia is the most common form of dystonia. In this instance, the dystonia involves the neck. There are four directions in which the head can be pulled: torticollis, or rotation of the head to the left or right, lateralcollis in which the head is pulled toward the shoulder, anterocollis with pulling of the head forward, and retrocollis in which the head is pulled back. Torticollis is the most common form of cervical dystonia; however, the majority of cases have a combination of directions. For example, rotation of the head with tilting of the head is a combination of torticollis and lateralcollis. Dystonic tremor may be seen in cervical dystonia and at times precedes the full development of the cervical dystonia. Generally, the tremor will occur when the head is attempting to maintain a neutral posture. Uncommonly, the cervical dystonia will consist of predominantly dystonic tremor also called tremulous cervical dystonia, and this may represent a clinical subtype of cervical dystonia of which a gene has recently been associated [18].

Sensory tricks found in cervical dystonia can include touching the side of the face or the back of the neck. Pain is associated with cervical dystonia in up to 70 % of patients and can be a major disabling factor [28].

Botulinum toxin injections are the most effective treatment for cervical dystonia. The goal of treatment is to improve the abnormal posture of the head, reduce associated pain, and to prevent the development of secondary complications such as contractures, cervical radiculopathy, and cervical myelopathy [16]. Medications can be used in addition to the injections to achieve greater muscle relaxation and pain reduction. Benzodiazepines such as diazepam or lorazepam and tricyclic antidepressants such as nortriptyline or amitriptyline are commonly prescribed. The targeted muscles depend on the patient and their specific neck position. Prior to giving injections, evaluation of the patient's head position and response to treatment should be noted. Injection patterns can change as the dystonia can evolve to include different muscle patterns. Proper identification of involved muscles is important to achieving a good result from the botulinum toxin injections. Identification of targeted muscles can be with palpation for more superficial muscles, EMG, and ultrasound [3, 15, 16]. For torticollis, the sternocleidomastoid (SCM) muscle contralateral to the direction of the head rotation in combination with the ipsilateral splenius capitis if the chin is elevated or the head pulled back is the most common set of muscles targeted. The trapezius and levator scapulae are commonly targeted in lateralcollis. Bilateral splenius capitis and bilateral SCM muscles are targeted in retrocollis and anterocollis, respectively. If bilateral muscles are targeted for botulinum toxin injections, the rule is to use smaller doses of toxin to prevent head drop. Anterocollis appears to be the type of cervical dystonia most resistant to treatment with botulinum toxin. This may be due to contraction of the deep prevertebral paraspinal muscles which cannot be reached without radiological guidance [18]. Botulinum toxin injections can also be used to treat the tremor in tremor-dominant cervical dystonia. Generally, smaller doses of toxin are needed to treat the tremor alone.

Side effects from botulinum toxin injections commonly include neck weakness resulting in head drop and dysphagia dependent upon the location of the injections. These effects are transient and oftentimes resolve within 2 weeks.

37.6 Writer's Cramp

Writer's cramp is an adult onset focal task-specific dystonia involving the hand and/or arm. It is a form of occupational dystonia in which the occupation requires repetitive and excessive fine motor activity. Patients have had such employment as draftsmen, insurance salesmen, dental hygienists, architects, and nursing. The symptoms of finger or hand posturing and at times arm flexion tend to occur when writing only. Other tasks requiring fine motor skill are unimpaired. Over time the symptoms may generalize to occur during performance of fine motor tasks.

Botulinum toxin injections can improve the symptoms; however, abstention from performing the offending task is generally accepted as helpful. It is thought that the dystonia will not spread or progress as much in severity if the patient stops writing with that hand. Depending upon the movement of the fingers, either the finger flexors or extensors are targeted. Should there be wrist flexion, the flexor carpi ulnaris and/or flexor carpi radialis can be injected as well. Doses of toxin tend to be smaller since the hand and arm function may be compromised with larger doses [9].

37.7 Limb Dystonia

Sometimes focal dystonia can involve the upper and/or lower extremities. In adults, focal onset dystonia most commonly involves the upper extremities. The majority of cases of limb dystonia are task specific, and writer's cramp is one example (see above). Musicians including guitar and piano players are other examples. It appears that any activity in which there is repetitive movement over long periods of time can induce task-specific dystonia [18]. The dystonia may remain task specific or generalize to occur during other activities. Treatment of the upper limb dystonia with botulinum toxin injections has variable results, and the targeted muscles depend on the presentation and the hand or finger position. In general, lower doses of botulinum toxin are used in the upper limb in order to maintain function.

Generalized and early onset dystonia commonly begins in the foot presenting as foot inversion. Sometimes foot dystonia is the most prominent dystonia seen in cases of generalized dystonia warranting treatment of the affected limb with botulinum toxin. Foot dystonia can be part of Parkinson's disease occurring more often during off times and can consist of toes curling and great toe extension. Leg dystonia may actually be a presenting symptom of Parkinson's disease preceding the onset of tremor or bradykinesia [18]. If the dystonia occurs a large amount of time, botulinum toxin injections can be helpful. In any case, botulinum toxin injections can help to improve the foot position which affects gait and balance. Targeted muscles depend on presentation and foot and/or toe position.

Potential side effects from botulinum toxin injections include limb weakness.

37.8 Truncal Dystonia

Truncal dystonia is uncommon as a focal form of dystonia in adults. It can be part of segmental or generalized dystonia. Sometimes it can be a part of Parkinson's disease or Parkinsonism; it can be a result of neuroleptic medication usage or as a part of scoliosis. When the trunk is bent forward, the condition is known as camptocormia; when bent backward, it is known as opisthotonus; and when bent sideways, it is known as the Pisa syndrome. Movements of the trunk can be fixed or spasmodic. Botulinum toxin injections can be performed, but the results from the injections are modest due to the large truncal muscle involvement. Targeted muscles include the paraspinal and abdominal muscles. Treatment of this condition with DBS is thought to be superior [18].

37.9 Laryngeal Dystonia

Spasmodic dysphonia is the most common form of laryngeal dystonia involving the vocal cords. The two forms of spasmodic dysphonia are the adductor and the less common abductor type. The voice is broken due to spasms of the laryngeal muscles in the adductor spasmodic dysphonia and breathy in abductor dysphonia from excessive opening of the vocal cords. Spasmodic dysphonia is a task-specific form of dystonia and occurs during speech. Patients can sing, whisper, or yell normally. Adductor dysphonia is more common, and botulinum toxin injections into the thyroarytenoid and sometimes the cricoarytenoid muscles are helpful to maintain speech. These injections are performed by specialists with the aid of a laryngoscope and/or EMG. Very small doses are necessary. Side effects from this procedure include hypophonia, hoarseness, and dysphagia with aspiration [18].

37.10 Hemifacial Spasm

Hemifacial spasm is characterized as involuntary irregular clonic or tonic movements of the facial muscles innervated by the seventh cranial nerve on one side of the face and is most often a result of vascular compression of the facial nerve at the root exit zone [30]. The twitches generally begin around the eye and then spread to involve one side of the face. It can uncommonly spread to involve the other side. Stress or emotion tends to exacerbate the condition. The twitching can persist during sleep and can induce eye closure thereby interfering with vision. The mouth can be pulled to the side or down. The movements are brief muscle twitches and not sustained pulling movements as seen in dystonia. Over time the symptoms can progress and facial weakness can develop. Hypertension is thought to be a risk factor for the development of the condition. The majority of cases are the result of a vascular compression of the facial nerve at the root exit zone. The goal with botulinum toxin injections is to reduce the muscle twitching at the level of muscle activity. Common muscles involved in hemifacial spasm include the corrugator, orbicularis oculi, zygomaticus major, orbicularis oris, depressor angularis oris, and risorius. Additional muscles can include the nasalis, frontalis, and platysma. At times, the contralateral side may require a few injections to maintain facial symmetry. Attention to avoidance of the orbicularis oris should be paid in order to avoid a lip droop. Lip droop will give an asymmetric smile and inhibit pursing the lips interfering with drinking from a straw and speech [11].

37.11 Sialorrhea

Sialorrhea or hypersalivation can be part of many disorders. Sialorrhea is commonly part of Parkinson's disease as there is excessive saliva production in combination with a reduction in swallowing. Other neurological conditions can also produce sialorrhea such as cerebral palsy, stroke conditions, traumatic brain injury, or neurodegenerative conditions such as ALS. Any condition or situation in which there is a reduction in swallowing can produce sialorrhea. Sialorrhea is socially embarrassing and can interfere with oral hygiene and is a risk factor for bronchial aspiration. Management of sialorrhea can be with gum or hard candy to induce swallowing. If this is not sufficient, botulinum toxin injections have been associated with improvement in this socially embarrassing condition. Botulinum toxin injections have been regarded as effective in the treatment of Parkinson's-associated sialorrhea [24]. Botulinum toxin injections are given in the parotid and/or submandibular salivary glands. Ultrasound localization of the salivary glands is used should palpation not be sufficient. Botulinum toxin injections do not appear to spread to adjacent musculature enough to interfere with the oropharyngeal swallowing dynamics of Parkinson's disease patients [20].

37.12 Synkinesis and Facial Palsy

Synkinesis commonly occurs following Bell's palsy or any peripheral paralysis of cranial nerve VII. Synkinesis is referred to as involuntary movement of facial muscles that accompanies voluntary movement of another set of muscles. The most common forms of synkinesis are oculo-oral (involuntary contraction of zygomaticus and/or orbicularis oris during voluntary eye closure) and oro-ocular (involuntary eye closure with voluntary mouth movement) [6]. Synkinesis is thought to be the result of aberrant nerve regeneration. Treatment with botulinum toxin involves the orbicularis oculi muscle of the affected eye. This reduces muscle activity preventing complete eye closure when chewing or talking.

Incomplete recovery of the facial paralysis results in facial asymmetry which can be more disabling than synkinesis. The apparent asymmetry can be treated by botulinum toxin injections to the contralateral side of the weakness. By injecting botulinum toxin in the unaffected side, the normal muscles become weaker, thereby matching the appearance of the affected side creating greater facial symmetry [7].

37.13 Tremor

Tremor can be treated with botulinum toxin when oral medications have poor efficacy or intolerable side effects. Botulinum toxin injections can be used in conjunction with medication for more optimal results [25]. Dystonic tremor has been mentioned previously. Essential tremor tends to involve the limbs and head. Reducing muscle activity can reduce the amplitude of the tremor allowing a more normal state. Botulinum toxin injections can be given in the neck for head tremor and tend to be more effective for lateral head tremor (no/no). Injection patterns are similar for dystonic tremors of the head and include bilateral splenius capitis muscles. For vertical tremor (yes/yes), bilateral sternocleidomastoid muscles are injected. Lower doses are used to treat the tremors and because of the bilaterality to avoid the head drop.

Essential tremor of the upper extremities can be treated according to the direction of the tremor – flexion/extension or pronation/supination. Be mindful of the dosing so as not to interfere with normal hand and arm functioning. Essential tremor tends to respond to medication, so botulinum toxin injections are not always necessary. In fact, deep brain stimulation therapy has been quite successful in controlling tremor with or without medication. In many cases, botulinum toxin injections are reserved for those who do not tolerate medications to treat tremor or do not respond to these medications, and deep brain stimulation is not favorable.

37.14 Tics

Tics are brief, sudden involuntary movements or sounds which are intermittent but may be repetitive and with variable intensity, frequency, and duration. Tics are divided into two categories: motor or vocal and simple or complex movements [27]. Examples of simple motor tics include eye blinking or shoulder shrugging, and simple vocal tics can be throat clearing or sniffing. Complex motor tics have the appearance of purposeful movement and include touching while coprolalia or repetitive words are examples of complex vocal tics. Tics tend to wax and wane, are exacerbated by stress, and can be voluntarily suppressed for a short period of time. Following suppression, the tics become more frequent as there is a buildup of tension that resolves after the tic is permitted to occur. Premonitory urges usually precede the tic are described as tension, pressure, tickle or itch that is relieved after performing the tic.

Treatment of tics is with psychological therapy such as cognitive therapy and medications. Medications tend to consist of neuroleptics which can be difficult to tolerate. Focal, repetitive, simple motor tics and sometimes vocal tics can be successfully treated with botulinum toxin. Botulinum toxin injections can alleviate the premonitory urge which may explain somewhat the reduction in tics. An evidence-based review has supported the use of botulinum toxin injections for the treatment of motor tics but is unsupported for the treatment of vocal tics [26]. Facial tics can involve contraction of the bilateral nasalis muscles, frontalis muscles, and sometimes the orbicularis oculi. The orbicularis oris is avoided so as not to produce a droopy lip resulting in difficulty with drinking, chewing, and using a straw. Tics involving the neck are also improved with botulinum toxin injections, and the targeted muscles are determined by the specific neck movement performed in the tic. Treating tics involving the extremities are similar in that it depends on the specific movement produced in performing the tic. Sometimes the trapezius is targeted with shoulder movements [25]. Vocal tics sometimes respond to botulinum toxin injection into the laryngeal folds. The frequency of vocal tics tends to be reduced with this treatment in part via a reduction of premonitory urges [27].

37.15 Spasticity

Spasticity is the result of upper motor neuron syndrome and consists of increased muscle tone, exaggerated reflexes, and clonus. Spasticity can be a result of cerebrovascular disease, stroke multiple sclerosis, cerebral palsy, traumatic brain, or spinal cord injury. Botulinum toxin injections can be useful when treating cases of spasticity provided the spasticity is limited. Botulinum toxin injections will reduce the muscle tone, prevent contractures, and can improve pain.

Botulinum toxin injections have been FDA approved for treatment of spasticity in the and lower extremities. The most common pattern of spasticity in the upper limb involves flexion of the fingers, wrist, and elbow; adduction with internal rotation at the shoulder; and sometimes thumb curling across the palm or fist [19]. Targeted muscles include flexor digitorum profundus and superficialis, flexor pollicis longus, and adductor pollicis [21]. With wrist flexion, flexor carpi ulnaris and/or radialis can be targeted. At times, there is significant elbow flexion, and the biceps or brachioradialis muscles can be injected. The goal of botulinum toxin injections in this case is to relax the hand in order to maintain palmar hygiene and to help with getting dressed. The addition of braces can be helpful to achieve the optimum response.

Significant spasticity can also occur in the lower extremities. The thighs can be too close together preventing hygiene. The knees are extended with plantar flexion of the ankle. The foot can turn in or the toes can be flexed or the great toe extended. Targeted muscles include the thigh adductors, the gastrocnemius, the soleus, the tibialis posterior, and the extensor hallucis longus [21]. The goals of treatment are to restore more normal foot posture which facilitates walking, allows hygiene, and facilitates ease of dressing.

In conclusion, botulinum toxin injections can be useful to treat a multitude of movement disorders by relaxing unwanted or overactive muscle activity. Dystonia continues to be a major disorder whose mainstay of treatment is with botulinum toxin injections. Many times spasticity can be improved with botulinum toxin injections allowing for maintenance of hygiene and facilitate dressing.

References

1. Albanese A, Bentivoglio AR, Colosimo C, Galardi G, Maderna L, Tonali P. Pretarsal injections of botulinum toxin improve blepharospasm in previously unresponsive patients. J Neurol Neurosurg Psychiatry. 1996;60: 693–4.
2. Albanese A, Bhatia K, Bessman SB, DeLong MR, Fahn S, Fung VSC, Hallett M, Jankovic J, Jinnah HA, Klein C, Lang AE, Mink JW, Teller JK. Phenomenology and classification of dystonia: a consensus update. Mov Disord. 2013;28(7):863–73.
3. Beneke R, Frei K, Comella C. Treatment of cervical dystonia. Manual of botulinum toxin therapy. Cambridge University Press; New York 2009. p. 29–41.
4. Cakmur R, Ozturk V, Uzunel F, Donmez B, Idiman F. Comparison of preseptal and pretarsal injections of botulinum toxin in the treatment of blepharospams and hemifacial spasm. J Neurol. 2002;249:64–8.
5. Cardoso F, Bhidayasiri, Truong D. Treatment of oromandibular dystonia. Manual of botulinum toxin therapy. Cambridge University Press; New York 2009. p. 53–60.
6. Cecini M, Pavese C, Comelli M, Carlisi E, Sala V, Bejor M, Toffola ED. Quantitative measurement of

evolution of postparetic ocular synkinesis treated with botulinum toxin type a. Plast Reconstr Surg. 2013; 132(5):1255–64.
7. Choi KH, Rho SH, Lee JM, Jeon JH, Park SY, Kim J. Botulinum toxin injections of both sides of the face to treat post-paralytic facial synkinesis. J Plast Reconstr Aesthet Surg. 2013;66(8):1058–63.
8. Colosimo C, Tiple D, Berardelli A. Treatment of blepharospam. Manual of botulinum toxin therapy. Cambridge University Press; New York 2009. p. 49–52.
9. Das CP, Truong DD, Hallett M. Treatment of focal hand dystonia. Manual of botulinum toxin therapy. Cambridge University Press; New York 2009. p. 61–75.
10. Dressler D, Bigalke H. Pharmacology of botulinum toxin drugs. Manual of botulinum toxin therapy. Cambridge University Press; New York 2009. p. 13–22.
11. Frei K, Roggenkamper P. Treatment of hemifacial spasm. Manual of botulinum toxin therapy. Cambridge University Press; New York 2009. p. 43–47.
12. Frucht SJ. Embouchure dystonia – portrait of a task-specific cranial dystonia. Mov Disord. 2009;24(12): 1752–62.
13. Frucht SJ, Fahn S, Greene PE, O'Brien C, Gelb M, Truong DD, Welsh J, Facotr S, Ford B. The natural history of embouchure dystonia. Mov Disord. 2001;16(5):889–906.
14. Fung VSC, Jinnah HA, Bhati K, Vidailhet M. Assessment of patients with isolated or combined dystonia: an update on dystonia syndromes. Mov Disord. 2013;28(7):889–98.
15. Hong JS, Sathe GG, Niyonkuru C, Munin MC. Elimination of dysphagia using ultrasound guidance for botulinum toxin injections in cervical dystonia. Muscle Nerve. 2012;46(4):535–9.
16. Jankovic J. Medical treatment of dystonia. Mov Disord. 2013;28(7):1001–12.
17. Jedynak CP, Bonnet AM, Agid Y. Tremor and idiopathic dystonia. Mov Disord. 1991;6.230–6.
18. Jinnah HA, Berardelli A, Comella C, DeFazio G, DeLong MR, Factor S, Galpern WR, Hallett M, Ludlow CL, Perlmutter JS, Rosen AR. The focal dystonias: current views and challenges for future research. Mov Disord. 2013;28(7):926–43.
19. Mayer NH, Esquenazi A, Childers MK. Common patterns of clinical motor dysfunction. Spasticity: etiology, evaluation, management, and the role of botulinum toxin. In: Mayer NH, Simpson DM, editors. WE MOVE. 2002:16-26.
20. Nobrega AC, Rodrigues B, Melo A. Does botulinum toxin injection in parotid glands interfere with the swallowing dynamics of Parkinson's disease patients? Clin Neurol Neurosurg. 2009;111(5):430–2.
21. Pathak MS, Brashear A. Spasticity. Manual of botulinum toxin therapy. Cambridge University Press; New York 2009. p. 101–13.
22. Satoh M, Narita M, Tomimoto H. Three cases of focal embouchure dystonia: classifications and successful therapy using a dental splint. Eur Neurol. 2011;66(2): 85–90.
23. Scott AB. Botulinum toxin injection into extraocular muscles as an alternative to strabismus surgery. Ophthalmology. 1980;87:1044–9.
24. Seppi K, Weintraub D, Coelho M, Perez-Lloret S, Fox SH, Katzenschlager R, Hametner EM, Poewe W, Rascol C, Goetz CG, Sampaio C. The Movement Disorder Society evidence-based medicine review update: treatments for the non-motor symptoms of Parkinson's disease. Mov Disord. 2011;26 Suppl 3:S42–80.
25. Sheffield JK, Jankovic J. Botulinum toxin in tic disorders and essential hand and head tremor. Manual of botulinum toxin therapy. Cambridge University Press; New York 2009. p. 195–204.
26. Simpson DM, Blitzer A, Brashear A, Comella C, Dubinsky R, Hallett M, Jankovic J, Karp B, Ludlow CL, Miyasaki JM, Naumann M, So Y. Assessment: botulinum neurotoxin for the treatment of movement disorders (an evidence-based review): report of the Therapeutics and Technology Assessment Subcommittee of the American Academy of Neurology. Neurology. 2008; 70(19):1699–706.
27. Singer HS. Treatment of Tics and Tourette's syndrome. Curr Treat Options Neurol. 2010;12:539–61.
28. Stamelou M, Edwards MJ, Hallett M, Bhatia KP. The non-motor syndrome of primary dystonia: clinical and pathophysiological implications. Brain. 2012;135: 1668–81.
29. Thompson PD, Obeso JA, Delgado G, Gallego J, Marsden CD. Focal dystonia of the jaw and the differential diagnosis of unilateral jaw and masticatory spasm. J Neurol Neurosurg Psychiatry. 1986;49: 651–6.
30. Wang A, Jankovic J. Hemifacial spasm: clinical findings and treatment. Muscle Nerve. 1998;21(12): 1740–7.

Pantothenate Kinase-Associated Neurodegeneration

38

Susanne A. Schneider

Pantothenate kinase-associated neurodegeneration (PKAN) is a rare clinically complex genetic disorder and the most common form of the syndromes with neurodegeneration with brain iron accumulation (NBIA) [1]. This group of disorders is characterized by progressive motor dysfunction (often complicated by other features) and excessive iron deposition in the brain, particularly affecting the basal ganglia, mainly the globus pallidus (GP), detected radiologically and on brain pathology. The worldwide prevalence of PKAN is about 1:1,000,000, but regional clustering occurs (i.e., in the Dominican Republic, 1:10,000) due to founder effects.

38.1 Clinical Presentation: The Typical and Atypical Form

Three quarters of patients present in childhood (typical form) at a mean age of 3–4 years [2, 3]. Conversely, the average age at onset of atypical PKAN is in teenagehood (age 14); even adult onset has been described [4]. Typical presenting features in classical PKAN are clumsiness, gait abnormalities, and motor/global neurodevelopmental delay with development of dystonia (generalized, often with predominant oro-lingual-mandibular involvement) and spasticity. Two thirds of typical PKAN patients develop visual disturbance due to retinitis pigmentosa. Atypical PKAN may present with speech difficulties or neuropsychiatric features with only subtle dystonia. Compared to the classical form, motor involvement tends to be less severe. PKAN takes a progressive course with affected children usually becoming wheelchair bound within 10–15 years of diagnosis. Late-onset cases may take a more benign course.

38.2 Neuroimaging in PKAN

Neuroimaging using MRI [5, 6] (particularly the iron-sensitive T2*- and SWI-weighted MR images) typically demonstrates a characteristic imaging pattern referred to as "eye of the tiger sign." There is hypointensity due to iron accumulation in the anterior-medial part of the globus pallidus with a central hyperintensity (Fig. 38.1). Additional internal capsule, subthalamic, and nigral iron may occur [7, 8]. The development of the MRI alterations appears to be a dynamic process, and there is debate regarding the correlation

Electronic supplementary material The online version of this chapter (doi:10.1007/978-3-7091-1628-9_38) contains supplementary material, which is available to authorized users.

S.A. Schneider
Department of Neurology, University of München and University of Kiel, Feodor-Lynen-Str 19, München (Munich) 81377, Germany
e-mail: s.schneider@ucl.ac.uk; susanne.schneider@med.uni-muenchen.de

C. Falup-Pecurariu et al. (eds.), *Movement Disorders Curricula*,
DOI 10.1007/978-3-7091-1628-9_38

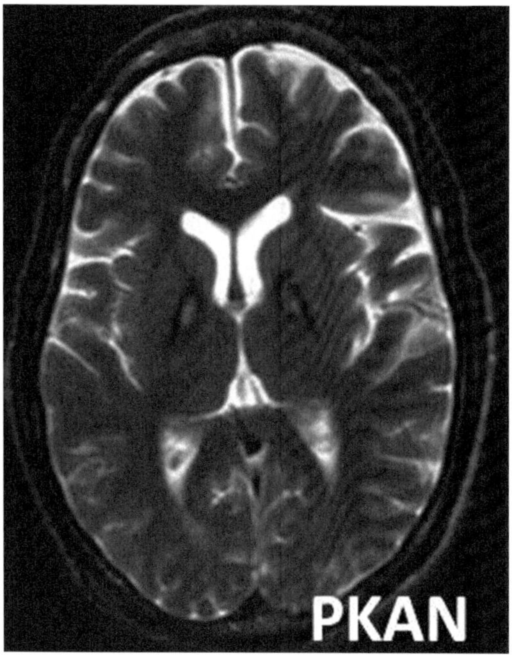

Fig. 38.1 Eye of the tiger sign as typically seen in PKAN patients on MRI

between the presence of the eye of the tiger sign and clinical findings. Imaging abnormalities may precede the development of clinical signs (i.e., in asymptomatic carriers of homozygous mutations) but, on the other hand, may also be absent in early disease stages, or the bright spot may vanish over time [1, 7, 9]. Thus, repeated MRI may be useful. Atypical globus pallidus calcifications on CT imaging have been reported in one case [10].

Diffusion tensor imaging showed increased fractional anisotropy and an abnormal mean diffusivity in globus pallidus and substantia nigra. Dopamine transporter (DaT) SPECT imaging is usually normal. Transcranial sonography demonstrates hyperechogenicity in the substantia nigra and lenticular nucleus.

38.3 Pathology in PKAN

Pathologically, PKAN affects the CNS, particularly the globus pallidus [11]. Cortex, brainstem, and remaining deep gray nuclei, optic nerves, and the cerebellum are spared, and there is only occasional peripheral manifestation. Key features are a significant burden of neuroaxonal spheroids (representing swollen dystrophic axons) and iron deposition (mainly as Fe^{3+} but also as Fe^{2+}). Notably, PKAN is not a synucleinopathy. Lewy bodies are absent.

38.4 Molecular Genetics of PKAN

PKAN is inherited in an autosomal recessive manner due to mutations in the *PANK2* gene located on chromosome 20p [12, 13]. Mutations, mostly missense, have been detected in all seven exons of the *PANK2* gene. Deletions, duplication, and splice site mutations as well as exon deletions have also been reported. Some mutations may be associated with milder phenotypes than others. Two common mutations (1231G > A and 1253C > T) account for about one third of all PKAN cases. Most of the remaining cases have "private mutations." Genotype-phenotype correlations for PKAN continue to be emerging.

38.5 Pathophysiology

The exact pathophysiology of PKAN remains poorly understood. The associated *PANK2*-encoded protein governs the first regulatory step of coenzyme A synthesis by catalyzing the phosphorylation of pantothenate (vitamin B5) to yield phosphopantothenate. Mitochondrial dysfunction and abnormal lipid metabolism may play a key role.

38.6 Therapy

Treatment remains symptomatic (i.e., anticholinergics, baclofen). Pantothenic acid (vitamin B5) does not produce benefit (personal communication) but a compound related to this pathway which may be more stable is under development [14]. Iron chelators (i.e., deferiprone) which reduce the amount of free iron are being explored [15] (for summary of use in PKAN, see [1]). However, while levels of brain iron may decrease as assessed by quantitative MRI, there is usually no or limited clinical benefit. Deep brain stimulation of the globus pallidus internus (DBS GPi) may produce some benefit by around 20 % in two thirds of patients but cannot influence the progressive nature of the disease (for review, see [1]).

References

1. Schneider SA, Dusek P, Hardy J, Westenberger A, Jankovic J, Bhatia KP. Genetics and pathophysiology of neurodegeneration with brain iron accumulation (NBIA). Curr Neuropharmacol. 2013;11:59–79.
2. Hayflick SJ. Neurodegeneration with brain iron accumulation: from genes to pathogenesis. Semin Pediatr Neurol. 2006;13:182–5.
3. Hayflick SJ, Westaway SK, Levinson B, et al. Genetic, clinical, and radiographic delineation of Hallervorden-Spatz syndrome. N Engl J Med. 2003;348:33–40.
4. Hayflick SJ. Unraveling the Hallervorden-Spatz syndrome: pantothenate kinase-associated neurodegeneration is the name. CurrOpinPediatr. 2003;15:572–7.
5. Kruer MC, Boddaert N, Schneider SA, et al. Neuroimaging features of neurodegeneration with brain iron accumulation. AJNR Am J Neuroradiol. 2012;33:407–14.
6. Amaral LL, Gaddikeri S, Chapman PR, et al. Neurodegeneration with brain iron accumulation: clinicoradiological approach to diagnosis. J Neuroimaging Off J Am Soc Neuroimaging. 2015;25:539–51.
7. Delgado RF, Sanchez PR, Speckter H, et al. Missense PANK2 mutation without "eye of the tiger" sign: MR findings in a large group of patients with pantothenate kinase-associated neurodegeneration (PKAN). J Magn Reson Imaging JMRI. 2012;35:788–94.
8. Fermin-Delgado R, Roa-Sanchez P, Speckter H, et al. Involvement of globus pallidus and midbrain nuclei in pantothenate kinase-associated neurodegeneration: measurement of T2 and T2* time. Clin Neuroradiol. 2013;23:11–5.
9. Hayflick SJ, Hartman M, Coryell J, Gitschier J, Rowley H. Brain MRI in neurodegeneration with brain iron accumulation with and without PANK2 mutations. AJNR Am J Neuroradiol. 2006;27:1230–3.
10. Wu YW, Hess CP, Singhal NS, Groden C, Toro C. Idiopathic basal ganglia calcifications: an atypical presentation of PKAN. Pediatr Neurol. 2013;49:351–4.
11. Kruer MC, Hiken M, Gregory A, et al. Novel histopathologic findings in molecularly confirmed pantothenate kinase-associated neurodegeneration. Brain. 2011;134:947–58.
12. Hartig MB, Hortnagel K, Garavaglia B, et al. Genotypic and phenotypic spectrum of PANK2 mutations in patients with neurodegeneration with brain iron accumulation. Ann Neurol. 2006;59:248–56.
13. Gregory A, Polster BJ, Hayflick SJ. Clinical and genetic delineation of neurodegeneration with brain iron accumulation. J Med Genet. 2009;46:73–80.
14. Srinivasan B, Baratashvili M, van der Zwaag M, et al. Extracellular 4′-phosphopantetheine is a source for intracellular coenzyme A synthesis. Nat Chem Biol. 2015;11:784–92.
15. Kalman B, Lautenschlaeger R, Kohlmayer F, et al. An international registry for neurodegeneration with brain iron accumulation. Orphanet J Rare Dis. 2012;7:66.

Movement Disorders of the Face

39

Mónica M. Kurtis

39.1 Motor Control of Facial Movements

In humans and primates, the orofacial motor region is represented in the primary motor cortex located on the lateral aspect of the precentral gyrus (Brodmann's area 4, M1). M1 is the main source of cortical motor output and utilizes somatosensory input from the primary somatosensory cortex located in the postcentral gyrus (Brodmann's areas 1, 2, 3a, and 3b) to control orofacial movements. These cortical areas are interconnected and function as a unit termed sensorimotor cortex. In their seminal work on the anatomy of the brain, Penfield and colleagues represented the somatotopic organization of the sensorimotor cortex with a homunculus that included a large orofacial region [1]. Recent studies with sensory evoked potentials, magnetoencephalography, positron-emission tomography, and functional magnetic resonance have confirmed these findings and provided more detailed mapping. Animal and human functional neuroimaging and neurophysiological investigations have also provided evidence for somatotopic organization at subcortical levels [2].

The complexity and variety of facial movements are the result of the integration of extensive face sensorimotor networks. The sensorimotor cortex receives both excitatory and inhibitory input from: (1) other cortical areas (premotor cortex, supplementary motor cortex, and cingulate cortex), (2) subcortical areas (thalamus, basal ganglia, and red nucleus), (3) the cerebellum, and (4) the brain stem (central generators; motor nuclei V, VII, and XII; and sensory nuclei V). Commissural fibers are responsible for bilateral coordination. Unlike skeletal muscles, most orofacial muscles have bilateral representations, thus projections to, and from, the sensorimotor cortex are mainly bilateral, with hemispheric dominance for some tasks and input reception.

It is well established that voluntary facial movements such as smiling, jaw opening, and closing are generated and under the control of M1. Evidence from the past two decades also points toward M1 involvement in automatic movements such as eye closing and semiautomatic movements such as chewing or swallowing (affected in many movement disorders), which classically have been considered under the control of brain stem generators. Mechanoreceptor input from the orofacial region S1 provides feedback that plays a crucial role for the control of elemental and semiautomatic

Electronic supplementary material The online version of this chapter (doi:10.1007/978-3-7091-1628-9_39) contains supplementary material, which is available to authorized users.

M.M. Kurtis
Movement Disorders Unit, Department of Neurology, Hospital Ruber Internacional,
Calle La Maso 38, Madrid 28034, Spain
e-mail: mkurtis@ruberinternacional.es

C. Falup-Pecurariu et al. (eds.), *Movement Disorders Curricula*,
DOI 10.1007/978-3-7091-1628-9_39

orofacial movements. Face S1 is connected with face M1 but also with subcortical motor circuits involved in orofacial motor function. These sensory motor circuits are dynamic and can undergo neuroplastic structural and functional changes induced by peripheral or central alterations as seen in dystonia [2].

39.2 Hypokinetic Movements

39.2.1 Hypomimia

Bradykinesia is a characteristic of Parkinson's disease (PD) and other parkinsonisms. When facial muscles are affected, the result is decreased spontaneous facial movements and loss of expression. Patients are described as having a "mask face" or "poker face" (since poker card players do not show any emotion during their game). The eyes develop a staring expression as the palpebral fissures become wider, the nasolabial folds are flattened, and the lips are involuntarily parted and the mouth left open (see Fig. 39.1a). Spontaneous orofacial movements such as smiling are reduced both in frequency and amplitude, and voluntary orofacial movements are also bradykinetic. With disease progression, the lips can remain open most of the time, and blink rate becomes severely decreased, leading to ocular problems such as dry eye. Clinical observation, neuroimaging, and neurophysiological studies indicate that separate, although partially overlapping, cortical and subcortical areas are involved in the generation of spontaneous, emotional, and voluntary facial movements. Thus, in hypomimia, it remains to be clarified whether the problem is purely motor or may also be related to depression, impairment in facial emotion imagery, or cognitive problems [3].

39.2.2 Hypomimia in Different Parkinsonian Syndromes

Neurophysiological studies have quantitatively characterized the kinematics of blinking in PD patients. Overall spontaneous blinking rate is reduced, and voluntary blinking is also impaired due to a prolonged interphase pause between the eye closing and opening phases. However, muscle contractions of the orbicularis oculi and levator palpebrae show normal velocity and amplitude [4]. In progressive supranuclear palsy (PSP), spontaneous blinking rate is markedly reduced and voluntary blinking is overtly bradykinetic. The interphase pause between the closing and opening of the eyes is prolonged not only during voluntary blinking as in PD but also during reflex blinking [5]. Neurophysiological data is lacking for other parkinsonian syndromes such as multiple system atrophy (MSA) or corticobasal degeneration. Increased blinking can also be seen in any type of parkinsonism, since blepharospasm can represent a form of secondary dystonia or of levodopa-induced dysinesias.

Detailed observation of the phenomenology of hypomimia can aid the differential diagnosis of PD and other types of parkinsonisms. In PD, hypomimia is usually bilateral and symmetrical, but hemihypomimia affecting the facial side homolateral to the body side where PD started and is most symptomatic has also been described [6] and is possibly under reported since it goes unnoticed in clinical practice [7] (see Fig. 39.1c). Hypomimia improves with dopaminergic therapy and also during the rapid eye movement sleep phase [8] while the effect of subthalamic deep brain stimulation on facial expression is unclear [3].

PSP patients also have an expressionless face; however, they show deep nasolabial folds due to dystonic facial contractions. They can also show contraction of the frontalis, procerus, and corrugator muscle giving them a surprised look, characterized by vertical wrinkles in the glabellar region and bridge of the nose that has been called the procerus sign [9] (see Fig. 39.1b). Patients with neuroferritinopathy can show frontalis and platysma contractions that give them a startled look similar to that seen in PSP patients [10]. Characteristically patients with Wilson's disease have a sardonic smile produced by involuntary facial grimacing. These tonic contractions of the risorius may also be seen in MSA. Finally, hypomimia is a sign that can also be seen in depressed patients and this differential diagnosis must be kept in mind.

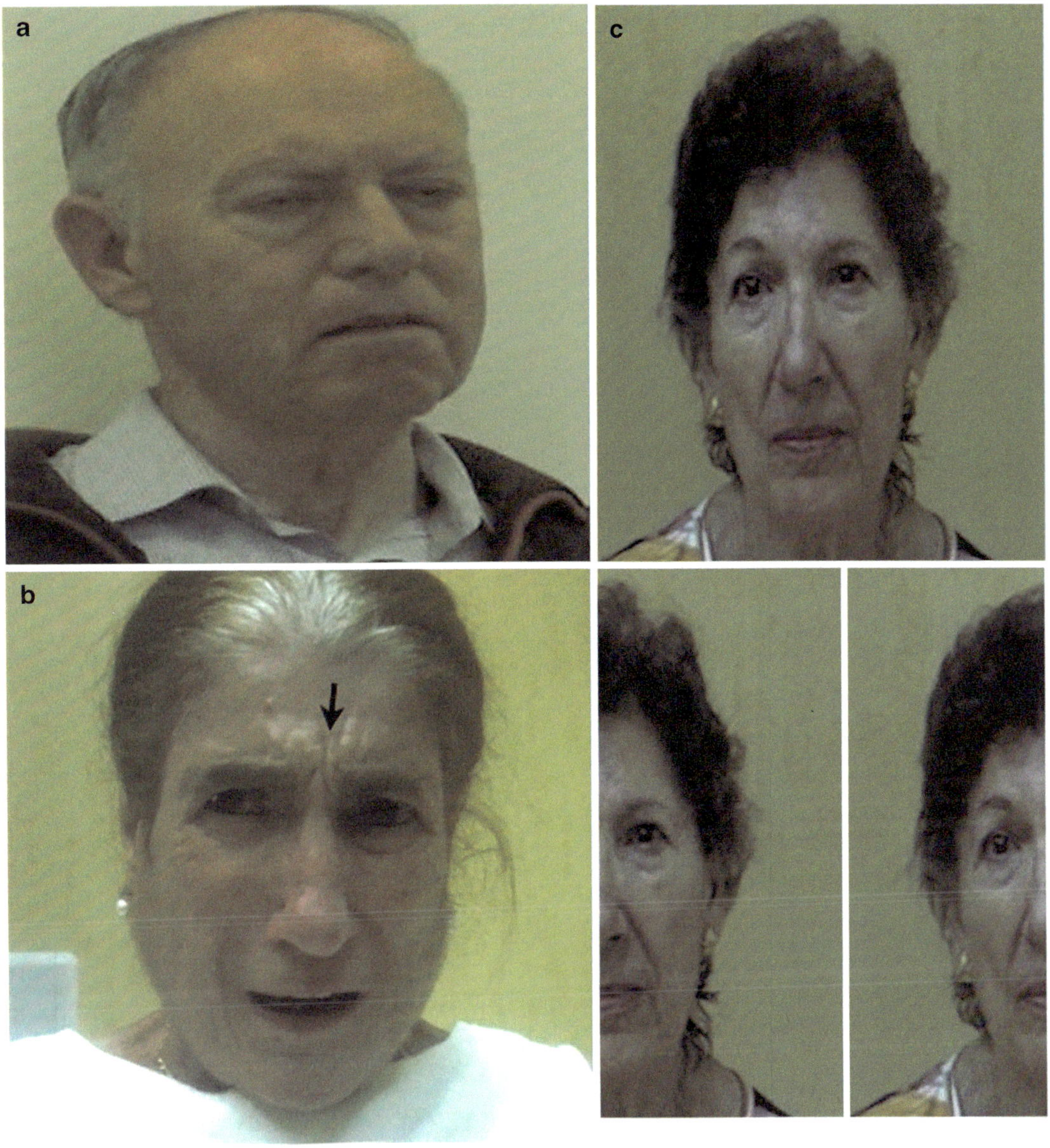

Fig. 39.1 Hypomimia. (**a**) PD patient, note the flattened nasolabial folds and involuntarily open mouth. (**b**) PSP parkinsonism patient, note the startled look and procerus sign. (**c**) PD Patient with hemihypomimia. The right nasolabial fold is less prominent in this woman with right-sided PD

39.3 Hyperkinetic Movements

39.3.1 Dystonia

Dystonia is characterized by intermittent or sustained muscle contractions that lead to stereotyped, repetitive, and twisting movements. This classic definition is based on limb and trunk phenomenology. When dystonia affects facial muscles, there are no twisting postures but stereotyped, intermittent, repetitive, and tonic contractions of the upper or lower facial muscles that can be unilateral or bilateral (see Tables 39.1 and 39.2).

Blepharospasm is defined as involuntary spasms of the muscles that close the eyes (orbicularis oculi, corrugator, and procerus). It is one of the most common focal dystonias with a reported

Table 39.1 Clinical features of hyperkinetic movements affecting the eyelids/eyebrows

Condition	Pattern	Activation	Typical features	Other features
Blepharospasm	Bilateral Repetitive Stereotyped	Spontaneous Bright light Walking	Charcot's sign Sensory trick	Dystonia of other body parts
Apraxia of eyelid opening	Bilateral Stereotyped	Voluntary eye opening Bright light Looking up	Drooping eyelids No obvious orbicularis oculi contraction with frontalis contraction	Sensory tricks Responds to pretarsal botulinum toxin injections
Apraxia of eyelid closing	Bilateral	Voluntary eye closing		
Hemifacial spasm	Unilateral Clonic or tonic Stereotyped	Lying down	Other Babinski sign Synkinesias	Primary (arterial loop) Secondary to facial palsy
Huntington's chorea	Bilateral Non-stereotyped		Forehead wrinkling Raising eyebrows	Slow saccades Chorea in other body parts Family history
Neuroferritinopathy	Bilateral Fixed	Spontaneous	Contraction of frontalis	Family history
PSP	Spontaneous Fixed	Spontaneous	Contraction of frontalis	

prevalence of 5–13 per 100,000 people. Age of onset is usually in the fifth to seventh decade and it affects women more than men by a 3:1 ratio [11]. It is usually bilateral, although it can be asymmetric, and severity can vary, ranging from mildly increased blinking rate to continuous forced closure leading to functional blindness. Patients report worsening with luminous stimuli (sunlight, television) and sometimes with motor tasks such as walking or driving. On the other hand, blepharospasm can improve with mouth movements such as talking, chewing gum, or humming and with sensory tricks like touching the temple or eyelid. A clinical sign to look for that may help differentiate blepharospasm from other involuntary eye closing movements is the Charcot's sign, in which the eyebrow descends below the superior orbital rim with each eye closure spasm (see Fig. 39.2a). The differential diagnosis should be made with other disorders that may show similar phenomenology such as eyelid opening apraxia, hemifacial spasm (see Fig. 39.2), motor tics, psychogenic movements, and muscle disorders like ocular myasthenia gravis and orbicularis oculi neuromyotonia.

The most common etiology is idiopathic (termed primary or essential blepharospasm) although approximately 20 % of cases have a positive family history of dystonia, supporting the hypothesis that focal dystonia is an autosomal disease with reduced penetrance [12, 13]. However, there are well-established secondary causes such as drug-induced tardive dystonia, Parkinson's disease and other forms of parkinsonism, and basal ganglia, thalamus, or brain stem lesions.

Apraxia of eyelid opening is characterized by drooping eyelids and the transient inability to voluntarily open the eyes in the absence of overt orbicularis oculi contraction. The use of this terminology is confusing and used to describe any patient who shows clinical difficulties in opening the eyes upon command or voluntarily, with preserved spontaneous opening. However, it is very rarely a true apraxia [14] as it generally represents a form of dystonia that can occur in isolation or coexist with blepharospasm. Like other forms of dystonia, it can be seen in the context of a parkinsonian syndrome (particularly PSP) and has been reported as a secondary effect of subthalamic deep brain stimulation [15]. In the isolated form, there is reduced blinking,

Table 39.2 Clinical features of hyperkinetic movements affecting the lower face ± upper face

Disorder	Movement pattern	Activation/suppression	Typical features	Other features
Oromandibular dystonia	Stereotypic Bilateral (can be asymmetric)	Spontaneous Triggered by eating, speaking	Dystonic tremor Sensory tricks	Jaw closing more frequent than jaw opening
Craniocervical dystonia	Stereotypic Bilateral	Spontaneous Triggered by eating, speaking	Sensory tricks Upper and lower face	Often spread from upper to lower face
Tardive dyskinesias	Stereotypic Bilateral	Spontaneous Improve with eating, speaking	Oro-buccolingual muscles	History of exposure to neuroleptics Dyskinesias in toes
Levodopa-induced dyskinesias in PD	Random Bilateral	Spontaneous Worsen with eating or speaking	Upper and lower facial muscles	Dyskinesias in other body parts Worse in young patients
Levodopa-induced dyskinesias in MSA	Stereotypic Bilateral	Worsen with speaking	Risus sardonicus	No dyskinesias in other body parts
Edentulous dyskinesias	Stereotypic Bilateral (can be asymmetric)	Disappear when dentures are removed	Loose dentures	No dyskinesias in other body parts
Neuroacanthocytosis McLeod syndrome	Random Bilateral	Worsen with eating	Oro-buccal dystonia and dyskinesias Tongue biting, mouth lesions	Possible family history Acanthocytes Myopathy
Tics	Stereotypic Unilateral or Bilateral	Spontaneous Sensory prodrome	Partial voluntary suppression	Tics in other body parts
Psychogenic movement disorders	Unilateral > Bilateral	Improve with speaking and distraction	Lower jaw/lip deviation Tonic spasms	Acute onset Precipitant Depression
Lgi1 antibody limbic encephalitis	Unilateral Alternating	Spontaneous	Faciobrachial jerks	Acute onset Precludes encephalitis

no evident forceful closure of the eyes, and frequent involuntary drooping of the eyelids. When trying to open the eyes, the patient contracts the frontalis muscle with secondary elevation of the brows and sometimes opens the mouth in a conscious effort to break eye closure (see Fig. 39.2b).

Many patients can use sensory tricks such as touching the eyelid to initiate eye opening and triggers such as bright light and certain actions have been described. Electrophysiological studies show that these patients exhibit co-contraction of the levator palpebrae and the pretarsal portion of the orbicularis oculi (thus it is sometimes called pretarsal or atypical blepharospasm) which impedes voluntary eye opening [16]. These patients are often refractory to traditional blepharospasm botulinum toxin regimens which involve the orbitary portion of the orbicularis oculi and should be injected in the pretarsal portion [13, 17]. However, a small percentage of patients with eyelid opening dysfunction do not exhibit dystonic features on EMG studies. These patients present inappropriate inhibition or delayed response of the levator palpebrae muscle without abnormal activity of any of the portions of the orbicularis oculi and thus do not respond to botulinum toxin injections.

Apraxia of eyelid closure is an uncommon movement disorder of the eyelids that is characterized by transient inability to close the eyelids voluntarily. It is considered a supranuclear lid

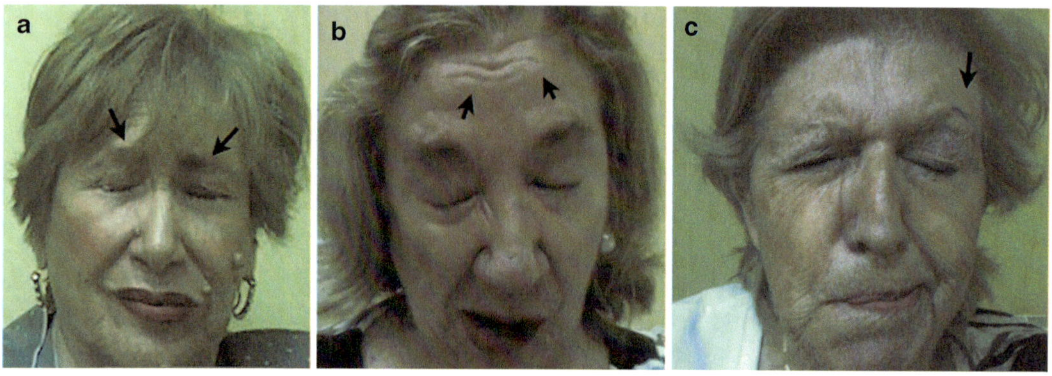

Fig. 39.2 Abnormal eyelid closure. (**a**) Blepharospasm. Depression of the brow (Charcot's sign, see *arrow*) during spasm. (**b**) Apraxia of eyelid opening. Contraction of the frontalis muscles (see *arrow*) with no obvious contraction of the orbicularis oculi. Attempting to open the eyes voluntarily, the person elevate eyebrows and open the mouth. (**c**) Hemifacial spasm. Contraction of the frontalis ipsilateral to the facial spasm (the other Babinski sign, see *arrow*)

dysfunction and can be seen in the context of parkinsonian syndromes (particularly PSP) and right-sided cortical frontal lesions. There is no effective treatment and patients overcome the difficulty by activating other muscles much like in apraxia of eyelid opening [10].

Oromandibular dystonia is characterized by spasms of the masticatory muscles (masseter, temporal, and pterygoid muscles) that produce repetitive, jaw-closing movements. As in other forms of dystonia, the movements characteristically worsen with action and can thus interfere with speaking, swallowing, and eating and can show concomitant dystonic tremor in the affected orolingual structures. Patients can respond to sensory tricks and in some, oral appliances that mimic these tricks can be useful. Less frequently, the lateral pterygoid and digastric muscles are affected, resulting in prominent jaw-opening dystonia. This less common form has a worse prognosis since the muscles involved are less accessible and show only a partial response to botulinum toxin [18]. The etiology is most commonly primary but it can also be found in certain choreas (neuroacanthocytosis), and drug-induced oromandibular mouth dystonia is the second most common drug-induced movement disorder in the geriatric population after oro-buccolingual dyskinesias (see below).

Craniocervical dystonia can occur in 50 % of patients with onset of dystonia in the eyelids (blepharospasm), as dystonia spreads to the lower facial, masticatory, lingual, pharyngeal, laryngeal, and/or cervical muscles [19]. The risk of spread is particularly increased within the first 3 years of initial symptoms. This segmental dystonia has been called various eponymic terms such as Meige and Brueghel syndromes but is probably best defined as craniocervical dystonia. As in other forms of dystonia, sensory tricks may be useful, such as touching the orbital region, biting a toothpick, or chewing gum.

As in blepharospasm, it is more prevalent in women (2 females to 1 male ratio) and the most common etiology is primary. However signs of spinocerebellar ataxia and PSP must be examined, and a careful medical history should rule out the possibility of a pharmacological origin (see Video 39.1). Primary genetic dystonias that may show some form of craniocervical dystonia include DYT1 (torsinA), DYT3 (TAF1), and DYT6 (THAP1) [20] and the recently discovered DYT24 (ANO·) and DYT25 (GNAL) [21].

39.3.2 Drug-Induced Dyskinesias

Oro-buccolingual dyskinesias are the most common form of tardive dyskinesias. They are characterized by involuntary, repetitive, stereotyped movements that affect the lower facial muscles resulting in a combination of frowning, smiling, lip puckering, lip smacking, sucking, and tongue protrusion. They tend to improve with voluntary muscle movements such as talking or eating (see Video 39.1) (see Table 39.1).

Levodopa-induced dyskinesias can also affect the facial muscles. They often coexist with dystonia such as blepharospasm and dyskinesias in other body parts. They are characterized by upper and lower face involvement producing excessive blinking, raising of the eyebrows, and orolingual movements. About 40 % of patients with Parkinson's disease develop dyskinesias after 5 years of treatment, and they are more prominent and disabling in young-onset patients [22]. In MSA patients, levodopa-induced dyskinesias tend to affect the lower face and platysma resembling risus sardonicus, and there is a notable absence of dyskinesias in other body parts [23] (see Table 39.1).

39.3.3 Chorea

From the Greek, to dance, chorea is characterized by irregular, sinusoidal, non-stereotypical movements anywhere in the trunk, limbs, or face that are superimposed on to voluntary movements.

Huntington's disease (HD) is the most frequent hereditary chorea, showing an autosomic dominantly inherited pattern with complete penetrance. It is produced by the expansion of CAG (>35 triplet repetitions) in gene IT15. It is characterized by slow saccades (loss of saccades as the disease progresses), dysarthria, dysphagia, chorea, dystonia, tics, parkinsonism, and psychiatric and behavioral problems that can be devastating. As far as facial movements, HD involves the forehead and eyebrows more than the perioral musculature (see Table 39.1).

Neuroferritinopathy is an autosomal dominantly transmitted condition with onset in adulthood characterized pathologically by neurodegeneration with brain iron accumulation. It is caused by a mutation of the gene encoding the ferritin light chain polypeptide, which causes an abnormal structure and function of ferritin. Resulting abnormal iron deposition can be visualized by brain magnetic resonance imaging in the substantia nigra, red nucleus, pallidum, and/or motor cortex. The most common clinical manifestations are chorea, followed by focal dystonia and parkinsonism, while cognition is relatively intact. Patients often show dystonic contractions of the frontalis muscles (similar to PSP). In the first years of the disease course, they develop hypophonia and dysarthria due to bulbar involvement and oro-buccal dyskinesias (particularly with slow tongue movement) [24] (see Table 39.1).

Neuroacanthocytosis is an autosomic recessively inherited condition due to mutations in the chorein gene. It is characterized by chorea, tics, dystonia, parkinsonism, dementia, seizures, and peripheral axonal neuropathy. Patients show characteristic oro-buccal dystonia and dyskinesias that result in grimacing movements, with lip biting, tongue protrusion, and vocalizations that can be very disabling since they interfere with feeding. Blood tests typically show elevated liver enzymes, elevated creatine-kinase, and the presence of acanthocytes on a blood smear. McLeod syndrome is an X-linked disease due to a mutation in the XK gene that shows similar neurological symptoms to neuroacanthocytosis with similar progressive oro-buccal dystonia. However, it can also lead systemic alterations with myocardiopathy, myopathy with muscle wasting, and anemia due to hemolysis (see Table 39.1).

39.3.4 Tics

Motor tics are sudden, abrupt, transient, and often repetitive coordinated movements (stereotypic) that resemble gestures and fragments of normal behavior. They vary in intensity and can occur at irregular intervals. They can occur in isolation or as part of Tourette syndrome, a neurological disorder with childhood onset that is manifested by motor and vocal tics as well as a realm of psychiatric-behavioral problems. Motor tics commonly involve facial muscles, producing blinking, raising of the eye brows, grimacing, tongue movements, nose twitching, and platysma contractions (see Video 39.2). In fact, the phenotype of adult TS is dominated by facial, neck, and trunk tics, when compared to children [25]. Blink reflex and startle reflex studies disclose an increased excitability of brain stem interneurons in patients with tics [26].

Facial tics can mimic any other movement disorder: stereotypies when they involve lip smacking/licking or facial grimacing, dystonia when movements involve sustained or repetitive contractions, dyskinesias when they affect the orobuccal region, hemifacial spasm if they involve half the face, or myoclonus when they are very brief and quick. Although they can occur in isolation, a clue to the diagnosis of tics is the presence of movements in other parts of the body or the eyes (darting of the eyes or sustained eye deviation), their partial or complete suppression with effort and their stereotyped pattern (see Table 39.1).

39.3.5 Myoclonus

Positive myoclonus is a phenomenologic term for sudden, brief, jerky, irregular involuntary movements caused by abnormal muscle contractions that can be seen in the face as well as other body parts. Facial myoclonus can originate from several levels of the neural axis: the cortex, subcortex (mainly the brain stem), and peripheral nerves. Neurophysiological characterization of myoclonic spasms is key in determining the topography of the myoclonic generator.

Cortical myoclonus is commonly generalized or multifocal and shows irregular 25–50 ms muscle activity on EMG recording. This type of myoclonus can be seen in postanoxic patients, where action myoclonus of the face, particularly during speech, and blepharoclonus during blinking are typical findings. Facial cortical myoclonus has also been described in Creutzfeldt-Jakob disease and the serotoninergic syndrome [10]. Facial myoclonus can also represent the main manifestation of focal epilepsy or the beginning of a generalized seizure.

Brain stem myoclonus can also generate facial twitching and generally show longer muscle activation patterns (100–400 ms). Brain stem reticular myoclonus starts in the muscles innervated by the lower brain stem and then spreads up the brain stem and down the spinal cord, and this can be detected by polymyography. Brain stem reticular myoclonus is commonly stimulus sensitive and is also referred to as reticular reflex myoclonus. In startle syndrome, the movement is an exaggerated form of a physiologic startle response. The physiologic startle response is a myoclonic movement that is triggered by unexpected auditory, somatosensory, or visual stimuli and involves facial muscles. It consists of a simultaneous blink, contortion of the face, flexion of the neck and trunk, and abduction and flexion of the arm and looks like a jump. In startle syndrome, the movement is an exaggerated form of physiologic startle response, and patients show increased sensitivity or lack of habituation to triggers. The movement of startle syndrome is thought to arise from the generator of the physiologic startle response in the medial bulbopontine reticular formation [27]. When the startle syndrome is hereditary, it is called hyperekplexia, of which most cases are caused by mutations in the gene encoding the α1 subunit of the inhibitory glycine receptor [28].

Hemifacial spasm is the best known example of peripherally generated myoclonus and consists of involuntary very brief contractions of the ipsilateral upper and lower facial muscles (clonic hemifacial spasms). In some cases, movements are more sustained, the duration is beyond the myoclonic range [29], and the term used is tonic hemifacial spasm. In this type of hemifacial spasm, the healthy side of the face may seem paretic, but voluntary movements reveal synkinesias on the affected side [10]. The other Babinski sign [30] can be a helpful diagnostic clue to differentiate this entity from other abnormal facial movements (see Fig. 39.2). It involves the ipsilateral eyebrow rising during eye closure due to simultaneous contraction of the orbicularis oculi and the external part of the frontalis.

Primary facial spasm is most commonly caused by compression of the facial nerve as it exits the pons by an arterial loop of one of the inferior cerebellar arteries. Clinical onset is generally in the eyelid muscles, progressing to the lower face over the following months. Secondary facial spasm can result from Bell palsy or facial nerve or brain stem pathology. In these cases, most patients report simultaneous involvement of the upper and lower face (see Table 39.1).

Hereditary chin myoclonus, hereditary chin trembling, or geniospasm is a rare hereditary condition that involves brief, shock-like, pseudorhythmic involuntary contractions of the mentalis muscle resulting in spontaneous chin movements (dimpling of the chin) and quivering of the lower lip. These tremor/myoclonic-like movements may occur spontaneously or be grouped in episodes lasting minutes to hours. They are exacerbated by emotions and attenuated by alcohol intake. The condition runs in families following an autosomal dominant pattern with high penetrance, although the clinical manifestations can be heterogeneous [31, 32].

39.3.6 Tremors

Tremors are defined as oscillatory, rhythmic, and regular movements that can affect the limbs, neck, vocal cord, or chin.

Parkinsonian tremor of the jaw shows a characteristic 4–6 Hz frequency, is present at rest (defined as the state where the jaw is closed or the tongue is at rest on the floor of the mouth), and disappears when the patient moves the jaw to speak or eat. It is frequent in PD and has been described in postencephalitic parkinsonism but not in atypical parkinsonisms such as MSA or PSP [33].

ET tremor of the jaw can range in frequency from 4 to 10 Hz and shows similar characteristics to tremor of the limbs as it is induced by actions such as speaking, swallowing, drinking, or eating. It is present in up to 20 % of patients with essential tremor [33].

Position or task-specific orolingual tremors have also been described. By definition the tremors appear exclusively during a task or certain position of the orolingual structures. Orthostatic tremor of the jaw showing high-frequency 13–18 Hz tremors has also been reported.

Rabbit syndrome is a form of tardive tremor that involves the perioral muscles at rest, showing vertical oscillations that mimic the chewing actions of a rabbit. Other tardive tremors can involve the jaw and vary in frequency from 2 to 6 Hz [33].

Myorhythmia of the jaw is a slow 1–2 Hz oscillation of the jaw. When synchronous with convergence oscillations of the eyes (oculomasticatory myorhythmia), it is pathognomonic of Whipple's disease.

39.4 Psychogenic Movement Disorders

The phenotype of psychogenic facial movement disorders is widely variable, but a recent multicenter retrospective study has given some insight on the most common characteristics of psychogenic movement disorders [34]. Of the 61 patients included in the study, all showed phasic or tonic spasms simulating dystonia, more often involving the lips and the eyelids than the perinasal region or the forehead. As in other psychogenic movements, onset was usually acute, and in more than half of the patients, a precipitating psychological stress was identified. The incidence was much higher in women (>90 %) and the most prevalent comorbidities were depression and tension headache.

The lower face was most commonly affected, with a characteristic fixed jaw and/or lip downward deviation pattern resembling unilateral oromandibular dystonia. The spasms occurred in isolation or with other facial, platysma, or limb spasms. Some psychogenic movement disorders with unilateral involvement may resemble hemifacial spasm, but these patients show asynchronous tonic contraction in the ipsilateral lower and upper face or synchronous contractions of the lower face, as opposed to the synchronous clonic or tonic contractions in the lower and upper face found in hemifacial spasm. In the series described by Fasano et al. [34], no patients showed the other Babinski sign.

Generally, the historical and clinical data are enough to make a positive diagnosis. Some useful clinical signs to keep in mind are that psychogenic facial movements generally do not increase with actions such as speaking, they do not improve with sensory tricks, and the clinical presentation is usually asymmetric (see Table 39.1).

39.5 Other Abnormal Facial Movements to Keep in the Differential Diagnosis

39.5.1 Affecting the Eyelids

Myokymia of facial muscles is characterized by a continuous, undulating, rippling motion that may be rhythmic and action induced. The most common form occurs in the lower orbicularis oculi and is associated with fatigue. But it has been described as a symptom of pontine lesions and can also be seen in spinocerebellar degenerations (SCA3) and neuromyotonia. It shows characteristic doublet or triplet motor unit discharges on EMG [10].

Myotonia is characterized by delayed muscle relaxation and can affect facial muscles as well as other body parts. Eyelid myotonia and delay in opening can be seen in myotonia congenita and in hypocalcemic periodic paralysis. On EMG, high-frequency muscle discharges are detected.

Neuromyotonia is characterized by continuous motor unit activity with impaired relaxation after contraction due to peripheral nerve hyperexcitability. It can affect facial muscles causing eye closure, grimacing, and platysma, as well as other limb muscles.

Eyelid myoclonia with absences, or Jeavons syndrome, is a generalized epileptic condition clinically characterized by eyelid myoclonia with or without absences, eye closure-induced electroencephalography paroxysms, and photosensitivity; in addition, rare tonic-clonic seizures may also occur.

39.5.2 Affecting the Mouth and Jaw

Edentulous oral dyskinesias are typical of older patients with ill-fitting dentures. They involve stereotypical movements of the lips, jaw, and sometimes the tongue that can resemble tardive dyskinesias. The diagnostic clue is that they disappear when the dentures are removed (see Video 39.3). Treatment involves denture insertion and occlusal treatment (see Table 39.1).

Voltage-gated potassium channel (VGKC) complex/leucine-rich glioma-inactivated-1 (Lgi1) antibody limbic encephalitis produces characteristic (possibly pathognomonic) faciobrachial movements [35]. With a distinctive adult onset, these patients show frequent (up to hundreds), brief dystonic attacks predominantly affecting the arm and ipsilateral face that have been termed "faciobrachial seizures." The contractions can be brief and shock-like, within the 50–200 ms duration of myoclonus, or present as longer duration dystonic-like spasms. They can occur bilaterally, but each event only involves one side. Most patients develop these movements prior to full-blown encephalitic symptoms like amnesia, sleep-wake cycle alterations, and confusion. In their seminal article, Irani et al. [35] found that only 25 % of their patients showed evidence of ictal or interictal epileptiform activity and that antiepileptic drugs were not efficacious. The debate is ongoing as to whether these movements represent seizures, thus having a cortical origin, or if they should be described as hemidystonia or myoclonus and probably involve a subcortical origin [36]. In any case, the very characteristic semiology should be recognized and followed by prompt testing for VGKC complex/Lgi1 antibodies in blood and spinal fluid and appropriate immunotherapy started to prevent cognitive decline and possible death (see Table 39.1).

Hemimasticatory spasm is a rare condition that is characterized by unilateral contraction and hypertrophy of the masseter and temporalis muscles causing bruxism, pain, and tongue biting. It can occur in isolation, with hemifacial atrophy, or concomitantly with scleroderma (Parry-Romberg syndrome). The clinical suspicion can be confirmed by EMG which shows high-frequency discharges. It generally shows a good response to botulinum toxin injections. In contrast to unilateral oromandibular dystonia, there are signs of connective tissue alterations, pain is a salient symptom, and it does not respond to sensory tricks [10].

References

1. Penfield W, Rasmussen T. The cerebral cortex of man. New York: Macamillan. 1950
2. Avivi-Arber L, Martin R, Lee JC, Sessle BJ. Face sensorimotor cortex and its neuroplasticity related to orofacial sensorimotor functions. Arch Oral Biol. 2011;56(12):1440–65.
3. Bologna M, Fabbrini G, Marsili L, Defazio G, Thompson PD, Berardelli A. Facial bradykinesia. J Neurol Neurosurg Psychiatry. 2013;84(6):681–5.
4. Agostino R, Bologna M, Dinapoli L, Gregori B, Fabbrini G, Accornero N, et al. Voluntary, spontaneous, and reflex blinking in Parkinson's disease. Mov Disord. 2008;23(5):669–75.
5. Bologna M, Agostino R, Gregori B, Belvisi D, Ottaviani D, Colosimo C, et al. Voluntary, spontaneous and reflex blinking in patients with clinically probable progressive supranuclear palsy. Brain. 2009;132(Pt 2):502–10.
6. Ozekmekci S, Benbir G, Ozdogan FY, Ertan S, Kiziltan ME. Hemihypomimia, a rare persistent sign in Parkinson's disease: follow up of 11 patients. J Neurol. 2007;254(3):347–50.
7. Crosiers D, Marechal E, van Ael Y, Cras P. Left-sided hemihypomimia in Parkinson's disease. Acta Neurol Belg. 2011;111(3):225–7.
8. De Cock VC, Vidailhet M, Leu S, Texeira A, Apartis E, Elbaz A, et al. Restoration of normal motor control in Parkinson's disease during REM sleep. Brain. 2007;130(Pt 2):450–6.
9. Romano S, Colosimo C. Procerus sign in progressive supranuclear palsy. Neurology. 2001;57(10):1928.
10. Fabbrini G, Defazio G, Colosimo C, Thompson PD, Berardelli A. Cranial movement disorders: clinical features, pathophysiology, differential diagnosis and treatment. Nat Clin Pract Neurol. 2009;5(2):93–105.
11. Ross AH, Elston JS, Marion MH, Malhotra R. Review and update of involuntary facial movement disorders presenting in the ophthalmological setting. Surv Ophthalmol. 2011;56(1):54–67.
12. Jankovic J, Orman J. Blepharospasm: demographic and clinical survey of 250 patients. Ann Ophthalmol. 1984;16(4):371–6.
13. Defazio G, Livrea P, De Salvia R, Manobianca G, Coviello V, Anaclerio D, et al. Prevalence of primary blepharospasm in a community of Puglia region. Southern Italy Neurol. 2001;56(11):1579–81.
14. Zadikoff C, Lang AE. Apraxia in movement disorders. Brain. 2005;128(Pt 7):1480–97.
15. Krack P, Batir A, Van Blercom N, Chabardes S, Fraix V, Ardouin C, et al. Five-year follow-up of bilateral stimulation of the subthalamic nucleus in advanced Parkinson's disease. N Engl J Med. 2003;349(20):1925–34.
16. Elston JS. A new variant of blepharospasm. J Neurol Neurosurg Psychiatry. 1992;55(5):369–71.
17. Forget R, Tozlovanu V, Iancu A, Boghen D. Botulinum toxin improves lid opening delays in blepharospasm-associated apraxia of lid opening. Neurology. 2002;58(12):1843–6.
18. Hallett M, Albanese A, Dressler D, Segal KR, Simpson DM, Truong D, et al. Evidence-based review and assessment of botulinum neurotoxin for the treatment of movement disorders. Toxicon. 2013;67:94–114.
19. Abbruzzese G, Berardelli A, Girlanda P, Marchese R, Martino D, Morgante F, et al. Long-term assessment of the risk of spread in primary late-onset focal dystonia. J Neurol Neurosurg Psychiatry. 2008;79(4):392–6.
20. LeDoux MS. Meige syndrome: what's in a name? Parkinsonism Relat Disord. 2009;15(7):483–9.
21. Balint B, Bhatia KP. Dystonia: an update on phenomenology, classification, pathogenesis and treatment. Curr Opin Neurol. 2014;27(4):468–76.
22. Luquin MR, Scipioni O, Vaamonde J, Gershanik O, Obeso JA. Levodopa-induced dyskinesias in Parkinson's disease: clinical and pharmacological classification. Mov Disord. 1992;7(2):117–24.
23. Wenning GK, Colosimo C, Geser F, Poewe W. Multiple system atrophy. Lancet Neurol. 2004;3(2):93–103.
24. Lehn A, Boyle R, Brown H, Airey C, Mellick G. Neuroferritinopathy. Parkinsonism Relat Disord. 2012;18(8):909–15.
25. Jankovic J, Gelineau Kattner R, Davidson A. Tourette's syndrome in adults. Mov Disord. 2010;25(13):2171–5.
26. Berardelli A, Curra A, Fabbrini G, Gilio F, Manfredi M. Pathophysiology of tics and Tourette syndrome. J Neurol. 2003;250(7):781–7.
27. Brown P. Neurophysiology of the startle syndrome and hyperekplexia. Adv Neurol. 2002;89:153–9.
28. Andermann F, Andermann E. Startle disorders of man: hyperekplexia, jumping and startle epilepsy. Brain Dev. 1988;10(4):213–22.
29. Nielsen VK. Electrophysiology of the facial nerve in hemifacial spasm: ectopic/ephaptic excitation. Muscle Nerve. 1985;8(7):545–55.

30. Stamey W, Jankovic J. The other Babinski sign in hemifacial spasm. Neurology. 2007;69(4):402–4.
31. Danek A. Geniospasm: hereditary chin trembling. Mov Disord. 1993;8(3):335–8.
32. Devetag Chalaupka F, Bartholini F, Mandich G, Turro M. Two new families with hereditary essential chin myoclonus: clinical features, neurophysiological findings and treatment. Neurol Sci. 2006;27(2):97–103.
33. Silverdale MA, Schneider SA, Bhatia KP, Lang AE. The spectrum of orolingual tremor – a proposed classification system. Mov Disord. 2008;23(2):159–67.
34. Fasano A, Valadas A, Bhatia KP, Prashanth LK, Lang AE, Munhoz RP, et al. Psychogenic facial movement disorders: clinical features and associated conditions. Mov Disord. 2012;27(12):1544–51.
35. Irani SR, Michell AW, Lang B, Pettingill P, Waters P, Johnson MR, et al. Faciobrachial dystonic seizures precede Lgi1 antibody limbic encephalitis. Ann Neurol. 2011;69(5):892–900.
36. Striano P. Faciobrachial dystonic attacks: seizures or movement disorder? Ann Neurol. 2011;70(1):179–80.

Drug-Induced Movement Disorders

40

Mário-Miguel Rosa and Ana-Marta Anes

40.1 Introduction

Drug-induced movement disorders (DIMD) are characterized by abnormal involuntary movements associated to drugs. Since the introduction in clinical practice of the first dopamine receptor-blocking agents (DRBA) in the 1950s and their widespread use in the decades after in psychiatric illness and other diseases or symptoms, they became relatively common neurological disorders. Moreover these adverse events become part of the complex disease we often need to treat, such as LDOPA-induced chorea or motor fluctuations in PD, leading to significant therapeutic challenges. There are no absolute figures on frequency of DIMD, as they depend upon the population treated (e.g., children vs elderly), the use of medication, classification criteria, and the easiness of reporting [1, 2]. In spite of these limitations, some publications report values as high as 60 % for parkinsonism signs in schizophrenia-treated patients [3, 4].

M.-M. Rosa (✉)
Laboratory of Clinical Pharmacology and Therapeutics, Lisbon Faculty of Medicine, University of Lisbon, Lisbon 1649-028, Portugal

Clinical Pharmacology Unit, Instituto de Medicina Molecular, Lisbon 1649-028, Portugal
e-mail: mrosa@medicina.ulisboa.pt

A.-M. Anes
Laboratory of Clinical Pharmacology and Therapeutics, Lisbon Faculty of Medicine, University of Lisbon, Lisbon 1649-028, Portugal
e-mail: anamartaanes@sapo.pt

40.2 Drug-Induced Adverse Events

The World Health Organization defines an adverse event as "a response to a drug which is noxious and unintended, and which occurs at doses normally used in man for the prophylaxis, diagnosis, or therapy of disease, or for the modifications of physiological function" [5]. Some regulatory agencies such as the European Medicines Agency have broadened the definition to include cases of overdose, self-administration, or off-label use, by just considering "a response to a medicinal product which is noxious and unintended" [6].

Drug-induced adverse events are usually classified by type [7]:

- Type A: Exaggerated pharmacological response (e.g., tetrabenazine-induced parkinsonism)
- Type B: Nonpharmacological, often allergic, or idiosyncratic response (e.g., clozapine-induced aplastic anemia or DRBA-induced NMS)

C. Falup-Pecurariu et al. (eds.), *Movement Disorders Curricula*,
DOI 10.1007/978-3-7091-1628-9_40

- Type C: Continuous or long term (time related) (e.g., weight gain or impulse control disorders on dopamine agonists for PD)
- Type D: Delayed (lag time) (e.g., LDOPA priming of motor fluctuations/chorea or tardive syndromes)
- Type E: Ending of use (withdrawal) (e.g., NMS-like upon abrupt LDOPA cessation in PD patients)
- Type F: Failure of efficacy (no response) (e.g., clonazepam failure to treat myoclonus)

Like all adverse events, most DIMD are type A. As such they are predictable and, in some cases, preventable. Early identification and implementation of counteracting measures may significantly decrease the burden of MIDM.

40.3 Drug-Induced Movement Disorder Mechanisms

Alterations in dopaminergic, cholinergic, serotonergic, gamma-aminobutyric acid (GABA), and sigma opiate receptor activity are believed to be responsible for most DIMD manifestations. This explains why there are several drug classes which are pointed as causal agents for these conditions.

For most DIMD dopamine pathways are consensually involved, but its role is not totally understood since it is unclear if dopamine activity is too low or too high in DIMD patients. If acute conditions associated with neuroleptic use seem to be caused by reduced dopaminergic transmission/blockade of dopamine receptors (especially D2 receptors), tardive signs and symptoms suggest dopaminergic excess caused by chronic dopamine blockade which can precipitate dopamine receptor hypersensitivity (by increased number and affinity of postsynaptic D2 dopamine receptors that occur after continued DRBA therapy). This proposed mechanism can also contribute to explain tardive chorea induced by levodopa in Parkinson disease patients. The atypical antipsychotics like clozapine and new-generation atypicals (risperidone, quetiapine, aripiprazole) are less likely to produce DIMD since they have a lower affinity to D2 receptors and a greater affinity to D1 and D4 receptors. New approaches such as metabotropic glutamate receptor 5 (mGlur5) agents may further decrease DIMD in psychiatric patients. Clinical experience, however, shows that DIMD risk, although decreased in frequency or intensity as compared to classic and older drugs, is not abolished. By the time of marketing authorization, all newly developed CNS agents have been related to some form of DIMD.

Complementary explanation regarding the pathophysiology of DIMD is that dopaminergic hypofunction results in a relative overactivity of cholinergic mechanisms. This is corroborated by the efficacy of anticholinergic drugs like biperiden or diphenhydramine (an antihistamine with anticholinergic properties) in reversing acute DRBA-induced dystonias [8, 9].

Additionally it is known that serotonin activity inhibits dopamine synthesis and dopaminergic neurons in the brain thereby contributing also to the installation of DIMD. This feature can explain movement disorders induced by antidepressants along to some ability of these agents like clomipramine to also block dopamine receptors. GABAergic hypofunction is also implicated in tardive dyskinesia, and adrenergic function influences movement and can explain tremor induced by β2-agonists.

Drug interactions are very frequent in the polymedicated and the elderly. They can be pharmacokinetic or pharmacodynamic in their nature and be implicated in the origin of DIMD. For instance, SSRI are frequently highly bound to proteins, and they may displace neuroleptics from their plasma binding freeing neuroleptics and consequent dopamine blockade, inducing parkinsonism when they are added to DRBA therapy [8]. Inhibition or induction of drug metabolism (such as specific CYP450 isoenzymes) is also another mechanism by which a medication may indirectly cause MD, by modification of the bioavailability of the agent.

For obvious reasons any combination of drugs whose mode of action enhances dopaminergic depletion or increase cholinergic or serotonergic activity may contribute to the onset of DIMD. Uptitration of drugs that share similar mechanisms of action may also be an important factor for the emergence of these conditions.

40.4 Risk Factors for DIMD

Risk factors for DIMD have been identified for some of the more frequent DIMD like tardive dyskinesias or parkinsonism. The most common patient-related identified risk factors are age, female gender, genetic (several Mendelian loci), past history of nervous system disorder, blood-brain barrier disruption, comorbidities, and non-compliance [10, 11].

40.5 Forms of DIMD

However difficult to describe DIMD, they are usually divided into several categories describing phenomenology. It should be stressed that the commonly used terms in pharmacovigilance and regulatory management of ADRs do not strictly correlate with the definitions currently in use by movement disorders specialists. They intend to be easily understood by healthcare professionals (not only neurologists or even clinicians) and sometimes approach lay language:

- Akathisia – subjective feeling of restlessness with inability to maintain a posture or objective manifestation of restlessness in the form of movements of the limbs with a tendency to change body position.
- Ballism/chorea and dyskinesia – brief, jerky, and unpredictable movements that flit from one body part to another.
- Dystonia – muscle contraction resulting in repetitive movements or abnormal postures.
- Myoclonus – brief, lightning-like jerk that can involve muscle contraction or inhibition of muscle activity. It may also be part of a wider syndrome, such as serotonin syndrome, with tachycardia, muscle stiffness, tremor fever, and dysautonomia).
- NMS – condition characterized by severe rigidity, fever, diaphoresis, labile or elevated blood pressure, autonomic dysfunction, and elevated creatinine phosphokinase. Note that this includes dopaminergic drugs' abrupt withdrawal as per regulatory agency definition.
- Parkinsonism (when we observe two or more of the following features: bradykinesia, resting tremor, muscle rigidity, gait with some degree of disability, or postural instability).
- Tics – brief, complex, and repetitive movements including gestures and sounds.
- Tremor – rhythmic oscillation of a body part.

These disorders can also be classified as to their time of onset as acute (dystonia, akathisia, or parkinsonism), chronic/delayed (tardive – dyskinesia, dystonia, akathisia, myoclonus, tics, and tremor), or miscellaneous (NMS) [8, 9]. Chronic or delayed (types C and D) DIMD are frequently undiagnosed, for the link between the drug and the disorder is not always evident. It took years to relate punding to dopamine agonists, to describe the dopamine dysregulation syndrome, and finally to include this adverse event in the label of dopamine agonists.

40.6 Drugs Frequently Involved in DIMD

The main class involved in DIMD is DRBA. Most of these agents are antipsychotic drugs like classic neuroleptics (e.g., haloperidol) but also atypicals such as risperidone, olanzapine, quetiapine, aripiprazole, and even clozapine. Other DRBA include dopamine receptor-blocking agents for other clinical conditions like vertigo or vomiting (metoclopramide, domperidone, etc.). The exponential drug use pattern explains the growing frequency of the phenomena in the past six decades.

Non-DRBA drugs like antiepileptics or antidepressants especially selective serotonin reuptake inhibitors (SSRI) and other agents like opiates, calcium channel blockers, or β2-agonists may also cause DIMD. A detailed pharmacological history of patients who present the most common features of drug-induced movement disorders is crucial for differential diagnosis, management, and prophylaxis of DIMD [12].

An abridged list of agents involved in different forms of DIMD is shown below (Table 40.1).

Table 40.1 Drugs that can cause or exacerbate movement disorders

DIMD	Therapeutic group/agent
Akathisia	Antidepressants (SSRI, tricyclics)
	Antiepileptic drugs (carbamazepine, ethosuximide)
	Buspirone
	Calcium channel blockers (cinnarizine, diltiazem, flunarizine)
	DRBAs
	Lithium
	Monoamine depletors (tetrabenazine)
Ballism/chorea and dyskinesia	Anticholinergics
	Antidepressants (SSRI, tricyclics)
	Antiepileptics (carbamazepine, gabapentin, phenytoin, valproate)
	Antihistamines
	Dopaminergic drugs (dopamine agonists, levodopa)
	Hormones (thyroid hormone, estrogen)
	Lithium
	Stimulants (amphetamines, cocaine, methylphenidate)
	Miscellaneous (aminophylline, baclofen, cimetidine, digoxin)
Dystonia (acute and tardive)	Antiepileptics (carbamazepine, phenytoin, ethosuximide)
	Antidepressants (SSRI)
	Antimalarials (amodiaquine, chloroquine)
	Dopaminergic drugs (dopamine agonists, levodopa)
	Diphenhydramine
	Disulfiram
	DRBAs
	Fentanyl
	Midazolam
	Ondansetron
	Monoamine depletors (tetrabenazine)
Myoclonus	Anesthetics (etomidate, enflurane, propofol, spinal anesthetics)
	Antibiotics/antimalarials (cephalosporins, fluoroquinolones, imipenem, mefloquine, penicillins)
	Anticholinergics
	Antiepileptics (carbamazepine, gabapentin, lamotrigine, phenytoin, pregabalin, retigabine, tiagabine, valproate, vigabatrin)
	Antidepressants (MAO inhibitors, SSRI, tricyclics)
	Antineoplastics (chlorambucil, ifosfamide)
	Calcium channel blockers (diltiazem, nifedipine, verapamil)
	Contrast agents
	DRBAs
	Dopaminergic drugs (dopamine agonists, levodopa)
	Gastrointestinal drugs (bismuth salts)
	MDMA (ecstasy)
	Opiates (methadone, meperidine, morphine, oxycodone, tramadol)
	Miscellaneous (gamma-hydroxybutyrate, tranexamic acid)

Table 40.1 (continued)

DIMD	Therapeutic group/agent
NMS	Antidepressants (desipramine, dothiepin)
	Dopaminergic drugs abrupt withdrawal (dopamine agonists, levodopa)
	DRBAs (including atypical antipsychotics and antiemetics)
	Lithium
	Monoamine depletors (tetrabenazine)
Parkinsonism	Amiodarone
	Antineoplastics (cyclophosphamide, cytosine arabinoside)
	Calcium channel blockers (verapamil, diltiazem, nifedipine, amlodipine)
	Disulfiram
	Lithium
	Methyldopa
	Opiates (meperidine)
	SSRI (citalopram, fluoxetine, paroxetine, sertraline)
	Valproate
	Miscellaneous (amphotericin B, cyclosporine)
Serotonin syndrome	Antidepressants (bupropion, MAOI, mirtazapine, SNRI, SSRI, tricyclics)
	Anti-migraine (carbamazepine, triptans, valproate)
	Antiemetics (granisetron, metoclopramide, ondansetron)
	Buspirone
	DRBAs (risperidone, olanzapine)
	Drugs of abuse (cocaine, hallucinogenic amphetamines, methamphetamine, MDMA, MDA, pentazocine, phentermine)
	Lithium
	Opiates (buprenorphine, dextromethorphan, fentanyl, hydrocodone, meperidine, oxycodone, tapentadol, tramadol)
	Stimulants (methylphenidate, sibutramine)
	Miscellaneous (LDOPA, linezolid, ritonavir)
Tics	Antidepressants (SSRI: escitalopram, fluoxetine, sertraline)
	Antiepileptics (carbamazepine, lamotrigine)
	Drugs of abuse (cocaine, heroin)
	Levodopa
	Stimulants (amphetamines, cocaine, methylphenidate)
Tremor	Antiarrhythmics (amiodarone, mexiletine, procainamide, propafenone)
	Antibiotics, antifungals (fluconazole, itraconazole, trimethoprim/sulfamethoxazole)
	Antidepressants (amitriptyline, SSRI, MAOI)
	Antiepileptics (valproate, lamotrigine)
	Antineoplastics (tamoxifen, ifosfamide, thalidomide)
	Bronchodilators (betamimetics)
	DRBAs
	Drugs of abuse (amphetamine, cocaine, ethanol, MDMA, nicotine)
	Gastrointestinal drugs (metoclopramide, cimetidine)
	Hormones (epinephrine, thyroxine, calcitonin, medroxyprogesterone)
	Immunosuppressants (tacrolimus, cyclosporine, α-interferon)
	Methylxanthines (theophylline, caffeine)

References

1. Naranjo CA, Busto U, Sellers EM, Sandor P, Ruiz I, Roberts EA, Janecek E, Domecq C, Greenblatt DJ. A method for estimating the probability of adverse drug reactions. Clin Pharmacol Ther. 1981;30(2):239–45.
2. Meyboom RHB, Royer RJ. Causality classification at pharmacovigilance centres in the european community. Pharmacoepidemiol Drug Saf. 1992;1:87–97.
3. Farde L, Wiesel FA, Halldin C, Sedvall G. Central D2-dopamine receptor occupancy in schizophrenic patients treated with antipsychotic drugs. Arch Gen Psychiatry. 1988;45(1):71–6.
4. Korczyn AD, Goldberg GJ. Extrapyramidal effects of neuroleptics. J Neurol Neurosurg Psychiatry. 1976;39(9):866–9.
5. WHO. Technical Report No 498. International drug monitoring: the role of national centres. Geneva: WHO; 1972.
6. European Medicines Agency/Heads of Medicines Agencies. Guideline on good pharmacovigilance practices. Annex I – Definitions. EMA/876333/2011 Rev. 1*. London, December 2012.
7. Aronson JK. Drug therapy. In: Haslett C, Chilvers ER, Boon NA, Colledge NR, Hunter JAA, editors. Davidson's principles and practice of medicine. 19th ed. Edinburgh: Elsevier Science; 2002. p. 147–63.
8. Wojcieszek J. Drug-induced movement disorders. In: Biller J, editor. Iatrogenic neurology. Oxford: Butterworth-Heinemann; 1998. p. 215–31.
9. Jain KK. Drug-induced neurological disorders. 3rd ed. Seattle: Hogrefe Publishing; 2012.
10. Yassa R, Nastase C, Dupont D, et al. Tardive dyskinesia in elderly psychiatric patients: a 5-year study. Am J Psychiatry. 1992;149:1206–11.
11. Wu RM, Chiu HC, Wang M, Chen RC. Risk factors on the occurrence of response fluctuations and dyskinesias in Parkinson's disease. J Neural Transm. 1993;5(2):127–33.
12. Rosa MM. Reacções adversas neuropsiquiátricas. In: Pinheiro L, Marques da Silva P, Carmona R, Maria VA, editors. Farmacovigilância em Portugal. Lisbon: INFARMED – Ministério da Saúde; 2003. p. 303–22.

Stereotypies

41

Subhashie Wijemanne and Joseph Jankovic

41.1 Introduction

Stereotypies are defined as coordinated, patterned, repetitive, rhythmic, and seemingly purposeless movements that can occur involuntarily or in response to or induced by inner sensory stimulus or unwanted feeling (involuntary) [24, 25, 37, 40, 62, 76]. Etiologically, stereotypies are also classified as primary or physiological, as seen in otherwise normal children [36, 54, 78], or secondary stereotypies caused by a variety of disorders including autistic or other pervasive developmental disorders [62, 77]. When stereotypies occur in children, they usually become evident within the first few years of life [36]. Stereotypies may also occur in adults with tardive dyskinesia (TD) [87]; catatonia [30]; schizophrenia [20, 61]; restless legs syndrome; encephalitis, particularly anti-N-methyl-D-aspartate receptor (NMDAR) encephalitis [9]; degenerative dementias [70] including frontotemporal dementia [55, 57, 64]; and obsessive-compulsive disorder [19] among others (Table 41.1).

S. Wijemanne, MD, MRCP • J. Jankovic, MD (✉)
Department of Neurology, Parkinson's Disease Center and Movement Disorders Clinic,
Baylor College of Medicine, 7200 Cambridge Street, Suite 9A, Houston, TX 77030, USA
e-mail: josephj@bcm.edu; http://www.jankovic.org

41.2 Phenomenology

Typical motor stereotypies encountered in children include a wide range of movements such as body rocking, head nodding, head banging, hand waving, covering ears, fluttering of fingers or hands in front of the face, repetitive and sequential finger movements, eye deviation, lip smacking, and chewing movements [25]. Phonic stereotypies can include grunting, moaning, humming, noncontextual phrases or words, and repetition of unintelligible sounds or some combination [6]. Each child has his or her own distinct repertoire of motor and phonic stereotypies which are usually intermittent and can last from a few seconds to several minutes and appear multiple times a day. Motor stereotypies usually have a fixed pattern and typically occur when the child is engrossed in stimulating activities, excited, stressed, or fatigued. They do not usually interfere with the ability to perform tasks, although they can occur during excited play and briefly interrupt the ongoing activity [76]. In contrast to intermittent nature of stereotypies in autistic disorders such as Rett syndrome [84], it can be continuous as in TD [87]. It can be simple such as foot tapping or body rocking or complex such as complicated rituals [54].

Stereotypy needs to be differentiated from tics, mannerisms, compulsions, akathisia, and automatisms of epileptic seizures. In contrast to stereotypies, motor tics are typically brief, jerk-like movements preceded by premonitory sensa-

C. Falup-Pecurariu et al. (eds.), *Movement Disorders Curricula*,
DOI 10.1007/978-3-7091-1628-9_41

Table 41.1 Causes of stereotypies

Physiologic
Normal developmental stereotypies
Leg stereotypy disorder in adults
Pathologic
Autism and other pervasive developmental disorders
Rett syndrome
Intellectual disability
Schizophrenia
Catatonia
Restless legs syndrome
Obsessive compulsive disorder
Tardive dyskinesia
Dementia including frontotemporal dementia
Encephalitis including anti-NMDA receptor antibody encephalitis
Structural lesions
Psychogenic

tion or urge [39]. When complex tics occur repetitively, they may resemble stereotypies. Mannerisms are gestures or sets of movements that are unique to the individual and generally attached to a normal activity. Compulsions are repetitive behaviors or rituals with an overwhelming irresistible urge to perform an act or ritual such as handwashing that are performed to relieve anxiety caused by obsessive thoughts or intrinsic rules. Akathisia refers to a feeling of inner, general restlessness that is reduced or relived by moving about [25]. Some of the restless movements, such as hair and face rubbing, picking at clothes, crossing and uncrossing legs, sitting down and standing up, and marching in place, can resemble complex stereotypies. Repetitive movements during frontal lobe seizures can resemble stereotypy, but the pattern is paroxysmal, reproducible, and unique for a given patient [56].

Punding is a peculiar stereotyped behavior characterized by an intense fascination with a complex, excessive, non-goal-oriented, repetitive activity such as manipulation of technical equipment, handling, examining or sorting through common objects, grooming, or hoarding [27, 80]. Some consider punding as a drug-induced stereotypy due to dopaminergic medications as in patients with Parkinson's disease treated with levodopa or dopamine agonists or in patients with addiction to cocaine or amphetamine [26, 27, 43].

41.3 Pathophysiology

The underlying pathophysiological mechanism and neuroanatomical substrate for stereotypies are not well understood. Involvement of the basal ganglia has been implicated in some stereotypy [83], and involvement of frontal subcortical circuits is also proposed [62]. Stereotypy-inducing drugs like amphetamines have been used to study possible mechanisms in animal models [50]. Rodents chronically treated with psychomotor stimulants have exhibited stereotyped movements, attributed to a dysfunction in prefrontal cortico-basal ganglia circuits [3, 15]. Peripheral injection of a low dose of raclopride or high-frequency stimulation of the subthalamic nucleus rapidly stops cocaine-induced motor stereotypy in rats, presumably by restoring the extracellular level of acetylcholine in the prefrontal territory of the dorsal striatum [2].

Genetic causes of stereotypies have been observed and in one study involving non-autistic children with motor stereotypies, 25 % showed a positive family history of motor stereotypies suggesting an underlying genetic abnormality [36]. A mouse model Ts65Dn of Down syndrome exhibited spontaneous stereotypies consisting of repetitive jumping compared to control mice [86]. One theory, proposed to explain mechanisms of stereotypies, suggests that the repetitive movements are self-stimulatory in response to boredom or a physical constraint. This is supported by the observation that stereotypies are almost never present in animals in the wild, but when these animals are placed in a constrained environment with low or no stimulation, such as the zoo, they often develop stereotypic behaviors [35]. Stereotypies are also seen in children and adults with sensory deprivation such as blindness [28, 85] and hearing impaired [7]. Another theory is that stereotypies are commonly maintained by automatic reinforcement as evidenced by the persistence of stereotypy in the absence of social consequences and reductions in stereotypy in the presence of alternative sources of automatic reinforcement [72].

41.4 Physiologic Stereotypy

Stereotypies in healthy children [11, 18, 51, 82] are typically seen before the age of 3 years. Common stereotypies include arm flapping, hand waving or rotating, finger wiggling, head nodding, body rocking, thumb-sucking, and nail-biting [54]. Some children, almost exclusively girls, exhibit stereotypic crossing and extending of legs, as a form of self-gratifying or masturbatory behavior [11, 88]. The fact that similar movements can be seen in children with autism and intellectual disability is often a source of concern for parents.

The prevalence of stereotypies in healthy children are unknown but has been estimated to be as high as 20 % [74]. Head banging is seen up to 15 % of normal children [74]. Although these children have an apparently normal development, studies have shown that associated conditions are common in this non-autistic motor stereotypy population, with nearly 50 % of children receiving at least one comorbid diagnosis [36, 73]. In subjects aged less than 7 years, beyond the expected age for the appearance of signs, 30 % demonstrated attention-deficit hyperactivity disorder, and 18 % demonstrated tics and obsessive-compulsive behaviors [36]. The long-term outcome of childhood-onset stereotypies has not been well studied, but most report a decline after age 4 years [53], but stereotypies may persist beyond childhood years [36, 65]. Studies conducted in college population have shown that stereotypic movements are common in a college population [18] and are associated with increased scores of obsessive-compulsive symptoms, of perfectionism, and of impulsive-aggressive traits [63]. Some of the common movements include repetitive touching of face; scratching scalp; biting nails; cracking knuckles; shaking legs; body rocking; rubbing personal objects, such as jewelry or clothing; and playing with hair [63]. Although stereotypies start as involuntary and seemingly purposeless, later in childhood and beyond, they may acquire a function of facilitating pleasurable fantasy and/or regulating arousal and thus be performed in a more conscious and deliberate manner [31, 71].

41.5 Autism and Autism Spectrum Disorder

Autism and autism spectrum disorder (ASD) are a biologically based neurodevelopmental disorder characterized by impairments in two major domains: (1) deficits in social communication and social interaction and (2) restricted repetitive patterns of behavior, interests, and activities. According to the Diagnostic and Statistical Manual of Mental Disorders V (DSM-V), the presence of restricted, repetitive, and stereotyped patterns of behaviors, activities, and interests is one of the essential diagnostic features of autistic disorder [4]. Common stereotypies observed in autistic children include hand flapping, body rocking, twisting, rocking, swaying, toe walking, spinning objects, sniffing, immediate and delayed echolalia, and running objects across one's peripheral vision. Other forms involve more complex behaviors, such as restricted and stereotyped patterns of interest or the obsessive need for sameness [21, 59]. Persistent fixation on certain parts of objects or an inflexible adherence to specific, nonfunctional routines or rituals is also seen. In children with intellectual disability and autism are often associated with self-injurious stereotypy [8, 23] which are sometimes repetitive and can be rhythmic. These behaviors range from mild hair pulling to much more severe actions such as head banging or autoextraction of teeth and are often performed in the absence of reporting pain [22]. Children with low functioning autism had a greater prevalence and an increased number and variety of stereotypies compared to those with high-functioning autism, developmental language disorder, and non-autism-related low intelligence quotient [16, 34, 67]. Symptoms of ASD most commonly are recognized in the second year of life

[48, 49], but may present earlier [60, 68]. There is evidence that the presence of repetitive behaviors can negatively impact the learning and socialization [52] of individuals with autism spectrum of disorders. Stereotypic behaviors are not isolated to autism, and they are common to individuals with other sensory, intellectual, or developmental disabilities [10, 34]. In one study primary stereotypies in developing children ($N=28$) were compared to secondary stereotypies, those occurring within autistic or mentally retarded children ($N=28$) [32]. The investigators found that primary stereotypies were predominantly motor, simple, of shorter duration, and of less frequency, whereas secondary stereotypies had more vocalization, complexity, longer durations, and higher frequencies.

41.6 Rett Syndrome

Rett syndrome is a neurodevelopmental disorder, classified as an autism spectrum disorder, and linked to a mutation in the *MECP2* gene in 75–95 % of cases [5, 75]. Children with Rett syndrome tend to have a normal development until 6–18 months of age which is followed by gradual regression of both motor and language skills, development of repetitive hand stereotypies, gait impairment, and other neurological and movement disorders [29]. The hand stereotypies, the dominant movement disorder, include hand clapping, wringing, clenching, washing, patting, rubbing, picking, and mouthing [84]. In one study of 144 females with Rett syndrome, 96.4 % of whom had a pathogenic mutation experienced stereotypies, and 61.8 % of participants who had a mutation in the *MECP2* gene displayed a midline hand-wringing stereotypy [17]. Based on the phenomenology, there are prominent differences in stereotypies between Rett syndrome and autism that help to differentiate the two conditions [33]. In Rett syndrome the hand stereotypies are continuous and predominantly seen in the midline, whereas in autism these stereotypies are typically intermittent and involving more distal body parts.

41.7 Tardive Dyskinesia

TD is a delayed-onset iatrogenic hyperkinetic movement disorder caused by dopamine receptor-blocking drugs, also referred to as neuroleptics [38, 81, 87]. Stereotypies are one of the key clinical manifestations of this syndrome. Classic TD manifests typically as involuntary stereotypic movements in the oro-bucco-lingual region, such as lip smacking or pursing, chewing, facial grimacing, and tongue movements inside the mouth or tongue protrusions, the so-called oro-bucco-lingual stereotypy. The term "tardive stereotypy" is often used to describe the seemingly purposeful, repetitive, and coordinated movement sometimes giving the appearance of ritualistic gestures or mannerisms. Although oro-bucco-lingual stereotypy of classic TD is the most common form of tardive stereotypy, some patients also have limb stereotypies, manifested as repetitive foot tapping, complex stereotypic piano-playing finger and toe movements, and hand rubbing. Trunk stereotypies are typically manifested by repetitive rocking and swaying body movements. Tardive akathisia is a feeling of inner restlessness involving the whole body or certain body parts; it is usually uncomfortable to the patients and sometimes disabling [14]. The patients often have repetitive and stereotypy movements (rocking in a chair, crossing/uncrossing of legs when sitting, pacing on a spot, shifting weight from one foot to another when standing, face or scalp touching or scratching) in an attempt to relieve feelings of restlessness. The restless movements sometimes resemble limb and trunk stereotypies of TD. In addition to sensory motor disorder seen in akathisia, TD may be associated with other sensory components such as pain or discomfort, particularly in the mouth (or vaginal area) [69].

41.8 Dementia

Elementary stereotypic behaviors are recognized in degenerative dementias such as Alzheimer's disease (AD) and particularly in frontotemporal dementia (FTD) [55, 64]. These may include simple actions such as grunting, hand rubbing, foot tapping to rituals relating to toileting or dressing, wandering, and pacing in a fixed route, perseverative responses, and stereotyped use of words and phrases [64]. The overall prevalence of stereotypic behaviors is higher in FTD than in Alzheimer's disease [13, 79].

41.9 Others

The leg stereotypy disorder (LSD) is manifested by stereotypic, 1–2 Hz rhythmical, flexion-extension movements of the hips while the individual is sitting with the toes of the foot pressed against the floor [41, 69]. It is often associated with an intense need to move the legs in response to an inner tension or state of anxiety or muscle ache, which is transiently relieved by the movement. Although frequently attributed to anxiety, LSD is often familial, thus indicating possible genetic etiology.

41.10 Therapy

Evidence-based therapy for the treatment of stereotypies is lacking. Behavioral therapies may be effective in both non-autistic and autistic children, but they require a high degree or compliance in order to provide sustained benefits [12, 58]. Stereotypies in an otherwise healthy child if not bothersome do not warrant treatment; however, proper diagnosis and differentiation from other disorders is important. There can be considerable parental anxiety concerning a possible underlying neurological or developmental cause [31]. On the other hand stereotypies that occur with coexisting conditions, or are severely restricting or include self-injurious behaviors, require therapeutic intervention. Miller et al. [58] demonstrated the effectiveness of a combination of modified habit reversal and differential reinforcement of other behaviors in non-autistic children with stereotypies. Lancioni et al. [47] provided an overview of studies from 1995 to 2007 that used behavioral strategies to reduce hand-related stereotypies in patients with severe to profound intellectual and multiple disabilities. Although various behavioral strategies were useful in reducing or eliminating hand stereotypies, some methods employ relatively drastic measures, such as mechanical restraints in rigid arm sleeves [46, 89]. Response interruption and redirection (RIRD) is a form of behavioral therapy that is increasingly used to pursue a dual goal of reducing the stereotyped behavior and increasing adaptive (alternative) responses that could produce preferred stimulation [1, 47].

Pharmacological options in the treatment of stereotypy are very limited. Citalopram was found to be ineffective in children with autism spectrum disorders and high levels of repetitive behavior [45]. The dopamine-depleting drugs reserpine and tetrabenazine that inhibit vesicular monoamine transporter (VMAT) at the presynaptic membrane of the nerve terminal are effective in treating stereotypy of TD [42, 44, 87]. Tetrabenazine has also been reported to be effective in stereotypies seen in patients with frontotemporal dementia [66].

References

1. Ahrens EN, Lerman DC, et al. Further evaluation of response interruption and redirection as treatment for stereotypy. J Appl Behav Anal. 2011;44(1):95–108.
2. Aliane V, Perez S, et al. Raclopride or high-frequency stimulation of the subthalamic nucleus stops cocaine-induced motor stereotypy and restores related alterations in prefrontal basal ganglia circuits. Eur J Neurosci. 2012;36(9):3235–45.
3. Aliane V, Perez S, et al. Cocaine-induced stereotypy is linked to an imbalance between the medial prefrontal and sensorimotor circuits of the basal ganglia. Eur J Neurosci. 2009;30(7):1269–79.
4. American, Psychiatric, et al. Diagnostic and statistical manual of mental disorders: DSM-V. Washington, DC: American Psychiatric Association; 2013.
5. Amir RE, Van den Veyver IB, et al. Rett syndrome is caused by mutations in X-linked MECP2, encoding methyl-CpG-binding protein 2. Nat Genet. 1999; 23(2):185–8.
6. Athens ES, Vollmer TR, et al. An analysis of vocal stereotypy and therapist fading. J Appl Behav Anal. 2008;41(2):291–7.
7. Bachara GH, Phelan WJ. Rhythmic movement in deaf children. Percept Mot Skills. 1980;50(3 Pt 1):933–4.
8. Baghdadli A, Pascal C, et al. Risk factors for self-injurious behaviours among 222 young children with autistic disorders. J Intellect Disabil Res. 2003;47(Pt 8):622–7.

9. Baizabal-Carvallo JF, Stocco A, et al. The spectrum of movement disorders in children with anti-NMDA receptor encephalitis. Mov Disord. 2013;28(4):543–7.
10. Bodfish JW, Symons FJ, et al. Varieties of repetitive behavior in autism: comparisons to mental retardation. J Autism Dev Disord. 2000;30(3):237–43.
11. Bonnet C, Roubertie A, et al. Developmental and benign movement disorders in childhood. Mov Disord. 2010;25(10):1317–34.
12. Boyd BA, McDonough SG, et al. Evidence-based behavioral interventions for repetitive behaviors in autism. J Autism Dev Disord. 2012;42(6): 1236–48.
13. Bozeat S, Gregory CA, et al. Which neuropsychiatric and behavioural features distinguish frontal and temporal variants of frontotemporal dementia from Alzheimer's disease? J Neurol Neurosurg Psychiatry. 2000;69(2):178–86.
14. Burke RE, Kang UJ, et al. Tardive akathisia: an analysis of clinical features and response to open therapeutic trials. Mov Disord. 1989;4(2):157–75.
15. Canales JJ, Graybiel AM. A measure of striatal function predicts motor stereotypy. Nat Neurosci. 2000; 3(4):377–83.
16. Carcani-Rathwell I, Rabe-Hasketh S, et al. Repetitive and stereotyped behaviours in pervasive developmental disorders. J Child Psychol Psychiatry. 2006; 47(6):573–81.
17. Carter P, Downs J, et al. Stereotypical hand movements in 144 subjects with Rett syndrome from the population-based Australian database. Mov Disord. 2010;25(3):282–8.
18. Castellanos FX, Ritchie GF, et al. DSM-IV stereotypic movement disorder: persistence of stereotypies of infancy in intellectually normal adolescents and adults. J Clin Psychiatry. 1996;57(3):116–22.
19. Chok JT, Koesler B. Distinguishing obsessive-compulsive behavior from stereotypy: a preliminary investigation. Behav Modif. 2014;38(3):344–73.
20. Compton MT, Fantes F, et al. Abnormal movements in first-episode, nonaffective psychosis: dyskinesias, stereotypies, and catatonic-like signs. Psychiatry Res. 2015;226(1):192–7.
21. Cunningham AB, Schreibman L. Stereotypy in autism: the importance of function. Res Autism Spectrosc Disord. 2008;2(3):469–79.
22. Duerden EG, Card D, et al. Self-injurious behaviours are associated with alterations in the somatosensory system in children with autism spectrum disorder. Brain Struct Funct. 2014;219(4):1251–61.
23. Duerden EG, Oatley HK, et al. Risk factors associated with self-injurious behaviors in children and adolescents with autism spectrum disorders. J Autism Dev Disord. 2012;42(11):2460–70.
24. Edwards MJ, Lang AE, et al. Stereotypies: a critical appraisal and suggestion of a clinically useful definition. Mov Disord. 2012;27(2):179–85.
25. Fahn S, Jankovic J, Hallett M. Stereotypies. Principles and practice of movement disorders. Elsevier. 2nd ed. 2011. p. 380–8.
26. Fasano A, Evans AH. Is punding a stereotypy? Mov Disord. 2013;28(3):404–5.
27. Fasano A, Petrovic I. Insights into pathophysiology of punding reveal possible treatment strategies. Mol Psychiatry. 2010;15(6):560–73.
28. Fazzi E, Lanners J, et al. Stereotyped behaviours in blind children. Brain Dev. 1999;21(8):522–8.
29. FitzGerald PM, Jankovic J, et al. Rett syndrome and associated movement disorders. Mov Disord. 1990;5(3):195–202.
30. Francis A. Catatonia: diagnosis, classification, and treatment. Curr Psychiatry Rep. 2010;12(3): 180–5.
31. Freeman RD, Soltanifar A, et al. Stereotypic movement disorder: easily missed. Dev Med Child Neurol. 2010;52(8):733–8.
32. Ghosh D, Rajan PV, et al. A comparative study of primary and secondary stereotypies. J Child Neurol. 2013;28(12):1562–8.
33. Goldman S, Temudo T. Hand stereotypies distinguish Rett syndrome from autism disorder. Mov Disord. 2012;27(8):1060–2.
34. Goldman S, Wang C, et al. Motor stereotypies in children with autism and other developmental disorders. Dev Med Child Neurol. 2009;51(1):30–8.
35. Gross AN, Richter SH, et al. Cage-induced stereotypies, perseveration and the effects of environmental enrichment in laboratory mice. Behav Brain Res. 2012;234(1):61–8.
36. Harris KM, Mahone EM, et al. Nonautistic motor stereotypies: clinical features and longitudinal follow-up. Pediatr Neurol. 2008;38(4):267–72.
37. Jankovic J. Stereotypies. In: Marsden CD, Fahn S, editors. Movement disorders. 3rd ed. London: Butterworth Heinemann; 1994. p. 501–17.
38. Jankovic J. Tardive syndromes and other drug-induced movement disorders. Clin Neuropharmacol. 1995; 18(3):197–214.
39. Jankovic J. Tourette's syndrome. N Engl J Med. 2001;345(16):1184–92.
40. Jankovic J. Tics and stereotypies. In: Freund HJ, Jeannerod M, Hallett M, Leiguarda R, editors. Higer-order motor disorders. Oxford England: Oxford University Press; 2005. p. 383–96.
41. Jankovic J. Leg stereotypy disorder. J Neurol Neurosurg Psychiatry. 2016;87(2):220–1.
42. Jimenez-Shahed J, Jankovic J. Tetrabenazine for treatment of chorea associated with Huntington's disease. Expert Opin Orphan Drugs. 2013;1:423–36.
43. Katzenschlager R. Dopaminergic dysregulation syndrome in Parkinson's disease. J Neurol Sci. 2011; 310(1-2):271–5.
44. Kenney C, Jankovic J. Tetrabenazine in the treatment of hyperkinetic movement disorders. Expert Rev Neurother. 2006;6(1):7–17.
45. King BH, Hollander E, et al. Lack of efficacy of citalopram in children with autism spectrum disorders and high levels of repetitive behavior: citalopram ineffective in children with autism. Arch Gen Psychiatry. 2009;66(6):583–90.

46. Lalli JS, Livezey K, et al. Functional analysis and treatment of eye poking with response blocking. J Appl Behav Anal. 1996;29(1):129–32.
47. Lancioni GE, Singh NN, et al. An overview of behavioral strategies for reducing hand-related stereotypies of persons with severe to profound intellectual and multiple disabilities: 1995–2007. Res Dev Disabil. 2009;30(1):20–43.
48. Landa R, Garrett-Mayer E. Development in infants with autism spectrum disorders: a prospective study. J Child Psychol Psychiatry. 2006;47(6):629–38.
49. Landa RJ, Gross AL, et al. Developmental trajectories in children with and without autism spectrum disorders: the first 3 years. Child Dev. 2013;84(2):429–42.
50. Le WP., Sayana et al. Animal models of Parkinson's disease: a gateway to therapeutics? Neurotherapeutics. 2014;11(1):92–110.
51. Leekam S, Tandos J, et al. Repetitive behaviours in typically developing 2-year-olds. J Child Psychol Psychiatry. 2007;48(11):1131–8.
52. Loftin RL, Odom SL, et al. Social interaction and repetitive motor behaviors. J Autism Dev Disord. 2008;38(6):1124–35.
53. MacDonald R, Green G, et al. Stereotypy in young children with autism and typically developing children. Res Dev Disabil. 2007;28(3):266–77.
54. Mahone EM, Bridges D, et al. Repetitive arm and hand movements (complex motor stereotypies) in children. J Pediatr. 2004;145(3):391–5.
55. Mateen FJ, Josephs KA. The clinical spectrum of stereotypies in frontotemporal lobar degeneration. Mov Disord. 2009;24(8):1237–40.
56. McGonigal A, Chauvel P. Prefrontal seizures manifesting as motor stereotypies. Mov Disord. 2013;29:1181.
57. Mendez MF, Shapira JS, et al. Stereotypical movements and frontotemporal dementia. Mov Disord. 2005;20(6):742–5.
58. Miller JM, Singer HS, et al. Behavioral therapy for treatment of stereotypic movements in nonautistic children. J Child Neurol. 2006;21(2):119–25.
59. Ming X, Brimacombe M, et al. Prevalence of motor impairment in autism spectrum disorders. Brain Dev. 2007;29(9):565–70.
60. Mitchell S, Brian J, et al. Early language and communication development of infants later diagnosed with autism spectrum disorder. J Dev Behav Pediatr. 2006;27(2 Suppl):S69–78.
61. Morrens M, Hulstijn W, et al. Stereotypy in schizophrenia. Schizophr Res. 2006;84(2-3):397–404.
62. Muthugovindan D, Singer H. Motor stereotypy disorders. Curr Opin Neurol. 2009;22(2):131–6.
63. Niehaus DJ, Emsley RA, et al. Stereotypies: prevalence and association with compulsive and impulsive symptoms in college students. Psychopathology. 2000;33(1):31–5.
64. Nyatsanza S, Shetty T, et al. A study of stereotypic behaviours in Alzheimer's disease and frontal and temporal variant frontotemporal dementia. J Neurol Neurosurg Psychiatry. 2003;74(10):1398–402.
65. Oakley C, Mahone EM, et al. Primary complex motor stereotypies in older children and adolescents: clinical features and longitudinal follow-up. Pediatr Neurol. 2015;52(4):398–403. e391.
66. Ondo WG. Tetrabenazine treatment for stereotypies and tics associated with dementia. J Neuropsychiatry Clin Neurosci. 2012;24(2):208–14.
67. Osterling JA, Dawson G, et al. Early recognition of 1-year-old infants with autism spectrum disorder versus mental retardation. Dev Psychopathol. 2002;14(2):239–51.
68. Ozonoff S, Losif AM, et al. A prospective study of the emergence of early behavioral signs of autism. J Am Acad Child Adolesc Psychiatry. 2010;49(3):256–66. e251-252.
69. Patel N, Jankovic J, et al. Sensory aspects of movement disorders. Lancet Neurol. 2014;13(1):100–12.
70. Prioni S, Fetoni V, et al. Stereotypic behaviors in degenerative dementias. J Neurol. 2012;259(11):2452–9.
71. Rafaeli-Mor N, Foster L, et al. Self-reported body-rocking and other habits in college students. Am J Ment Retard. 1999;104(1):1–10.
72. Rapp JT, Vollmer TR. Stereotypy I: a review of behavioral assessment and treatment. Res Dev Disabil. 2005;26(6):527–47.
73. Robinson S, Woods M, et al. Intense Imagery Movements (IIM): more to motor stereotypies than meets the eye. Eur J Paediatr Neurol. 2016;20(1):61–8.
74. Sallustro F, Atwell CW. Body rocking, head banging, and head rolling in normal children. J Pediatr. 1978;93(4):704–8.
75. Samaco RC, Neul JL. Complexities of Rett syndrome and MeCP2. J Neurosci. 2011;31(22):7951–9.
76. Sanger TD, Chen D, et al. Definition and classification of hyperkinetic movements in childhood. Mov Disord. 2010;25(11):1538–49.
77. Singer HS. Motor stereotypies. Semin Pediatr Neurol. 2009;16(2):77–81.
78. Smith EA, Van Houten R. A comparison of the characteristics of self-stimulatory behaviors in "normal" children and children with developmental delays. Res Dev Disabil. 1996;17(4):253–68.
79. Snowden JS, Bathgate D, et al. Distinct behavioural profiles in frontotemporal dementia and semantic dementia. J Neurol Neurosurg Psychiatry. 2001;70(3):323–32.
80. Spencer AH, Rickards H, et al. The prevalence and clinical characteristics of punding in Parkinson's disease. Mov Disord. 2011;26(4):578–86.
81. Stacy M, Cardoso F, et al. Tardive stereotypy and other movement disorders in tardive dyskinesias. Neurology. 1993;43(5):937–41.
82. Tan A, Salgado M, et al. The characterization and outcome of stereotypical movements in nonautistic children. Mov Disord. 1997;12(1):47–52.
83. Tanimura Y, King MA, et al. Development of repetitive behavior in a mouse model: roles of indirect and

striosomal basal ganglia pathways. Int J Dev Neurosci. 2011;29(4):461–7.
84. Temudo T, Ramos E, et al. Movement disorders in Rett syndrome: an analysis of 60 patients with detected MECP2 mutation and correlation with mutation type. Mov Disord. 2008;23(10):1384–90.
85. Troster H, Brambring M, et al. Prevalence and situational causes of stereotyped behaviors in blind infants and preschoolers. J Abnorm Child Psychol. 1991;19(5):569–90.
86. Turner CA, Presti MF, et al. Spontaneous stereotypy in an animal model of Down syndrome: Ts65Dn mice. Behav Genet. 2001;31(4):393–400.
87. Waln O, Jankovic J. An update on tardive dyskinesia: from phenomenology to treatment. Tremor Hyperkinet Mov (NY) 2013;3.
88. Yang ML, Fullwood E, et al. Masturbation in infancy and early childhood presenting as a movement disorder: 12 cases and a review of the literature. Pediatrics. 2005;116(6):1427–32.
89. Zhou L, Goff GA. Effects of increased response effort on self-injury and object manipulation as competing responses. J Appl Behav Anal. 2000;33(1):29–40.

42 Movement Disorders in Children

Teresa Temudo and Inês Carrilho

42.1 Introduction

Movement disorders (MDs) in children have some peculiarities compared with adults. In front of a pediatric patient with a specific type of movement disorder, usually the etiologies are different from those considered in an adult, and by the other hand, the clinical manifestations are different because they are influenced by the age of onset of a certain disease. In children with movement disorders, hyperkinetic movements predominate; in adults bradykinesia is much more prevalent. Moreover, certain disorders occur almost exclusively in children, as is the case of transient movement disorders, or are much more frequent as metabolic and autoimmune diseases.

In this chapter we will only describe the group of movement disorders that are more frequent in children.

T. Temudo, MD, PhD (✉)
Serviço de Neuropediatria, Departamento da criança e Adolescente, Centro Hospitalar do Porto, Porto, Portugal

Instituto de Ciências Biomédicas Abel Salazar, Universidade do Porto, Porto, Portugal
e-mail: ttemudo11@gmail.com

I. Carrilho, MD
Serviço de Neuropediatria, Departamento da criança e Adolescente, Centro Hospitalar do Porto, Porto, Portugal

42.2 Transient Benign Movement Disorders in Children (TBMDC)

They are underdiagnosed but represent about 20% of cases of movement disorders (tics excluded) seen in a neuropediatric department [1]. Dystonia, tremor, and myoclonus are the most common.

Transient movement disorders in children include:

- Jitteriness
- Palatal essential tremor
- Shuddering
- Transient idiopathic dystonia of infancy
- Spasmus nutans
- Benign paroxysmal torticollis of infancy
- Benign paroxysmal tonic upgaze
- Benign myoclonus of infancy
- Gratification behavior
- Sandifer syndrome
- Stereotypies

This group of disorders is idiopathic and unassociated with other neurologic diseases. The outcome is favorable, although developmental abnormalities can be occasionally observed. Full spontaneous remission is the rule, even if some disorders occasionally persist into adulthood. TBMDC are mainly diagnosed

C. Falup-Pecurariu et al. (eds.), *Movement Disorders Curricula*,
DOI 10.1007/978-3-7091-1628-9_42

and classified on the basis of physical examination and detailed history taking. Video recordings are very useful to make the diagnosis. The investigation of these children is normal and the diagnosis is made only based on clinical experience. Transient movement disorders are quite common but the pathogenic basis and prevalence are unknown.

In Table 42.1, the clinical characteristics, diagnostic testing, and treatment of TBMDC are presented.

42.3 Movement Disorders in Neuro-Metabolic Diseases

Inborn errors of metabolism (IEM) are a group of genetic disorders characterized by the dysfunction of an enzyme or other protein involved in the cellular metabolism. Most IEM involve the nervous system (neuro-metabolic diseases or NMDs), and they often present with a complex neurologic clinical picture as a consequence of the involvement of multiple cerebral and cerebellar structures. Movement disorders (MDs) are more frequently only part of this complex neurologic picture than a predominant symptom. However, in some NMDs, the movement disorder is the predominant sign and the red flag to obtain the diagnosis.

Other than ataxia, movement disorders in children may be divided into rigid akinetic syndrome (parkinsonism) and dyskinetic movements (dystonia, athetosis, tremor, chorea, myoclonus, tic, and stereotypy) [16]. Tics are very rarely related to IEMs. Important MDs in IEMs are dystonia, secondary parkinsonism, chorea, tremor, and myoclonus (Table 42.2). In children with an IEM, movement disorders emerge during the evolution of the disease but they may be present at onset. Movement disorders are often dystonic but different MD may coexist in the same patient [20]. The presence of one single movement disorder tends to be a specific diagnostic clue. In general, diseases causing parkinsonism in adults may present with dystonia in children [21]. The pattern of movement disorders tends to evolve with age, with the evolution of the disease.

Features suggesting NMD are consanguinity, childhood onset, familial cases, MDs not explained by other classical etiologies, and associated clinical signs and symptoms (neurological and systemic).

Main NMD-causing MDs are metal storage diseases, neurotransmitter synthesis defects, energy metabolism disorders, and lysosomal storage diseases (Table 42.3). The onset of MD can be acute, paroxysmal, or chronic progressive (Table 42.4).

Acute MD in NMD is most often due to nonketotic hyperglycinemia, glutaric acidemia type I, Leigh disease, methylmalonic acidemia, biotin-responsive basal ganglia disease, and creatine deficiency.

Paroxysmal MD in NMD can be due to Glut1 deficiency and leucinosis (intermediary form).

Chronic MD in NMD can be classified according to the presence or absence of basal ganglia lesions on cerebral MRI (Fig. 42.1).

Treatable diseases (Table 42.5) should be always kept in mind even if clinical symptoms or radiological signs are not typical [24]. Movement disorders that appear acutely can reveal emergencies, especially when they appear in the context of an acute encephalopathy with confusion or coma. Failure to accurately diagnose and manage the patient may result in significant morbidity or mortality. Diseases in this group include acute Wilson disease, nonketotic hyperglycinemia, pyruvate dehydrogenase deficiency, or biotin-responsive basal ganglia disease. Paroxysmal movement disorders (usually paroxysmal dystonia), spontaneous or induced by exercise, can also be a presenting feature of glucose transporter deficiency and less frequently by L-dopa-responsive dystonia or intermediary forms of leucinosis [22].

42.4 Movement Disorders in Autoimmune Diseases

Some movement disorders previously considered idiopathic or degenerative are now recognized as immunologically mediated.

Table 42.6 shows the main movement disorders associated with autoimmune diseases in

Table 42.1 Transient and benign movement disorders in childhood: clinical characteristics, investigation, and treatment

Disorder	Description	Age at onset	Age at resolution	Diagnostic testing	Treatment
Neonatal jitteriness [2]	Paroxysmal, stimulus sensitive, bilateral tremor of the chin and extremities	Neonatal period	<1 month (2 months–1 year)	Video EEG	No
Neonatal sleep myoclonus [3, 4]	Paroxysmal bilateral diffuse and synchronous jerks occurring only during sleep. Immediate cessation with arousal	Neonatal period	<6 months	Video EEG	No
Benign myoclonus of infancy [5]	Paroxysmal brief or sustained limb contraction	6 months (up to 1 year)	<2 years (up to 3 years)	Video EEG, brain MRI	No
Sleep-related rhythmic movement disorders [6]	Rhythmic stereotyped movements of large groups of muscles typically reported during the pre-sleep period	<3 months	Up to adulthood	Video EEG	No
Spasmus nutans [7, 8]	Paroxysmal head nodding associated with nystagmus	4–18 months	1–2 years after onset	Video EEG, brain MRI	No clinical follow-up Ophthalmologic examination, visual-evoked potential
Benign paroxysmal torticollis of infancy [9, 10]	Recurrent paroxysmal abnormal head posture associated or not with irritability, nausea, vomiting, pallor, ataxia	1–30 months	<4 years	Video EEG, brain MRI	No
Benign paroxysmal tonic upgaze [11, 12]	Conjugate upward deviation of the eyes with neck flexion	5 months	<4 years	Video EEG, brain MRI Ophthalmologic examination, visual-evoked potential, electroretinography	L-dopa? Clinical follow-up

(continued)

Table 42.1 (continued)

Disorder	Description	Age at onset	Age at resolution	Diagnostic testing	Treatment
Transient idiopathic dystonia of infancy [13, 14]	Paroxysmal abnormal posture of one limb that disappears with movement	5–10 months	3 months–5 years	Video, brain MRI	No
Shuddering attacks [15]	Paroxysmal shuddering of the head and shoulders	<1 year	<4 years	Video EEG	No
Gratification behavior [6]	Paroxysmal hip flexion, thigh adduction, rhythmic pelvic movements, staring eyes, grunting, facial flushing. Suppressible by distraction	4 months	NA	Video EEG	No
Stereotypies [6]	Paroxysmal repetitive and patterned purposeless movements. Triggered by excitement and suppressible by distraction	<3 years	Can persist until adolescence	Video EEG	No
Sandifer syndrome [6]	Cervical dystonia related to food intake	3 weeks–14 years	No resolution if left untreated	pH metering	Medical and/or surgical treatment of GER

Modified from: Bonnet et al. [6]

NA non applicable, *EEG* electroencephalography, *MRI* magnetic resonance imaging, *GER* gastroesophageal reflux disease

Table 42.2 Type of movement disorder in specific NMD

Dystonia	Glutaric aciduria I
	Leigh syndrome
	MSDU
	Disorders of dopamine metabolism
	Niemann–Pick C
	Gangliosidosis
	PKAN
	Pyruvate dehydrogenase deficiency
	Metachromatic leukodystrophy
Myoclonus	Mitochondrial disorders
	MERFF, MELAS, POLG
	Lysosomal disorders
	Neuronal ceroid lipofuscinosis
	Sialidosis
	GM1, GM2
	Niemann–Pick C
Chorea	Mitochondrial disorders
	Organic acidurias
Tremor	Wilson disease
	Vitamin E deficiency
	Glutaric acidemia I
Stereotypies	PKU
	Lesch–Nyhan disease
Rigid-akinetic syndrome	Disorders of dopamine metabolism (synthesis and transport) [17, 18]
	Early-onset disorders of energy metabolism [19]
	Wilson disease
	Neurodegeneration with brain iron accumulation
	Lysosomal disorders:
	Batten disease
	Gaucher disease

Table 42.3 Main metabolic diseases causing MD

Metal storage diseases	Wilson disease
	PANK2
Neurotransmitter synthesis defects	
Energy metabolism disorders	Respiratory chain disorders (RCDs)
	Pyruvate dehydrogenase
	Biotin deficiency
	Creatine deficiency
Aminoacidopathies and organic acidurias	Glutaric aciduria
	Methylmalonic aciduria
	Propionic aciduria
	MSDU
	Fenilcetonuria
Lysosomal storage diseases	NPC
	Gaucher disease
	GM1, GM2
Defects of transport	Glut1
	Dopamine

children and Table 42.7 the several categories of neuronal autoantibody targets.

42.4.1 Sydenham's Chorea (SC)

Sydenham's chorea (SC) is the commonest form of acquired chorea in children [27]. It is considered the prototype of disorders in which an infectious agent, group A beta-hemolytic *Streptococcus* (GABHS), triggers an autoimmune response [28]. Children with SC have elevated serum antineuronal antibody titers, indicating that the condition is a humorally mediated autoimmune condition [29, 30].

The usual age of onset is 8–9 years, although there are reports in the third decade [28]. The main clinical features of SC are presented in Table 42.8.

The distribution of chorea is usually asymmetrical, and pure hemichorea can be seen in 20 % of patients [31]. Children may have severe chorea and/or hypotonia with few psychiatric symptoms or mild chorea with pronounced psychiatric symptoms [32].

The diagnosis of SC should be considered in all children with an acute onset of chorea.

Table 42.9 shows possible treatments of SC.

42.4.2 Systemic Lupus Erythematosus (SLE) and Primary Antiphospholipid Syndrome (APS)

Chorea usually appears within the first year after the onset of SLE and often precedes the clinical diagnosis of SLE [33]. Chorea has been reported

Table 42.4 Types of NMD according to the way of presentation

Mode of presentation	Neuro-metabolic disorder
Acute	Leigh syndrome
	Glutaric aciduria type I
	Methylmalonic aciduria
	Nonketotic hyperglycinemia
	Creatine deficiency
Paroxysmal	Maple syrup urine disease (intermediary form) [22]
	Glut1 deficiency syndrome [23]
	PDH deficiency
	L-Dopa responsive dystonia (less frequently)
Chronic progressive (Fig. 42.1)	
1. With normal basal ganglia on MRI	
2. With abnormal basal ganglia on MRI	

Modified from: Gouider-Khouja et al. [25]

in 1.3 % of patients with APS and is more common in those patients with APS onset younger than 15 years of age [34]. Chorea has been described as an isolated clinical manifestation in children with APS or in association with SLE [35–37]. Assessment of the true pediatric prevalence of APS is difficult because current diagnostic criteria are based on adult population studies. The features of APS have been increasingly recognized in children, and since APL-related thrombosis can affect any organ, pediatricians of different subspecialties must be aware of this syndrome and associated complications [38, 39].

42.4.3 N-Methyl-D-Aspartate Receptor (NMDA-R) Encephalitis Syndrome

MDs have been described for many years in encephalitis syndromes. NMDA-R encephalitis syndrome was typically described in young women as a paraneoplastic syndrome; it is now recognized in young children and is typically idiopathic or postinfectious. Almost half of the patients are children. In teenage girls, approximately one third have a teratoma. Girls under age 14 and adult men and boys infrequently have a tumor [40, 41]. Table 42.10 show main clinical aspects.

The acute stage of the disease is followed by a prolonged phase of recovery, during which executive functions are altered and psychiatric symptoms often resurface. The treatment involves a multidisciplinary approach, dealing with the acute symptoms of the disease, removal of any underlying causative tumor, induction of immunosuppressive therapy, and management of long-term residual deficits following the remission of the autoimmune process.

42.4.4 Opsoclonus–Myoclonus–Ataxia Syndrome (OMAS)

OMAS in children can occur as a paraneoplastic (neuroblastoma, ganglioneuroma) or nonparaneoplastic (viral infections) syndrome. In both cases, an autoimmune pathophysiology has been proposed.

The presenting symptoms are opsoclonus (involuntary, rapid, multidirectional, conjugate eye movements), myoclonus (muscle jerks), and ataxia. In children, there may be additional features, such as behavioral disturbances, irritability, and cognitive impairment [53].

About 40–50 % of the childhood OMAS are paraneoplastic and vice versa; about 1.5–3.0 % of children with neuroblastoma develop OMAS [54].

Treatment of pediatric OMAS involves resection of the neuroblastoma, if present, and immunotherapy (corticosteroids, plasmapheresis, rituximab, or cyclophosphamide) [55].

The eye movement disorder often improves or resolves, but patients are frequently left with motor, speech, behavioral, and sleep disorders. Relapses are frequent, usually during intercurrent illnesses or attempts to reduce immunotherapy.

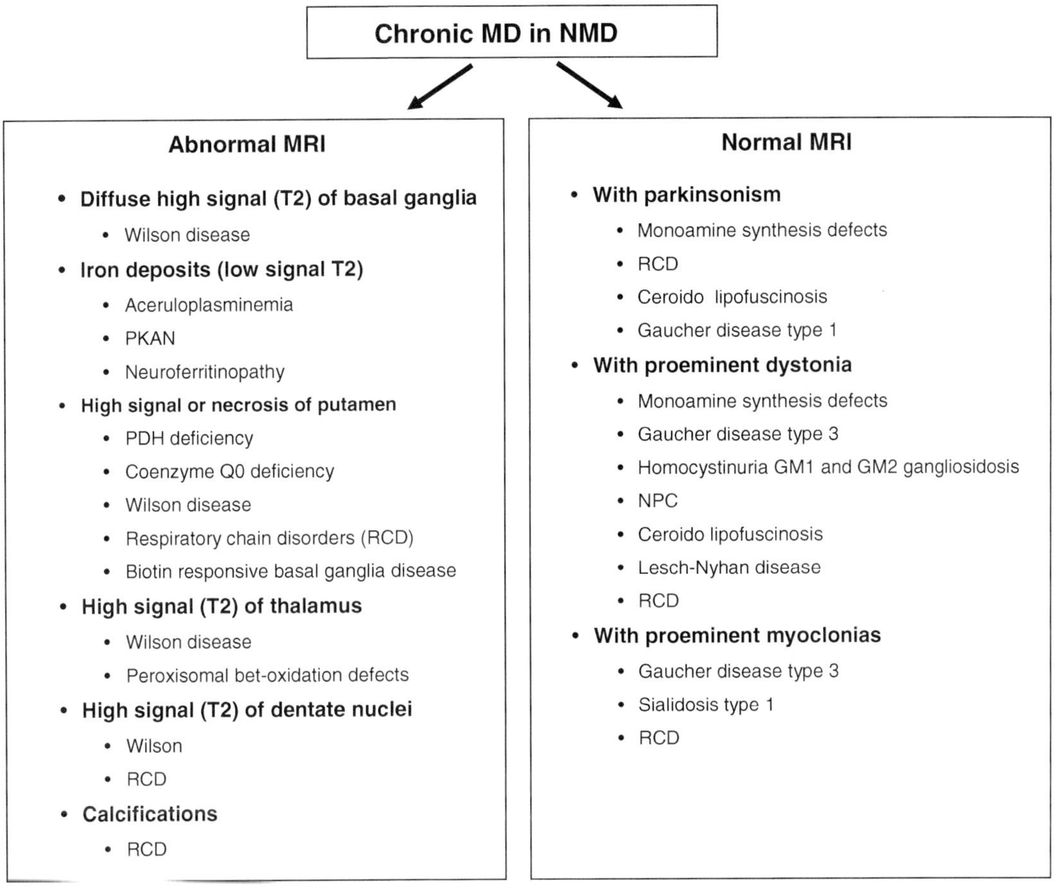

Fig. 42.1 Classification of chronic MD in NMD according to the presence or absence of basal ganglia lesions on cerebral MRI (Modified from: Sedel et al. [24])

Table 42.5 Treatable neuro-metabolic disorders

Wilson disease
Disorders of monoamine metabolism
Biotin-responsive basal ganglia [26]
Pyruvate dehydrogenase deficiency
Glucose transporter type I deficiency
Glutaric aciduria type I
Propionic aciduria
MSDU
Gaucher disease

42.4.5 Progressive Encephalomyelitis, Rigidity, and Myoclonus (PERM)

PERM is a rare neurological disorder, until recently classified as part of the stiff person syndrome (SPS) spectrum. PERM is characterized by limb and truncal rigidity, painful muscle spasms, hyperekplexia, and brain stem signs.

Glycine receptor (GlyR) alpha 1 antibodies have been described in some adult patients with PERM and related disorders, who generally had good outcomes if treated [56].

Actually there is only one report of a child with severe PERM positive for GlyR antibodies. The disease started acutely at the age of 14 months, had periods of exacerbation, and showed a clear response to steroids and other immunotherapies. The features ranged from mild segmental dystonia, auditory sensitive myoclonus and rigidity, and spinal cord and brain stem signs (ocular motor disturbance, hemifacial spasm) to episodes of widespread severe hyperekplexia, rigidity, and myoclonus that affected her respiratory function [57].

Table 42.6 Movement disorders associated with autoimmune disease in children

Main movement disorder	Autoimmune diseases	Other manifestations
Chorea	Sydenham chorea (SC)	See text
	Antiphospholipid syndrome (APS)	
	Systemic lupus erythematosus (SLE)	
	Paraneoplastic chorea	
Dystonia	NMDA-receptor encephalitis	See text
Myoclonus	Opsoclonus myoclonus syndrome (OMS)	See text
	Progressive encephalomyelitis, rigidity, and myoclonus (PERM)	
Tics	PANDAS	See text
Parkinsonism	Anti-NMDA-R encephalitis	See text
	Anti-Ma2 encephalitis	
Miscellaneous of movement disorders	Steroid-responsive encephalopathy associated with autoimmune thyroiditis (SREAT)	Cerebellar ataxia [42, 43] dystonia, tremor, oculogyric crises, parkinsonism, chorea
	Celiac disease and gluten sensitivity	Psychiatric features, sleep disturbance, and brainstem dysfunction [44]
	Dopamine-2 receptor (D2R) antibody-positive encephalitis	

Table 42.7 Neuronal autoantibody targets in some encephalopathy with MDs

Intracellular antigens–antibodies (commonly paraneoplastic)	Anti-Ma2	Testicular cancers	*Upper brain stem* (cranial neuropathies, ophthalmoparesis), *diencephalic* (daytime sleepiness, parkinsonism, or choreatiformic MDs), *limbic symptoms* (seizures, confusion, and short-time memory disturbances)
	Anti-CV2/CRMP5	Small cell lung cancer (SCLC), thymoma	In adults: chorea, dystonia, ballism, cerebellar syndrome
Membrane antigens–antibodies (less commonly paraneoplastic)	Anti-VGKC	SCLC, thymoma	Parkinsonism, chorea, tremor, myoclonus, SPS-like
	Anti-NMDA-R	Ovarian teratoma	See text
Other antigens–antibodies (rarely or nonparaneoplastic)	Antiglycine	Lung, thymoma	SPS, PERM (see text), hypereklepsia
	Anti-TPO, anti-NAE		See text

42.4.6 PANDAS

The term PANDAS (pediatric autoimmune neuropsychiatric disorders associated with streptococcal infections) was coined in 1997. The proposed criteria include (1) onset between 3 years of age and puberty, (2) presence of OCD and/or tic disorder, (3) abrupt onset of symptoms and/or course with recurrent exacerbations and remissions, (4) abnormal neurological examination without frank chorea, and (5) temporal association of symptom exacerbation with *Streptococcus* infection [58].

Treatment with antibiotics has yielded inconclusive results. IVIg and plasmapheresis have been reported to be beneficial in a small number of patients. These treatments, however, have potential serious adverse effects and are generally not recommended.

Table 42.8 Main clinical features of Sydenham chorea

Main symptoms and signs	Neurological abnormalities
	Chorea (4–8 weeks after GABHS pharyngitis but it may develop over hours or days and may occur several months after GABHS infection) [45]
	Muscular weakness and hypotonia (in severe cases this is so pronounced that children may be confined to a wheelchair, termed chorea mollis or chorea paralytica)
	Psychiatric disorders (emotional lability, hyperactivity, distractibility, anger, obsessions, and compulsions) [6]
Investigations	Demonstration of a previous GABHS infection
	Throat cultures
	Anti-streptolysin O or anti-DNAse antibodies (supports the diagnosis, but these tests are not specific)
	Heart examination and echocardiogram (may demonstrate asymptomatic carditis)

Table 42.9 Treatment of Sydenham chorea

Elimination of the *Streptococcus*	Acute phase
	Penicillin 500 mg twice daily (10 days) [46]
	Secondary prophylaxis
	IM benzylpenicillin or daily oral penicillin (penicillin VK 250 mg twice daily) [47, 48]
Treatment of the involuntary movements and psychiatric symptoms	Risperidone, tetrabenazine, haloperidol, pimozide [47, 48] valproic acid, carbamazepine
Treatment of the immune and inflammatory response	Corticosteroids, plasmapheresis, and intravenous immunoglobulin can be considered in severe refractory cases [49]
Supportive measures	Supportive psychotherapy, family therapy, and educational interventions [47]

Table 42.10 Main clinical features of N-methyl-D-aspartate receptor (NMDA-R) encephalitis syndrome

Main symptoms and signs	Prodromal symptoms resembling a viral illness (headache, low-grade fever, fatigue or irritability, upper respiratory tract symptoms, or diarrhea and vomiting)
	Psychiatric symptoms (in children hyperactivity or irritability are more frequent than psychosis), catatonia, agitation
	Seizures, decreased level of consciousness
	Abnormal movements
	Dyskinesias (86 %) of face, trunk, abdomen, prominent orobuccolingual dyskinesias (lip smacking, chewing) [50]
	Chorea, ballismus
	Opisthotonic postures
	Autonomic instability (tachycardia, hyperthermia, and hypertension)
Investigations	Abnormal MRI in 30–50 % of the patients: mild or transient T2/FLAIR signal hyperintensity in the hippocampi, cerebellum, cerebral cortex, subcortical regions, basal ganglia, or brainstem [41]
Treatment	Tumor resection
	Immunotherapy
	First line: methylprednisolone, immunoglobulins
	Second line: cyclophosphamide or rituximab
	Plasmapheresis
	Immunosuppression can be continued for at least 1 year with a steroid-sparing agent [40, 51]
Outcome	About 75 % of patients ultimately recover, usually slowly, over a period of months [40, 52]

42.4.7 Steroid-Responsive Encephalopathy Associated with Autoimmune Thyroiditis (SREAT)

SREAT formerly known as Hashimoto's encephalopathy is rarely described and is underdiagnosed. In a retrospective study with 42 children, Hashimoto's encephalopathy was recognized in 19 % of children with an acute onset of behavioral disturbances, neuropsychiatric features with or without seizures, focal deficits, and dystonia in the absence of other diagnoses and presence of elevated antibodies to thyroperoxidase (anti-TPO antibody) titers (>800 IU/mL) [59, 60]. Tremor and myoclonus are frequently seen on clinical examination.

Antibodies to TPO and thyroglobulin are suggestive of SREAT in the appropriate clinical setting. The complete or near-complete return to the patient's neurological baseline status following corticosteroid treatment is one of the diagnostic criteria.

References

1. Fernandez-Alvarez E. Transient movement disorders in children. J Neurol. 1998;245:1.
2. Shuper A, Zalzberg J, Weitz R, Mimouni M. Jitteriness beyond the neonatal period: a benign pattern of movement in infancy. J Child Neurol. 1991;6(3):243–5.
3. Kaddurah AK, Holmes GL. Benign neonatal sleep myoclonus: history and semiology. Pediatr Neurol. 2009;40:343–6.
4. Maurer VO, Rizzi M, Bianchetti MG, Ramelli GP. Benign neonatal sleep myoclonus: a review of the literature. Pediatrics. 2010;125(4):e919–24.
5. Caraballo RH, Capovilla G, Vigevano F, Beccaria F, Specchio N, Fejerman N. The spectrum of benign myoclonus of early infancy: clinical and neurophysiologic features in 102 patients. Epilepsia. 2009;50(5):1176–83.
6. Bonnet C, Roubertie A, Doummar D, Bahi-Buisson N, Cock VC, Roze E. Developmental and benign movement disorders in childhood. Mov Disord. 2010;25(10):1317–34.
7. Gottlob I, Wizov SS, Reinecke RD. Spasmus nutans. A long-term follow-up. Invest Ophthalmol Vis Sci. 1995;36(13):2768–71.
8. Wizov SS, Reinecke RD, Bocarnea M, Gottlob I. A comparative demographic and socioeconomic study of spasmus nutans and infantile nystagmus. Am J Ophthalmol. 2002;133:256–62.
9. Drigo P, Carli G, Laverda AM. Benign paroxysmal torticollis of infancy. Brain Dev. 2000;22(3):169–72.
10. Giffin NJ, Benton S, Goadsby PJ. Benign paroxysmal torticollis of infancy: four new cases and linkage to CACNA1A mutation. Dev Med Child Neurol. 2002;44(7):490–3.
11. Campistol J, Prats JM, Garaizar C. Benign paroxysmal tonic upgaze in childhood with ataxia: a neuro-ophthalmological syndrome of familial origin? Dev Med Child Neurol. 1993;35:436–9.
12. Ouvrier R, Billson F. Paroxysmal tonic upgaze of childhood-a review. Brain Dev. 2005;27(3):185–8.
13. Good WV, Hou C, Carden SM. Transient, idiopathic nystagmus in infants. Dev Med Child Neurol. 2003;45:304–7.
14. Calado R, Monteiro JP, Fonseca MJ. Transient idiopathic dystonia in infancy. Acta Paediatr. 2011;100(4):624–7.
15. Vanasse M, Bedard P, Andermann F. Shuddering attacks in children: an early clinical manifestation of essential tremor. Neurology. 1976;26:1027–30.
16. Fernandez-Alvarez E, Aicardi J, Bathien N. Movement disorders in children. New York: Cambridge University Press; 2001.
17. Pons R. The phenotypic spectrum of paediatric neurotransmitter diseases and infantile parkinsonism. J Inherit Metab Dis. 2009;32:321–32.
18. Kurian MA, Zhen J, Cheng SY, Li Y, Mordekar SR, Jardine P, Morgan NV, Meyer E, Tee L, et al. Homozygous loss-of-function mutations in the gene encoding the dopamine transporter are associated with infantile parkinsonism-dystonia. J Clin Invest. 2009;119(6):1595–603.
19. Garcia Cazorla A, Rabier D, Touati G, Chadefaux-Vekemans B, Marsac C, de Lonlay P, Saudubray JM. Pyruvate carboxylase deficiency: metabolic characteristics and new neurological aspects. Ann Neurol. 2006;59:121–12.
20. Assmann B, Surtees R, Hoffmann GF. Approach to the diagnosis of neurotransmitter diseases exemplified by the differential diagnosis of childhood-onset dystonia. Ann Neurol. 2003;54 Suppl 6:S18–24.
21. Garcia-Cazorla A, Wolf NI, Serrano M, Perez-Duenas B, Pineda M, Campistol J, et al. Inborn errors of metabolism and motor disturbances in children. J Inherit Metab Dis. 2009;32:618–29.
22. Temudo T, Martins E, Poças F, Cruz R, Vilarinho L. Maple syrup disease presenting as paroxysmal dystonia. Ann Neurol. 2004;56(5):749–50.
23. Suls A, Dedeken P, Goffin K, Van Esch H, Dupont P, Cassiman D, et al. Paroxysmal exercise-induced dyskinesia and epilepsy is due to mutations in SLC2A1, encoding the glucose transporter GLUT1. Brain. 2008;131(Pt 7):1831–44.
24. Sedel F, Saudubray J-M, Roze E, Agid Y, Vidailhet M. Movement disorders and inborn errors of metabolism

in adults: a diagnostic approach. J Inherit Metab Dis. 2008;31:308–18.
25. Gouider-Khouja N, Kraoua I, Benrrhouma H, Fraj N, Rouiissi A. Movement disorders in neuro-metabolic diseases. Eur J Paediatr Neurol. 2010;14:304–7.
26. Ozand PT, Gascon GG, Al Essa M, Joshi S, Al Jishi E, Bakheet S, et al. Biotin-responsive basal ganglia disease: a novel entity. Brain. 1998;121(Pt 7):1267–79.
27. Demiroren K, Yavuz H, Cam L, Oran B, Karaaslan S, Demiroren S. Sydenham's chorea: a clinical follow-up of 65 patients. J Child Neurol. 2007;22:550–4.
28. Cardoso F, Silva CE, Mota CC. Sydenham's chorea in 50 consecutive patients with rheumatic fever. Mov Disord. 1997;12:701–3.
29. Paz JA, Silva CAA, Marques-Dias MJ. Randomized double-blind study with prednisone in Sydenham's chorea. Pediatr Neurol. 2006;34:264–9.
30. Swedo SE. Sydenham's chorea. A model for childhood autoimmune neuropsychiatric disorders. JAMA. 1994;272:1788–91.
31. Baizabal-Carvallo JF M.D., M.Sc., Jankovic J M.D. Movement disorders in autoimmune diseases. Mov Disord. 2012;27(8):935.
32. Garvey MA, Swedo SE. Sydenham's chorea clinical and therapeutic update. Adv Exp Med Biol. 1997;418(2):115–20.
33. BaizabalCarvallo JF, Alonso-Juarez M, Koslowski M. Chorea in systemic lupus erythematosus. J Clin Rheumatol. 2011;17:69–72.
34. Cervera R, Asherson RA, Font J, et al. Chorea in the antiphospholipid syndrome: clinical, radiologic, and immunologic characteristics of 50 patients from our clinics and the recent literature. Medicine (Baltimore). 1997;76:203–12.
35. Angelini L, Zibordi F, Zorzi G, et al. Neurological disorders, other than stroke, associated with antiphospholipid antibodies in childhood. Neuropediatrics. 1996;27:149.
36. Kiechl-Kohlendorfer U, Ellemunter H, Kiechl S. Chorea as the presenting clinical feature of primary antiphospholipid syndrome in childhood. Neuropediatrics. 1999;30:96.
37. Watanabe T, Onda H. Hemichorea with antiphospholipid antibodies in a patient with lupus nephritis. Pediatr Nephrol. 2004;19:451.
38. Avcin T, Cimaz R, Meroni PL. Recent advances in antiphospholipid antibodies and antiphospholipid syndromes in pediatric populations. Lupus. 2002;11:4.
39. Ravelli A, Martini A. Antiphospholipid syndrome. Pediatr Clin North Am. 2005;52:469.
40. Dalmau J, Lancaster E, Martinez-Hernandez E, et al. Clinical experience and laboratory investigations in patients with anti-NMDAR encephalitis. Lancet Neurol. 2011;10:63–74.
41. Dalmau J, Tuzun E, Wu HY, et al. Paraneoplastic anti-N-methyl-D-aspartate receptor encephalitis associated with ovarian teratoma. Ann Neurol. 2007;61:25–33.
42. Kieslich M, Errázuriz G, Posselt HG, et al. Brain white-matter lesions in celiac disease: a prospective study of 75 diet-treated patients. Pediatrics. 2001;108:E21.
43. Zelnik N, Pacht A, Obeid R, et al. Range of neurologic disorders in patients with celiac disease. Pediatrics. 2004;113:1672–6.
44. Dale RC, Merheb V, Pillai S, Wang D, Cantrill L, Murphy TK, Ben-Pazi H, Varadkar S, Aumann TD, Horne MK, Church AJ, Fath T, Brilot F. Antibodies to surface dopamine-2 receptor in autoimmune movement and psychiatric disorders. Brain. 2012;135:3453–68.
45. Zomorrodi A, Wald ER. Sydenham's chorea in western Pennsylvania. Pediatrics. 2006;117:e675–9.
46. Walker KG, Lawrenson J, Wilmshurst JM. Neuropsychiatric movement disorders following streptococcal infection. Dev Med Child Neurol. 2005;47:771–5.
47. Walker KG, Wilmshurst JM. An update on the treatment of Sydenham's chorea: the evidence for established and evolving interventions. Ther Adv Neurol Disord. 2010;3(5):301–9.
48. Cardoso F. Sydenham's chorea. Curr Treat Options Neurol. 2008;10:230–5.
49. Garvey MA, Snider LA, Leitman SF, Werden R, Swedo SE. Treatment of Sydenham's chorea with intravenous immunoglobulin, plasma exchange, or prednisone. J Child Neurol. 2005;20:424–9.
50. Dalmau J, et al. Anti-NMDA-receptor encephalitis: case series and analysis of the effects of antibodies. Lancet Neurol. 2008;7:1091–8.
51. Ferdinand P, Mitchell L. AntiNMDA receptor encephalitis. J Clin Cell Immunol. 2012;S10:007. doi:10.4172/2155-9899.S10-007.
52. Irani SR, Bera K, Waters P, et al. N-methyl-D-aspartate antibody encephalitis: temporal progression of clinical and paraclinical observations in a predominantly non-paraneoplastic disorder of both sexes. Brain. 2010;133:1655–67.
53. Krug P, Schleiermacher G, Michon J, et al. Opsoclonus-myoclonus in children associated or not with neuroblastoma. Eur J Paediatr Neurol. 2010;14:400–9.
54. Tate ED, Allison TJ, Pranzatelli MR, et al. Neuroepidemiologic trends in 105 US cases of pediatric opsoclonus-myoclonus syndrome. J Pediatr Oncol Nurs. 2005;22:8–19.
55. Blaes F. Paraneoplastic brain stem encephalitis. Curr Treat Options Neurol. 2013;15:201–9.
56. Turner MR, Irani SR, Leite MI, Nithi K, Vincent A, Ansorge O. Progressive encephalomyelitis with rigidity and myoclonus: glycine and NMDA receptor antibodies. Neurology. 2011;77(5):439–43.
57. Damásio J, Leite MI, Coutinho E, Waters P, Woodhall M, Santos MA, Carrilho I, Vincent A. Progressive encephalomyelitis with rigidity and myoclonus: the first pediatric case with glycine receptor antibodies. JAMA Neurol. 2013;70(4):498–501.
58. Swedo SE, Leonard HL, Mittleman BB, et al. Identification of children with pediatric autoimmune

neuropsychiatric disorders associated with streptococcal infections by a marker associated with rheumatic fever. Am J Psychiatr. 1997;154:110–2.
59. Mamoudjy N, Korff C, Maurey H, Blanchard G, Steshenko D, Loiseau-Corvez M-N, Husson B, Brauner R, Tardieu M, Deiva K. Hashimoto's encephalopathy: identification and long-term outcome in children. Eur J Paediatr Neurol. 2013;17:280e287.
60. Erol I, Saygi S, Alehan F. Hashimoto's encephalopathy in children and adolescents. Pediatr Neurol. 2011;45:420e2.

Systemic Illnesses That Cause Movement Disorders

43

Ovidiu A. Bajenaru

As the brain network of circuits related to the cortical and subcortical structures involved in the control of motor behavior is structurally and functionally extremely complex, implying a multisynaptic activity and an intracellular metabolic signaling system using multiple biochemical pathways, its vulnerability to various pathogenetic mechanisms related to many of the systemic diseases with CNS involvement is increased. This vulnerability is related to both structural lesions and biochemical alterations, and the large variability of systemic diseases and their particular mechanisms explain why different movement disorders, among chorea and dystonia, are probably the most frequent [1], being part of the clinical symptomatology of these diseases, usually in association with other neurological and specific non-neurological symptoms suggestive for a particular etiology.

In this review, we shall try to describe in a concise and systematized manner these abnormalities related to the most frequent systemic diseases, grouped in etiologic categories.

43.1 Infectious Diseases

43.1.1 HIV Infection

Neurological disorders associated with HIV infection are due to lesions which may appear at all levels of both central and peripheral nervous system, in all stages and forms of the disease (both the primary HIV-associated illness and the secondary neurologic complications determined by immunosuppression as the opportunistic infections – toxoplasmosis, tuberculosis, cryptococcosis, syphilis, progressive multifocal leukoencephalopathy, or primary lymphoma of the CNS). In particular, in HIV encephalopathy the basal ganglia have a particular susceptibility, probably because of the high density of microglia (those cells infected by the virus, which mediate subsequent neuronal death) and due to the intrinsic properties of the neurons in this brain area [2]. In rare cases, spinal myoclonus has been associated with HIV infection [3]. Also the secondary effects of some of the specific drugs used in the current era of HAART may contribute to some clinical particularities of the secondary movement disorders that might become apparent in this illness. Not only parkinsonism and dystonia but also chorea–ballismus, myoclonus, tremor,

O.A. Bajenaru, MD, PhD
Department of Neurology, University Emergency Hospital Bucharest, 169, Splaiul Independentei, sectorul 5, Bucharest RO-050098, Romania

Department of Neurology, Neurosurgery and Psychiatry, University of Medicine and Pharmacy "Carol Davila" Bucharest, Bucharest, Romania
e-mail: alstov9157@gmail.com

C. Falup-Pecurariu et al. (eds.), *Movement Disorders Curricula*,
DOI 10.1007/978-3-7091-1628-9_43

akathisia, neuroleptic malignant syndrome, oculomasticatory myorhythmia (associated with Whipple's disease), and paroxysmal dyskinesias have been reported in HIV-infected patients [1, 4–16]. Also tardive dyskinesia may be seen in these patients [17]. Drug interactions with ritornavir, indinavir, and risperidone have been related to the appearance of a dystonic syndrome in some patients [18]. In several cases, dystonia in HIV-infected patients has been correlated to the presence of bilateral striatal lucencies on MR images [19]. The presence of hyperkinesias in patients with AIDS seems to be most often correlated with *Toxoplasma gondii* abscesses [16].

43.1.2 Other Viral Infections

The clinical manifestations and severity of many of the systemic viral infections are due to their particular neurotropism and become apparent mainly by an encephalitic picture which often includes movement disorders. Among these, in the Japanese encephalitis parkinsonism, chorea, dystonia, tremor, and myoclonus have been reported [20–24]. Also other viral encephalitis produced by the arboviruses, enteroviruses, herpes simplex virus, varicella virus, cytomegalovirus, mumps, measles, Epstein–Barr virus, rubella, and postvaccination complications, which appear especially among children, can be associated in the course of the infection with abnormal movements [25–28].

Transient choreoathetosis has been reported in cases of acute encephalitis determined by influenza virus A infection [29]. For a more detailed description of these conditions, see [1].

43.1.3 Bacterial Infections

The CNS lesions in bacterial infections either are mediated by autoimmune mechanisms, due to the production of antibodies which cross-react to structures of the CNS, without a nervous system direct infection, or produced by direct infection of the nervous structures. In the first group of illnesses, the most typical is *Sydenham chorea* – one of the major manifestations of rheumatic fever, caused by the group Aβ-hemolytic streptococcus infection. Anti-basal ganglia antibodies (antineuronal antibodies) can be detected with a high sensitivity and specificity [30]. The movement disorders have often an insidious onset, with a delay of some months after the causative infection, and they typically progress over some weeks, but generally spontaneously disappear within 6 months [3]. Most often, the motor signs consist in generalized chorea, but in a minority of cases hemichorea has been reported and even more rarely a later clinical form of paralytic chorea [1]. Other movement abnormalities reported in Sydenham chorea are ballismus, facial grimacing, dysarthria, tics, dystonia and dystonic choreoathetosis, oculomotor abnormalities, and motor impersistence; the motor abnormalities are in most cases associated with other neuropsychiatric manifestations as hyperactivity, attention deficit, obsessive–compulsive disorders, anxiety, and less frequent psychosis [1, 31–37].

In less than 20 % of *CNS tuberculosis* cases, tremor, chorea–ballismus, dystonia, myoclonus, and parkinsonism may also be present [1]. The first case of parkinsonian tremor related to a mesencephalic lesion has been described by G. Marinescu and P. Blocq in 1893, in a case of tuberculoma localized in the substantia nigra [38]; this observation has been at the origin of the subsequent research of Brissaud [39] who in 1895 reported that parkinsonism is a consequence of lesions in the substantia nigra. Chorea, myoclonus, and dystonia have also been reported in cases with tuberculous meningitis [40, 41]. Beyond the above historical observations, the actual reported data in such patients do not allow the evidence of a clear correlation between neurological findings and focal lesion on imaging studies [42].

Movement disorders have also been reported in patients with *meningitis* caused by numerous other bacterial agents (*Salmonella*, *Legionella pneumophila*, *Borrelia burgdorferi*, *Treponema pallidum*, Streptococcus viridans, *Haemophilus influenzae*, *Streptococcus pneumoniae*, and *Neisseria meningitidis*) [1]. Dystonia has been reported in cases of infections caused by

Mycoplasma pneumoniae who had acute bilateral thalamic necrosis [43, 44]. In rare cases, spinal myoclonus has been associated with Lyme disease [3].

43.1.4 Parasitic Diseases

Symptomatic movement disorders have been reported mainly in patients with *malaria* and *neurocysticercosis* [1] but also in *African trypanosomiasis* [45] and *paracoccidioidomycosis* [46].

In patients with *malaria*, motor abnormalities may appear both in the acute phase of the disease and as component of the clinical picture of the post-malaria neurological syndrome. They may manifest as tremor and opsoclonus, opsoclonus–myoclonus syndrome, chorea, dystonia, and parkinsonism [1]. There is no clear relationship between the specific mechanisms of the disease and these motor abnormalities.

In *neurocysticercosis*, parkinsonism and tremor are the most common movement disorders, but in rare cases also chorea, dystonia, myoclonus, and hemifacial spasm have been reported [1]. Hydrocephalus seems to be the main cause of parkinsonism and tremor, but the presence of perimesencephalic cysts and the lacunar ischemic lesions might be due to the satellite vasculitis complicating severe forms of neurocysticercosis.

43.2 Autoimmune Inflammatory Systemic Diseases

The most typical disease in this group which clinical manifestations include sometimes movement disorders is *systemic lupus erythematosus (SLE)* when impairment of CNS is present; also the *antiphospholipid antibody syndrome*, which may appear associated with SLE or independently, may clinically manifest with different movement disorders when CNS impairment is associated, both in adults and children. These motor abnormalities may appear after some years from the onset of the disease and are usually associated with other neurologic manifestations as seizures, psychosis, and myelitis, but rarely they may be the initial symptoms [1]. In particular, asymmetric or unilateral chorea has been most often reported in association with these nosologic entities [47]. A special mention is related to the apparition of chorea in pregnant women which in certain situations could be the first clinical manifestation of SLE and implies a differential diagnosis with a clinical recurrence of Sydenham chorea or drug-related chorea. In rare cases of SLE in children, an associated parkinsonian syndrome has been described [48]. In a report [49], blepharospasm has been associated with the presence of collagen diseases in a group of patients.

43.3 Paraneoplastic Disorders

Movement disorders have been associated to some of the neurological paraneoplastic disorders, usually associated with other neurologic manifestations. In *anti-NMDA encephalitis* (which may also be a primary autoimmune disease, not always being the clinical expression of a paraneoplastic syndrome), different types of dyskinesias have been described, more commonly but not exclusively in young women and children [50, 51]. In the paraneoplastic *opsoclonus–myoclonus syndrome*, the motor abnormalities usually consist in myoclonus of the trunk, limbs, or head, associated with opsoclonus. In children, this clinical syndrome has been most often associated with neuroblastoma, while in adults small-cell lung carcinoma, breast cancer, and ovary cancer are the most frequent causes. In rare cases, this clinical syndrome has not a paraneoplastic origin, but may be related to other inflammatory diseases as viral encephalitis [50, 52]. *Paraneoplastic stiff-person syndrome* has been associated with small-cell lung carcinoma, renal cancer, breast cancer, non-Hodgkin lymphoma, or other types of cancer [1, 51]. Other paraneoplastic syndromes manifesting with movement disorders have also been reported: *paraneoplastic chorea* (associated with small-cell lung carcinoma, renal cancer, non-Hodgkin lymphoma), *paraneoplastic parkinsonism–dystonia* (associated with ductal cell breast carcinoma), *Holmes tremor* (associated with ovarian cancer), and paraneoplastic myoclonus (associated with cancer, carcinoma of the kidney, pulmonary carcinoma) [1].

43.4 Hematologic Disorders

Iron-deficiency anemia is one of the conditions which may be the cause of a secondary *restless legs syndrome* (see Chap. 36). Even though the primary restless syndrome is probably more frequent, always for the differential etiologic diagnosis in patients with this syndrome, the iron-deficiency anemia and *diabetes mellitus*, *amyloidosis*, *uremia*, *gastrectomy*, *cancer*, *chronic obstructive pulmonary disease*, *peripheral vascular diseases*, *rheumatoid arthritis*, *hypomagnesemia*, and *hypothyroidism* have to be taken into account [53]. In *pernicious anemia*, cases with stiff-person syndrome have been reported [3].

In the *hemolytic disease of the newborn* caused by different blood group incompatibility, the unconjugated bilirubin reaches very high serum levels and cross the blood–brain barrier causing the so-called "nuclear jaundice" or "kernicterus" due to its toxic neuronal effects mainly in the basal ganglia, cerebellum, hippocampus, and cranial nerve nuclei. This disease has a high mortality; the survivors develop a chronic neurologic syndrome manifested by the *choreoathetoid* form of *cerebral palsy* [54].

Chorea, reversible if the hematologic condition is effectively treated, has been reported in cases of *polycythemia* [47]. The CNS leukocytoclastic IgA-mediated vasculitis which appears in patients (most often children) with *Henoch–Schönlein purpura*, as a particular expression of a multisystem vasculitis, may cause brain lesions. These lesions may be clinically expressed in some cases by *chorea* associated or not with other neurologic manifestations, such as *ataxia*, *motor weakness*, or *seizures*; in these patients, the CNS vasculitis is sometimes associated with lesions of the peripheral nerves manifesting as peripheral neuropathy [54].

In some rare genetic diseases associated with *red cell abnormalities* manifesting as *acanthocytosis*, *neuroacanthocytosis* (with autosomal recessive transmission), and *McLeod syndrome* (X-linked transmission), movement disorders are present and important for the clinical suspicion of the etiologic diagnosis in the context of particular clinical pictures (see also Chap. 44). In *neuroacanthocytosis*, the clinical expression manifests in young patients by progressive movement disorders (*dystonia*, predominantly *orofacial with dystonic tongue protrusion*, *chorea*, *tics*, and, in more advanced stages, *parkinsonism*) associated with cognitive and behavioral modifications [3]. In *McLeod syndrome*, which has its clinical onset in more advanced age patients (around 50 years old), *limb chorea* is more frequent than *oral movements* and *limb and tongue biting* [3] are sometimes associated with peripheral axonal neuropathy. Among the non-neurologic clinical manifestations, cardiomyopathy and hemolytic anemia seem to be most often present [3, 55].

43.5 Hypoxic–Ischemic Causes

Global cellular hypoxia of the brain is the consequence of multiple etiologic conditions which may appear essentially in two categories of patients: in newborns, due to perinatal anoxia and at any age after the perinatal period, due to cardiopulmonary diseases, asphyxia, drugs, and intoxications. The metabolic consequences at the neuronal level and other cells in the CNS may be diffuse but usually nonhomogeneous due to different biological factors: cellular susceptibility to anoxic aggression, local density of the microvascular network, preexisting vascular subclinical abnormalities, etc. Particularly, the striatum components have a higher vulnerability to hypoxic–ischemic conditions due to their intense oxidative metabolism and to their functional organization, implying a very rich and highly interconnected synaptic network activity, which is mediated by a high number of neurotransmitters and neuromodulators, dependent on an extremely complex metabolic activity. This activity is in turn regulated by enzymatic regulation related to the synthesis, intracellular transport, storage, synaptic release, receptor binding, and activation of these neurotransmitters, triggering numerous and specific postsynaptic cellular signaling pathways, reuptake, metabolism, and recycling. These events are only a part of the pathophysiological premises for the appearance of abnormal movements related to the brain hypoxic–ischemic lesions.

In *perinatal anoxia* cases, the abnormalities manifest most often as *dystonia* in different variants: generalized, focal, or segmental [56]; the onset of dystonia is usually delayed, so that in any case of delayed-onset dystonia in children, perinatal anoxia has to be taken into account for the etiologic differential diagnosis [57]. Delayed-onset *choreoathetosis* has been reported as well [58]. The most typical pathologic condition in these cases is *status marmoratus of the striatum* [1, 25, 59]. Parkinsonism has also been reported as a consequence of perinatal anoxia [60].

The "*post – pump chorea*" has been described in children who had surgery necessitating controlled circulatory arrest, cardiopulmonary bypass, and hypothermia [1, 25, 61] which caused important neuronal loss and gliosis in particular in the globus pallidus [25]. The clinical consequences of these lesions are chorea or ballismus, episodic eye deviations, and hypotonia after a short initial asymptomatic period [25], in some cases very severe and irreversible.

At any age, *cardiorespiratory arrest,* which is resuscitated after a more or less prolonged delay, is the most common cause of brain hypoxic–ischemic injury, determined by different etiologic conditions: cardiac arrest (occurring by primary or secondary paroxysmal dysrhythmia), general anesthesia, pulmonary asthma, drowning, and drug overdoses. In these cases, *myoclonus* may be present very early, even during the comatose phase (often associated with seizures) and/or during the recovery from the acute hypoxia (the Lance–Adams syndrome). After recovery, myoclonic jerks accompanying voluntary movements and extending to body parts not directly involved in voluntary movements can appear [3]. *Dystonia* with onset after a variable delay (months–years) has often been reported. A different clinical and pathophysiological condition than acute hypoxia is *encephalopathy* which appears as a consequence of *chronic pulmonary insufficiency* and may manifest by *postural tremor*, *myoclonus*, *asterixis*, and brisk tendon reflexes with or without papilledema [47].

Stroke is a brain-specific disorder, but taking into account its causes (which in most instances are different to a primary CNS pathology) and the acute/subacute pathophysiologic consequences on the cardiovascular and neuroendocrine homeostatic regulatory systems of the organism, it may also be considered as a systemic disorder. In 3.7 % of cases of patients who had a stroke, different movement disorders have been reported [62]. In most instances, poststroke movement disorders are related to deep vascular lesions in the striatum, thalamus, and their connections, but more rarely the lesions have been reported in cortical areas or in the brain stem (mainly in the mesencephalic nuclei) and spinal cord [1]. The clinical manifestations may be variable, related to the etiology and location of the vascular lesions, their number and combinations (mainly for the deep infarcts or hemorrhages), and possibly other structural, genetic susceptibilities and biologic particularities of the brain for each individual patient: parkinsonism (see Chap. 22), focal or segmental dystonia, focal choreoathetosis, ballism (most often hemiballism), myoclonus, tremor, tourettism, and asterixis [1, 63–65].

43.6 Metabolic Disorders

The metabolic encephalopathies, as a group of neurological disorders, generally manifest by an association of an altered mental status – often with delirium, slight increase in muscle tone, and particular movement abnormalities [66] which are mentioned below, in relation to different etiologic forms.

A. The *portal systemic encephalopathy* which appears as a complication of liver diseases may manifest early by a quite suggestive neurological sign: the *flapping tremor* or *asterixis*, which in certain cases may be the only neurological sign [67]. This clinical sign is due to a sudden loss of the postural tone which may be seen most often as a sudden flexion of the wrist followed by a rapid return to extension, but it may also be noticed at the knees in patients in prone position. Sometimes, this sign manifests earlier at the level of the fingers in a more discrete manner, as small lateral movements [66]. Even if the most probable clinical condition related to the appearance of asterixis is the portal systemic encephalopathy, this abnormal movement has also been noticed in other etiologic conditions, such as other metabolic encephalopathies, drug intoxications, or stroke [63].

B. *Chronic hepatocerebral degeneration* is a concept referring to a non-Wilsonian neurologic syndrome caused by a chronic acquired parenchymal liver disease (with different etiologies) in the absence of the portal systemic encephalopathy. The neurologic clinical picture has similarities with the one in Wilson disease; more types of movement abnormalities have been reported including *action tremor*, *buccolingual masticatory dyskinesias* (which are particularly common), *generalized chorea* [68], *choreoathetosis* [47], *dystonia* [69], *parkinsonism* (in some patients it may be prominent) [70], *ataxia*, and *dysarthria* [47].

C. *Wilson disease* (*hepatolenticular degeneration*) is a systemic, autosomal recessive inherited, metabolic condition leading to the impossibility of the hepatocyte to use cooper ions for the normal integration in the structure of ceruloplasmin and the impossibility to evacuate excessive copper content from hepatocyte to the biliary pathways; as a consequence, a massive hepatocyte destruction will appear with progressive development of hepatic fibrosis and cirrhosis followed by systemic copper deposition in other organs: CNS, eye (cornea, crystalline), kidney, pancreas, heart, muscles, and blood cells. Secondary iron metabolism abnormalities are present, due to the incapacity of the abnormal ceruloplasmin to exert its function of oxidase for the ferrous form to ferric form of the iron ion. The neurologic picture due to the CNS lesions is dominated by movement abnormalities associated with psychiatric and behavioral manifestations and specific laboratory abnormalities (a detailed description of this disease is the subject of Chap. 33). The movement abnormalities are mainly related to a characteristic *extrapyramidal rigidity* and abnormal movements: *postural* and *action tremor*, *progressive dystonia* (*focal*, *segmental*, *or generalized*, sometimes leading to invalidating *dystonic postures*), *parkinsonism*, *ataxia*, *titubation*, *chorea*, *dysarthria*, and *seizures* [3].

D. *Uremic encephalopathy* is caused by severe renal failure, which causes are quite diverse (chronic arterial hypertension, diabetes mellitus, autoimmune systemic disorders, infective diseases of the kidney, others). Due to the interferences between these different etiologic conditions which often result in direct lesions in the nervous system and the metabolic consequences of the renal failure itself, sometimes enhanced by the secondary effects of the treatment, the neurologic manifestations of the so-called "uremic encephalopathy" are not strictly dependent of the patient's renal function. Among the movement abnormalities which usually accompany an altered mental status and appear quite frequent related to this type of encephalopathy, the most often reported are *asterixis*, *tremor*, *myoclonus*, *tetany*, *and spontaneous carpopedal spasms* [66].

E. *Electrolyte disturbances*

   1. Movement disorders related to *sodium disturbances* are mainly noticed in very severe *hypernatremia* (sodium serum level over 155 mEq/L) with abrupt increase of hyperosmolarity and consist in *asterixis*, *myoclonus*, *seizures*, *choreoathetotic movements* associated with impairment of consciousness [66]. This clinical picture is more often present in children [71]. In *hyponatremia* (serum sodium levels below 135 mEq/L), which may be the result of numerous etiologic circumstances,

movement disorders are not specific; in these cases, there is an important impairment of consciousness often associated with *convulsions*. One particular pathology is related to the rapid therapeutic correction of hyponatremia, leading to the development of an *osmotic demyelination syndrome* (which may also be related to other etiologies) [72] with more pathologic forms: *central pontine myelinolysis* and *extrapontine osmotic demyelination* (including the impairment of *basal ganglia* that has been reported). Movement disorders related to the osmotic demyelination syndrome have usually a delayed onset and manifest as *generalized dystonia during voluntary movements* (in some cases improved by trihexyphenidyl), *choreoathetosis*, *parkinsonism* [73–77], and *myoclonus* [60]. *Painful dystonia of the facial muscles and lower limbs* has also been reported [60]. An *acute rigid–akinetic syndrome responsive to levodopa* has also been described, in contrast to the *delayed-onset movement disorders* which usually are not treatment responsive [73]. Not in all cases with movement disorders related to an osmotic demyelination syndrome, MRI lesions in the basal ganglia have been detected [74, 76], while in other cases, such lesions were evident [75].

2. In contrast to serum sodium abnormalities, neurologic manifestations of serum *potassium disequilibrium* are rare and nonspecific, but in these cases the severe life-menacing cardiac dysrhythmia is most important. In rare cases, a *generalized muscle weakness* has been reported [71].
3. Movement disorders related to serum calcium abnormalities will be described in the next section of this chapter (related to endocrine disorders).

F. *Vitamin deficiencies*. Motor abnormalities have also been related to some chronic vitamin deficiency usually associated with more specific neurological signs, as *cobalamin* (rare cases of *chorea*), *nicotinamide* (*paratonia, startle myoclonus*), genetic mutations related to *tocopherol* activity nonresponsive to vitamin E supplementation (*ataxia, dystonic movements*), or tocopherol deficiency related to small bowel disease, which are responsive to vitamin E supplementation (*ataxia*) [60, 78].

G. In *Whipple disease* movement abnormalities, such as *oculomasticatory myorhythmia* (pendular vergence oscillations of the eyes with concurrent contractions of masticatory muscles), *oculofacial–skeletal myorhythmia*, *myoclonus*, *cerebellar ataxia*, and *seizures* [47] may be present in association with progressive cognitive impairment leading to dementia (which is the most common neurologic feature).

H. *Abnormalities of iron metabolism*. Iron overload diseases may imply multiorgan pathology manifesting as systemic diseases or as organ-specific disorders, including CNS (this group of diseases formerly known as "Hallervorden–Spatz syndrome" is discussed in Chap. 38; it includes four subtypes causing progressive extrapyramidal movement disorders: pantothenate kinase gene mutation-associated neurodegeneration, neuroferritinopathy, infantile neuroaxonal dystrophy, and aceruloplasminemia). *Hemochromatosis* is an inherited systemic disease which is related to dysregulation of iron metabolism resulting in deposition of abnormal quantities and eventually secondary lesions in the cells of a wide range of organs (including CNS). *Secondary iron overload* which can lead to similar pathologic and clinical features as hemochromatosis refers to an acquired condition determined by some iron-loading types of anemia as thalassemia or sideroblastic anemia [79]. In some cases of hemochromatosis, neurologic manifestations have been reported, including *tremor*, *myoclonus*, *parkinsonism*, and *dystonia* associated with multiple hyperintensities on T2-weighted MRI in hemispheric white matter and cerebral and cerebellar atrophy [60].

I. *Genetic metabolic diseases*. Due to the limited dimensions of this chapter, in this section, we shall mention just some of the very numerous entities included in this large group of diseases, in which some movement abnormalities have been reported as significant clinical manifestations [cited by 60]:

- *Niemann–Pick disease type C*: *ataxia* and *vertical gaze palsy*
- *Glutaric aciduria type I*: *acute dystonia*
- *Methylmalonic aciduria, propionic aciduria, pyruvate dehydrogenase deficiency*: *episodic dystonia*
- *Triosephosphate isomerase deficiency*: *dystonic movements, tremor*
- *GLUT 1 gene mutation*: *ataxia, dystonia, choreoathetosis*
- *GM1 gangliosidosis*: *early-onset generalized dystonia*
- *GM2 gangliosidosis*: *juvenile progressive dystonia*, *choreoathetosis*, and *ataxia*
- *Homocystinuria*: *progressive generalized dystonia*
- *Hartnup disease*: *intermittent dystonic posturing of the lower extremities*

43.7 Endocrine Diseases

A. *Diabetes mellitus* is the most frequent endocrine and metabolic disorder in the modern world. Apart from its vascular complications of the CNS manifested as silent or clinical stroke, abnormal movements may also appear in relation with hyperglycemia or hypoglycemia. In *nonketotic hyperglycemia*, such neurologic abnormalities accompanying most often a progressive alteration of the mental status and sometimes seizures and/or motor weakness may manifest as *chorea*, *ballism*, or other *hyperkinetic movement disorders* associated with focal hyperintensities in the putamen and caudate nuclei on T1-weighted brain MRI [47, 80].

B. *Hypoglycemia* may be related to cases of diabetes mellitus treated with insulin or oral antidiabetic drugs but who do not respect the food schedule, or to other etiologic conditions different to diabetes, like insulin-producing tumors. In these cases, *tremor* may be a very early sign, even before the alteration of the mental status with or without other clinical signs of sympathetic reactive overactivation. In patients who had repeated episodes of hypoglycemia, *chronic persistent choreatic movements* have also been reported [81], while in certain cases *paroxysmal kinesigenic choreoathetosis*, accompanying acute hypoglycemic episodes have been noticed [82, 83]. Episodes manifesting as postprandial *restless legs syndrome* have been suggested to be correlated with hypoglycemia [84].

C. *Hyperthyroidism*. The most prominent motor abnormality in hyperthyroidism is an *enhanced physiological tremor* associated with *myotatic hyperreflexia* [85]. Other abnormal movements reported in association with this disease are *chorea* and *paroxysmal choreoathetosis* [47] and *episodic relapsing paroxysmal kinesigenic dystonia* which remitted once the euthyroid status is obtained [86].

D. In *Hashimoto's thyroiditis*, *tremor*, *multifocal myoclonus*, and *gait ataxia* have been reported [87]. Myoclonus may be aggravated by antiepileptic drugs [88]. Also *opsoclonus*, *chorea*, and a *rigid–akinetic syndrome* have been noticed. *Palatal tremor* and *myorhythmias* have rarely been described [89].

E. *Hypoparathyroidism* (idiopathic or postthyroidectomy) and *pseudohypoparathyroidism* due to peripheral resistance to the physiological effects of the parathyroid hormone (PTH) are associated with neurological manifestations probably related at least in part to *hypocalcemia* and abnormal calcium and phosphorus metabolism. The abnormal tissue utilization of calcium in the absence of the PTH effects determines at the level of the brain calcium accumulation predominantly in the basal ganglia, but in most cases, this pathology does not determine any clinical manifestation. The idiopathic *basal ganglia calcification* frequently associated with calcifications in the dental nuclei of the cerebellum (*Fahr's disease* or *bilateral striato–pallido–dentate calcification*) is most often not related to abnormalities of the parathyroid hormone utilization; it is estimated that in up to 1 % of all CT brain scans, this represents an incidental finding without a definite etiologic significance, but other causes have also been related to this pathology (metabolic, infectious, genetic disorders) [3]. In the symptomatic patients, the development of a *progressive parkinsonism* with delayed onset up to 30 years after thyroidectomy [1] associated with mental changes has been described [90–92]. Other reported motor manifestations in such cases are *Chvostek's sign, painful spasms, carpopedal spasms, generalized spasms, grand mal seizures, mild choreatic movements* [1, 47], *dystonia, athetosis, tremor*, and *orofacial dyskinesia* [3].

F. *Panhypopituitarism* has been associated in cases with the presence of a *stiff-person syndrome* which remitted with the hormonal substitution treatment [93, 94].

43.8 Intoxications

Many types of intoxications are associated with CNS pathology. These are drug-related intoxications or related to environmental chemical or physical agents. In this chapter, we shall just mention the *toxic-induced parkinsonism* (which is detailed in Chap. 21) related to some *pesticides, MPTP (1-methyl-4-phenyl-1,2,3,6-tetrahydropyridine), post-acute carbon monoxide intoxication*, and *manganese chronic intoxication* [3]. In the *manganese chronic intoxication*, not only parkinsonism may develop but also other neurologic manifestations as headache, behavioral modifications, and cognitive impairment followed by motor abnormalities: *parkinsonism, dystonia, retropulsion*, and *gait impairment* (a characteristic *cock walk*) [95, 96]. Apart from the parkinsonian syndrome, in the survivors of *carbon monoxide intoxication* a *delayed-onset dystonia* has also been noticed [60]. *Myoclonus, ataxia, seizures*, and *tremor* associated with headache, mental changes, nausea, and visual disturbances have been related to acute exposure to *lower concentrations of methyl bromide* (used as refrigerant, insecticide, fire extinguisher, fumigant) [95, 97, 98]. Secondary movement disorders may also develop as adverse reactions to many drugs (see Chap. 40); here we just mention that in certain systemic diseases, some specific drugs used for their specific treatment may be related to some movement disorders: in patients treated by *lamivudine (acute dystonic reactions)* [99], *cinnarizine (parkinsonism, buccolingual masticatory syndrome, dystonia)* [100], *flunarizine (dystonia)* [100], and antitussive medication containing *dextromethorphan* or *codeine (dystonic reactions*, mainly in children) [101]. In patients using stimulant substances as cocaine, amphetamine, dextroamphetamine, methamphetamine, methylphenidate, and 3,4-methylenedioxymeth amphetamine (MDMA, ecstasy), the presence of movement abnormalities has often been reported: *hyperkinetic movement disorders (dystonia, acute dystonic reactions to neuroleptics, chorea*, and *motor and vocal tics*) which sometimes may be persistent for months after abstinence [95, 102]. In patients using amphetamine, *oromandibular stereotypical movements* have been reported [95].

IX. *Tardive dyskinesia* and other *tardive syndromes* are discussed in Chap. 27 of this book.

References

1. Alarcon F, Gimenez-Roldan S. Systemic diseases that cause movement disorders. Review. Parkinsonism Relat Disord. 2005;11:1–18.
2. Boisse L, Gill J, Power C. Neurological disorders associated with human immunodeficiency virus infection. In: Schapira AHV, Byrne E, DiMauro S, Frackowiack RSJ, Johnson RT, Mizumo Y, Samuels MA, Silberstein SD, Wszolek ZK, editors. Neurology and clinical neuroscience. Philadelphia: Mosby Elsevier; 2007. p. 1261–72.
3. Jankovic J. Movement disorders. In: Daroff RB, Fenichel GM, Jankovic J, Mazziotta JC, editors. Bradley's neurology in clinical practice. 6th ed. Philadelphia: Elsevier Saunders; 2012. p. 1762–801.
4. Lees AJ. Odd and unusual movement disorders. J Neurol Neurosurg Psychiatry. 2002;72 Suppl 1:117–21.
5. Brew BJ. HIV neurology. New York: Oxford University Press; 2001.
6. Nath A, Jankovic J, Pettigrew C. Movement disorders and AIDS. Neurology. 1987;37(1):37–41.

7. Mirsattari SM, Roke Berry ME, Holden JK, Ni W, Nath A, Power C. Paroxysmal dyskinesias in patients with HIV infection. Neurology. 1999;52(1): 109–14.
8. Elder G, Sever JL. Neurologic disorders associated with AIDS retroviral infection. Rev Infect Dis. 1988;10(2):286–302.
9. Berger JR, Moskowitz L, Fisch L, Kelley RE. The neurologic complications of the acquired immunodeficiency syndrome. Neurology. 1984;34 Suppl 1: 134–5.
10. Metzer WS. Movement disorders with AIDS encephalopathy: case report. Neurology. 1987;37(8):1438.
11. Piccolo I, Causarano R, Sterzi R, Sberna M, Oreste PL, Maioli C, Caggese L, Girotti F. Chorea in patients with AIDS. Acta Neurol Scand. 1999;100(5): 332–6.
12. Piccolo I, Sterzi R, Thiella G, Minazzi MS, Caraceni T. Sporadic choreas: analysis of a general hospital series. Eur Neurol. 1999;41(3):143–9.
13. Carranza EJ, Rossitch E, Samuels MA. Parkinsonian symptoms in a patient with AIDS and cerebral toxoplasmosis. J Neurol Neurosurg Psychiatry. 1989; 52(12):1445–7.
14. Hirose G. Parkinsonism in a patient with AIDS. Intern Med. 2000;39(12):1006–7.
15. Maggi P, de Mari M, Moramarco A, Fiorentino G, Lamberti P, Angarano G. Parkinsonism in a patient with AIDS and cerebral opportunistic granulomatous lesions. Neurol Sci. 2000;21(3):173–6.
16. Mirsattari SM, Power C, Nath A. Parkinsonism with HIV infection. Mov Disord. 1998;13(4):684–9.
17. Factor SA, Troche-Panetto, Weaver SA. Dystonia in AIDS: report of four cases. Mov Disord. 2003; 18(12):1492–8.
18. Kelly DV, Beique LC, Bowmer MI. Extrapyramidal symptoms with ritonavir/indinavir plus risperidone. Ann Pharmacother. 2002;36(5):827–30.
19. Abbruzzese G, Rizzo F, Dall'Agata D, Morandi N, Favale E. Generalized dystonia with bilateral striatal computed-tomographic lucencies in a patient with human immunodeficiency virus infection. Eur Neurol. 1990;30(5):271–3.
20. Kalita J, Misra UK. Markedly severe dystonia in Japanese encephalitis. Mov Disord. 2000;15(16): 1168–72.
21. Misra UK, Kalita J. Prognosis of Japanese encephalitis patients with dystonia compared to those with Parkinsonian features only. Postgrad Med J. 2002; 78(918):238–41.
22. Murgod UA, Muthane UB, Ravi V, Radhesh S, Desai A. Persistent movement disorders following Japanese encephalitis. Neurology. 2001;57(12):2313–5.
23. Pradhan S, Pandey N, Shashank S, Gupta RK, Mathur A. Parkinsonism due to predominant involvement of substantia nigra in Japanese encephalitis. Neurology. 1999;53(8):1781–6.
24. Kalita J, Das BK, Misra UK. SPECT studies of regional cerebral blood flow in 8 patients with Japanese encephalitis in subacute and chronic stage. Acta Neurol Scand. 1999;99(4):213–8.
25. Janavs JL, Aminoff MJ. Dystonia and chorea in acquired systemic diseases. J Neurol Neurosurg Psychiatry. 1998;65(4):436–45.
26. Gollomp SM, Fahn S. Transient dystonia as a complication of varicella. J Neurol Neurosurg Psychiatry. 1987;50(9):1228–9.
27. Hargrave DR, Webb DW. Movement disorders in association with Herpes Simplex virus encephalitis in children: a review. Dev Med Child Neurol. 1998; 40(9):640–2.
28. Verma A, Brozman B. Opsoclonus–myoclonus syndrome following Epstein-Barr virus infection. Review. Neurology. 2002;58(7):1131–2.
29. Ryan MM, Procopis PG, Ouvier RA. Influenza A encephalitis with movement disorders. Pediatr Neurol. 1999;21(3):669–73.
30. Dale RC, Church AJ, Benton S, Surtees RA, Lees A, Thompson EJ, Giovannoni G, Neville BG. Poststreptococcal autoimmune dystonia with isolated bilateral striatal necrosis. Dev Med Child Neurol. 2002;44(7):485–9.
31. Church AJ, Cardoso F, Dale RC, Lees AJ, Thompson EJ, Giovannoni G. Anti-basal ganglia antibodies in acute and persistent Sydenham's chorea. Neurology. 2002;59(2):227–31.
32. Swedo SE. Sydenham's chorea: a model for childhood autoimmune neuropsychiatric disorders. JAMA. 1994;272(22):1788–91.
33. Cardoso F, Eduardo C, Silva AP, Mota CC. Chorea in fifty consecutive patients with rheumatic fever. Mov Disord. 1997;12(5):701–3.
34. Cardoso F, Vargas AP, Oliveira LD, Guerra AA, Amaral SV. Persistent Sydenham's chorea. Mov Disord. 1999;14(5):805–7.
35. Murphy TK, Petitto JM, Voeller KK, Goodman WK. Obsessive compulsive disorder. Is there an association with childhood streptococcal infections and altered immune function? Semin Clin Neuropsychiatry. 2001;6(4):266–76.
36. Murphy TK, Goodman WK, Ayoub EM, Voeller KK. On defining Sydenham's chorea: where do we draw the line? Biol Psychiatry. 2000;47(10): 851–7.
37. Dale RC, Heyman I, Surtees RA, Church AJ, Giovannoni G, Goodman R, Neville BG. Dyskinesias and associated psychiatric disorders following streptococcal infections. Arch Dis Child. 2004;89(7): 604–10.
38. Blocq P, Marinesco G. Sur un cas de tremblement parkinsonien hemiplegique symptomatique d'une tumeur du pedoncle cerebral. CR Soc Biol. 1893;5: 105–11.
39. Brissaud E. Lecons sur les maladies nerveuses (Salpetriere 1893–1894). Paris: G. Masson; 1895. p. 469–501.
40. Alarcón F, Tolosa E, Muñoz E. Focal limb dystonia in a patient with a cerebellar mass. Arch Neurol. 2001;58(7):1125–7.

41. Tey HL, Seet RC, Lim EC. Tuberculomas causing cervical dystonia. Intern Med J. 2005;35(4):261–2.
42. Alarcon F, Duenas G, Cevallos N, Lees AJ. Movement disorders in 30 patients with tuberculous meningitis. Mov Disord. 2000;15(3):561–9.
43. Ashtekar CS, Jaspan T, Thomas D, Weston V, Gayatri NA, Whitehouse WP. Acute bilateral thalamic necrosis in a child with Mycoplasma pneumoniae. Dev Med Child Neurol. 2003;45(9):634–7.
44. Green C, Riley DE. Treatment of dystonia in striatal necrosis caused by Mycoplasma pneumoniae. Pediatr Neurol. 2002;26(4):318–20.
45. Kumar A. Movement disorders in the tropics. Parkinsonism Relat Disord. 2002;9(2):69–75.
46. Sawhney IMS, Singh G, Lekhra OP, Mathuriya SN, Parihar PS, Prabhakar S. Uncommon presentations of neurocysticercosis. J Neurol Sci. 1998; 154(1):94–100.
47. Aminoff MJ, Josephson A. Neurological complications of systemic disease: adults. In: Daroff RB, Fenichel GM, Jankovic J, Mazziotta JC, editors. Bradley's neurology in clinical practice. 6th ed. Philadelphia: Elsevier Saunders; 2012. p. 894–915.
48. Kwong KL, Chu R, Wong SN. Parkinsonism as unusual neurological complication in childhood systemic lupus erythematosus. Lupus. 2000; 9(6):474–7.
49. Jankovic J, Patten BM. Blepharospasm and autoimmune diseases. Mov Disord. 1987;2(3):159–63.
50. Florance-Ryan N, Dalmau J. Update on anti-N-methyl-D-aspartate receptor encephalitis in children and adolescents. Curr Opin Pediatr. 2010; 22(6):739–44.
51. Rosenfeld MR, Dalmau J. Cancer and the nervous system. Paraneoplastic disorders of the nervous system. In: Daroff RB, Fenichel GM, Jankovic J, Mazziotta JC, editors. Bradley's neurology in clinical practice. 6th ed. Philadelphia: Elsevier Saunders; 2012. p. 1200–10.
52. Panzer J, Dalmau J. Movement disorders in paraneoplastic and autoimmune disease. Curr Opin Neurol. 2011;24(4):346–53.
53. Chokroverty S, Avidan AY. Sleep and its disorders. In: Daroff RB, Fenichel GM, Jankovic J, Mazziotta JC, editors. Bradley's neurology in clinical practice. 6th ed. Philadelphia: Elsevier Saunders; 2012. p. 1634–702.
54. Hamati AI. Neurological complications of systemic disease: children. In: Daroff RB, Fenichel GM, Jankovic J, Mazziotta JC, editors. Bradley's neurology in clinical practice. 6th ed. Philadelphia: Elsevier Saunders; 2012. p. 916–30.
55. Jeren-Strujić B, Jeren T, Thaller N, Zivković Z, Raos V. A case of McLeod syndrome with chronic renal failure. Blood Purif. 1998;16(6):336–40.
56. Jimenez-Jimenez FJ, Burguera JA, Catalan MJ, Vazquez A, Vaamonde J, Vela-Desajo L, Martınez-Martin P, Balseiro J, Pondo-Sordo M, Domingo J, Garcıa-Ruiz PJ, Munoz-Vazquez A, Molina JA, Ceballos-Hernansont MA, Arcaya J, Duarte J. Delayed onset dystonia in patients with antecedents of perinatal asphyxia. Parkinsonism Relat Disord. 1997; 3(1):21–5.
57. Burke RE, Fahn S, Gold AP. Delayed-onset dystonia in patients with "static" encephalopathy. JNNP. 1980;43(9):789–97.
58. Roland EH, Poskitt K, Rodriguez E, Lupton BA, Hill A. Perinatal hypoxic-ischemic thalamic injury: clinical features and neuroimaging. Ann Neurol. 1998;44(2):161–6.
59. Carpenter MB. Athetosis and the basal ganglia. Arch Neurol Psychiatry. 1950;63(6):875–901.
60. Dalvi A, Lyons KE, Pahwa R. Secondary dystonia. In: Stacy MA, editor. Handbook of dystonia. 2nd ed. London: Informa Healthcare; 2012. p. 251–75.
61. Kupsky WJ, Drozd MA, Barlow CF. Selective injury of the globus pallidus in children with post-cardiac surgery choreic syndrome. Dev Med Child Neurol. 1995;37(2):135–44.
62. Alarcon F, Zijlmans JCM, Duenas G, Cevallos N. Post-stroke movement disorders: report of 56 patients. J Neurol Neurosurg Psychiatry. 2004;75(11):1568–740.
63. Siniscalchi A, Gallelli L, Di Benedetto O, De Sarro G. Asterixis as a presentation of cerebellar ischemic stroke. West J Emerg Med. 2012;13(6):507–8.
64. Mejia NI, Jankovic J. Secondary tics and tourettism. Rev Bras Psiquiatr. 2005;27(1):11–7.
65. Kwak CH, Jankovic J. Tourettism and dystonia after subcortical stroke. Mov Disord. 2002;17(4):821–5.
66. Lockwood AH. Toxic and metabolic encephalopathies. In: Daroff RB, Fenichel GM, Jankovic J, Mazziotta JC, editors. Bradley's neurology in clinical practice. 6th ed. Philadelphia: Elsevier Saunders; 2012. p. 1321–39.
67. Cadranel JF, Lebiez E, Di Martino V, Bernard B, El Koury S, Tourbah A, Pidoux B, Valla D, Opolon P. Focal neurological signs in hepatic encephalopathy in cirrhotic patients: an underestimated entity? Am J Gastroenterol. 2001;96(2):515–8.
68. Thobois S, Giraud P, Debat P, Maurizi A, Pret-Liaudet A, Kopp NB, Rusolle E. Orofacial dyskinesias in a patient with primary biliary cirrhosis: clinicopathological case report and review. Mov Disord. 2002;17(2):415–9.
69. Demarquay G, Setiey A, Morel Y, Trepo C, Chazot G, Broussolle E. Clinical report of three patients with hereditary hemochromatosis and movement disorders. Review. Mov Disord. 2000; 15(6):1204–9.
70. Federico P, Zochodne DW. Reversible Parkinsonism and hyperammonemia associated with portal vein thrombosis. Acta Neurol Scand. 2001; 103(3):198–200.
71. Ropper AH, Samuels MA. Adams and Victor's principles of neurology. 9th ed. New York: McGrawHill Medical; 2009. p. 1081–107. Chapter 40, The acquired metabolic disorders of the nervous system.
72. Bajenaru O. Osmotic demyelination syndromes. In: Lisak RP, Truong DD, Carroll WM, Bhidayasiri R,

editors. International neurology. A clinical approach. Oxford: Wiley-Blackwell; 2009. p. 386–9.
73. de Souza A. Movement disorders and the osmotic demyelination syndrome. Parkinsonism Relat Disord. 2013;19(8):709–16.
74. Wu CL, Lu CS. Delayed-onset dystonia following recovery from central pontine myelinolysis. J Formos Med Assoc. 1992;91(10):1013–6.
75. Maraganore DM, Folger WN, Swanson JW, Ahlskog JE. Movement disorders as sequelae of central pontine myelinolysis: report of three cases. Mov Disord. 1992;7(2):142–8.
76. Tison FX, Ferrer X, Julien J. Delayed onset movement disorders as a complication of central pontine myelinolysis. Mov Disord. 1991;6(2):171–3.
77. Seah AB, Chan LL, Wong MC, Tan EK. Evolving spectrum of movement disorders in extrapontine and central pontine myelinolysis. Parkinsonism Relat Disord. 2002;9(2):117–9.
78. So YT, Simon RP. Deficiency diseases of the nervous system. In: Daroff RB, Fenichel GM, Jankovic J, Mazziotta JC, editors. Bradley's neurology in clinical practice. 6th ed. Philadelphia: Elsevier Saunders; 2012. p. 1340–52.
79. Powell LW. Hemochromatosis. In: Longo DL, Kasper DS, Jameson JL, Fauci AS, Hauser SL, Loscalzo J, editors. Harrison's principles of internal medicine. 18th ed. New York: McGrawHill Medical; 2012. p. 3162–7.
80. Ahlskog JE, Nishino H, Evidente VGH, Tulloch JW, Forbes GS, Caviness JN, Gwinn-Hardy KA. Persistent chorea triggered by hyperglycemic crisis in diabetics. Mov Disord. 2001;16(5):890–8.
81. Hefter H, Mayer P, Benecke P. Persistent chorea after recurrent hypoglycemia. Eur Neurol. 1993; 33(3):244–7.
82. Newman, Kinkle WR. Paroxysmal choreoathetosis due to hypoglycemia. Arch Neurol. 1984;41(3):341–2 RP.
83. Schmidt BJ, Pillay N. Paroxysmal dyskinesia associated with hypoglycemia. Can J Neurol Sci. 1993; 20(2):151–3.
84. Kurlan R. Postprandial (reactive) hypoglycemia and restless legs syndrome: related neurologic disorders? Mov Disord. 1998;13(3):619–20.
85. Milanov I, Georgiev D, Todorov T. Clinical and electromyographic characteristics of tremor in patients with depression. Parkinsonism Relat Disord. 2000;6(2):101–5.
86. Yen DJ, Shan DE, Lu SR. Hyperthyroidism present as recurrent short paroxysmal kinesigenic dyskinesia. Mov Disord. 1998;13(2):361–3.
87. Castillo P, Woodruff B, Caselli R, Vernino S, Lucchinetti C, Swanson J, Noseworthy J, Aksamit A, Carter J, Sirven J, Hunder G, Fatourechi V, Mokri B, Drubach D, Pittock S, Lennon V, Boeve B. Steroid-responsive encephalopathy associated with autoimmune thyroiditis. Arch Neurol. 2006; 63(2):197–202.
88. Ghika-Schmid F, Ghika J, Regli F, Dworak N, Bougousslavsky J, Stadler C, Portman L, Despland PA. Hashimoto's myoclonic encephalopathy: an underdiagnosed treatable condition? Mov Disord. 1996;11(5):555–62.
89. Erickson JC, Carrasco H, Grimes JB, Jabbari B, Cannard KR. Palatal tremor and myorrythmias in Hashimoto's encephalopathy. Neurology. 2002;58(3):504–5.
90. Klawans HL, Lupton M, Simon L. Calcification of the basal ganglia as a cause of levodopa-resistant Parkinsonism. Neurology. 1976;26(3):221–5.
91. Berger JR, Ross DB. Reversible parkinsonian syndrome complicating postoperative hypoparathyroidism. Neurology. 1981;31(7):881–2.
92. Gálvez-Jiménez N, Hanson MR, Cabral J. Dopa-resistant Parkinsonism, oculomotor disturbances, chorea, mirror movements, dyspraxia, and dementia: the expanding clinical spectrum of hypoparathyroidism. A case report. Mov Disord. 2000;15(6):1273–6.
93. Chroni E, Papadimitriou A, Avramidis T, Terentiou AE, Tzioras C, Divari R. Stiff-person like syndrome in a patient with multiple pituitary hormone deficiencies. Acta Neurol Scand. 2000;102(6):403–5.
94. Lee MT, Lee TI, Won JG, Chau WK, Yang HJ, Li JC, Lin HD, Tang KT. Primary hypothalamic lymphoma with panhypopituitarism presenting as stiff-man syndrome. Am J Med Sci. 2004; 328(2):124–8.
95. Aminoff MJ, So YT. Effects of toxins and physical agents on the nervous system. In: Daroff RB, Fenichel GM, Jankovic J, Mazziotta JC, editors. Bradley's neurology in clinical practice. 6th ed. Philadelphia: Elsevier Saunders; 2012. p. 1353–76.
96. Ono K, Komai K, Yamada M. Myoclonic involuntary movement associated with chronic manganese poisoning. J Neurol Sci. 2002;199(1–2):93–6.
97. de Souza A, Narvencar KP, Sindhoora KV. The neurological effects of methyl bromide intoxication. J Neurol Sci. 2013;335(1–2):36–41.
98. Suwanlaong K, Phanthumchinda K. Neurological manifestation of methyl bromide intoxication. J Med Assoc Thai. 2008;91(3):421–6.
99. Song X, Hu Z, Zhang H. Acute dystonia indu ced by lamivudine. Clin Neuropharmacol. 2005; 28(4):193–4.
100. Fabiani G, Pastro PC, Froehner C. Parkinsonism and other movement disorders in outpatients in chronic use of cinnarizine and flunarizine. Arq Neuropsiquiatr. 2004;62(3B):784–8.
101. Polizzi A, Incorpora G, Ruggieri M. Dystonia as acute adverse reaction to cough suppressant in a 3-year-old girl. Eur J Paediatr Neurol. 2001; 5(4):167–8.
102. Weiner WJ, Rabinstein A, Levin B, Weiner C, Shulman LM. Cocaine-induced persistent dyskinesias. Neurology. 2001;56(7):964–5.

44 Neuroacanthocytosis Syndromes

Andreas Hermann

44.1 Introduction

Initial reports of neuroacanthocytosis syndromes appeared in the late 1970s by Levine and Critchley [1–3]. Neuroacanthocytosis (NA) syndromes are defined by neurological abnormalities in combination with misshaped acanthocytic red blood cells affecting only one person in three million inhabitants. NA syndromes are characterized by a wide variety of dysfunction of the nervous system including epileptic seizures and basal ganglia-related movement disorder symptoms, dementia, psychosis, and speech/swallowing difficulties all together leading to a markedly reduced life-span [4–6]. No curative treatment approach is available; only fairly effective symptomatic treatment is available for NA syndromes so far.

44.2 Classification

NA syndromes can be classified into [7, 8]:

I. Core NA syndromes:
   (a) Chorea-acanthocytosis (ChAc, OMIM #200150), autosomal recessive
   (b) McLeod syndrome (MLS; OMIM #300842), X-chromosomal recessive
II. Degenerative disorders where acanthocytosis is occasionally seen:
   (a) Pantothenate kinase-associated neurodegeneration (PKAN; OMIM #234200), autosomal recessive
   (b) Huntington disease-like 2 (HDL 2; OMIM #606438), autosomal dominant
III. Disorders with reduced blood lipoproteins and acanthocytosis:
   (a) Bassen-Kornzweig syndrome (OMIM #200100), autosomal recessive
   (b) Hypobetalipoproteinemia (OMIM #615558), autosomal recessive

44.3 Chorea-Acanthocytosis

ChAc is an autosomal recessive disorder caused by loss-of-function mutations in the *VPS13A* gene encoding chorein. Neuropathology showed that basal ganglia, mainly the striatum and substantia nigra, are mainly affected [5, 9]. The striatum suffers from a pronounced atrophy that correlates with extensive striatal neuronal loss and reactive astrogliosis. Clinical symptoms are variable most often with a progressive movement disorder with involuntary movements, oromandibular dyskinesias,

A. Hermann, M.D., Ph.D.
Department of Neurology, Technische Universität Dresden, Fetscherstraße 74, 01307 Dresden, Germany

DZNE, German Centre for Neurodegenerative Diseases, Research Site Dresden, 01307 Dresden, Germany
e-mail: Andreas.Hermann@uniklinikum-dresden.de

C. Falup-Pecurariu et al. (eds.), *Movement Disorders Curricula*,
DOI 10.1007/978-3-7091-1628-9_44

which often change to parkinsonism in the course of the disease. Epilepsy is common and often appear prior to the movement disorder. Creatine kinase is elevated in serum (CAVE, often wrongly attributed to the epilepsy), and blood acanthocytosis of 7–50% is seen in almost all patients [10]. Mean age of onset of chorea-acanthocytosis is in the early 30s, although it has been reported appearing from the first to the seventh decade [5, 11] (Table 44.1).

The disorder, originally known as "Levine-Critchley syndrome," has been confirmed to be ChAc, at least in Critchley's original Kentucky family [12].

Recent new data suggest the disturbance of the Lyn kinase pathway in patient erythrocytes [13, 14]. Mice carrying upregulated Lyn develop blood cell acanthocytosis [15]. Furthermore, we recently described chorein as an upstream regulator of cortical actin depolymerization in erythrocytes and thrombocytes through the PI3K-RAC-PAK pathway [16, 17]. Whether this holds true for neurons is as yet unknown.

44.4 McLeod Syndrome

McLeod syndrome is an X-linked recessive disorder, mutations are found in the *XK* gene, and heterozygous females only rarely show symptoms. There is significant overlap to ChAc including the movement disorder, neuropsychiatric disturbances, acanthocytosis, and creatine kinase elevation [4]. It is seen typically in middle-aged males [4], therefore sometimes called "ChAc of old men" [11]. Nevertheless, there are some differences. Neuropathy is not that prominent, whereas myopathic changes in neuropathology and myography are common. Compensated hemolysis, splenomegaly, and hepatomegaly are

Table 44.1 Differential diagnosis

Main symptom/syndrome	Differential	Red flags (pointing toward a core NA syndrome)
Chorea	Huntington	Acanthocytosis
		Neuropathy (ChAc)
		Myopathy (McLeod)
		Epilepsy
		CK↑, ALAT↑, ASAT↑
	Wilson	Acanthocytosis
		Epilepsy
		CK↑, ALAT↑, ASAT↑
Dystonia	Wilson	Acanthocytosis
		Epilepsy
		CK↑, ALAT↑, ASAT↑
	PKAN	No iron deposits in cMRI
		Epilepsy
		CK↑, ALAT↑, ASAT↑
Epilepsy	Familial epileptic syndromes	Acanthocytosis
	Sporadic epileptic syndromes	Involuntary movements (not always drug induced)
		CK ↑(not always due to seizures)
		ASAT, ALAT↑ (not always drug induced)
Psychiatric disturbances	Tourette syndrome	Acanthocytosis
	Obsessive-compulsive disorder	Involuntary movements (not always drug induced)
		Parkinsonism (not always neuroleptic induced)

frequently seen in McLeod. There are several reports of severe transfusion reactions [6, 18]. Patients should bank their own blood in case of need for transfusion, to avoid the production of anti-Kell antibodies. Cardiomyopathy is a common feature of McLeod (>60 % of patients) and needs to be monitored on a regular basis.

MLS is diagnosed by decreased expression of Kell and Kx antigens on erythrocytes, known as the "McLeod phenotype." (A report of "Kell negative" is not adequate.) Abnormalities of cation transport may underlie at least some of the erythrocyte manifestations [19].

44.5 Pantothenate Kinase-Associated Neurodegeneration (PKAN)

PKAN, an autosomal recessive disease with mutations in the *PANK2* gene, normally affects young children (disease onset before the age of 6 years). Atypical forms also appear in adolescence or early adulthood. PKAN belongs to the group of neurodegeneration with brain iron accumulation (NBIA syndromes) which are characterized by increased iron deposits within the basal ganglia. Therefore, cMRI is the crucial diagnostic instrument showing the "eye of the tiger" sign. The phenotype is typically a progressive generalized dystonia, but also features of hypokinesia and rigidity do appear (especially in the atypical forms). Pigmentary retinopathy is common in the typical young onset form, while acanthocytosis is only seen in approximately 10 % of PKAN patients [20]. HARP syndrome is allelic with PKAN (hypobetalipoproteinemia, acanthocytosis, retinitis pigmentosa, and pallidal degeneration) [5].

44.6 Huntington Disease-Like 2 (HDL2)

HDL2 is due to a CTG/CAG trinucleotide repeat expansion within junctophilin-3 (JPH3) on chromosome 16q24.3 [21] and up to now only reported in individuals of African ancestry. Affected individuals have repeat expansions of 41–58 triplets. Acanthocytosis is reported in about 10 % of cases [22]. It shows a similar clinical picture as ChAc or HD and manifests in young-mid adulthood, with an age of onset inversely related to size of the trinucleotide repeat expansion [23]. Dystonia and parkinsonism appear to be more prominent than in HD and are unrelated to repeat size [24]. As in HD, early signs may be personality change and psychiatric symptoms.

44.7 Hypolipoproteinemia (HLP) and Abetalipoproteinemia (ALP)

Acanthocytosis was long known occurring together with spinocerebellar degeneration and neuropathy in ALP (Bassen-Kornzweig syndrome). Patients normally lack basal ganglia movement disorders but suffer from steatorrhea, pigmentary retinopathy, and significant vitamin E deficiency. ALP is inherited in an autosomal recessive manner; HLP can be symptomatic in heterozygote or homozygote patients [5].

Acknowledgment The author is supported by the Advocacy for Neuroacanthocytosis Patients and by the Federal Ministry of Education and Research (BMBF, 01GM1303) under the frame of E-Rare-2, the ERA-Net for Research on Rare Diseases (www.emina2.de).

References

1. Estes JW, Morley TJ, Levine IM, Emerson CP. A new hereditary acanthocytosis syndrome. Am J Med. 1967;42(6):868–81. Epub 1967/06/01. eng.
2. Levine IM, Estes JW, Looney JM. Hereditary neurological disease with acanthocytosis. A new syndrome. Arch Neurol. 1968;19(4):403–9. Epub 1968/10/01. eng.
3. Critchley EM, Clark DB, Wikler A. Acanthocytosis and neurological disorder without betalipoproteinemia. Arch Neurol. 1968;18(2):134–40. Epub 1968/02/01. eng.
4. Danek A, Rubio JP, Rampoldi L, Ho M, Dobson-Stone C, Tison F, et al. McLeod neuroacanthocytosis: genotype and phenotype. Ann Neurol. 2001;50(6):755–64. Epub 2002/01/05. eng.
5. Dobson-Stone C, Rampoldi L, Bader B, Velayos Baeza A, Walker RH, Danek A, et al. In: Pagon RA,

Adam MP, Bird TD, Dolan CR, Fong CT, Stephens K, editors. Chorea-acanthocytosis. Seattle: GeneReviews; 1993.
6. Jung HH, Danek A, Walker RH. Neuroacanthocytosis syndromes. Orphanet J Rare Dis. 2011;6:68. Pubmed Central PMCID: 3212896, Epub 2011/10/27. eng.
7. Walterfang M, Evans A, Looi JC, Jung HH, Danek A, Walker RH, et al. The neuropsychiatry of neuroacanthocytosis syndromes. Neurosci Biobehav Rev. 2011;35(5):1275–83. Epub 2011/01/18. eng.
8. Hermann A, Chapter 3: Chorea-acanthocytosis, in Chorea, F.E. Micheli, P.A. LeWitt (eds.), Springer; p.31–55.
9. Danek A, Dobson-Stone C, Velayos Baeza A, Monaco AP. The phenotype of chorea-acanthocytosis: a review of 106 patients with VPS13A mutations. 2nd International Neuroacanthocytosis Symposium: Movement Disorders; 2005. p. 1678.
10. Storch A, Kornhass M, Schwarz J. Testing for acanthocytosis A prospective reader-blinded study in movement disorder patients. J Neurol. 2005;252(1):84–90. Epub 2005/01/18. eng.
11. Rampoldi L, Danek A, Monaco AP. Clinical features and molecular bases of neuroacanthocytosis. J Mol Med (Berl). 2002;80(8):475–91. Epub 2002/08/20. eng.
12. Velayos-Baeza A, Holinski-Feder E, Neitzel B, Bader B, Critchley EM, Monaco AP, et al. Chorea-acanthocytosis genotype in the original critchley kentucky neuroacanthocytosis kindred. Arch Neurol. 2011;68(10):1330–3. Epub 2011/10/12. eng.
13. De Franceschi L, Scardoni G, Tomelleri C, Danek A, Walker RH, Jung HH, et al. Computational identification of phospho-tyrosine sub-networks related to acanthocyte generation in neuroacanthocytosis. PLoS One. 2012;7(2):e31015. Pubmed Central PMCID: 3280254, Epub 2012/02/23. eng.
14. De Franceschi L, Tomelleri C, Matte A, Brunati AM, Bovee-Geurts PH, Bertoldi M, et al. Erythrocyte membrane changes of chorea-acanthocytosis are the result of altered Lyn kinase activity. Blood. 2011;118(20):5652–63. Pubmed Central PMCID: 3217364, Epub 2011/09/29. eng.
15. Slavova-Azmanova NS, Kucera N, Satiaputra J, Stone L, Magno A, Maxwell MJ, et al. Gain-of-function Lyn induces anemia: appropriate Lyn activity is essential for normal erythropoiesis and Epo receptor signaling. Blood. 2013;122(2):262–71. Epub 2013/05/23. eng.
16. Foller M, Hermann A, Gu S, Alesutan I, Qadri SM, Borst O, et al. Chorein-sensitive polymerization of cortical actin and suicidal cell death in chorea-acanthocytosis. FASEB J. 2012;26(4):1526–34. Epub 2012/01/10. eng.
17. Schmidt EM, Schmid E, Munzer P, Hermann A, Eyrich AK, Russo A, et al. Chorein sensitivity of cytoskeletal organization and degranulation of platelets. FASEB J. 2013;27(7):2799–806. Epub 2013/04/10. eng.
18. Russo DC, Oyen R, Powell VI, Perry S, Hitchcock J, Redman CM, et al. First example of anti-Kx in a person with the McLeod phenotype and without chronic granulomatous disease. Transfusion. 2000;40(11):1371–5. Epub 2000/12/02. eng.
19. Rivera A, Kam SY, Ho M, Romero JR, Lee S. Ablation of the Kell/Xk complex alters erythrocyte divalent cation homeostasis. Blood Cells Mol Dis. 2013;50(2):80–5. Pubmed Central PMCID: 3540154, Epub 2012/11/06. eng.
20. Hayflick SJ, Westaway SK, Levinson B, Zhou B, Johnson MA, Ching KH, et al. Genetic, clinical, and radiographic delineation of Hallervorden-Spatz syndrome. N Engl J Med. 2003;348(1):33–40. Epub 2003/01/03. eng.
21. Holmes SE, O'Hearn E, Rosenblatt A, Callahan C, Hwang HS, Ingersoll-Ashworth RG, et al. A repeat expansion in the gene encoding junctophilin-3 is associated with Huntington disease-like 2. Nat Genet. 2001;29(4):377–8. Epub 2001/11/06. eng.
22. Walker RH, Rasmussen A, Rudnicki D, Holmes SE, Alonso E, Matsuura T, et al. Huntington's disease – like 2 can present as chorea-acanthocytosis. Neurology. 2003;61(7):1002–4. Epub 2003/10/15. eng.
23. Margolis RL, Holmes SE, Rosenblatt A, Gourley L, O'Hearn E, Ross CA, et al. Huntington's disease-like 2 (HDL2) in North America and Japan. Ann Neurol. 2004;56(5):670–4. Epub 2004/10/07. eng.
24. Walker RH, Jankovic J, O'Hearn E, Margolis RL. Phenotypic features of Huntington's disease-like 2. Mov Disord. 2003;18(12):1527–30. Epub 2003/12/16. eng.

Index

C. Falup-Pecurariu et al. (eds.), *Movement Disorders Curricula*,
DOI 10.1007/978-3-7091-1628-9